Complementary Medicine in Clinical Practice

Integrative Practice in American Healthcare

Edited by
David Rakel, MD
Director, University of Wisconsin Integrative Medicine

Assistant Professor
Department of Family Medicine
University of Wisconsin Medical School
Madison, WI

Nancy Faass, MSW, MPH
Health Writing and Communications
Director, WordWorks and
the Health Writers' Group
San Francisco, CA

JONES AND BARTLETT PUBLISHERS
Sudbury, Massachusetts
BOSTON   TORONTO   LONDON   SINGAPORE

World Headquarters

Jones and Bartlett Publishers
40 Tall Pine Drive
Sudbury, MA 01776
978-443-5000
info@jbpub.com
www.jbpub.com

Jones and Bartlett Publishers
Canada
6339 Ormindale Way
Mississauga, Ontario L5V 1J2
CANADA

Jones and Bartlett Publishers
International
Barb House, Barb Mews
London W6 7PA
UK

Jones and Bartlett's books and products are available through most bookstores and online booksellers. To contact Jones and Bartlett Publishers directly, call 800-832-0034, fax 978-443-8000, or visit our website www.jbpub.com.

Substantial discounts on bulk quantities of Jones and Bartlett's publications are available to corporations, professional associations, and other qualified organizations. For details and specific discount information, contact the special sales department at Jones and Bartlett via the above contact information or send an email to specialsales@jbpub.com.

Production Credits
Executive Editor: Jack Bruggeman
Production Director: Amy Rose
Editorial Assistant: Katilyn Crowley
Associate Production Editor: Tracey Chapman
Marketing Manager: Emily Ekle
Manufacturing Buyer: Amy Bacus
Composition: Auburn Associates, Inc.
Text Design: Auburn Associates, Inc.
Cover Design: Anne Spencer
Printing and Binding: Malloy, Inc.
Cover Printing: Malloy, Inc.

Library of Congress Cataloging-in-Publication Data
Complementary medicine in clinical practice : integrative practice in
  American healthcare / [edited by] David Rakel, Nancy Faass.
    p. ; cm.
  Includes bibliographical references and index.
  ISBN 0-7637-3065-3 (pbk.)
  1. Alternative medicine. 2. Integrative medicine.   I. Rakel, David.
II. Faass, Nancy.
  [DNLM: 1. Complementary Therapies. 2. Referral and Consultation.   WB 890 C7376 2005]
  R733.C6553 2005
  615.5—dc22

                        2005002448

Printed in the United States of America
09 08 07 06 05   10 9 8 7 6 5 4 3 2 1

Dedication

To patients everywhere and the millions of dedicated health care professionals who serve them.

Brief Contents

Contents

Foreword

Complementary and alternative medicine (CAM) and integrative medicine (IM) continue to emerge as key areas in the future of health care. Popular use of CAM continues to increase. Professional interest in IM is expanding and government interest in establishing policy and practice is becoming more prominent.

Over the past century, conventional medicine has been tremendously successful in treating acute disease and saving people from dying. As a result, people are living longer and developing more chronic diseases. Part of the interest in IM arises from the failure of conventional medicine to adequately treat these chronic conditions. Therefore, significant challenges remain in developing a new model of medicine for care of the chronically ill. A number of questions will need to be addressed if a new model of medicine appropriate for chronic care is to be developed.

- Can we expand the continuum of care to include prevention?
- Can low-tech care be brought into a sub-specializing, highly technical system?
- How much and what kind of evidence is enough to adopt a practice?
- Does the type of evidence we need for approving practices differ when risks are low?
- Who is qualified to practice integrative medicine? And, how do we tell?

These and other issues are succinctly addressed in this compilation of information on integrative medicine. *Complementary Medicine in Clinical Practice* has done an admirable job of capturing the essential features of integrative medicine from some of the country's leading thinkers on the subject. Concise and comprehensive, this volume is essential reading for all who want to explore the primary themes, trends, and current information on CAM and IM. Here you will find information on research, practices, products, public use, the business of integrative medicine, nutrition, exercise, mind-body medicine, self-care, and the main systems of complementary and alternative approaches to health care.

In seeking the threads of healing, our challenge is to integrate these practices in a way that efficiently merges them with the best of biomedicine. *Complementary Medicine in Clinical Practice* provides fundamental information to meet that challenge and helps us lay out a path toward optimal healing environments.

Wayne B. Jonas, MD
Director
Samueli Institute

Contributor List

Sidney MacDonald Baker, MD
Associate Editor, *Integrative Medicine*
Clinical Practice
Sag Harbor, New York

Brian Berman, MD
Chair, Steering Committee
Consortium of Academic Medical Centers
Founder and Director
University of Maryland Center for
   Integrative Medicine
Baltimore, Maryland

Clement Bezold, PhD
President, Institute for Alternative Futures
President, Alternative Futures Associates
Alexandria, Virginia

Stephen Birch, PhD, LAc
Cofounder
Society for Acupuncture Research
Clinical Practice
Amsterdam, Netherlands

Aat Bos, PhD
Private Practice
Amsterdam, Netherlands

Brian Bouch, MD
Associate Clinical Professor
Medical Acupuncture
University of California, Los Angeles
School of Medicine
Cofounder, Hill Park Medical Center
Petaluma, California

Lex M. Bouter, PhD
Institute for Research in Extramural
   Medicine
Vrije University Medical Center
Amsterdam, Netherlands

Francis J. Brinker, ND
Clinical Assistant Professor
Program in Integrative Medicine
University of Arizona College of Medicine
Tucson, Arizona

Gert Bronfort, PhD, DC
Research Professor
Director of the Neck and Back Research
   Program
Northwestern Health Sciences University
Bloomington, Minnesota

Cedric X. Bryant, PhD, FACSM
Chief Exercise Physiologist
Vice President of Educational Services
American Council on Exercise
San Diego, California

Carlo Calabrese, ND, MPH
Senior Investigator
Helfgott Research Institute
Research Professor
National College of Naturopathic Medicine
Portland, Oregon

Claire Cassidy, PhD, LAc
Director, Windpath Healing Works Clinic
Director
Paradigms Found Consulting Services
Bethesda, Maryland

David Chapman-Smith, LLB
Secretary-General
World Federation of Chiropractic
Editor, *The Chiropractic Report*
Toronto, Ontario, Canada

Ronald A. Chez, MD
Deputy Director
Samueli Institute
Alexandria, Virginia

Linda Chrisman, MA, CMT
Clinical Massage Practice
Founding Associate
Health Medicine Institute
Lafayette, California

Michael Devitt
Managing Editor
Acupuncture Today
Huntington Beach, California

C. James Dowden
Executive Administrator
American Board of Medical Acupuncture
Los Angeles, California

Roni L. Evans, DC, MS
Northwestern Health Sciences University
Bloomington, Minnesota

Nancy Faass, MSW, MPH
Writer and Editor
Director
Health Writers' Group
San Francisco, California

Tiffany M. Field, PhD
Director, Touch Research Institutes
University of Miami School of Medicine
Miami, Florida

Leo Galland, MD
Clinical Practice
President, Applied Nutrition Inc.
New York, New York

James S. Gordon, MD
Founder and Director
Center for Mind-Body Medicine
Washington, DC

Joy Kettler Gurgevich
Nutritionist, Private Practice
Sabino Canyon Integrative Medicine, LLC
Preceptor, Program in Integrative Medicine
University of Arizona
Tucson, Arizona

Steven Gurgevich, PhD
Psychologist, Private Practice
Sabino Canyon Integrative Medicine, LLC
Assistant Professor
University of Arizona College of Medicine
Tucson, Arizona

Mitchell Haas, DC, MA
Associate Professor
Center for Outcome Studies
Western States Chiropractic College
Portland, Oregon

Richard Hammerschlag, PhD
Research Director
Oregon College of Oriental Medicine
Portland, Oregon

Patrick Hanaway, MD
Medical Director
Great Smokies Diagnostic Laboratory
Founder and Medical Director
Family to Family Clinic
Asheville, North Carolina

Debra Harris, RN, BSN
Health Coach, Private Practice
Cofounder, Harris 2 Consulting
Bend, Oregon

Thecla A.M. Hekker, MD
Microbiology
Free University Hospital
Amsterdam, Netherlands

Jan Keppel Hesselink, MD, PhD, FFPM
Department of Pharmacology
University of Witten
Herdecke, Germany

Vickie Ina, MBA
Mill Valley, California

Roger Jahnke, OMD
CEO, Health Action Consulting
Santa Barbara, California

Wayne B. Jonas, MD
Director
Samueli Institute for Information Biology
Alexandria, Virginia

David S. Jones, MD, President
Institute for Functional Medicine
Gig Harbor, Washington

Fokke A.M. Jonkman, MD, PhD
Private Practice
Amsterdam, Netherlands

Efrem Korngold, LAc, OMD
Co-director, Clinical Practice
Chinese Medicine Works
Adjunct Faculty
American College of Traditional Chinese
    Medicine
San Francisco, California

William J. Lauretti, DC, FICC
Assistant Professor
New York Chiropractic College
Seneca Falls, NY

Whitney Lowe
Founding Member
National Certification Board for
    Therapeutic Massage and Bodywork
Director
Orthopedic Massage Education &
    Research Institute
Sisters, Oregon

Victoria Maizes, MD
Executive Director
Program in Integrative Medicine
Associate Professor of Medicine
Family and Community Medicine, and
    Public Health
University of Arizona
Tucson, Arizona

Douglas Mann, PhD
Professor of Neurology
University of North Carolina School of
    Medicine
Medical Director
UNC Neurology Clinics and
UNC Program on Integrative Medicine
Chapel Hill, North Carolina

Donna Manning, MS
Exercise Physiologist
ValleyCare Health System
Livermore, California

M. Caroline Martin, MHA, RN
Appointee
Governor's Council for Healthy Virginians
President and CEO, NurseWorks
Suffolk, Virginia

Rebecca McLean
National Director
Circle of Life Coaches Training
Santa Barbara, California

J. Michael Menke
Health Services Researcher
Evaluation Group for the Analysis of Data
Faculty Member
Program in Integrative Medicine
University of Arizona
Tucson, Arizona

Ryan Milley
Research Associate
Oregon College of Oriental Medicine
Portland, Oregon

Robert D. Mootz, DC
Associate Medical Director for
    Chiropractic
Washington State
Department of Labor and Industries
Olympia, Washington

Michael T. Murray, ND
Clinical Practice
Board of Trustees, Bastyr University
Seattle, Washington

Patricia Norris, PhD
Clinical Director
Life Sciences Institute of Mind-Body
    Health
Topeka, Kansas

Sister Mary Elizabeth O'Brien, PhD, MTS,
    RN, FAAN
Spiritual Advisor
Professor of Nursing
Catholic University of America
Washington, DC

Karin Olsen, BA, LMP
Appointed Member
Washington State Massage Examining
    Board
Owner and Director
Kaleidoscope Massage Therapy
Shelton, Washington

Kelli Pearson, DC, DABCO, FICC
Clinical Coordinator
Pearson & Weary Pain Relief Clinics
Spokane, Washington

James A. Peterson, PhD, FACSM
Fellow, American College of Sports
    Medicine
CEO, Healthy Learning
Monterey, California

Joel G. Pickar, DC, PhD
NIH Advisory Council, NCCAM
Professor
Palmer Center for Chiropractic Research
Davenport, Iowa

Bruce Pomeranz, MD, PhD
Researcher
Professor Emeritus
Program in Neuroscience
University of Toronto
Toronto, Canada

David P. Rakel, MD
Medical Director
Integrative Medicine Program
Assistant Professor
Department of Family Medicine
University of Wisconsin
Madison, Wisconsin

John C. Reed, MD, MD(H)
Vice President for Medical Affairs
American WholeHealth
Sterling, Virginia
Senior Consultant in Integrative Medicine
University of Maryland Integrative
    Medicine LLC
Baltimore, Maryland

Susan Rosen
Founding Member
National Certification Board for
    Therapeutic Massage and Bodywork
Director, Susan Rosen and Associates
Olympia, Washington

Martin L. Rossman, MD, Dipl Ac
Clinical Associate, Department of
    Medicine
University of California, San Francisco
Founder, The Healing Mind
Mill Valley, California

Charles A. Simpson, DC, DABCO
Vice President, Medical Director
Complementary Healthcare Plans
Beaverton, Oregon

Neil Sol, PhD, FACSM, FALCHP
Vice President of Outpatient Services
ValleyCare Health System
Livermore, California

Jill Stansbury, ND
Chair, Assistant Professor
Botanical Medicine Department
National College of Naturopathic Medicine
Portland, Oregon
Clinical Practice
Battle Ground Healing Arts
Battle Ground, Washington

John Triano, DC, PhD
Research Professor
Biomedical Engineering Program
University of Texas
Codirector, Conservative Medicine
Director, Chiropractic Division
Texas Back Institute
Plano, Texas

Melvyn Werbach, MD
Associate Editor
*Alternative Therapies in Health and
    Medicine*
Author
Third Line Press
Tarzana, California

PART I

Expanding the Continuum of Care

Chapter

CHAPTER 1

Perspectives on Integrative Practice

David Rakel, MD

PERSPECTIVES ON INTEGRATIVE MEDICINE

The resources in this book are offered to empower you through greater access to evidence-based therapies of complementary medicine—those with the greatest acceptance by physicians and most widely utilized by consumers. The relevance and effectiveness of the disciplines in this book have been established in a growing body of research over the past two decades. As health care practitioners, we all benefit from resources that help us do our jobs better, and when we expand our knowledge of therapeutic modalities, our patients benefit as well.

This information is also intended to expand communication between the professions, and aid physicians and practitioners in identifying other providers with whom they would like to share mutual referrals or collaborate on care. We encourage you to begin by exploring an area in which you have the deepest interest—one you believe will best serve the needs of your patients.

David Rakel, MD, is director of the University of Wisconsin Integrative Medicine Program and assistant professor in the Department of Family Medicine at the UW Medical School. A graduate of the 2-year fellowship program in integrative medicine at the University of Arizona Health Sciences Center with Andrew Weil, MD, Dr. Rakel is currently involved in two National Institutes of Health grants to study the placebo effect and to incorporate complementary and alternative therapy education into medical school curriculums. He is editor of the text *Integrative Medicine*, is board certified in family and holistic medicine, holds certifications in sports medicine and interactive guided imagery, and sits on the American Board of Holistic Medicine.

Research shows that on any given day, approximately 75% of people who see a primary care provider have a condition without a clear diagnosis (Kroenke et al., 1989). Nationwide, 44.5% of our population has one or more chronic conditions (Hoffman et al., 1996). In an overlay to chronic illness, excessive weight gain now affects 65% of our population—and half these people have obesity, with its potential for a range of sequelae. Clearly the issues facing medicine are significant. Expanding the continuum of care to include lifestyle approaches and complementary medicine can provide us with additional tools and resources to address the health concerns that challenge our patients.

PERSPECTIVES ON INTEGRATIVE PRACTICE

Access to healing. How can we promote healing? How can we access the underlying process that results in the body's ability to heal? What are the primary factors that sustain or enhance resiliency and host resistance? Underlying influences may involve physiological, psychological, or psychospiritual aspects of the patient's life.

Early intervention. Preventive medicine has been an important aspect of primary care for decades. It is also a cornerstone of integrative and holistic medicine. For example, the identification of patients with insulin resistance syndrome can potentiate therapeutic and lifestyle changes that may prevent the progression to overt diabetes and heart disease. In metabolic syndrome, tissues in the body develop resistance to the effects of insulin in stimulating glucose uptake. Initially, the body secretes more insulin to manage blood sugar. Eventually this adaptation is lost and the body is unable to sustain the insulin demand, resulting in diabetes.

The diagnosis of insulin resistance usually precedes the diagnosis of Type 2 diabetes by years, or even decades. This syndrome (also known as prediabetes, metabolic syndrome, or syndrome X) is associated with hyperinsulinemia, glucose intolerance, central obesity, elevated blood pressure, elevated triglycerides, and reduced HDL—processes that set the stage for heart disease.

Metabolic syndrome is an important illness to treat in the primary care setting, because if the progression is halted, diabetes can actually be prevented. Identifying the symptoms early enough and motivating the patient to make lifestyle changes can reverse the disease process (Lindstrom et al., 2003). Early intervention is significant, because once there is end-stage organ damage, the body is frequently unable to heal itself. The beauty—and challenge—of our work is to detect the problems before that degenerative process occurs.

Lifestyle medicine. We know from the evidence that lifestyle is a major factor in the development of insulin resistance. In one diabetes-prevention trial, evidence for the importance of exercise and nutrition became so compelling that it was deemed unethical to deny exercise and good nutrition to the control group, and the study was halted (Tuomilehto et al., 2001).

As a result of this type of data, we no longer take lifestyle for granted. For example, in the 27-center study cited above, researchers found that when patients at risk for diabetes lost just 8 pounds through regular exercise the incidence of Type 2 diabetes was reduced by approximately 58% (Tuomilehto et al., 2001). The epidemic of obesity has made it clear that if we do not begin paying more attention to lifestyle factors in health, we could potentially spend a great deal of money on disease-oriented care in response to the subsequent rise in diabetes, heart disease, and their sequelae.

Increasing the focus on health can provide a very exciting perspective to your practice. In a clinical context, when we expand the focus to include health and wellness, it creates more options and supports a broader perspective of health and illness. These are the basic elements every human being needs to facilitate health: good nutrition, exercise, healthy habits and lifestyle choices, spiritual connection, mind/body balance, supportive relationships, and good stress management. Lifestyle therapies are relevant to everyone, but need to be individualized based on the health, energy, resources, and personality of the patient.

Genetic expression. We now know that lifestyle also influences genetics. Over the past decade, the field of epigenetics has expanded its focus from genetic make-up to include the influence of environmental factors. Research shows that the lifestyle we create for ourselves can influence the phenotypic expression of our genotype. A gene can be turned on or off by the environment in which it is exposed. Genetic expression is affected by the foods we eat, the stresses we encounter (and how we cope with them), our spiritual connection, and our degree of social isolation. All these factors can influence how disease is expressed or whether it is expressed at all. For example, by simply adding fresh fruits and vegetables to the diet, people can decrease their risk of cancer by approximately 50% (Block et al., 1992). In general, the management of metabolic syndrome, diabetes, and heart disease all reflect the importance of patients' intention and behavior—reflected in their lifestyle (Koertge et al., 2003). Lifestyle can be modified to create good health, even if we have a certain genetic predisposition.

We know from the work of Dean Ornish on lifestyle and heart disease that even patients who have an incurable disease benefit from a lifestyle approach (Ornish et al., 1998). This is another example of how lifestyle medicine is providing us with a broader range of options to offer patients. As a practitioner, knowing that you can influence patients' genetic expression can enable you to provide a genuine sense of hope and optimism, which empowers them to make changes to improve and stabilize their health.

In another era, we might have said that there was nothing more we could do for patients. Now we know that there is always something that can be done.

Using evidence-based complementary therapy. In some cases, we may want additional options to assist our patients with chronic conditions. Migraine headaches provide a good example. A study of 400 patients, conducted in Britain (Vickers et al., 2004), evaluated the potential effects of acupuncture in the treatment of migraines. Both the control group and the acupuncture group received standard therapy and could use additional medication to abort headaches as needed. The acupuncture group also received acupuncture treatments weekly. The research found 35% improvement in headaches in the acupuncture group after 12 months, versus 16% in the control group. Patients receiving acupuncture experienced 22 fewer headaches over the course of a year, compared with the controls. Those in the acupuncture group also required 15% fewer

medications, 26% fewer physician visits, and had fewer days missed from work. Additional evidence indicates that this therapy was also cost-effective (Wonderling et al., 2004).

Employing an integrative approach. In conventional medicine, when patients have a complex, unresolved, or recurring condition, we frequently enlist the help of a specialist. Integrative medicine can also be used strategically and synergistically in a team approach. For example, some of our patients with migraines may have a genetic susceptibility to headaches and a lower threshold to pain.

To reduce the frequency of headaches, we need to explore a number of different factors. However, it is important to evaluate these approaches sequentially, to avoid overwhelming the patient, fragmenting care, and expending health resources. Our initial approach is often low-tech and cost-effective—for example, a dietary assessment. Patients can begin with an elimination diet, removing the most common foods known to trigger headaches such as aspartame, caffeine, chocolate, MSG, sulfite additives, and tyramine.

If the headache is due to muscle tension, manual therapy may be effective. Clinically, we find that chiropractic, osteopathic, or craniosacral therapy can be instrumental in relieving muscle tension that can trigger headaches. If these approaches do not resolve the headaches, we would also evaluate emotional triggers and the effects of stress.

The role of stress in illness. As clinicians, we have all experienced situations in which nothing seems to work. Consider the case of a patient with chronic daily headaches that have not resolved. At some point, we may have tried every available intervention—ordered all the appropriate studies, evaluated possible headache triggers, and recommended an elimination diet, but nothing seems to help.

One promising approach is to refer the patient to massage and counseling. Massage, as a form of short-term therapy, offers relief for the sore muscles and spasms. Counseling provides the patient the opportunity to work toward deeper insight into the causes of tension. Is there stress at work or at home? The counselor can facilitate the patient's health by increasing his or her awareness of the influence of lifestyle, habits, and behaviors. Then the patient is not just a passive recipient of temporary benefit, but also an active contributor to their own well-being.

If tension is the underlying cause, resolution of the symptoms requires introspection on the part of the patient to explore why the symptoms are recurring. Relief derived from manual therapy provides a useful indication that the symptoms can be improved (and an initial indication that the pain is not being caused by a structural or neurological condition). Combining this technique with encouragement to explore the source of tension offers the most efficient path to healing. Repeated treatments with manual therapy alone would not have produced this insight and would probably have led to symptom suppression. This approach also provides the patient with greater opportunity to participate in his or her own health and to become more adept at self-care. All healing is ultimately self-healing.

THE IMPORTANCE OF INTEGRATIVE MEDICINE

A decade ago, physicians were concerned that their patients were choosing complementary therapies instead of the services they provided. However, Astin's research (1998) found that only approximately 5% of patients used complementary therapies such as acupuncture in isolation. Of those who used complementary therapies, approximately 95% were also seen by a conventional physician. Although a sizable number of patients see complementary practitioners, the vast majority of these patients continue to see their primary care physician. This indicates that many patients want truly integrative care. Yet, until recently, it has been up to patients to integrate their own health care (Simpson, 2001).

This type of fragmented care may not be an issue when patients are well; however, if they lose their health, they need a more integrative approach. The patient's journey can be compared to climbing a mountain. When you hike in the local woods, it would never occur to you to hire a guide. However, if you go trekking in the Himalayas, you would not consider making the trip without one. Similarly, when patients develop serious illness, they want and need highly knowledgeable guidance. In this context, we consider it vital that physicians become genuinely well informed about complementary therapies, especially since many patients seek alternative care for serious conditions. We see it as equally important that complementary practitioners become skilled at communicating with conventional doctors. Effective referrals and good patient co-management ultimately serve health care providers and patients alike.

PRACTICAL APPROACHES TO COMPLEMENTARY MEDICINE

To educate yourself in greater depth about complementary medicine, we encourage a systematic approach to learning. Identify a discipline of greatest relevance to your practice and your patients' needs—one that is congruent with your own interests and style of clinical practice. Begin educating yourself by reading and attending workshops and conferences. Develop a strategy for learning. Some practitioners may wish to focus on a particular discipline such as mind-body medicine or botanical therapy. That strategy could have a very specific goal—for example, applications in managing pain or inflammatory conditions. Others may want to explore resources most relevant to the needs of a specific patient population, such as diabetes care or the treatment of rheumatoid arthritis. Whether you are exploring a particular discipline or focusing on the treatment of a specific diagnosis, there are several immediate approaches that can support greater access to complementary care.

1. Experience complementary therapies first-hand. The best way to actually learn about any given modality is to personally experience that therapy. This is also an excellent place to begin building relationships with practitioners to whom you would like to refer patients. The personal experience and understanding of another discipline, and its benefits help develop insight into what that therapy may or may not have to offer. An experiential approach provides the foundation for making effective referrals and for good professional communication. Many complementary practitioners are willing to provide a treatment free of charge to promote greater understanding between the disciplines and establish sources of mutual referral.

2. Make strategic referrals. To maintain your focus on the goal of healing, ask yourself:
   • Will this referral help resolve the problem?
   • Is there the potential for harm (physical or financial)?
   • Is there an evidence basis for this therapy?
   • How relevant is it to the patient's diagnosis?
   • Will it lead to symptom resolution or symptom suppression?
   • Will it empower the patient to be more active in self-care?
   • Will it support the most efficient use of health care resources?

3. Identify the most highly skilled practitioners for mutual referrals. It is important to know the practitioners to whom you refer patients. This is one of the reasons we encourage you to experience a treatment. You will also want to inquire about where the practitioners were trained and the type of licensure or certification they carry. Most important of all, you want to be sure they are skilled in what they do. Good sources of referrals include meetings, workshops, or conferences that could provide access to a network of practitioners. Feedback from your patients can also be quite useful. For example, there is a massage practitioner to whom I frequently send patients. Every patient I send gets better in some way, and my patients always have positive things to say about the care they receive.

4. Exchange information and collaborate to optimize patient care. Good collaboration improves our ability to coordinate care effectively. We are also more effective in a team approach when we have an understanding of other disciplines, their basic principles and vocabulary, and the strengths they have to offer our patients. Good communication supports further insight into the success of a particular treatment.

An integrative approach expands the options available to patients—and to the physicians and practitioners who provide their care. This could mean strategic referrals to a virtual network or a multidisciplinary approach within an integrative medicine center. Health care practitioners who expand their continuum of care to include lifestyle and complementary therapies are able to provide a wider range of treatment strategies and to implement care management more effectively. At every phase of care, it is important to ask ourselves: What is the most effective therapy? How can we best set healing in motion?

REFERENCES

Astin J. Why patients use alternative medicine: results of a national study. *JAMA*. 1998;279(19):1548–1553.

Block G, Patterson B, Subar A. Fruit, vegetables, and cancer prevention: a review of the epidemiological evidence. *Nutr Cancer*. 1992;18(1):1–29.

Hoffman C, Rice D, Sung HY. Persons with chronic conditions: their prevalence and costs. *JAMA*. 1996;276(18):1473–1479.

Koertge J, Weidner G, Elliott-Eller M, et al. Improvement in medical risk factors and quality of life in women and men with coronary artery disease in the Multicenter Lifestyle Demonstration Project. *Am J Cardiol*. 2003;91(11):1316–1322.

Kroenke K, Arrington ME, Mangelsdorff D. Common symptoms in ambulatory care: incidence, evaluation, therapy and outcome. *Am J Med*. 1989;86:262–266.

Lindstrom J, Louheranta A, Mannelin M, et al., and the Finnish Diabetes Prevention Study Group. The Finnish Diabetes Prevention Study (DPS): Lifestyle intervention and 3-year results on diet and physical activity. *Diabetes Care*. 2003;26(12):3230–3236.

Ornish D, Scherwitz LW, Billings JH, et al. Intensive lifestyle changes for reversal of coronary heart disease. *JAMA*. 1998;280(23):2001–2007.

Simpson CA. Pursuing integration: a model of integrated delivery of complementary and alternative medicine. In: Faass N, ed. *Integrating Complementary Medicine into Health Systems*. Gaithersburg, MD: Aspen; 2001.

Tuomilehto J, Lindstrom J, Eriksson JG, et al., and the Finnish Diabetes Prevention Study Group. Prevention of type 2 diabetes mellitus by changes in lifestyle among subjects with impaired glucose tolerance. *N Engl J Med*. 2001;344(18):1343–1350.

Vickers AJ, Rees RW, Zollman CE, et al. Acupuncture of chronic headache disorders in primary care: randomised controlled trial and economic analysis. *Health Technol Assess*. 2004;8(48):1–50.

Wonderling D, Vickers AJ, Grieve R, McCarney R. Cost effectiveness analysis of a randomised trial of acupuncture for chronic headache in primary care. *BMJ*. 2004 Mar 27;328(7442):747. Epub 2004 Mar 15.

CHAPTER 2

Who Uses Complementary Medicine?

Nancy Faass, MSW, MPH

RESEARCH DATA

In 1993 a seminal article in the *New England Journal of Medicine* changed the way we view American medicine. A research team affiliated with Harvard Medical School and led by Eisenberg (1993) estimated that in 1990, Americans made 425 million visits to practitioners of complementary and alternative medicine (CAM). The researchers projected expenditures for CAM in the United States at more than $13.6 billion. In that same year, out-of-pocket expenditures on hospitalization totaled $12.8 billion.

A second study by Eisenberg and colleagues (1998) found an almost 50% increase in the number of total visits to CAM practitioners (629 million), with expenditures in 1997 as high as $47.5 billion. Of this amount more than $12 billion was paid out-of-pocket for CAM health care providers such as chiropractors, acupuncturists, and massage therapists. These fees were more than the US public paid out-of-pocket for all hospitalizations in 1997, and about half that paid by consumers for physician services (Center for Medicare and Medicaid Services, 1997).

Nancy Faass, MSW, MPH, is a writer and editor in San Francisco who provides book and project development in health and medicine (www.HealthWritersGroup.com). With an MPH from the University of California at Berkeley and an MSW from Catholic University, Washington, DC, she has worked as a science editor, an archivist, and in scholarly publishing. Ms. Faass is co-author or co-editor of seven books and developer and editor of *Integrating Complementary Medicine into Health Systems*, voted 2001 Book of the Year by Doody's Publishing, a library review service.

The three major studies conducted in 1997 were in approximate agreement that 40–42% of the general population used CAM in some form (Eisenberg et al., 1998; Astin, 1998; InterActive Solutions, 1998). Two federal surveys of much larger populations using inperson interviews found comparable utilization somewhat lower, at approximately 29% in 1999 (Ni et al., 2002), and 36% in 2002 (Barnes et al., 2004). Table 2–1 summarizes major studies on CAM use conducted over the past 15 years.

ALTERNATIVE, COMPLEMENTARY, OR INTEGRATIVE CARE?

The National Institutes of Health (NIH) has defined complementary medicine as that used adjunctively to conventional care. "Alternative medicine" indicates therapies used in place of conventional interventions, while integrative medicine implies complementary and conventional care used in tandem. This raises the question: To what extent do patients use alternative therapies exclusively? Or do they seek *both* conventional and complementary care? The data indicate that the vast majority of patients who use complementary medicine also use conventional care.

A study by Astin (1998) at Stanford University found that only 4.4% of patients relied primarily on CAM. "The vast majority of individuals appear to use alternative therapies in conjunction with, rather than instead of, more conventional treatment." A

Table 2-1 Data on the Utilization of CAM Therapies

Source and Universe Surveyed	% use in past year
Utilization of CAM Lifestyle Therapies and Practitioners	
Harvard University, Center for Alternative Medicine Research. Random sample (N = 2,055) surveyed by telephone, 1997 (Eisenberg et al., 1998)	42.1
Stanford Center for Research. Subset (N = 1,035) of representative panel, written survey, 1997 (Astin, 1998)	40.0
National Center for Complementary and Alternative Medicine, NIH. Subset (N = 31,044) of 2002 National Health Interview Survey, in-person interviews (Barnes et al., 2004)	36.0
Harvard University, Center for Alternative Medicine Research. Nationally representative random sample (N = 1,539) surveyed by phone, 1990 (Eisenberg et al., 1993)	33.8
National Center for Health Statistics, CDC. Subset (N = 30,801) of 1999 National Health Interview Survey, in-person interviews (Ni et al., 2002)	28.1– 29.7
Utilization of CAM Practitioners	
Robert Wood Johnson Foundation. Subset (N = 3,450) of 1994 National Access to Care Survey, in-person interviews (Paramore, 1997)	9.4
Yale University, Departments of Psychiatry and Public Health (Druss and Rosenheck, 1999) and *University of Maryland, Complementary Medicine Program* (Bausell et al., 2001). Subset (N = 16,068) of 1994 Medical Expenditure Panel Survey, in-person interviews	8.3– 9.0

federal survey in 1994 funded by the Robert Wood Johnson Foundation reported, "Users of alternative therapies made almost twice as many visits to conventional (or orthodox) medical providers as nonusers made (8.3 and 4.2 respectively). [Yet these patients] still reported much higher levels of unmet need for medical care" (Paramore, 1997: 83). A number of studies have estimated the percentage of consumers who use complementary therapies and also use conventional medicine:

- Lafferty et al. (2004)—97.9%
- Eisenberg et al. (1998)—96.0%
- Astin (1998)—95.6%
- National Market Measures (1999)—86.0%
- Druss and Rosenheck (1999)—78.3%

Two perspectives are suggested by these data. First, the high utilization of conventional care among CAM users reflects appreciation of the value of technological Western medicine. The other implication is that the vast majority of patients are not neglecting conventional care for alternative treatment. A primary concern has been that patients might forgo necessary treatment or that serious health conditions might not be detected by CAM practitioners. The fact that the vast majority of CAM patients continue to use conventional services does not provide an automatic conclusion to the question of safety, but it does indicate that patients continue to avail themselves of biomedical services.

WHY PATIENTS USE COMPLEMENTARY MEDICINE

Professional Care or Self-Care?

Complementary medicine attracts multiple markets (R. Jahnke, written communication, 6/99, 8/04). One population consists of proactive individuals who use complementary approaches for prevention and health

enhancement. Another major segment consists of individuals with chronic disorders or pain conditions. The needs of these two populations overlap in their use of lifestyle therapies, nutrition, vitamins, and herbs. However, data confirm that the use of conventional practitioner services is much higher in the group with chronic conditions.

Self-care. In 1997, out-of-pocket expenditures on wellness were $14.8 billion for supplements, books, classes, and equipment (Eisenberg et al., 1998). By 1999 data from the natural products industry showed that expenditures on supplements, natural foods, and products totaled $28.2 billion (Traynor, 2000) and by 2003, totaled $42.8 billion, including at least $20 billion in sales for nutritional and herbal supplements (Spenser & Rae, 2004). Interest in health enhancement and self-care is now ubiquitous in consumer media and American culture (Barnes et al., 2004). (See Table 2–2.)

Table 2–2 Number of Adults (in Millions) Who Used Complementary and Alternative Medicine During the Past 12 Months: United States, 2002

Practitioner Care (in millions)		Self-Care (in millions)	
Chiropractic care	15	Deep-breathing exercises	23
Massage	10	Yoga	10
Acupuncture	2	Tai chi and Qigong	3
Homeopathic treatment	2	Natural products (nonvitamin,	
Naturopathy	0.2	nonmineral)	38
Folk medicine	0.2	Diet-based therapies	7
Ayurveda	0.1	Megavitamin therapy	6
Guided imagery	2	Meditation	15
Biofeedback	0.3	Progressive relaxation	6
Hypnosis	0.2		
Total	**32**	**Total**	**108**

Source of data: Barnes et al., 2004.

Professional care. A great deal of research over the past decade has focused on consumer use of CAM services. "Nearly one-tenth of the US population saw a professional for some type of alternative therapy in 1994. Most users of alternative therapies seek this type of care as an intervention for a specific health condition, rather than as a general health measure not connected to a particular disease or condition. Users seem to recognize the limitations of alternative medicine as they tend to seek this type of help for pain, stress, and anxiety; and see traditional medical providers for treatment as well" (Paramore, 1997: 88).

Data on current use of complementary practitioners from a recent analysis by the National Center for Complementary and Alternative Medicine (NCCAM) (Barnes et al., 2004) is summarized in Table 2–2.

DEMOGRAPHICS

What do we know about who uses complementary medicine? A number of trends have emerged from research on representative populations (see Table 2–3). Although people of all education levels and income levels use complementary medicine, the primary utilizers tend to have some college and higher income. This probably reflects out-of-pocket costs of care and lack of insurance coverage, which are clearly economic barriers to use for those at lower income levels. Approximately 40% to 50% of women (ages 30 to 59) use CAM lifestyle or therapies, compared with 30% to 40% of men. Utilization tends to be higher in western states at 43% compared with 36% in the Northeast and 37% in the Midwest. Southern utilization is projected at 30% (Barnes et al., 2004).

Table 2–3 Who Uses Complementary Medicine?

- Higher education (50% or more college graduates or beyond)
- Higher income (more than 50% earn more than $50K)
- Age group 30 to 59 has highest utilization
- More than 50% with poor health, comorbidities, or chronic pain
- Those with chronic illness utilize more conventional care than nonusers of CAM

Sources of data: Astin, 1998; Barnes et al., 2004; Bausell et al., 2002; Druss & Rosenheck, 1999; Eisenberg et al., 1993; Eisenberg et al., 1998; Gordon et al., 2004; Ni et al., 2002; Paramore, 1997.

CAM Use by Cohort

The data suggests an increasing demand. "Analyses of lifetime use and age at onset showed that 67.6% of respondents had used at least one CAM therapy in their lifetime. Lifetime use steadily increased . . . across three age cohorts" (Kessler et al., 2001: 262).

The percentage of respondents using some type of CAM therapy by age 33:

- Pre-baby boom cohort—30%
- Baby boom cohort (born 1945 to 1964)—50%
- Post-baby boom cohort—70%

"The trend of increased CAM therapy use across all cohorts since 1950, coupled with the strong persistence of use, suggests a continuing increased demand for CAM therapies that will affect all facets of health care delivery over the next 25 years" (Kessler et al., 2001: 267).

MOTIVATION FOR USE

Health Issues

The Astin survey at Stanford (1998) found that the two most frequently cited reasons for using complementary medicine were "relief for symptoms" and "efficacy for a particular health problem." This trend is echoed throughout the research:

- The "heaviest users of CAM therapies tend to be individuals with comorbid, non-life-threatening health problems" (Bausell et al., 2001: 2).
- The likelihood of CAM use among respondents with chronic pain was found to be twice that of respondents not reporting chronic pain (Astin, 1998).
- Back, neck, and shoulder pain were the most frequently cited reasons for visits to an alternative medicine provider (Borkan et al., 1994).
- Individuals suffering from mental, metabolic, or musculoskeletal complaints were more than three times as likely to have visited a CAM provider during the previous year (Bausell et al., 2001).
- A survey by the Kaiser Foundation of HMO members who experienced severe musculoskeletal pain reported that 21.5% used chiropractic, and 19.4% used massage therapy (Gordon et al., 2004).
- Respondents who reported anxiety were three times as likely as the average survey respondent to use CAM (Astin, 1998).
- A survey by American WholeHealth of CAM utilization at an integrative medicine center found that more than 90% of patients seeking complementary care had one or more co-morbidities (J. Reed, written communication, 12/04).
- A literature review of CAM utilization by health condition, from Wootton and Sparber (2003), reported use ranging from 9% to 100% when lifestyle therapies were included.

Prevalence of Chronic Conditions in the United States

This aspect of CAM use reflects a major trend. Chronic illness can now be considered a silent epidemic in the United States. Surprisingly, more than 44.5% of Americans—88.5 million individuals—have one or more chronic conditions (Hoffman et al., 1996). Their direct health care costs in 1987 accounted for three-fourths of all US health care expenditures—$425 billion. Indirect costs totaled an additional $234 billion.

Recent data from the National Center for Chronic Disease Prevention and Health Promotion at the CDC (2004) indicates that the treatment of chronic and degenerative diseases accounted for more than 75% of the nation's $1.4 trillion medical costs. This included $300 billion in health care costs for cardiovascular diseases. What is not fully reflected in the data is lost productivity and quality of life, as well as the impact on the individual, the family, and the community.

CONDITIONS TREATED IN COMPLEMENTARY MEDICINE

The Robert Wood Johnson survey of practitioner use found that in the majority of cases, CAM services were sought for the treatment of a specific condition (Paramore, 1997). Astin's study (1998) also found that higher use of CAM correlated with the presence of specific health conditions. The data from Astin (1998), Eisenberg et al. (1998), and Barnes et al. (2004) reflect general agreement in their findings on the conditions for which respondents most often seek CAM therapies (see Table 2–4).

Additional insight is provided by the analysis of Bausell, Lee, and Berman (2001). Health conditions of CAM users were determined by re-evaluating data from the 1996 Medical Expenditure Panel Survey (N = 16,038). Conditions reported most often in conjunction with CAM use by Bausell and colleagues (2001) were:

- Osteoarthritis, back conditions, and joint disorders

- Alcohol and drug use, anxiety, and other affective disorders; acute reaction to stress; and other nervous system disorders
- Malaise/fatigue, diabetes, and endocrine-metabolic-nutritional disorders

UTILIZATION OF CAM THERAPIES

Use of Specific Therapies

Which therapies are most widely used in complementary medicine? The research of Eisenberg and colleagues (1998) indicates

Table 2–4 Conditions for Which Complementary and Alternative Medicine Was Used in the United States, 1997 and 2002

Conditions for which CAM was used	Number using CAM for each condition	Percentage of people with these conditions who used CAM	
	NIH NCCAM, 2002	Harvard, 1997	Stanford, 1997
	in millions	in percentage	
Back pain or problem	12	48	
Neck pain or problem	5	57	
Joint pain or stiffness	3		
Sprains and strains		24	26
Anxiety	3	43	31
Depression		41	
Arthritis, gout, lupus, fibromyalgia	3	27	25
Stomach or intestinal illness	3	27	
Severe headache or migraine	2	32	24
Recurring pain	2		37
Insomnia	2	26	
Sinusitis	0.9		
Elevated cholesterol	0.8		
Asthma	0.8		
Hypertension	0.7		
Menopause	0.7		
Fatigue		27	
Addiction (alcohol or drugs)			25
Allergies		17	

Sources of data: Barnes et al., 2004; Eisenberg et al., 1998; Astin, 1998.

that five of the most popular CAM therapies involve the use of a practitioner. The most frequently utilized, chiropractic and massage, account for approximately 70% of all CAM visits to practitioners.

Total estimated annual visits in 1997 to CAM practitioners (in millions):

- Chiropractic   192
- Massage   114
- Self-help groups   80
- Commercial diet   27
- Imagery   22
- Megavitamins   22
- Herbal medicine   10
- Acupuncture   5
- Biofeedback   4

PHYSICIAN REFERRAL

Referrals to complementary therapies by American physicians appear to be increasing steadily. Research suggests that more than a third of physicians refer patients to acupuncture and chiropractic practitioners. The 2002 National Health Interview Survey indicates that 26% of patients who used complementary medicine were referred by a conventional provider (Barnes et al., 2004).

A Denver survey (Winslow & Shapiro, 2002), of predominantly primary care physicians (N = 302) reported that recommendations to patients for CAM were associated with physician self-education in CAM, belief in CAM efficacy, or physician use. Reporting on their experience with CAM:

- 76% indicated they had patients who used CAM
- 59% had patients who inquired about specific CAM treatments
- 48% had recommended CAM to patients
- 24% had personally used CAM

A survey of rheumatologists (N = 924) published the same year indicated similar findings (Berman et al., 2002). "On average, the respondents reported knowing enough to discuss 10 (of 22) therapies with patients, considered 9 to be part of legitimate medical practice, and had referred patients to someone else for 8 of the 22 therapies." Correlates of use and/or referral included a belief in the legitimacy of the therapies and self-reported knowledge.

The rheumatology study (Berman et al., 2002) indicated even higher rates of knowledge, acceptance, and referral. The percentage of these specialists who reported referring patients to specific therapies included:

- Exercise intervention—75%
- Biofeedback—65%
- Dietary prescription—65%
- Electromagnetic applications (TENS)—65%
- Behavioral medicine—58%
- Acupuncture—57%
- Massage or manual healing—51%

The rheumatology survey reported "an openness [among physicians] toward a number of CAM treatment modalities that they consider to be a legitimate medical practice" (Berman et al., 2002). In the Denver study, the majority of physicians surveyed (84%) expressed an interest or need to learn more about complementary medicine. Reasons cited were the desire to dissuade patients from undergoing an unsafe or ineffective modality, to recommend safe and effective CAM modalities, to obtain factual information about CAM modalities, and to be able to respond knowledgeably to patient inquiries (Winslow & Shapiro, 2002).

DISCUSSION

At this point, many physicians appear receptive to complementary medicine, while others want further research to support evidence-based practice. Actuaries, insurers, and employers want additional data to determine the economic feasibility of complementary medicine. To what extent will CAM offset the cost of other forms of treatment or drive up overall expenditures? Will reimbursement for programs offset the expense of providing them in more elaborate, conventional environments? Will the attractiveness of these programs expand market share to an extent that makes them worth offering?

The research indicates that the public is willing to pay out-of-pocket to expand its options for medical care. High levels of satisfaction with CAM are reported by consumers (Simpson, 2001; Trompeter, 2001). Improved health outcomes have been documented for massage (Chapters 34 and 36), acupuncture (Chapters 38, 40, and 41), and chiropractic (Chapters 49 and 52). There is

also a substantial body of research indicating cost-effectiveness for chiropractic (Branson, 2001). These data suggest the potential for health improvement and cost savings if CAM health insurance coverage became more widely available.

In the context of cost-effectiveness, would the inclusion of wellness programming and complementary medicine in health systems improve the overall health of clients? Will these therapies provide new tools for prevention and the management of chronic disorders? Do they provide meaningful options for treatment? Does complementary medicine improve health outcomes?

Existing data suggest positive outcomes, affordability, and cost-effectiveness, but the health care community awaits further confirmation. This book is offered to provide a range of perspectives and continue the dialogue on these important questions.

REFERENCES

Astin J. Why patients use alternative medicine: results of a national study. *JAMA*. 1998;279(19):1548–1553.

Astin JA, Marie A, Pelletier KR, Hansen E, Haskell WL. A review of the incorporation of complementary and alternative medicine by mainstream physicians. *Arch Intern Med*. 1998;158:2303–2309.

Barnes PM, Powell-Griner E, McFann K, Nahin R. Complementary and alternative medicine use among adults: United States, 2002. *Adv Data*. 2004;(343):1–16.

Bausell RB, Lee WL, Berman BM. Demographic and health-related correlates to visits to complementary and alternative medical providers. *Med Care*. 2001;39(2):190–196.

Berman BM, Bausell RB, Lee WL. Use and referral patterns for 22 complementary and alternative medical therapies by members of the American College of Rheumatology: results of a national survey. *Arch Intern Med*. 2002;162:766–770.

Berman BM, Singh BB, Hartnol SM, et al. Primary care physicians and complementary-alternative med-

icine: training, attitudes, and practice patterns. *J Am Board Fam Pract*. 1998;11:272–281.

Borkan J, Neher JO, Anson O, Smoker B. Referrals for alternative therapies. *J Fam Pract*. 1994;39:545–550.

Branson RA. Cost comparison of chiropractic and medical treatment: a literature review. In: Faass N, ed. *Integrating Complementary Medicine into Health Systems*. Sudbury, MA: Jones and Bartlett/Aspen, 2001.

Center for Medicare and Medicaid Services. 1997 National Health Expenditures Survey. Available at: http://www.cms.hhs.gov/statistics/nhe. Accessed December 1, 2004.

Druss B, Rosenheck R. Association between use of unconventional therapies and conventional medical services. *JAMA*. 1999;282(7):651–656.

Eisenberg D, Davis R, Ettner S, et al. Trends in alternative medicine use in the United States, 1990–1997: Results of a follow-up national survey. *JAMA*. 1998;280(18):1569–1575.

Eisenberg DM, Kessler RC, Foster C, et al. Unconventional medicine in the United States. *N Engl J Med*. 1993;328(4):246–252.

Gordon NP, Lin TY. Use of complementary and alternative medicine by the adult membership of a large northern California health maintenance organization. *J Ambulatory Care Manager*. 2004;27(1):12–24.

Gordon N, Sobel D, Tarazona E. Use of and interest in alternative therapies among adult primary care clinicians and adult members in a large health maintenance organization. *WJM*. 1998;169(3):153–161.

Hoffman C, Rice D, Sung HY. Persons with chronic conditions: their prevalence and costs. *JAMA*. 1996;276(18): 1473–1479.

InterActive Solutions. *Landmark Report I on Public Perceptions of Alternative Care*. Sacramento, CA: Landmark Healthcare; 1998.

Kessler RC, Davis RB, Foster DF, et al. Long-term trends in the use of complementary and alternative medical therapies in the United States. *Ann Intern Med*. 2001;135(4):262–268.

Lafferty WE, Bellas A, Baden AC, Tyree PT, Standish LJ, Patternson R. The use of complementary and alternative medical providers by insured cancer patients in Washington State. *Cancer*. 2004;100:1522–1530.

National Center for Chronic Disease Prevention and Health Promotion (NCCDPHP). Chronic disease overview. Atlanta, GA: CDC. Web site:www.cdc.gov/nccdphp/overview.htm. Accessed August 1, 2004.

National Market Measures. *The Landmark Report II*. Sacramento, CA: Landmark Healthcare; 1999.

Ni H, Simile C, Hardy AM. Utilization of complementary and alternative medicine by United States adults: results from the 1999 national health interview survey. *Med Care*. 2002;40(4):353–358.

Paramore L. Use of alternative therapies: estimates from the 1994 Robert Wood Johnson Foundation National Access to Care Survey. *J Pain Symptom Manage*. 1997;13:83–89.

Rooney B, Fiocco G, Hughes P, Halter S. Provider attitudes and use of alternative medicine in a midwestern medical practice in 2001. *WMJ*. 2001;100(7):27–31.

Simpson CA. Utilization data: chiropractic utilization and cost-effectiveness. In: Faass N, ed. *Integrating Complementary Medicine into Health Systems*. Sudbury, MA: Jones and Bartlett/Aspen, 2001.

Spenser MT, Rae P. Natural products sales top $42 billion. *Natural Foods Merchandiser*. 2004;25(6):1.

Traynor M. Natural products market tops $28 billion. *Nat Foods Merchandiser*. 2000;21(6):1, 21.

Trompeter T. Perspective: community health centers of King County. In: Faass N, ed. *Integrating Complementary Medicine into Health Systems*. Sudbury, MA: Jones and Bartlett/Aspen, 2001.

Winslow LC, Shapiro H. Physicians want education about complementary and alternative medicine to enhance communication with their patients. *Arch Intern Med*. 2002;162:1176–1181.

Wooten JC, Sparber AG. Surveys of complementary and alternative medicine usage: a review of general population trends and specific patient populations. *Seminars in Integrative Med*. 2003;1(1):10–24.

CHAPTER 3

Four Levels of Integrative Practice

Martin L. Rossman, MD, Dipl. Ac.

Integrative medicine is a systems-based medicine that acknowledges the importance of not only physical, but emotional, psychological, social, and spiritual dimensions in health, and seeks to support the patient in exploring these dimensions. It combines the best of conventional medicine with the best of complementary or traditional practices in a rigorously considered way. An integrative approach encourages patient self-care through personal growth and the development of greater health awareness.

There is a growing need for physicians knowledgeable in complementary medicine and skilled in the psychological and emotional aspects of patient care. Physician acceptance of such practices seems to be relatively high, although the knowledge level has not kept pace. Several studies in the United States, Canada, and Israel demonstrate that almost 60% of primary care physicians refer to complementary practitioners, and that many physicians use these services for themselves and their families. Yet the same studies suggest that only 8% of these physicians have in-depth knowledge about these alternative practices.

Training in integrative medicine could expand the cadre of physicians who can intelligently guide their patients through a sophisticated understanding of complementary practices. Training would ideally provide insight into the most relevant applications of complementary therapies and their effective coordination with biomedicine. There is a need for programs that will allow practicing physicians to upgrade their skills and attain certification without taking time away from their ongoing practices.

EXPANDING THE CONTINUUM OF CARE

In ancient China there were five levels of physicians, ranked according to their healing skills. The first was the veterinarian, next the acupuncturist, the surgeon, and then the equivalent of an internist, a doctor who used nutrition and herbal medicine. Yet none of these physicians were believed to be able to cure illness. The only doctor who could potentially effect a cure was the highest-level physician, whose role was to teach people how to live in order to sustain health.

This tradition is part of Western culture as well. The word "doctor" stems from the Latin root *docere*—to teach. Physicians in our time are still considered the ultimate authorities in health-related matters. However, the advent of technology, surgery, and pharmacology has

Martin L. Rossman, MD, Dipl. Ac. (NCCAOM) is a recognized leader in the fields of complementary medicine and health psychology. He is cofounder, with David E. Bresler, PhD, of the Academy for Guided Imagery, an accredited postgraduate institute in Malibu, California. Over the past 7 years, the academy has provided training and workshops to more than 10,000 psychologists, physicians, social workers, nurses, and other health professionals. Dr. Rossman received his medical degree from the University of Michigan and serves as a clinical associate in the Department of Medicine, University of California at San Francisco Medical School.

Level Four

At this level, education consists of in-depth training in one specific complementary clinical discipline compatible with integrative medicine. An appropriate specialization would include one of the following:

- Acupuncture
- Nutrition
- Botanical medicine
- Manual therapy
- Mind-body medicine

This type of training can be obtained through an existing organization such as the American Academy of Medical Acupuncture, Bastyr University, or the Academy for Guided Imagery. Training on this level ideally includes in-depth consideration of case history analysis, clinical conferencing, and review with role play and live-patient evaluations. Training is reinforced through ongoing resources for continued learning and the development of a personal network of integrative health professionals (see Table 3–1).

Table 3–1 Experiential Aspects of Integrative Medicine Training

Personal inventory	Beliefs about medicine and healing, purpose, vision, hopes, intention, resistance, and resources
Practice inventory	Patient's beliefs and needs, partner's beliefs, staff beliefs, resources, and barriers
Community inventory	Available services, community attitudes, community needs, community resources, and community barriers
Personal explorations	Bodywork, acupuncture, homeopathy, herbal exploration, tai chi, yoga, cognitive therapy, and interactive imagery
Personal practices	Imagery and visualization, the relaxation response, mindfulness meditation, prayer, and exercise

Courtesy of Martin Rossman, MD, Mill Valley, CA.

RESOURCES

Overviews of Integrative Medicine

Gordon, J. *Manifesto for a New Medicine.* Saddle River, NJ: Addison Wesley/Pearson Education; 1997.

Kligler B, Lee R. *Integrative Medicine: Principles for Practice.* New York: McGraw-Hill; 2004.

Micozzi, MS. *Fundamentals of Complementary and Alternative Medicine.* 2nd ed. Edinburgh, Scotland: Churchill Livingstone; 2001.

Novey, DW. *Clinician's Complete Reference to Complementary/Alternative Medicine.* St. Louis, MO: Mosby; 2000.

Weil, A. *Health and Healing.* Boston, MA: Houghton Mifflin; 1998.

Clinical Texts

Pizzorno, JE, Jr, Murray, MT, Joiner-Bey, H. *The Clinician's Handbook of Natural Medicine.* Edinburgh, Scotland: Churchill Livingstone; 2002.

Rakel, D. *Integrative Medicine.* Philadelphia: Saunders; 2003.

CHAPTER 4

Phasing in Integrative Medicine

Roger Jahnke, OMD

Medicine is at a profound juncture. Break-throughs are occurring simultaneously in new technologies and contemporary approaches to natural healing. In medical practices and clinical settings across the country, patients are inquiring about complementary medicine. You may be considering making referrals to complementary providers in your community or including them in your own practice.

If the integration of complementary therapies is of interest, you may find it helpful to incorporate these programs and services in phases. A phased or modular approach can be accomplished gradually over time. In this model, you and your clinical associates can evolve through the integrative process in stages, as appropriate to the needs of your patients and your practice. This can eliminate some of the pitfalls known to occur in implementing any new model of service too

Roger Jahnke, CEO of Health Action, Santa Barbara (www.HealthAction.net), has been engaged in health care and medical innovation since 1971, designing advanced delivery systems for individual practitioners, medical groups, clinics, and hospitals. As a consultant and futurist, he assists practices, institutions, and agencies initiating projects and programs in wellness, prevention, health promotion, disease management, and integrative and complementary medicine. He has presented to the American Medical Association, American College of Healthcare Executives, American Hospital Association, Catholic Health Association, and National Wellness Institute, and is a contributing author to numerous edited volumes on complementary and integrative medicine.

Courtesy of Roger Jahnke, OMD, Director, Health Action, Santa Barbara, California.

hastily. The phases can be introduced in any order or in parallel, in response to the level of interest and the pace that suits you, your colleagues, and your community:

Phase 1—Maximizing wellness, lifestyle, and health promotion.
Phase 2—Enhancing your practice infrastructure.
Phase 3—Referring patients to complementary therapies.
Phase 4—Integrating complementary medicine.

In most practices and clinics the inclusion of integrative medicine services is occurring gradually. Experience has shown that the transition to a more comprehensive and integrated health care delivery system is a developmental process that continues to evolve over time.

An initial emphasis on prevention, health improvement, and disease management can provide a window of opportunity for expanding the continuum of care in your practice. With that foundation, the later inclusion of complementary medicine can occur in a context that emphasizes wellness, healthy lifestyle, and appropriate self-care. Health improvement is a perspective inherent in integrative medicine and most systems of holistic or natural healing. This perspective is evident in a wide array of complementary therapies including Chinese medicine and clinical nutrition. Health improvement is also a prominent focus in disease management programs such as the Ornish model for heart disease and integrative oncology. As the evidence of positive treatment outcomes continues to build, it is logical that numerous complementary methodologies will be integrated more robustly with conventional approaches to treatment.

INVENTORY YOUR EXISTING PROGRAMS AND SERVICES

To expand the range of services you deliver and refer to in your practice, first evaluate the resources you currently have in place that reflect a focus on wellness and health enhancement. As you assess the programs and services available to your patients, you may find that some of the components of health improvement or complementary programming are already present. For example, many physicians already refer patients to resources for exercise, nutrition, or stress management.

In addition, inventory programs available to your patients in mind-body medicine, such as support groups, biofeedback, or health education. Survey your staff to determine who already has expertise and training in some aspect of health enhancement or complementary therapeutics. You may also wish to identify other resources:

- Programs in health promotion and wellness such as fitness centers
- Risk-reduction interventions such as cardiac prevention
- Disease management such as comprehensive cancer programs or diabetes prevention

The next step is to assess the needs and desires of your patients, your practice, and the community. The goal is to remain open and responsive to new information. This planning phase also includes input from partners in practice, administrators, and staff. One of the surprises in this process may be the discovery of assets that already exist within your practice or organization and among affiliates in the health plans in your community. In many regions, a dynamic community of complementary medicine providers and wellness services now exists and is a rich resource for referrals.

Then apply the principles of good strategic planning. If you have already implemented one or more of these phases, you can move ahead to the later phases. The most significant tool in the design of delivery for the emerging new era of health care is not just the addition of alternative therapies, but the application of "alternative thinking" to expand the continuum of care.

PHASE 1—MAXIMIZING HEALTH PROMOTION

In Phase 1, health-promotion programming is enhanced on several levels.

1-1. Maximizing and promoting referrals, resources, and programs
1-2. Participating in community health campaigns and marketing your expanded practice

Phase 1-1. Maximizing and promoting referrals, resources, and programs. First, upgrade your referral resources in wellness, lifestyle, and health promotion to include the most current, state-of-the-art programs available in your area (Babor et al., 2004). In organizations where there is resistance to complementary medicine or a misunderstanding of its benefits, referrals can simply focus on wellness, prevention, and disease management. Complementary therapies can always be introduced at a later stage, as the benefits of a more comprehensive approach become apparent. This phased integration can increase receptivity. It also provides the opportunity to strengthen organizational infrastructure—to support the coordination of multidisciplinary referrals. The introduction of complementary therapies can be reserved for Phase 3 or 4 and paced according to the mission of the practice and the needs of the community.

Programs for wellness and health promotion that are of potential benefit to your patients include:

- Exercise classes, such as yoga, tai chi, Qigong, movement therapy, and therapeutic exercise
- Nutritional counseling, cooking classes, and weight-loss programs
- Exercise and nutrition classes for those with special needs, such as cardiac rehabilitation
- Health education courses, such as childbirth coaching or diabetes management
- Support groups for people with conditions such as breast cancer, prostate cancer, or chronic illness
- Risk-reduction classes (for example, smoking cessation, blood pressure reduction, and osteoporosis management)
- Additional support for those at risk such as teens, people with addictions, or isolated seniors, through services involving group participation, health coaching, and/or case management
- Relaxation and stress-reduction classes, including meditation
- Mind-body services, such as counseling or biofeedback
- Therapeutic massage

The emphasis on health improvement is actually more important to patients than the inclusion of any single complementary therapy or technique. Consumers want a focus on health even more than they want alternative medicine. The seminal studies on complementary medicine (Eisenberg et al., 1993, 1998; Astin, 1998) suggest that more than two-thirds of reported CAM utilization focused on self-care such as nutrition, exercise, and relaxation techniques. Significantly less utilization involved complementary therapies such as acupuncture or chiropractic. Similar findings were reported in the 2002 analysis by the National Center for Complementary and Alternative Medicine (Barnes et al., 2004). Practitioners who respond to this consumer interest in health and wellness offer a means of increasing satisfaction for current patients and an avenue for attracting new ones.

Phase 1-2. Participating in community health campaigns and marketing your expanded practice. Provide information to your community on the services you currently offer that are patient-centered and holistic. Advertise any new health promotion services and, in tandem, promote any complementary services you offer such as mind-body therapies or massage. In this way, your organization can expand its emphasis on health and on familiar complementary therapies. Also market any services that are unique, widely utilized, or specific to your region, through your Web site, participation in community events, local presentations, or other noncommercial strategies. These are good ways to provide community service, attract customers who are interested in self-care and natural healing, differentiate your services, and gain market share.

PHASE 2—EXPANDING THE INFRASTRUCTURE

Phase 2 involves the expansion of infrastructure to support comprehensive services.

2-1. Proactive triage and referral
2-2. Case management, health coaching, and group support

The most genuine integration of services can be promoted through careful development of the infrastructure. At a later phase, this new infrastructure could also support in-house health promotion programs or patient services for holistic medicine.

Phase 2-1. Proactive triage and referral. Triage takes on a new meaning in the context of the health promotion and wellness paradigm. Traditionally, triage is the decision-making process used to evaluate what to do and when to do it, in clinical situations (Bristow & Herrick, 2002). It asks questions such as, "Does this person need to be treated immediately?" and "What is the most appropriate form of treatment?" In the emerging new paradigm, medical decision making focuses earlier in the delivery continuum (Richards et al., 2004). Rather than limiting triage to acute cases, the new emphasis is on implementing medical decision making to manage risk or prevent disease before it occurs. Optimally, this means that resources are identified to address patients' need for health care when they are first identified as "at risk." This could also mean intervening while they still have their health, through wellness activities focused on peak performance.

Systematically develop new care pathways for your practice—and identify resources that proactively address health issues at an earlier stage. This points to new opportunities for physicians to gain cross-disciplinary training and expertise in prevention, health improvement, and eventually in complementary clinical treatment.

Phase 2-2. Case management, health coaching, and group support. Upgraded case management, sometimes called care co-ordination, expands the domain of disease management (Cosby, 1996; Dzyacky, 1998). Rather than managing only the patient's medical case, care coordination also has the capacity to link the client with a coordinated interaction of primary care, prevention services, health promotion, mind/body wellness, and, potentially, complementary medicine.

These added services are relevant to patients with a range of needs—those who are relatively well and want to maximize their health, those who are at risk, and those who want assistance in coordinating their medical treatment with health promotion activities. Through the work of Dean Ornish (Ornish et al., 2001; Koertge et al., 2003) and others, we now know that lifestyle interventions can be used effectively even by those with conditions such as cardiovascular disease if they are provided with medical supervision, expanded case management, and group support. This range of approaches can provide clients access to cost-effective resources that involve them in health promotion, educational programs, health coaching, and various types of mind-body interventions.

PHASE 3—REFERRING TO COMPLEMENTARY THERAPIES

As the research evidence grows, it has become increasingly clear that many complementary therapies meet the criteria of safety, clinical effectiveness, and cost-effectiveness. For example, pain management using acupuncture (NIH, 1997) or therapeutic massage (Field, 2002; Field et al., 2002) can improve outcomes and patient satisfaction. The preparation in Phases 1 and 2 provides a foundation for more integrative care delivery and utilization of complementary therapies.

In Phase 3, the administrative goals include a series of dynamic action steps:

3-1. Selecting key therapies for referral
3-2. Developing protocols for screening and credentialing complementary practitioners
3-3. Identifying potential practitioners and applying credentialing protocol

Practices that currently refer patients to complementary practitioners may be ready to expand to Phase 4 and offer integrative medicine "in house." Referrals can initially focus on complementary therapies for which there is broad consensus, such as clinical massage, acupuncture, or biofeedback. The first steps to greater inclusion of complementary medicine involve vision and planning, plus careful design and timing.

Phase 3-1. Select key therapies for referral. Identify the therapies of greatest relevance to your particular practice and the needs of your patients. By performing a survey throughout the organization and community, you or your planning group can prioritize the list of therapies most requested. In general, it is also important that these therapies are agreed upon by primary stakeholders both within the organization and in the community (Barnes et al., 2004; Ni et al., 2002).

You may want to focus on the inclusion of one particular discipline at a time. Carefully prioritize the preferred therapies, especially those for which there is solid research evidence. For example, surveys of integrative medicine centers have found that one of the first modalities to be added is acupuncture. The Consensus Statement on Acupuncture of the NIH (1997) has significantly increased physician confidence in the safety and efficacy of this form of treatment. A survey by Landmark Healthcare also found that 31%

of HMOs offered acupuncture (National Market Measures, 1999).

To select the complementary therapies most appropriate for patient referrals, there are a number of questions that need to be answered:

- What is the research evidence for safety and effectiveness?
- Is this therapy central to the needs of your patients and your practice?
- How great is the demand?
- Is there existing insurance coverage for these services?
- Is coverage available through core benefits, a rider, a discounted program, or on a fee-for-service basis?
- If coverage is limited, is this a service consumers are willing to pay for out-of-pocket?

Phase 3-2. Developing protocols for screening and credentialing complementary practitioners. This phase involves developing screening and credentialing protocols. In some cases, a consultant may be helpful in clarifying credentialing protocol for CAM providers. The use of an outside credentialing resource is not an unrealistic possibility. In a 1999 survey, Landmark Healthcare found that 50% of all health plans providing complementary therapies used adjunctive organizations to credential complementary practitioners (National Market Measures, 1999).

The design of credentialing and screening requires attention and patience. The variety of disciplines typically evaluated for integrative medicine encompass a wide range of philosophies; each includes its own knowledge base, protocols, and practice wisdom. Acupuncturists, osteopaths, chiropractors, massage therapists, and naturopathic physicians are all involved in practices that are quite different from one another, with a wide range of research evidence and cultural biases. (For additional information, refer to Chapter 64 on credentialing.)

Phase 3-3. Identifying potential practitioners and applying credentialing protocols. Practitioners can be invited to apply for participation. In many cases, networking in your community will identify skilled complementary medicine professionals. An appropriate staff member can be assigned to perform the credentialing. Develop a process for monitoring clinical outcomes and reporting from practitioners to whom you make referrals.

PHASE 4—INTEGRATING COMPLEMENTARY MEDICINE ON-SITE

This phase is a continuum of Phase 3. If you elect to move ahead with an in-house CAM or integrative medicine program, without the phase of referring out to practitioners in the community, be sure to combine the steps from Phase 3 with Phase 4.

4-1. Developing consensus within your practice and customizing the business model
4-2. Bringing complementary practitioners on staff
4-3. Developing the integrative, multidisciplinary team

Phase 4-1. Developing consensus within your practice and customizing the business model. The first priority in establishing consensus is the identification and involvement of key players and stakeholders. Probably the worst error that can be made in the development of an integrative medicine prac-

tice or center is to proceed without a broad base of support. If you or your colleagues are not at a complete state of readiness, an immense amount of energy and money can be wasted.

Research your business model rigorously. Consider the legal structure and its implications. Joint venture, partnership, contract, or rental are all models that have had success in centers across the country. Each has unique reimbursement and liability factors. This is another situation in which a consultant can aid in the development of your practice model.

Phase 4-2. Bringing complementary practitioners on staff. In some practices or organizations, the inclusion of a complementary provider may simply involve provision of office space. For example, a clinical massage therapist could be made available to your patients certain days of the week. In a practice that includes many patients with arthritic or cancer pain, a skilled massage therapist with a clinical background can make an important contribution to patient care. Numerous other types of providers fit into an integrative model as well. Outcomes and feedback on patient satisfaction can be obtained through a quality assurance program, ideally implemented in tandem with your new services.

Phase 4-3. Developing the integrative, multidisciplinary team. In most medical service delivery, physicians, nurses, and other providers work together as a team. Integrative medicine reconceptualizes the multidisciplinary team. For example, in innovative cancer treatment programs such as those of the Integrative Medicine Service at Memorial Sloan-Kettering Cancer Center (2004), acupuncturists and massage therapists provide adjunctive services for pain management. In your redesigned delivery model, it is important to carefully develop care pathways as well as mechanisms for service coordination and team communication. This upgraded approach to health care delivery by teams creates the foundation for the genuine integration of complementary services (Scherwitz et al., 2003).

It is important to determine policy and procedures that define how the team will perform and collaborate. In some integrative centers, practitioners meet weekly to discuss complex cases. In other practices, the primary provider basically manages patient flow and referrals. Regardless of the model, communication is enhanced if there are clear pathways for patient flow, information sharing, referrals, and coordinated decision making. It is also critical to have a system for updating protocols and procedures—to incorporate refinements in care pathways and patient services.

CONCLUSION

The research, the media, and consumer trends continue to reflect growing interest in complementary and integrative medicine. The conventional medical community, many of the most respected journals, and the NIH National Center for Complementary and Alternative Medicine have supported major CAM research. Consumers are practicing tai chi and yoga, and seeking acupuncture and massage. At the same time they continue to have immense respect for their physicians. Many patients indicate the desire that more comprehensive health care services become available through their medical provider. In response to this interest, phasing in complementary or integrative medicine services offers a powerful business opportunity and will ultimately help to create a more comprehensive, meaningful, and clinically efficient health care delivery system.

REFERENCES

Astin J. Why patients use alternative medicine: results of a national study. *JAMA*. 1998;279(19):1548–1553.

Babor TF, Sciamanna CN, Pronk NP. Assessing multiple risk behaviors in primary care: screening issues and related concepts. *Am J Prev Med*. 2004;27(Suppl 2):42–53.

Barnes PM, Powell-Griner E, McFann K, Nahin R. Complementary and alternative medicine use among adults: United States, 2002. *Adv Data*. 2004;(343):1–16.

Bristow DP, Herrick CA. Emergency department case management: the dyad team of nurse case manager and social worker improve discharge planning and patient and staff satisfaction while decreasing inappropriate admissions and costs: a literature review. *Lippincotts Case Manag*. 2002;7(6):243–251.

Cosby C. *Case Management: Cost, Collaboration, Critical Paths, a Dynamic Process*. Park Ridge, IL: Emergency Nurses Association; 1996.

Dzyacky SC. An acute care case management model for nurses and social workers. *Nurs Case Manag*. 1998;3:208–215.

Eisenberg D, Davis R, Ettner S, et al. Trends in alternative medicine use in the United States, 1990–1997: results of a follow-up national survey. *JAMA*. 1998;280(18):1569–1575.

Eisenberg DM, Kessler RC, Foster C, et al. Unconventional medicine in the United States. *N Engl J Med*. 1993;328(4):246–252.

Field T. Massage therapy. *Complement Altern Med*. 2002;86:163–171.

Field T, Diego M, Cullen C, et al. Fibromyalgia pain and substance P decrease and sleep improves after massage therapy. *J Clin Rheumatol*. 2002;8:72–76.

Koertge J, Weidner G, Elliott-Eller M, et al. Improvement in medical risk factors and quality of life in women and men with coronary artery disease in the Multicenter Lifestyle Demonstration Project. *Am J Cardiol*. 2003;91(11):1316–1322.

Memorial Sloan-Kettering Cancer Center. Web site: www.mskcc.org. Accessed August 15, 2004.

National Institutes of Health. *Acupuncture. NIH Consensus Statement Online*. 1997 Nov 3–5;15(5): 1–34.

National Market Measures. *The Landmark Report II*. Sacramento, CA: Landmark Healthcare; 1999.

Ni H, Simile C, Hardy AM. Utilization of complementary and alternative medicine by United States adults: results from the 1999 national health interview survey. *Med Care*. 2002;40(4):353–358.

Ornish DM, Lee KL, Fair WR, Pettengill EB, Carroll PR. Dietary trial in prostate cancer: early experience and implications for clinical trial design. *Urology*. 2001;57(4 Suppl 1):200–201.

Richards DA, Meakins J, Godfrey L, Tawfik J, Dutton E. Survey of the impact of nurse telephone triage on general practitioner activity. *Br J Gen Pract*. 2004;54(500):207–210.

Scherwitz L, Stewart W, McHenry P, et al. An integrative medicine clinic in a community hospital. *Am J Public Health*. 2003;93(4):549–552.

CHAPTER 5

Strategic Business Planning for Your Practice

M. Caroline Martin, MHA, RN

MAJOR STEPS IN STRATEGIC PLANNING

- Defining mission, vision, and values
- Evaluating the options
- Surveying the needs of your patients and your community
- Assessing your environment
- Inventorying resources
- Decision making
- Implementing strategic action planning
- Ongoing evaluation

The provision of health care is both an act of service and a business. Without a humanistic mission, there may be little profit margin—but without that margin, the mission will not be possible. Consequently, like any other business, it is vital that health care practitioners utilize strategic planning. This process becomes especially important when presented with the opportunity to enhance your practice. Strategic planning allows a health care practice to address opportunities and transform strategic challenges into strategic advantages.

In good business planning, that process begins with the development and clarification of your mission, vision, and values. If you have been in practice for some time, strategic planning may also involve reevaluating or redefining your mission. If your goal is to expand your practice, planning will help you evaluate the wants and needs of your present patients and the opportunities to attract new patients within the community. The strategic planning process will enable you to assess the readiness of your practice to meet these needs and identify the resources you need to bring to that effort.

An assessment is a logical first step if you decide, for example, that you want to organize your practice to promote wellness and health enhancement. This involves determining where you are right now and where you want to be in the future. Whether you are starting a new practice or expanding an existing one, you want to deepen your understanding of what you want to achieve. As you become clear about the type of practice you have and develop a vision for its future, you will attract both staff and patients who also embrace your vision.

M. Caroline Martin, RN, MHA, is president and CEO of NurseWorks, a consulting firm whose mission is to advance the nursing profession through support for strategic planning, program development, advocacy, and motivational seminars. With a degree in nursing, Phi Beta Kappa, from the University of Maine, and a graduate degree from the Medical College of Virginia, she has extensive experience in health care administration, and for two decades served in a leadership capacity in Riverside Health System, one of the largest nonprofit hospital groups and health care providers in Virginia. Mrs. Martin is a diplomate of the American College of Healthcare Executives and an appointee to the Governor's Council for Healthy Virginians.

Courtesy of M. Caroline Martin, MHA, RN, NurseWorks, Inc., Suffolk, Virginia.

DEFINING MISSION, VISION, AND VALUES

What is the mission that drives your work?

- Your mission defines why you are here—your business.
- The vision explains what you aspire to be—the hope.
- The values describe what you want to be known for—your principles.

A well-written mission statement is a broad, powerful, and futuristic description of the ideal state of your practice, program, or organization. Defining your mission requires some effort—if you are a sole practitioner, this may involve soul searching and conversations with colleagues, patients, or community members. If you are in a partnership or part of a larger organization, it means developing consensus among your partners and staff. This consensus will support the development of guidelines for planning and implementation.

Any major shift in the focus of your organization necessitates a reassessment of your mission to evaluate how well you are achieving that mission. This may require taking a closer look at your current practice and where it is in comparison with where you want it to be. For example, is your mission to go beyond episodic sick care by increasing your emphasis on preventive medicine?

To effectively implement your goals through strategic planning, the process is initially more important than the results. That process answers fundamental questions about "who, what, when where, and how" to support the development of action plans. This provides the basis for future initiatives. Consider the following as you go through this process:

- Defining your stakeholders: This could include your board of directors, physicians, practitioners, key managers, and the entire staff. Other major stakeholders who might benefit from the process are funders, major vendors, or representatives from organizations with a similar mission.
- Facilitated decision making: You may want to consider enlisting a skilled facilitator to lead this analysis. This will allow you to be a full participant. In addition, a good facilitator, skilled in group dynamics, can draw on the very best from each participant to define the organization's greatest strengths.
- Developing consensus: Creating a clearly defined mission statement can set the stage for your organization's development.
- Involving your staff in the process: The most effective assessments include not only board and leadership, but also key staff members, enabling them to be knowledgeable participants in the implementation and evaluation phases.
- Defining your organizational culture: An effective mission statement supports the evolution of a unique, pervasive culture that will differentiate your practice from competitors.
- Establishing a service ethic: Awareness of your mission and strengths will guide the provision of superior service to your patient population.

This same approach to consensus can be utilized throughout the planning process to define your practice's strengths, opportunities, limitations, and challenges. Once this process has been used to develop the vision and values statements, you are ready to devise guidelines for implementation.

EVALUATING THE OPTIONS

The key questions to ask at this stage of your evaluation are:

- Do you want to expand?
- What is your level of readiness?
- Do you have the resources for expansion?

An evaluation of the readiness of your practice or organization to expand services or programs can take a number of forms:

- This discussion might emerge in the process of defining your mission.
- It could take place at a later planning session, as you determine the practical implications of your mission. This is the stage at which you operationalize your values, translating your vision into blueprints for future programs and services in your practice.
- For a large organization or an ambitious undertaking, the next step might be a feasibility study, which could be preliminary or comprehensive in nature, in response to the level of readiness of your organization and the scope of the project.

SURVEYING THE NEEDS OF YOUR PATIENTS AND YOUR COMMUNITY

A needs assessment involves understanding the wants and needs of your current patient population and the greater community (potential patients). If you are considering expanding your practice, it will be important to know more about your patients in terms of their demographics and their health status. The first step is to assess your own patient population by applying the perspective of population-based, health risk management. Ideally, this research also includes epidemiology and utilization patterns. Then apply this same approach to your potential patient population, assessing these factors in your community or service area.

Patient Demographics

In your initial planning, determine which patient populations are the focus of your practice:

- Do you serve primarily older patients, adults, and/or families?
- What are your patients' demographics and needs in terms of gender, education, economic status, ethnicity, and culture?

What is the level of need, within each of these subsets of your patient population, for various patient services such as:

- Wellness and health enhancement
- Risk management
- Disease management
- Management of chronic conditions

Patient Epidemiology

Gather in-depth epidemiological information on the health risks and most prevalent diseases and disorders within your patient population.

- Organize that information according to major health issues.
- Group your patients into targeted populations so you can better define their needs and focus your services.
- Develop care pathways, services, and/or referral resources for the most significant and prevalent health conditions you treat.
- Assess the needs that all your patients have in common.
- Identify cost-effective programs that can be developed in-house or to which you can refer patients, such as classes or programs in basic wellness, nutrition, exercise, or stress management.

Patient Utilization Patterns

There is value in reviewing consumer patterns and customer satisfaction data for your practice:

- What is the average length of time your patients have been with your practice?
- Do you know why those who leave do so?
- Do you know how your patients selected your practice?
- Is your practice full, growing, downsizing, or seeking new patients?

In addition to a classic epidemiological analysis, you also want to know the services of greatest interest to patients:

- What, from their perspective, are their needs and wants, segmented by patient type, age, disease category, and other key factors?
- Which services are the highest priority for them?
- Are there services for which they would be willing to pay out-of-pocket?

Community Profile

Defining your community may mean focusing on your local area or on the region in which your practice is located. If you offer specialized care or technology that meet specific needs within your region, patients may be willing to travel an hour or so to have access to your services. For example, an affluent county in California has one of the highest breast cancer rates in the country. There is a need in that region for a program that provides adjunctive testing, screening, counseling, and follow-up, especially a program that utilizes an integrative medicine approach. Have you had the opportunity to identify the specific needs within your community or metropolitan area?

- What are the demographics of the population within the larger community that you serve (your potential customers)?
- What is the epidemiological profile in your county and the surrounding counties? (Public health departments in each county usually have this type of information, which may be accessible through the Internet.)
- Could you obtain additional information on the community through focus groups, a series of interviews with key stakeholders, or market driven data?
- You can also use your own clinical practice data to identify and address community health problems.
- Apply your knowledge of planning information and methodology. What are the current health care delivery patterns in your region?

If your project involves the investment of capital (and it may or may not), you might consider enlisting the services of a consultant to provide a market analysis through focus groups or obtain data on consumer health care expenditures. Ultimately, you want the clearest possible picture of the needs and wants of potential patients in your region.

Example: If your dream is to provide disease management programs through patient support groups, is this a program your practice is ready to develop? Although you may sense a real need, it is only through an epidemiological analysis and a study of existing competition that you can obtain hard data on the level of need in your community.

If you understand both the individual medical issues in your own patient population and the prevalence of various disease and health issues in the broader community, you will be in a better position to decide where to put your emphasis, energy, and resources.

This process will be achieved through an ongoing or periodic assessment of your patient population. Maintaining and updating this database of demographic information will allow you to refine your services based on your customers' wants and needs.

ASSESSING YOUR ENVIRONMENT

Once you and your leadership have a clear vision for your practice, the next step is to assess the strengths, limitations, opportunities, and challenges of your practice or organization. Typically, strengths and limitations focus on the internal environment of the business, and challenges and opportunities are external. Begin by examining the current environment within which your practice operates.

Opportunities and Challenges

Environmental factors. Quality planning becomes a top priority as a practice expands to meet the evolving wants and needs of patients and the community. Success requires knowledge of multiple regulatory, financial, legal, and competitive factors in the context of the practice's current and developing strengths.

Fiscal challenges. It is vital to know who pays for the services within your practice, and the profit margin for each of those services.

- Competing for market share: Who competes for that portion of your business?
- Competing for reimbursement: Third party payers have ways of selecting who will be in their provider networks and which services they will pay for. Do your services meet their profiles?
- Competing for patient dollars: When a practice provides services for which patients pay out-of-pocket, then they compete not only with other practices, but also with all the other financial obligations and priorities of their patients. Understanding what your patients will and will not pay for requires that you monitor consumer trends and key market indicators on an ongoing basis.

Example: Is weight loss a priority for your patients? What types of services are most effective? Which are most appealing to your patients? Are these services covered by insurance, or are they services patients would be willing to pay for out-of-pocket?

Based on this information, from a financial perspective, do you want to expand your practice, and if so, what form would that expansion take? This is a matter of margin as well as mission. Fiscal considerations in complementary health practice are not to be taken lightly. Many integrative medicine centers have found that wellness programming, although ethically satisfying, did not provide a substantial level of economic support. Complementary medicine continues to be a field in which sustainable business models are still in development. They do exist, but the last word on economic and organizational feasibility in this field is not yet in.

INVENTORYING RESOURCES

Internal Resources

Identify the resources you already have in place (in-house) and those that will be needed in order to expand or upgrade certain aspects of your practice and your referral network. An inventory of your current resources will also help you identify the greatest strengths of your practice. It is also important to determine internal limitations that might be turned into strengths. In the context of your mission, your goals, the needs of your patients, and your environmental context, where are your strengths? What other resources will be necessary for you to accomplish your goals? Areas that merit careful consideration when identifying your resources include:

- Leadership
- Fiscal resources/capital
- Allies or funders
- Material resources (space, equipment, protocols, policies/procedures)
- Staff skills and strengths
- Relevant programs or services already in place
- Referral and community resources

This type of assessment also means exploring all major facets of your practice:

- Strengths: What do you already do really well?
- Programs and protocols: Do you have a process for gathering health assessment information?
- Staff expertise: Which staff have specialized training, for example as a health educator?
- Current services: Do you already provide wellness services or programs such as a diabetes education service?
- Are there services that should be strengthened or expanded?
- Is there a need for quality improvement in some aspect of your practice?
- Are additional resources required?

Example: In the assessment process, you might ask yourself key questions about your program or goals such as: I would like to teach diabetes education but I cannot get paid for it (an external challenge). I would like to offer diabetes education but I do not have anyone on staff trained to provide that service (an internal limitation). We would like to offer more patient support groups or patient education but we know that it is labor intensive to set up these groups. If we make a commitment to provide those services, do we have the administrative resources necessary? How might we retool in order to provide those groups efficiently and cost-effectively?

You may find that you can achieve a wellness-focused practice with only minor adjustments, for example, by:

- Evaluating and adding new patient education materials
- Relying on your well-trained personnel to provide patients with resources and links
- Expanding your referral network, after thoroughly investigating key referrals and resources that will make the greatest difference in the health of your patients
- Identifying the resources that will address the health issues of greatest concern (from your perspective as well as those of your patients)
- Emphasizing services most valued by your patients
- Determining if services can be brought in-house to meet any of these needs

Referral Opportunities

Exploring potential referrals to adjunctive health care providers and community resources involves asking key questions such as:

- Are there services you are now providing that could more appropriately be referred out?
- Would your patients benefit from wellness programming; if so, what resources are available in your community?
- Are there services or discount programs available to your patients, for example, through your affiliation with a health plan?

- Do you know of existing services within your community or within your practice that could meet the needs shared by all your patients, or the needs of a targeted group within your practice, based on age, diagnosis, or culture?
- Are there adjunctive complementary therapies that could address some of these needs?
- Do you already have a referral program with successful exercise and weight-reduction groups or smoking cessation programs for your patients who need these services?
- How accessible (financially and geographically) are your referral resources?
- How efficient is the referral process for your staff? Is it difficult for your patients?
- How comprehensive is your current community referral network? What is the quality of those resources?
- Do you have a practical process for obtaining feedback from those referrals, both from the practitioner or organization and from your patients?
- Do you receive good follow-up from those to whom you make referrals?
- Are there potential alliances with the practitioners to whom you refer? What may begin as a simple referral source could develop into an alliance and even a partnership over time.

Example: Do you have access to discounts for your patients to a community or hospital-based fitness center? Is there a good Phase 3 outpatient cardiac rehab program to which you can refer patients at risk who need exercise?

DECISION MAKING

The process that supports decision making returns you to your first step, the definition of your mission, vision, and values. Fol-lowing through with each of the stages of your assessment ideally has provided you with the data, information, and insight you will need to make informed decisions about your practice. In summary, the major steps of this process have involved:

- Defining mission, vision, and values
- Data gathering: demographics, current epidemiology (and projections of need) and a complete market analysis
- Environmental assessment, including regulatory considerations
- Competitive analysis
- Financial analysis, including the impact of managed care and other reimbursement patterns, such as new payment for technology or patient education
- Internal assessment of strengths and current limitations

Equipped with this information, the decision makers are ready to reconvene, often in a retreat environment, to initiate the decision-making process. The organization's mission is revisited, confirmed, or possibly modified, based on the insights that have emerged from the analysis. While all the data must be reviewed, key factors with regard to any new project focus on:

- Relevance of the new direction or project to the organization's mission
- Directions suggested by the data
- Magnitude of the need for the new services
- Financial viability of the project

These factors may be evaluated through a particular method, such as weighted analysis. At the end of the day, a decision is made to move forward, continue on the same course, or modify current operations in some way. At this point, guidelines and goals for implementation can be defined and the organization can take the next step.

IMPLEMENTING STRATEGIC ACTION PLANS

The development of your strategic action plan involves a series of steps that can manifest your vision, translating values and ideas into practical health care services or programs. Your resources (staff, time, and materials) are allocated best when they are highly focused:

- Targeted to clearly articulated goals
- Employed to address specific well-defined priorities
- Have demonstrated opportunities for synergy
- Are supported by an infrastructure that facilitates smooth, efficient referrals and an integrated continuum of care
- Promote referrals to programs and resources of the highest quality

Begin with four to five strategic action plans and measurable goals against which to benchmark progress. Tracking this implementation means very specifically identifying:

- Broad goals
- Specific objectives
- Action steps
- Target date(s)
- Cost and budget
- Personnel responsible and resource requirements
- Timeline and date to be completed

For example, action steps might include:

- An assessment of how to improve the educational process with patients. This might involve a review of current educational materials with regard to content on self-care and wellness practices.
- Creation of new health assessment tools and measures to use within your patient base.
- Building in a system for ongoing data gathering so you can trend the data as to the effectiveness of various services and activities

Once the goals and objectives have been written as specific action plans that include (for each activity) the required steps, resources, completion date, and an assigned person to be responsible, it will be relatively easy to track the implementation of each strategic goal. You may want to measure each goal against the following key results areas to determine if implementation has been successful with regard to:

- Improved clinical outcomes
- Cost, benefit, and financial viability of program(s)
- Quality of care and patient services

ONGOING EVALUATION

A robust set of listening and learning tools will enable you to audit your staff, patient, and community wants and needs on an ongoing basis. The implementation and evaluation phases can be managed on a cyclical timeline. Flexibility and adjustments in processes and services are essential. Ongoing analysis and continual feedback enables you to focus on the future and respond to a competitive and rapidly changing environment with agility. A simple way to describe this process of continual performance improvement from the Joint Commission on Accreditation of Healthcare Organizations is "Plan, Do, Check, Act." This continuous process enables you to plan and take action. At that point, you see how well you are doing and then act again to revise or expand your efforts. Use the initial assessment as a baseline to help you measure the time and energy of your various efforts against that initial plan.

The identification of key strategies and measurable goals that support the vision and the development of an operational plan include the definition of tactics, responsible parties, and associated time frames for each goal. If the fiscal year is the same as the calendar year, your planning year might look like this:

- April—Convene an educational retreat for key leadership to examine trends in the marketplace; review status of practice in light of trends.
- June—Assemble staff to discuss progress on existing goals and to begin setting new goals, tactics, and objectives for the coming year to identify needed resources.
- September—Develop capital and operational draft budgets for the upcoming year, with a goal or objective tied to each new revenue and expense item.
- November—Approve the annual strategic plan and the capital and operational budgets for the new year.

- February—Review prior year in terms of accomplishments and the readiness to repeat the process.

This ongoing evaluation can provide the basis for a 3- to 5-year budget and strategic plan. The process is continuous and can be plotted out on a revolving calendar. Ideally, this type of needs evaluation can be built into your organizational calendar to provide the feedback, information, and data you require for good practice management, and positions your practice to adapt and respond to emerging opportunities.

SUMMARY

Ultimately, the goal of these efforts is to promote wellness and good self-care in your patients through consistent, quality, personalized service. Strategic planning can serve as a basis for efficiently implementing this philosophy. This approach also supports an initial assessment of the readiness of your practice to expand wellness programming or referrals to adjunctive services. By evaluating the information obtained through this analysis, the practice leadership will be able to develop strategic business plans that will effectively guide the efforts of the entire organization.

CHAPTER 6

Preventable Causes of Disease

Clement Bezold, PhD

Complementary approaches to health and medicine are among the fastest growing aspects of health care in the United States. In 2002, more than one third (36%) of the US population used some form of complementary therapy or wellness activity, excluding vitamins and prayer, and approximately one half (49.8%) had used it at one time (Barnes et al., 2004). By 2010, it is likely that at least two thirds will be using one or more of the approaches now defined as complementary medicine.

In some contexts, these therapies will supplement current forms of treatment, and in other situations they will be applied instead of conventional treatment. These modalities also extend beyond treatment; in the future, they will be applied as viable methods of prevention and health promotion. This parallel use of various complementary approaches is already a significant aspect of their demand and is likely to grow.

In the United States and other industrial nations, as much as 90% of morbidity and mortality is now associated with lifestyle, genetic, and environmental factors. The focus of health care is expanding to include these factors, particularly lifestyle. This new scope of practice will increasingly favor prevention and treatment approaches with core components that are nutritional, physical, psychological, or spiritual. One reason for the growing interest in complementary medicine is that it includes or reinforces these components of care (Jonas & Chez, 2004).

INFLUENCES ON HEALTH

The work of McGinnis and colleagues suggests that the greatest long-term influence medical systems have on patients is through a focus on behavior and lifestyle. More than a decade ago McGinnis and Foege (1993) proposed that over the life course, 50% of the variance in premature morbidity was attributable to behavior and 20% to genetic factors. The two other primary factors were environment, 20%, and medical care, 10% (particularly in the context of a health episode or hospitalization). In 2002, that thesis was updated to suggest that primary influences are 40% behavior and 30% genetic factors (McGinnis et al., 2002) as shown in Table 6–1. Based on a review of the research,

Clement Bezold, PhD, is the President of the Institute for Alternative Futures (IAF) and its for-profit subsidiary Alternative Futures Associates (AFA). He received his doctorate in political science from the University of Florida and has authored or served as editor for 11 books and numerous articles focused on the future of health, health care, and the health professions, as well as government and the justice system. A well-known speaker on the future, he has given presentations to voluntary organizations, national and international corporations, health care organizations, and education groups and has taught at the University of Florida, Antioch University, and American University.

The IAF is a nonprofit research and educational organization founded in 1977 that specializes in aiding organizations and individuals to more wisely choose and create their preferred futures. IAF and its for-profit subsidiary, AFA, are leading providers of training and services in vision development and scenario planning to large associations, governments, and corporations.

Table 6–1 Factors Shaping Health and Premature Mortality

	1993	2002
	%	%
Behavior	50	40
Genetics	20	30
Environment	20	20
Social		(15)
Physical		(5)
Health Care	10	10

Sources of data: McGinnis & Foege, 1993; McGinnis et al., 2002.

it has been proposed that up to 70% of all potential genetically associated conditions could be averted through healthy lifestyle choices (Bland, 2002). These analyses suggest that lifestyle is now the major influence on health in industrialized nations.

This perspective suggests that one of the greatest points of leverage of a physician or health care provider is through influence on patients' health-related behavior and their environment. Given that smoking, diet, and physical inactivity now account for more than one third of all mortality, the data seem to bear out this thesis. A review of the statistics on the leading causes of mortality in 2002 indicates that only 11.96% of deaths in the United States were directly due to infectious illness (Kochanek & Smith, 2004). All the other major causes of mortality—chronic and degenerative disorders, accidents, suicide, and homicide—reflect the influence of lifestyle to some degree. A simple example of the influence of lifestyle is the finding that the inclusion of fresh fruits and vegetables in the diet cuts cancer risk by approximately 50% (Block et al., 1992) and cardiovascular disease by 20% (National Center for Chronic Disease Prevention and Health Promotion,

2004). These data suggest the increasing relevance of lifestyle approaches.

PREVALENCE OF CHRONIC DISORDERS

Chronic illness can be considered a silent epidemic in the United States. Surprisingly, more than 44.5% of Americans—90 million people—have one or more chronic conditions (Hoffman et al., 1996). Their direct health care costs in 1987 accounted for three fourths of all US health care expenditures. The total associated costs for chronic conditions projected to 1990 amounted to $659 billion. This figure includes $425 billion in direct health care costs.

The prevalence of chronic and degenerative disease is also reflected in the causes of mortality. Federal data for 2002 for the 15 leading causes of death (Kochanek and Smith, 2004), when aggregated, indicates the following incidence of mortality:

- Chronic and degenerative disease—1,637,819
- Infectious illness—243,058
- Accidents—102,303
- Self-inflicted harm and assault—47,691

Of these four causal domains, all but infectious illness can be influenced by addressing lifestyle and related risk factors. In effect, almost 90% of the causes of death in 2002 were related to preventable causes. The largest population with medical needs were those with chronic and degenerative diseases, which accounted for more than 75% of the nation's $1.4 trillion medical costs, including $300 billion in expenditures on cardiovascular diseases (National Center for Chronic Disease Prevention and Health Promotion, 2004).

The majority of chronic conditions experienced by Americans are not totally disabling, allowing them to lead relatively normal lives (Hoffman et al., 1996). However, people with chronic disorders must cope with the threat of recurrent episodes of illness, higher personal health care costs, more days lost from work, and the risk of long-term disabilities. Those with chronic illness are also reported to be at greater risk for being underinsured. This population is likely to continue to increase, given declining mortality rates across the entire life span, advances in medical technology, and higher survival rates associated with life-threatening conditions.

The Hoffman analysis points out that Western health care delivery is still essentially designed to provide acute care. We know from the research of Eisenberg et al. (1998) and Astin (1998) that complementary medicine is frequently sought out for the management of chronic disorders such as chronic pain (including back and neck pain and headaches), as well as arthritis, digestive disorders, fatigue, and allergies.

As the size of the population with chronic conditions approaches critical mass, this may further increase utilization of complementary and integrative medicine. Multidisciplinary approaches to disease management are likely to be expanded, such as the work of Dean Ornish in the management of heart disease (Koertge et al., 2003) and the Texas Back Institute for back pain and orthopedic conditions (Triano et al., 2001). Comprehensive cancer care, utilizing complementary therapies in coordination with oncology services, is another potential area of expansion.

SPECIFIC PREVENTABLE ASPECTS OF DISEASE

The pattern of disease is shifting in the US and worldwide. Data from the Centers for Disease Control (Mokdad et al., 2004) and World Heath Organization (Murray & Lopez, 1996; WHO, 2003) indicate that the primary causes of preventable morbidity and early mortality include:

- Tobacco-related deaths
- Obesity, poor diet, and inactivity
- Accidental injury
- Psychosocial disorders

Tobacco-Related Deaths

Tobacco use is anticipated to cause more premature deaths and disability than any other single risk factor; by the year 2020, it may be responsible for as much as 10% of the adult disease burden (US Department of Health and Human Services, 2004). According to a recent report by the CDC, smoking is the cause of death of 435,000 Americans annually. For men, smoking shortens lifespan by 13.2 years on average, and for women, by 14.5 years. The costs include $75 billion in direct medical care and $82 billion in lost productivity, as well as 18% of preventable deaths. An estimated 46.2 million adults in the US smoke, even though this behavior will result in death or disability to half of all regular smokers. Tobacco use is a causal factor in approximately 20% of cardiovascular diseases and has been linked to at least 9 forms of cancers (including leukemia), as well as cataracts and abdominal aortic aneurysms.

Prevention and therapeutics. It is encouraging to note that smoking among high school students has begun to decline and dropped by more than 6% over a 2-year period, to 28.5% (Schenker, 2004). A number of conventional strategies appear to be effective, including the nicotine patch. Complementary strategies that can be utilized in combination with other approaches in smoking cessation programs include group support, stress reduction, and other mind-body approaches; detoxification and nutrient therapy; acupuncture; and exercise.

Obesity, Poor Diet, and Inactivity

The incidence of obesity is increasing in the United States and, after smoking, is the second leading underlying cause of death (Mokdad et al., 2004). Together, these two aspects of lifestyle contribute to more than one third of all mortality in the US (34.7%). Obesity and inactivity increase the risks for heart disease, cancer, and cerebrovascular disorders, as well as diabetes, the sixth leading cause of death. The CDC report indicates, "These findings, along with escalating health care costs and aging population, argue persuasively that the need for a more preventive orientation in the U.S. health care and public health systems has become more urgent" (Mokdad et al., 2004). Obesity is a major cause of morbidity and mortality throughout industrialized nations worldwide.

Ironically, in the developing nations malnutrition and deficiencies of micronutrients remain one of the most significant influences on health. According to the WHO there are 10.8 million child deaths globally a year. The number attributed to deficiencies of zinc, vitamin A, and iron is more than 2 million, or approximately 20% of the total (Black, 2003).

Nutritional therapy. In the West efforts to improve nutrition in complementary, clinical, and functional nutrition have focused on diet with a consistent emphasis on healthy complex carbohydrates and healthy fats (essential fatty acids). A *moderate* approach to glycemic regulation is based on extensive research on the role of carbohydrate consumption in health. This perspective has also emerged in mainstream research such as the 50-year Framingham study (Kannel, 2000). Complementary approaches to weight loss include nutrient therapy, medical fitness, and behavioral support, and *balanced* carbohydrate diets such as *The Zone* (1992) by Barry Sears, PhD. The relevance of this approach has not been lost on the mainstream media and the fast food industry, which have begun to demonstrate major interest in fitness and nutrition issues over the past several years.

Accidental Injury

By 2020, trauma may rival infectious diseases as a major source of ill health. Worldwide, among people 15 to 44, traffic accidents were found to be the leading cause of death for men (Murray and Lopez, 1996). In the US, in 2001 and in previous years, accidents were the leading cause of death for those under 34 (Kochanek and Smith, 2004).

One important aspect of this problem is stress-related accidents and injuries. Mind-body medicine offers practical tools for coping with stress. We know from the work of Gordon in Kosovo and other war-torn regions that mind-body techniques can be quickly learned by people of all ages and can be effective tools for personal stress reduction even under highly adverse circumstances (Gordon et al., 2004).

Psychosocial Disorders

Disorders such as depression are among the fastest growing forms of morbidity. Psychosocial factors also have an impact on mortality. In the United States, for Caucasian males aged 15 to 34, the two top causes of death in 2001 were accidents and suicide; for African-American males in the same age group, homicide and accidents were the top causes (US Department of Health and Human Services, 2004b). Overall, Americans with the highest suicide rate are Caucasian males over 85.

Although we now know that depression has biochemical and physiological components, mood disorders also result from an unsatisfactory social context and loss of personal meaning. Mood disorders and mental illness are likely to increase as the world's population becomes concentrated in crowded, isolating urban enclaves, in megacities with populations that range from 4 to 20 million or greater.

Mind-body therapies. Approaches relevant to this sense of disconnectedness include spirituality, meditation, and meditative exercise such as yoga, tai chi, and Qigong. Complementary practitioner-based interventions include counseling, coaching, group support, and biofeedback. Of special interest is the empowerment that comes with teaching these therapies to consumers as a form of self-care. For example, simple methods of biofeedback can easily be learned by most people, enabling them to shift out of the stress response/sympathetic mode (Green & Green, 1977). Other techniques that can be adapted to self-care include imagery, self-hypnosis, and various stress-reduction techniques. Extensive research on psychoneuroimmunology provides a rational evidence basis for these approaches. In the future, with the increasing prevalence of depression and diseases of meaning, health care providers who are skilled in mind-body medicine are likely to be sought for their expertise.

Additional complementary approaches to depression include clinical nutrition, which has been used to treat a range of mood disorders (Werbach, 1999). For patients with mild depression, exercise can also be beneficial. Physicians can find information on writing exercise prescriptions using a "green prescription card" available from the Canadian Health Association on the Web at www.goforgreen.ca (2004).

IMAGES OF THE FUTURE

Within a decade, we predict that health care will be likely to operate within a new paradigm—one oriented to prevention, self-care, and holism. It will be capable of addressing an individual's unique status from the microscopic (genotype) to the macroscopic (environment). Outcomes will increasingly drive better prevention and therapeutics, including the integration of complementary approaches into standard health care. Treatment options will also be far more numerous, but resolving health conditions could also extend to social and environmental interventions aimed at uprooting problems at their source. Much health care will be self-care, with the services of health care professionals applied more strategically and even more effectively. Individuals will experience a greater range of options for managing personal health, through expanded options, resources, and supporting tools.

Pessimistic images exist as well. Any of a variety of wildcards could intrude and redirect US health care into less-desirable channels—environmental, economic, or social dislocations; slowdown or reversal of health care's movement toward monitoring outcomes and accountability; or the failure to ensure greater health equality in terms of both access and outcomes.

To sustain a positive vision of the future, alternative images are important for our thinking, to clarify what we want. We create the future all the time by what we do and what we fail to do. One aspect of creating the future is hope and the prospects of visionary possibilities. Hope is a way of manifesting those possibilities. A number of major trends provide hope that a healthier, more integral future could emerge:

- One positive sign is the continued growth of public interest in complementary and alternative health approaches.
- A second is the integration of these approaches in many areas of health care, albeit slow.

- Third is the gradual but steady development of an evidence-based foundation for care, one in which the rules for evidence are becoming progressively less prejudiced toward holistic approaches.
- There are also signs that health care is approaching a period of dramatic change. Although change is not always comfortable, it provides opportunities for progress.
- Likewise, the pressures of aging, aging care, long term care, and Medicaid all indicate that the status quo will not hold. In that context, the inventiveness of individuals pursuing more integral lives and better health will become increasingly more important.
- Technologies to support self-care, personal health monitoring, and behavioral change will become more ubiquitous and more user friendly, less expensive, and better integrated into electronic medical record data and our personal knowledge tools.
- Innovative technologies will continue to emerge, including new testing, devices, and interventions. More accessible testing, for example, is likely to take many forms, such as simple saliva, breath, and urine tests. Some of these tests will provide early indicators for the onset of disease, including many chronic disorders. Such testing is already becoming more widely available. The prospect is that these technologies could be developed in ways that make them accessible to all.
- There is also continued movement towards a greater sense of equity in health policy. Europe tends to be ahead of the United States, but even in the US there has been a greater commitment since 1998, to eliminate health disparities. This has continued in the Bush administration. The larger disparity issues reflect social and economic conditions that make life more difficult, and make healthy lifestyle and good nutrition less accessible.

These are all improvements that will take time to achieve; consequently they require greater patience and a sustained focus. However, even in the marketplace there are important developments, for example in the fast food industry, that give us hope that we can improve the determinants of health. Society will continue to be faced with choices about how healthy we want our lives to be and how accessible health care should be. If we make the right choices, individually and as a society, 2010 will be far healthier.

REFERENCES

Astin J. Why patients use alternative medicine: results of a national study. *JAMA.* 1998;279(19):1548–1553.

Barnes PM, Powell-Griner E, McFann K, Nahin R. Complementary and alternative medicine use among adults: United States, 2002. *Adv Data.* 2004;(343): 1–16.

Black R. Micronutrient deficiency: an underlying cause of morbidity and mortality. *Bull World Health Organ.* 2003;81(2).

Bland JS. *Genetic nutritioneering.* New York: Keats/ McGraw-Hill; 1999.

Block G, Patterson B, Subar A. Fruit, vegetables and cancer prevention: a review of the epidemiological evidence. *Nutr Cancer.* 1992;18:1–29.

Eisenberg D, Davis R, Ettner S, et al. Trends in alternative medicine use in the United States, 1990–1997: results of a follow-up national survey. *JAMA.* 1998;280(18):1569–1575.

Gordon JS, Staples JK, Blyta A, Bytyqi M. Treatment of posttraumatic stress disorder in postwar Kosovo high school students using mind-body skills groups: a pilot study. *J Trauma Stress.* 2004;17(2):143–147.

Green E, Green A. *Beyond biofeedback.* New York: Delacorte Press; 1977.

Hoffman C, Rice D, Sung HY. Persons with chronic conditions: their prevalence and costs. *JAMA.* 1996; 276:1473–1479.

Jonas WJ, Chez RA. Implementing and evaluating optimal healing environments. In Research on paradigm, practice, and policy. *J Altern Complement Med.* 2004;10(suppl 1):S1–S6.

Kannel WB. The Framingham Study: Its 50-year legacy and future promise. *J Atheroscler Thrombosis.* 2000;6(2):60–66.

Kochanek KD, Smith BL. Deaths: preliminary data for 2002. *National Vital Statistics Reports.* 2004;52(13): 1–48. Epub 2004 Feb 12.

Koertge J, et al. Improvement in medical risk factors and quality of life in women and men with coronary artery disease in the Multicenter Lifestyle Demonstration Project. *Am J Cardiol.* 2003;91(11): 1316–1322.

McGinnis JM, Foege WH. Actual causes of death in the United States. *JAMA.* 1993;270(18):2207–2212

McGinnis JM, Williams-Russo P, Knickman JR. The case for more active policy attention to health promotion. *Health Aff.* 2002;21(2):78–93.

Mokdad, AH, et al. Actual causes of death in the United States, 2000. *JAMA.* 2004;291(10):1238–1241.

Murray C, Lopez AD, eds. The global burden of disease. In: *The Global Burden of Disease and Injury Series.* Vol 1. Cambridge, MA: Harvard University School of Public Health; 1996:990–994.

National Center for Chronic Disease Prevention and Health Promotion (NCCDPHP). Chronic disease overview. Atlanta, GA: CDC. available at: www.cdc.gov/nccdphp/overview.htm. Accessed August 1, 2004.

Schenker M. Targeting tobacco use: the nation's leading cause of death. Atlanta, GA: CDC. Available at: www.cdc.gov/nccdphd/aaag/aag_osh.htm. Accessed August 1, 2004.

Sears B. *The zone: A dietary road map to lose weight permanently.* New York: ReganBooks; 1995.

Triano JJ, Rashbaum RF, Hansen DT, Raley B. The integrative multidisciplinary spine center: the Texas Back Institute. In: Faass N, ed. *Integrating Complementary Medicine into Health Systems.* Sudbury, MA: Jones and Bartlett/Aspen, 2001.

US Department of Health and Human Services (USHHS). (2004a). New surgeon general's report expands list of diseases caused by smoking. Available at: http://www.hhs.gov/news/press/2004pres/20040527a.html. Accessed August 1, 2004.

US Department of Health and Human Services (USHHS). (2004b). Violence prevention. Available at: www.healthgap.omhrc.gov/violence_prevention.htm. Accessed August 1, 2004.

Werbach MR. *Nutritional Influences on Mental Illness: a Sourcebook of Clinical Research.* 2nd ed. Tarzana, CA: Third Line Press; 1999.

World Health Organization (WHO). Causes of death (2001). Geneva, Switzerland: WHO. Available at: www.who.int/bod; Epub 2003. Accessed August 1, 2004.

CHAPTER 7

Lifestyle and Disease Management

Nancy Faass with Wayne B. Jonas

This chapter is based on interviews with Dr. Jonas.

THE CHANGING DEMOGRAPHICS OF DISEASE

The primary therapeutics of modern medicine were developed to treat acute conditions. One hundred years ago, infectious disease was one of the primary causes of morbidity and mortality. The other major challenges in medicine were dealing with the consequences of trauma. We have found very effective ways to treat such conditions and have developed a model of health care that has been extremely successful. That model is now acknowledged and used all over the world.

One of the consequences of the success of that model is that we are no longer dying as often from acute conditions. This system has been so successful that it has shifted the epidemiology of human illness to diseases of

Wayne B. Jonas, MD, is the director of the Samueli Institute for Information Biology in Alexandria, Virginia, and a family practice physician. He has served as director of the Office of Alternative Medicine at the National Institutes of Health and the director of Medical Research Fellowship at Walter Reed Army Institute of Research. He has also participated as chair of the Program Advisory Council for the NIH office of Alternative Medicine, as director of the WHO Collaborating Center for Traditional Medicine, and as a member of the Cochrane Collaboration. Dr. Jonas has authored more than 140 publications and 4 books, made hundreds of presentations around the world, is on the editorial board of 8 peer-reviewed journals, and was a member of the White House Commission on Complementary Medicine.

aging. Consequently, the focus of medicine has also shifted to conditions for which the model is less successful. As a result of these changes in disease and population characteristics, we now have more people who live for longer periods of time with multiple chronic conditions. The acute care model does not work as well for the management of chronic illness. The treatment of chronic illness involves a fundamentally different perspective. Thus, we must develop new approaches to the types of illnesses that now predominate. It is not that we should abandon the acute care model; rather, we should focus the technologies and range of treatments that are available to address the majority of conditions now facing our health care system.

MANAGING CHRONIC ILLNESS

We currently have additional resources available that we can apply to the management of chronic disease.

Behavioral Approaches

In behavioral medicine we have considerable knowledge about what motivates and discourages people and how to bring about behavioral changes. That is a foundation to be built into the management of chronic disease. The marketing and advertising industries have done considerable research on what influences human behavior. We have not yet fully incorporated this knowledge into health care delivery.

Preventive Medicine

We know the basic elements involved in prevention, but it appears to be fairly difficult for individuals to implement these. Many people tend not to engage in healthy lifestyles. Interventions such as the Ornish program use diet, yoga, and a group support model as a means of helping people maintain healthy behavior. The group dynamic sustains people through the process of change.

Lifestyle Interventions

There are limitations in our ability to implement Ornish-style programs broadly, however. The infrastructure and resources are not yet in place to offer comprehensive lifestyle interventions. In contemporary medicine, we do have some resources available; for example, we are trained in certain areas of nutrition. However, if I send patients to the nutritionist, they will be covered for only two or three visits. In terms of the exercise component of the program, I can prescribe the services of an exercise therapist to work with my patients and get them started on a therapeutic exercise program. However, at most hospitals, that type of program is not available.

Support for Change

In addition to a new diet or exercise program, patients need to better understand how to manage their lives in a way that promotes health and stimulates the body to heal itself. They need support to make new habits part of their daily lives in order to maintain the benefits. Although there are support groups available, they are typically not targeted toward the needs of individuals in a lifestyle program. Thus, there is usually no infrastructure in place to support these types of programs on a broad scale.

Lifestyle Medicine

Lifestyle management is the foundation of many alternative healing systems such as Chinese medicine, Ayurveda, and naturopathic medicine. These systems each apply lifestyle management through its own unique cultural approach. They ask, "What is this person's life about, and how is his or her lifestyle causing health problems? What can be done to manage lifestyle in a way that promotes health, and how does that management fit into his or her behavior?"

Most traditional health systems also have components that focus on therapeutic diet, exercise, social support, and spiritual connections. Only on that foundation does the traditional physician add supportive treatment with herbs, acupuncture, or some other form of medical intervention. Such therapies are used against specific, targeted problems in the context of a healthy lifestyle.

Consequently, we are well served by expanding the continuum of our chronic disease management systems to include lifestyle programs and health promotion. If lifestyle interventions are effective in correcting advanced disease states, it is likely that they are also effective in preventing the development of the underlying problem. However, prevention is very difficult to measure. If we can collect the data showing that lifestyle programs can make a difference for people who are ill, we will have data that will likely apply to prevention. In both populations, the focus is on self-healing and the correction of underlying causes.

EXPANDING THE CONTINUUM TOWARD OPTIMAL HEALING ENVIRONMENTS

The first step in this process is to develop a clear understanding of the model on which chronic disease management must be based and how it is different from the curative model on which acute disease management has been so successfully built. We must also initiate more programs that support the development of health. This could include core lifestyle programs that are offered to everyone with chronic disease. The challenge is to determine how to do this in a cost-efficient manner and to engage patients' commitment in the process.

The future of medicine will include provision of integrative treatments within the context of optimal healing environments (Jonas & Chez, 2004). Such environments will address both the personal, inner aspects of healing, and the community and physical aspects that promote healing. At a minimum, optimal healing environments will involve methods that address the following 5 domains:

1. Conscious development of intention, awareness, expectation, and belief in improvement and well-being
2. Self-care practices that facilitate the experience of wholeness and well-being and foster greater compassion, love, and awareness of interconnectivity
3. Development of listening and communication skills, and service-oriented, altruistic behaviors that cultivate social support and trust, including the *therapeutic alliance*, in the health care setting
4. Instruction and practice in health-promoting behaviors in lifestyle to support self-healing such as proper diet, exercise, the balance of leisure and work, and addiction management
5. Responsible use of integrative medicine via the collaborative application of conventional and complementary practices in a manner supportive of healing processes

REFERENCES

Jonas WJ, Chez RA. Implementing and evaluating optimal healing environments. In: Research on Paradigm, Practice, and Policy: Toward Optimal Healing Environments in Health Care. *Journal of Alternative and Complementary Medicine.* 2004; 10(suppl 1):S1–S6.

CHAPTER 8

Creating a Virtual Integrative Practice

John C. Reed, MD, MD(H)

INTRODUCTION

Growing interest in complementary and alternative health care has led to greater access to complementary service providers. The practical challenge of integrating these therapies into patient treatment and prevention programs now means that both complementary providers and orthodox medical and allied health professionals need to learn how to work together. One model for achieving this is the "referral panel" or "virtual team practice."

While the advice in this chapter is directed to medical and osteopathic physicians who are seeking to broaden their referrals to complementary practitioners, the process described applies equally to complementary practitioners who are ready to build referral relationships with conventional health providers.

As a conventional physician, your decision to refer patients to complementary treatment may be based on upcoming changes in the standards of care in your profession, indicating that a practice such as acupuncture or clinical massage would be helpful for your patients. It may also be in response to patient requests for these types of therapies.

On the other hand, if you are a complementary care provider seeing patients, you will need one or more medical generalists to whom you can refer clients for biomedical diagnosis, emergency care, and drug management to meet the needs of those with chronically unstable health conditions. In addition, most patients will accept—and expect—lifesaving biomedical care in a real crisis, even if they prefer a "lighter touch" in their chronic outpatient care.

COMPLEMENTARY MEDICINE IN SPECIALTY PRACTICE

In making referrals, the choice of practitioner (whether conventional or complementary) depends on the type of practice and the patient population being served.

If you are in a specialist care practice—for example, an orthopedic surgeon, a cancer specialist, a hematologist, or a psychiatrist—the usefulness of complementary practitioners on your "virtual team" relates to the specific needs of your patient population. Patients come to specialists with the expectation that a particular kind of health problem is going to be resolved efficiently. By

John C. Reed, MD, MD(H) is the national medical director of American WholeHealth, a position he has held for a decade, where he has directed the formation of a large, multicity, interdisciplinary complementary health care group and provides oversight for a national network program of more than 25,000 complementary health care practitioners. A board-certified family physician graduated from the University of Pennsylvania School of Medicine, he is founding vice president of the American Academy of Medical Acupuncture, and a founding member of the American Holistic Medical Association. He has been a faculty member of the UCLA Medical Acupuncture course (1985 to 2001), a consultant for the NIH Office of Alternative Medicine, and is currently a senior consultant at the University of Maryland Integrative Medicine program.

Courtesy of John C. Reed, MD, MD(H), Sterling, Virginia.

and large they are not going to question the biomedical model; their interest is in how well your expertise and therapeutic approach will work for them. In this case you need to be informed as to which complementary therapies are most likely to improve the outcomes for your patients, based on the research evidence with regard to their specific diagnoses.

- Orthopedics—For example, if you are an orthopedic surgeon, you may want to expand your referral network beyond physical medicine specialists, podiatrists, and physical therapists to include chiropractors, acupuncturists, personal trainers, and yoga instructors. This could broaden the options and results for the management of the nonsurgical orthopedic patients you see who are not appropriate for immediate or eventual surgery.
- Oncology—If you are an oncologist, you may want to include an acupuncturist on your referral list to provide additional pain management or nausea control for patients undergoing treatment, as well as a mind-body therapist and a nutritionist.
- Internal medicine subspecialist—If you are an internal medicine subspecialist such as a cardiologist, it may be helpful to have a clinical nutritionist, an herbal consultant, or a naturopath for patients who are sensitive to medication or who request dietary alternatives to multiple pharmaceutical therapy.
- Pediatrics—If you are a pediatrician or child psychiatrist, you might want to have a working relationship with a clinical nutritionist, an auricular (ear) acupuncturist, or a biofeedback specialist to provide care for children with ADD whose families are not yet ready to place them on medication.
- Internal medicine generalist—An internist or a physician whose practice includes a

great many patients with diabetes will want a good nutritionist and possibly an herbalist to help patients manage food cravings.
- Fertility services—If you are a fertility specialist, you might include the "low-tech" services of an acupuncturist, a mind-body skills instructor or hypnotherapist, and a manual therapist on your treatment team to complement the high-tech tools that people use to reach their dream of parenthood.

COMPLEMENTARY MEDICINE IN PRIMARY CARE

In contrast to specialty practice, the practice of a primary care physician typically involves a great deal of evaluation and diagnostic work, whether in family medicine, pediatrics, gynecology, or internal medicine.

Meeting Specific Patient Needs

Chronic illness. Currently in American culture, we have many people with complex chronic health problems. We have a highly motivated population that does not readily accept physical illnesses and symptoms, even in cases in which standard medicine has nothing to offer in terms of relief or solace. In these circumstances, the evaluation process of a complementary therapy such as traditional Chinese medicine can provide a way of looking at the patient's health problem that is systemically different than the conventional focus on disease and pathological diagnosis of biomedicine.

This additional viewpoint often provides either (1) an approach to treatment that is not available in Western biomedicine, or (2) an alternative explanation of the patient's experience of disease that better fits the patient's belief system.

Recurring illness. Consider the situation of a patient whose chief complaint is, "I come down with a cold whenever I sit in a draft or an air-conditioned room." A standard workup to rule out chronic bronchitis, chronic sinusitis, or a cellular immune deficiency disorder could be nicely complemented by a diagnosis from the perspective of Chinese medicine and treatment with herbs and acupuncture to support the immune system and the body's natural defenses (described as *wei chi*).

Preference for alternatives to medication. There are also a number of patients who avoid drug treatment because of a metabolic sensitivity to certain types of pharmaceuticals (in biomedicine we are learning about genetic variation in liver p450 enzymes related to this problem). Others have cultural values or religious beliefs that man-made drugs interfere with the nature of the body.

Exposure to an alternative model of illness does not negate the biomedical physician's role or treatment options, but often allows the patient to accept and follow an integrative treatment plan. The family physician or internist who understands how to effectively refer to a competent CAM practitioner in these circumstances will earn the respect and loyalty of these patients.

Personal Practice Style

If you are a health care generalist, you will also want to choose practitioners for your "virtual team" who are compatible with your practice style and the expectations of your patients.

- If you are the kind of person who likes to coach patients, you are probably going to want a complementary practitioner with a coaching style.
- If you tend to be a little more directive with patients, you will want to find a complementary practitioner who is also somewhat

directive and would like to work with you in creating integrative treatment plans for patients.
- If your practice is built around social friendliness and common community values with your patients, find a CAM practitioner who reflects similar social and community values in their dealings with their clients

BUILDING REFERRAL RELATIONSHIPS WITH COMPLEMENTARY PROVIDERS

Credentialing for Practitioners

How does one go about finding highly skilled complementary practitioners? In health systems, hospitals, and other institutional environments, credentialing programs focus on the complementary professions that are licensed and/or governed by health care regulations. This includes chiropractors, licensed acupuncturists, massage therapists, naturopathic physicians, and certain mind-body practitioners, such as biofeedback therapists (those who are not already licensed as psychologists). To find practitioners who have already been credentialed, a good place to start would be health care organizations and major health plans with national scope such as Aetna, Anthem, Cigna, Guardian, Humana, Pacificare, Prudential, United Health Care, Wellpoint, or the various regional Blues plans. They may have credentialing programs for some or all of the complementary professionals you seek. This will enable you to develop an initial list of people who have already been credentialed by another reputable organization.

Credentialing for Wellness Services

If you have a wellness component associated with your practice, you may find that many of these practitioners do not have formal state or local licensure (for example fitness instructors), yet can potentially provide significant benefits for some of your patients. These practitioners include providers who deal with musculoskeletal problems and movement disorders, such as Feldenkrais and Pilates instructors. A wellness focus in your practice may also involve personal trainers and instructors in yoga, tai chi, or Qigong.

For these providers, there is typically no health care industry credentialing in place, although some health plans are beginning to develop networks of these practitioners. If you are looking for practitioners who are not currently part of a health care system, explore your community, ask your patients, and perhaps experience some of these practices yourself. You can also obtain potential referrals through the recommendations of your colleagues and friends, your own personal research, and the review of practitioner listings on professional association Web sites.

Evaluating Practitioners

Once you obtain the names of potential referrals, how does one evaluate them? Having identified practitioners in the community, it would be useful to meet with them. Have lunch or meet them over coffee (or herbal tea!). Invite them to your office or go visit them at their offices. Receive a pro-bono treatment or schedule an informal presentation to staff—this can provide a clearer idea of who the practitioners are and what they do, as well as their style of communication. For example, in the massage profession, practitioners who are establishing a new practice and want to obtain referrals from physicians often provide a massage to the physician or someone on his staff—gratis. Physical therapists or acupuncturists

who are interested in working with pain management patients are frequently willing to give a brief presentation to clinics or group practices about their specialties. In the final analysis, you will want to talk with the practitioners to understand their practice philosophy and to explain to them your expectations for referrals.

Contacting Potential Candidates

If you are interested in establishing a referral network, you can send letters to practitioners you have identified and request a description of their practice and background. This is a reasonable request. Typically, if a provider does not have their practice organized well enough to send you a coherent letter about their background or to forward a CV or resume, they are probably not going to be organized enough to share adequate communication with you about the progress of your patients. Communication is relevant, even with the nonlicensed professions. For example, if you are going to refer a patient for an exercise program and are concerned about some type of medical or physical limitations, you need to be able to confer with the personal trainer or exercise specialist. If you have concerns, for example, that the patient may become overheated, have difficulty maintaining stable blood sugar, or experience side effects of medication, you need to be able to communicate that type of information to your referral and know that it will be acknowledged and acted upon.

INITIATING REFERRALS

Referral protocol in complementary medicine is not much different than referral protocol in standard medicine. Some managed health plans have specific paperwork and procedural requirements when referring to specialists, including CAM practitioners. Most practices find it useful to have a brief formatted notepad or form that referring physicians fill out for their patients. The form includes the reason for the referral and the name(s) of the specialists the patient is to contact.

Developing a Referral List

Initially, include several options on your trial referral list based on clinical expertise and patient accessibility. In some ways, building a referral list to complementary practitioners is not that different from developing other types of medical referrals. In conventional practice, for example, a family practitioner or an internist may recognize that they will periodically have patients who need to be seen by an orthopedist for a particular situation. Practitioners who do not already have a skilled orthopedist in mind may call one or two colleagues to determine the best choice for that patient, and then make the referral. If there are several specialists in town who have been personally recommended, the referring doctor will typically send the patient to one or more of their practices and see what kind of response they receive from the specialist: Do they get a note or a call back? Was the patient pleased with the clinical outcome?

Referring Your Focus

Another consideration for your practice referral plan is the question of whether the majority of your referrals are focused on prevention or treatment:

- To what degree does your own practice emphasize wellness or maintenance?

- Are you looking most frequently for a clinical outcome to resolve a disability, to rehabilitate a patient from an injury, or restore function that has been lost due to accident or injury?

Some complementary practices are wellness oriented and want to build a practice base of people who will come and see them once a month or every two weeks to deal with the everyday stresses of life that inconvenience and affect people. In this type of practice, patients are often asked to commit to an ongoing series of services or a structured plan, similar to enrolling as a member of a health club or gym. There is nothing wrong with the wellness-oriented practices that are managed by those CAM practitioners. However, referring to such a practice might not be a good fit if you have a disease-focused practice. In that case, you will want to be referring to practitioners oriented toward resolving problems, who think in terms of creating a treatment plan with a definable end point. You also want a practitioner who will discharge this patient back to your clinical care when maximum benefit has been achieved.

In contrast, if you are making a referral for wellness and you know the patient simply needs an exercise program, then you want them to go to a physical therapist, trainer, health coach, or health club that will work with them over the next 6 months or year to help them stay on their program. That is one of the primary differences to be discerned when you are making referrals.

Tracking Referral Outcomes

In building your referral panel, listen to what your patients say about their experience in the specialty practitioner's office, clinic, or studio. Does the communication style of the practitioner match your communication style and your expectations? Are the management of their office and their hours appropriate for your patients' lifestyles? These are the subtleties of referral that make a difference— and that your patients will appreciate.

Ultimately, the most important aspect of the referrals is the outcomes you observe in the course of follow-up. Did the surgery go better when the patient used the mind-body imagery tapes and practiced relaxation skills? Did the herbal prescription address the perimenopausal symptoms effectively? If you find, for example, that a patient with chronic pain has gone to a chiropractor, acupuncturist, massage therapist, or biofeedback specialist for 6 to 12 treatments and the patient is not noticing any improvement in their level of pain, it is time to reevaluate. If the practitioner has not called you to communicate about progress, then perhaps the skill set of that person is not up to the level of problem solving you need for that patient. This does not mean that the practice of chiropractic, acupuncture, or specialty physical

therapy is not appropriate for your referral network; it may simply mean that you need to find someone with a higher skill set.

CONCLUSION

In summary, you want to be clear about what your own goals are in your health care practice. This enables you not only to select the right specialists for your team, but also to build good relationships with those who share your motivations, beliefs, and style of patient care. Ultimately, you are developing a patient care team. Your goal is to match the needs of your patients with the resources that are available within the greater health care system and the complementary health care community. Our hope is that the resources and information in this book will expand the resources and treatment options you offer patients. After reviewing the rest of the book you will have a better idea of the types of practitioners who would round out your own practice. Revisit this chapter as you use the charts in Chapter 63 to help you clarify potential specialties for your own referral network.

PART II

Clinical Nutrition

Chapter

CHAPTER 9

Clinical Nutrition

Leo Galland, MD

Nutritional therapy can address many of the problems that physicians encounter in their practice on a daily basis. Research has shown that clinical nutrition can be effective in the treatment of mild acute conditions; chronic disorders; and in some cases, even advanced disease. For physicians who want an integrative approach, nutrition is a good entry point. The principals of nutrition are biochemical and physiological, founded in the knowledge base of Western medicine. This is not a mystical approach to healing—nutrition is ultimately the realm of molecular biology.

Clinical nutrition is a practical tool for improving the health of patients. Diet is an area over which patients have a significant amount of control. In fact, whenever doctors can involve patients in taking a greater role in their own health, we enhance their ability to influence their health positively. Nutritional therapy also provides an opportunity to partner with our patients. To be fully effective in these collaborations, one of the major focuses of our efforts must be to motivate them.

Many physicians notice that when patients begin to take control of their diet, they change psychologically as well. In many cases, they are not only changing their diets, they are also changing their relationship to the process of health and healing. Consequently, nutrition can provide patients with the experience of better self-care. Since we all eat several times a day, this change does not require engaging in an unfamiliar activity. Rather, patients are simply approaching a familiar activity from a different perspective.

ASSESSMENTS: INTERVIEWS AND QUESTIONNAIRES

In my own practice, I begin my work with patients by increasing their awareness of food and the process of eating. Good nutrition and diet change has to begin with increased consciousness. The first step for a physician who wants to work nutritionally with patients is to learn what your patient is already eating. Even before ordering laboratory tests, you want to learn the patient's dietary habits and practices.

The Interview

There are several methods that can be used for nutritional assessment by health care professionals. One approach is to simply ask questions. This is what I have done for 25 years—I ask patients about what they eat, when, and how: Do you usually eat break-

Leo Galland, MD, is an internist practicing in New York City, received his undergraduate degree at Harvard University and his medical training at New York University. He has served as director of medical research at the Gesell Institute for Human Development, and is currently director of the Foundation for Integrative Medicine, and of Applied Nutrition, Inc. Dr. Galland is author of two books on nutrition, *Superimmunity for Kids* and *Power Healing*, and developer of software for nutritional assessment, *The Drug-Nutrient Workshop* and *The Nutrition Workshop*, www.NutritionWorkshop.com.

fast? If so, what do you typically eat for breakfast? What do you drink at breakfast? What do you usually have at lunchtime? And for dinner? Where do you usually eat dinner? Do you have snacks during the day? What do you drink during the day? Do you tend to have desserts? What about late night snacks?

It is also important to know *how* people eat. It is one thing to know what they eat, but it is another to know about their relationship to food: How much do they eat out? Do they eat with other people? Are they obsessed with food? There is a whole series of important questions related to food that involve the psychosocial aspects of patients' lives. If you are going to support people in the process of change, it is important to know their underlying attitudes and beliefs, their habits, and the social conditions under which they live.

This can give you a very broad picture of a patient's dietary pattern and attitudes toward food, but the problem in asking those questions is that it only gives you a qualitative assessment, not quantitative information. However, this is a good place to start.

Food-Frequency Questionnaires

Much of the research on nutrition, health, and disease has involved the use of food frequency questionnaires (FFQs). One of these assessment tools was developed by Walter Willett, MD (1985, Willet et al., 1994), and has been used in all of the major nutritional studies from Harvard, including the Harvard Nurses Study and the Harvard Physicians Study. That entire immense body of work has relied upon the Willett food frequency questionnaire. Another instrument, developed by Gladys Block, PhD (1986), of the University of California, Berkeley, is a food frequency questionnaire that has been adopted by the National

Cancer Institute (NCI). In my own work, I have been adapting the NCI software for clinical use, so practitioners can obtain a more quantitative assessment of their patients' nutritional status.

Applying the Assessment

Once you have gathered information about your patients' dietary habits, you need some type of structure for organizing it and determining what is important. Those priorities depend, in part, on what is important about each individual patient. What matters for one person is not necessarily what is going to matter for another. The nutritional assessment is then integrated with the information on their family health history, personal health history, their goals, and whether they need to lose weight.

There are certain aspects of diet that we now know are important. From the perspective of preventive medicine, we know that some of the most significant nutritional factors include:

- Diversity of foods in the diet
- Adequacy of micronutrients and protein
- Level of fiber
- Consumption of fruits and vegetables
- Specific foods and food families that are rich in functional phytochemicals, such as tomato products, cruciferous vegetables, and allium family vegetables
- Consumption of fish and omega-3 fatty acids

If the first step in clinical assessment is to determine what your patients are eating, the next step is to compare that information with nutritional standards that have a scientific basis. When you perform this analysis, you will find that most patients are not eating the recommended levels of fruits and vegetables. Rather, they are consuming excessive quantities of sodium and possibly fat, generally too little of the omega-3 essential fatty acids, and an excess of junk food.

Recently released data suggests that the majority of Americans obtain approximately 35% of their calories from junk food (Block, 2004). Most people are simply not active enough to burn 35% of their caloric intake. In fact, even if they only consume 10% of their calories from junk food, most people are still likely to gain weight (Dong et al., 2004). This explains why 65% of US adults are over-weight and half that number are obese. Junk food consumption makes a significant contribution to both obesity and its sequelae. Obesity and obesity-related diseases have now emerged as the second leading cause of death in this country. Tobacco use is still the number one cause, but obesity is gaining on it fast (US Department of Health and Human Services, 2004; Mokdad et al., 2004). Consequently, any meaningful nutritional assessment includes questions about the patient's activity level. This enables the physician to determine the relationship between calories consumed and calories expended.

Effects of Disease and Medication on Micronutrient Levels

Most patients are taking medications. Medication can have an impact on nutritional requirements. A review by the author of approximately 900 of the most frequently used medications in the US indicates that more than 400 of these drugs have effects on nutrient requirements—effects that can produce deficiencies of specific nutrients. Clearly, the physician needs to know whether the patient is taking medication and the impact of that medication on his or her nutritional status.

In observing the patient, you may not see the symptoms of nutritional deficiency because they are usually quite subtle unless there is severe malnutrition. However, deficiencies can be a factor in a range of conditions:

- Frequent illness, suggesting poor immune function
- Impaired wound healing
- Possible growth impairment in children
- Sexual dysfunction or infertility
- Symptoms of fatigue
- Disturbances of mood or sleep

These are common problems. Nutritional deficiencies can result in low energy, one of the most frequent complaints of patients. In a great many cases, there is no obvious explanation for the fatigue. There are also many patients who are frequently ill, with no apparent cause for their impaired immunity. In my experience, particularly with children, these infections can almost always be reversed with nutritional measures.

Not only do nutritional deficits contribute to common symptoms, but diseases and their symptoms can cause nutritional deficits. Gastrointestinal disorders, in particular, may decrease appetite, cause patients to avoid food groups that are important sources of specific nutrients, or cause maldigestion, malabsorption, or nutrient losses through the intestinal wall. Chronic inflammation of any type may alter the availability of nutrients, producing zinc, iron, or protein deficiency, even if the diet is apparently adequate.

In summary, a comprehensive analysis can provide a physician with an understanding of patients' nutritional intake and whether it is affected in any way by the diseases they have or the medications they are taking.

THE PHYSICAL EXAMINATION

The physical exam can be helpful, but for the most part it does not shed as much light on the patient's nutritional status as laboratory testing. However, there are certain findings in the exam that may reflect basic nutritional issues or deficiencies:

- Insulin resistance: You certainly want to know about a person's weight, their body mass index, and their waist circumference. Waist circumference is probably a better measure of insulin resistance than body mass index.
- Blood pressure: You also want to know about their blood pressure and how it changes when they stand up, particularly from a position of lying down. A change, whether blood pressure drops or is elevated, may suggest a need for minerals.
- Sodium intake: Most people consume an excess of sodium, but there are people (frequently women) on a low sodium diet who are suffering from fatigue and have low blood pressure. These people may actually need more sodium in their diet and feel better if they use salt.
- Essential fatty acids: There are findings on the physical exam that may be suggestive of the need for more essential fatty acids in the diet. Dry skin or dry hair might be a response to a deficiency of fatty acids.

LABORATORY TESTING

Laboratory evaluations can be very helpful. It is not necessary to use special labs. The following basic tests for nutritional assessments can be obtained through any laboratory.

Blood Chemistry

- The CBC and chemistry panel
- Liver enzymes: Low levels of liver enzymes (ALT or AST) are sometimes the result of a deficiency of vitamin B_6, which is a cofactor for those enzymes. Low levels of alkyline phosphotase, another liver enzyme, could be a sign of magnesium deficiency. If a patient has a low level of those enzymes, you can recommend a supplement and a month later repeat the test to determine if the levels have normalized.

Mineral Levels

- Iron levels: Relevant testing includes both serum ferritin and iron/iron binding capacity. Iron levels are important to test for two reasons. Many people have iron deficiencies; however, another portion of the population is subject to iron overload (hemochromatosis). Frequently this occurs due to genetic factors and is more prevalent among people of western European background. Hemochromatosis can be fatal, and patients may not know they have this condition until significant damage has occurred to the liver, heart, or pancreas. Therefore, everyone should have their iron level tested.

- Zinc: The measurement of plasma or serum zinc can be quite useful. There are many people with zinc deficiency, particularly among those with current or chronic infections. Zinc intake in the US is quite marginal. Correcting zinc deficiency with supplementation can have a significant impact on immune function. Iron levels can also affect immunity.

- Magnesium: Magnesium should be evaluated in terms of both the serum level of magnesium and red blood cell level. Most magnesium is intracellular. Consequently, there are many people who have intracellular magnesium depletion, and yet their test results for serum magnesium are normal. A wide range of symptoms are associated with these deficiencies, including fatigue, irritability, muscle cramping and spasms, abdominal pain, and migraine headaches. Again, most Americans consume significantly less than the RDA for magnesium. Supplementing with magnesium can be very beneficial.

Vitamin Levels

- Vitamin A: This nutrient should be measured, particularly for people with recurrent infections and skin problems. Vitamin A is another of the nutrients for which the intake in this country is relatively low. Usually I do not favor vitamin A supplementation, but prefer to have people increase their dietary intake as a way of raising their levels of this nutrient. However, in some cases, it is important to use supplements. Vitamin A levels have an impact on immunity and wound healing, the quality of skin, and the mucous membranes.

- Folic acid: There are several options for evaluating this nutrient. One is to check homocysteine levels in the blood, because they are fairly sensitive to the adequacy of folic acid and become elevated when folic acid levels drop. In other cases, it is worth measuring serum folic acid and vitamin B_{12} levels independently of homocysteine. This is especially relevant for people who are suffering from immune problems, anemia, or depression.

  There is research indicating that people whose folic acid levels are low or relatively low do not respond well to antidepressant medication. The goal in these cases is to raise folic acid levels enough to lower homocysteine levels (even if homocysteine is not in the abnormal range). At that point, their response to antidepressant drugs usually improves significantly. This is especially true for women.

- Vitamin D: The best measure of this nutrient is 25 hydroxy vitamin D, the vitamin D that is absorbed from food. The vitamin D made in your skin must be converted into 25 hydroxy vitamin D (calcidiol), so that form is considered the best measure of the nutritional adequacy of vitamin D. The kidney then converts that form of the nutrient to 1,25 dihydroxy vitamin D (calcitriol), which is a hormone. However, it is possible to be vitamin D deficient and still have a normal level of the kidney-derived hormone. When this occurs, nutrient levels are being maintained because kidney enzymes are compensating by overproducing it, which is potentially harmful.

  There are a great many people with vitamin D deficiency in the US, particularly in the northern regions. Yet even in southern California, there are numerous people with these deficiencies because they use sun block on a constant basis. Sunlight is still the most efficient way to raise vitamin D levels. Ironically, in the effort to avoid skin cancer, people deprive themselves of sunlight, which is an essential nutrient. Supplementation may be necessary to achieve optimal vitamin D levels. I do not measure vitamin D in people who are obviously suntanned. However, a great many of my patients initially have either low or suboptimal vitamin D levels. Vitamin D deficiency is important; it not only has an impact on calcium absorption and bone health, it also affects immune function and can be a factor in cancer risk. A range of diseases have been linked to vitamin D deficiencies. There is a great deal of evidence that low levels of vitamin D deficiency are associated with colon cancer, multiple sclerosis, and Type 1 diabetes.

These tests for essential nutrients are available through any commercial laboratory. The results can reveal a tremendous amount of nutritional information, so this is an excellent place to begin. Nutrient levels are frequently low in patients with chronic illness. For example, those with diabetes, high blood pressure, chronic kidney disease, and inflammatory bowel disease tend to be nutrient deficient. Consequently, testing nutrient levels can be quite meaningful and relevant to treatment. The information from this testing provides a rational basis for recommending specific nutrients. It is not necessary to use special labs to order these tests, and their use can be justified to insurance companies.

Laboratory tests for these nutrients are quite reliable, which is one of the reasons why they are so widely available. However, there are subtleties to their use. For example, when testing for zinc levels, the results can indicate a normal level, even when there actually is a zinc deficiency. In this case, the test may simply not be sensitive enough. In contrast, a chronic inflammatory disease may cause a low level of zinc in the plasma or the serum without producing an actual zinc deficiency. Clinical nutrition involves more than a cookbook approach.

There are other situations that require your discernment as well. If I see a patient with symptoms of deficiency and the lab test comes back normal, but in the low-normal range, I frequently treat them. For example, if a patient has a borderline level of zinc on the lab work and they have a chronic infection that has not resolved, I recommend zinc supplements.

CLINICAL APPLICATIONS

At this point in the assessment process, I have obtained the patient's dietary profile and used that to make recommendations for changes in diet. I have ordered blood tests to measure some of the nutrients I think are most important for this particular patient and used those results as a basis for making specific recommendations about nutritional supplements. There are also certain nutrients that I do not measure but recommend for most all patients:

• Multivitamins: The majority of my patients take multivitamins.

• Essential fatty acids: Most Americans have an inadequate intake of essential fats, so I generally recommend a fatty acid supplement: Fish oil: usually approximately 2 to 3 grams per day. Flax seed oil: approximately 5 grams of oil or a tablespoon of ground flax seeds. The research has shown higher levels of fish oil supplements to be beneficial for disorders such as arthritis, inflammatory bowel disease, and bipolar disorder. For the most part, a complete nutritional assessment is not necessary before making this particular recommendation.

For patients who have specific disorders, I may suggest higher doses of particular supplements. The therapeutic use of nutrients requires a more advanced level of understanding on the part of the practitioner.

CONCLUSION

In applying clinical nutrition, it is important to remember that there is no fast track to this field. Practitioners almost always find that it is helpful (and essential) to read as broadly as possible. However, regardless of the approach, a certain amount of time is necessary to acquire this knowledge and gain proficiency in applying it clinically.

RESOURCES

Software for Clinical Practice

- *The Drug-Nutrition Workshop* is software intended for use by health professionals as a clinical management tool, which provides an analysis and a report for individual patients of potential interactions between drugs, nutrients, supplements, and foods they are consuming. The searchable database includes approximately 900 medications (by generic and brand name), 600 nutritional and herbal supplements, and information on more than 2000 documented interactions.

- *The Nutrition Workshop* is a dietary analysis tool, designed to provide health practitioners with both quantitative and descriptive information about their patients' diets. The software includes a food frequency questionnaire, and one on physical activity, that can be downloaded from a CD or from the Web. Information on the *Drug-Nutrient Workshop* and the *Nutrition Workshop* by Leo Galland, MD, can be obtained through Applied Nutrition, Inc., www.NutritionWorkshop. com.

Books. Another resource for physicians is a series of books, *Nutritional Influences on Illness*, developed by Melvyn Werbach, MD. These books contain a great deal of useful clinical information, based on the research literature and this is a good place to begin one's self-education. Information on the Werbach books can be obtained from Third Line Press in Tarzana, California or on the web at www.third-line.com.

Courses. *Food as Medicine* is a course on clinical nutrition sponsored by the Center for Mind-Body Medicine, which provides a step-by-step approach for physicians and other health care providers who want to expand the use of nutrition in their practice. More information regarding this course can be obtained by contacting the Center for Mind-Body Medicine in Washington, DC www.cmbm.org.

Seminars and conferences. Information on advanced seminars, an annual conference, and publications on a biochemical and technical approach to clinical nutrition can be obtained through the Institute for Functional Medicine in Gig Harbor, WA, or online at www.functionalmedicine.org.

REFERENCES

Block G. Foods contributing to energy intake in the US: data from NHANES III and NHANES 1999–2000. *J Food Composition and Analysis.* 2004;17:439–447.

Block G, Hartman AM, Dresser CM, Carroll MD, Gannon J, Gardner L. A data-based approach to diet questionnaire design and testing. *Am J Epidemiol.* 1986;124(3):453–69.

Dong L, Block G, Mandel S. Activities contributing to total energy expenditure in the United States: results from the NHAPS Study. *Int J Behav Nutr Phys Act.* 2004;1(1):4.

Mokdad AH, Marks JS, Stroup DF, Gerberding JL. Actual causes of death in the United States 2000. *JAMA.* 2004;291(10):1238–1241.

US Department of Heatlh and Human Services (USHHS). New surgeon general's report expands list of diseases caused by smoking. Available at: http://www.hhs.gov/news/press/2004pres/20040527 a.html. Accessed August 1, 2004.

Willett WC. Future directions in the development of food-frequency questionnaires. *AM J Clin Nutr.* 1994;(1 Suppl):171S–174S.

Willett WC, Sampson, L, Stampfer MJ, et al. Reproductibility and validity of a semiqualitative food frequency questionnaire. *Am J Epidemiol.* 1985;122(1):51–65.

CHAPTER 10

Research on Nutritional Therapy for Anemia

Melvyn Werbach, MD

INTRODUCTION

A great amount of literature exists documenting the impact of nutrients in relation to various disease states. However, to what extent can the results obtained in research studies be directly extrapolated to the clinical setting? Much of the promotional material on nutritional supplements certainly seems to suggest that everybody could benefit from taking supplements of almost every conceivable nutrient.

If you take the time to read the studies, researchers readily admit that this is rarely the case. Even those studies that find a particular nutrient to be highly effective will usually show that a significant percentage of the

Melvyn Werbach, MD, has served as faculty in psychiatry at the UCLA School of Medicine, sits on the editorial boards of several journals, and is associate editor for the journal, *Alternative Therapies in Health and Medicine*. He received his education at Columbia College, Tufts University School of Medicine, the National Institute of Mental Health, and the Cedars-Sinai Medical Center, and has served as consultant to the Pain Center, City of Hope National Medical Center and director of Clinical Biofeedback and Psychological Services, UCLA Pain Control Unit. Dr. Werbach is a diplomate of the American Board of Psychiatry and Neurology and author of the *Textbook of Nutritional Medicine*, *Nutritional Influences on Illness*, *Nutritional Influences on Mental Illness* (winner of the Book of the Year Award), and, with Michael Murray, ND, *Botanical Influences on Illness*.

Courtesy of Melvyn R. Werbach and Third Line Press. In: Werbach MR, Moss J. *Textbook of Nutritional Medicine*. Tarzana, CA: Third Line Press, Inc.; 1999.

study group did not respond positively, demonstrating that not everyone in a particular diagnostic group responds the same when supplemented with a nutrient.

INTEGRATIVE MEDICINE: A COMPREHENSIVE PARADIGM

During the last few years, a more comprehensive approach to determining nutritional requirements has arisen that comes closer to accurately identifying the needs of today's chronically ill patient. This method takes what we already know about clinical nutrition and places it in a different perspective, a perspective that maintains that *no* physiologic process, including one relating to nutrition, can be fully understood when examined as an isolated entity. The true significance of nutritional factors can only be comprehended when considered in conjunction with the physiologic processes which are, in turn, impacted by those factors.

Is it necessary to know the many physiologic interrelationships of nutritional factors to successfully employ nutrition clinically? For treating many patients, direct application of nutritional protocols derived from the research will be enough. However, for treating other chronically ill patients who "have been everywhere and tried everything," an understanding of the integrative principles discussed below may be necessary.

Of the many names this comprehensive approach has been given, we prefer "integrative medicine." Although nutrition is only one aspect of a comprehensive integrative approach, we did not choose "integrative nutrition" because the integrative model is more than just nutritional evaluation and treatment; it represents a different way of looking at patients.

In terms of evaluating the needs of the chronically ill patient, integrative medicine assumes that they are suffering due to a variety of causes that are working together in sometimes intricate ways to create the clinical picture. For decades, modern medicine has employed a "single cause, single cure" approach to disease that, as can be seen from the massive amount of studies on the effects of single nutrients on illness, has largely been adopted by clinical nutrition as well. Unfortunately, while this philosophy of health care was quite successful in the days when infection and gross nutrition deficiency were common, it is yielding diminishing returns now.

A discussion of the broad range of factors—including, for example, physical fitness and mental health—which are encompassed in the concept of integrative medicine is well beyond the scope of this text. Instead, we will limit ourselves to the most common nutritionally-relevant causes of chronic illness. These can be divided into five broad categories:

1. Neuroendocrine imbalance: This category primarily includes the stress response and its numerous downstream effects on endocrine function.

2. Improper nutrition: Micronutrient imbalances need to be considered when evaluating the chronic patient. Also, we will demonstrate that another aspect of nutritional imbalance, macronutrient imbalance, is epidemic yet much less appreciated in the chronically ill population.

3. Chemical and/or heavy metal toxicity: The evidence that environmental toxins are playing a major role in creating chronic illness is compelling. The ultimate clinical toxicity of xenobiotics can vary greatly in different individuals.

4. Compromised mucosal barriers: Improper function of the gastrointestinal tract can be a major cause of chronic illness due to poor digestive capacity, suboptimal absorption, and/or increased absorption of toxic substances, whether their origin is exogenous or endogenous. Factors such as poor diet, elevated stress hormones, and dysbiotic organisms can work together to make a major contribution to much of the chronic illness that exists today.

5. Genetics: This area has traditionally received little attention because genes were believed to be impermeable to environmental influences. Exciting new research is suggesting, however, that genetic expression is quite responsive to external surroundings. Furthermore, this research demonstrates that nutrients have a powerful impact on both gene expression and the function of DNA repair mechanisms.

According to this proposed model, in order to properly address the needs of the chronic patient, the following points must be kept in mind:

• These major causes of chronic illness rarely work in isolation to create ill health. Rather, they interact in often intricate ways to create the clinical picture.
• All five causes may be of etiologic importance. This represents a key difference be-

tween a disease-oriented model and the integrative model. Using the integrative approach, diagnostic procedures continue beyond simply putting together sufficient data to fit the patient with a disease label. Instead, they continue until the causative factors can be reasonably determined. What follows is the exploration of a single diagnosis, anemia, utilizing an integrative model.

OVERVIEW OF ANEMIA TREATMENT

The microcytic anemia of iron deficiency, and the megaloblastic anemia of folate or vitamin B_{12} deficiency, are widely known. While nutritional pharmacotherapy does not appear to be indicated in the treatment of anemia, many anemias are fostered by deficiencies of any of a variety of vitamins and minerals, repletion of which will often result in active blood regeneration. (See Tables 10–1 and 10–2.)

Hydrochloric acid deficiency should be considered as a cause of iron-deficiency and sickle cell anemias. Gluten sensitivity may present as anemia, while milk sensitivity may cause an iron deficiency by provoking intestinal bleeding.

VITAMIN DEFICIENCIES

Vitamin A Deficiency

Anemia gradually develops several months after starting a diet deficient in vitamin A. Serum hemoglobin begins to decline well before the loss of night vision or the development of "deficient" serum levels of the vitamin (Hodges et al., 1978). The anemia, which is due to impaired hemoglobin synthesis, is reversible with supplementation (West & Roodenburg, 1992). Vitamin A may

also be deficient in sickle cell anemia (Sindel et al., 1990).

Vitamin B Complex Deficiencies

Folic acid deficiency is a well-known cause of megaloblastic anemia. Deficiency can also be related to sickle cell anemia (Pierce & Rath, 1962) that, in turn, is responsive to supplementation (Reed et al., 1987). When deficient, folate supplementation may also be beneficial in treating aplastic anemia (Branda et al., 1978) or red cell aplasia (Gothoni, et al., 1995). When deficient, pantothenic acid supplementation can be helpful in alleviating anemia (McCurdy, 1973).

Riboflavin deficiency can cause a normochromic, normocytic anemia and reticulocytopenia that responds to supplementation (Lane & Alfrey, 1965). Riboflavin deficiency also may be associated with sickle cell anemia, usually in conjunction with other deficiencies (Sindel et al., 1990).

A 53-year-old black female was admitted with anorexia, weight loss, lethargy, incontinence and hypochromic anemia with increased iron storage in the bone marrow. After an unsuccessful trial of pyridoxine, all symptoms and signs improved dramatically following the administration of pantothenic acid (pantothenyl alcohol 50 to 200 mg IM daily).

Several years later, a similar clinical picture developed and there was a clinical, but probably not a hematologic, response to a multivitamin preparation containing large amounts of pantothenic acid (McCurdy, 1973).

Thiamine deficiency may be associated with a megaloblastic anemia (Mangel et al., 1984) which, in turn, may respond to supplementation.

Table 10–1 Nutritional Treatment Guide

✓ = Efficacy generally accepted.
* = Efficacy *demonstrated* by controlled human trials.
[+] = Efficacy *suspected* from uncontrolled human trials.
[−] = Efficacy *suspected* from indirect data.
? = Efficacy *challenged* in a study of similar design.

Nutritional Factors
✓ **Folic acid deficiency:** 800 mcq/daily
✓ **Iron deficiency:** 30 mg/twice daily; then minimal possible dosage
✓ **Vitamin B$_{12}$ deficiency:** 1000 mcq/intramuscularly weekly initially and monthly afterwards

---

* **Vitamin A deficiency:** 50,000 IU daily for 6 weeks (10,000 IU daily during pregnancy)
* **Zinc deficiency:** Zinc sulfate 220 mg twice daily *and* **Copper** 2 mg daily

---

[+] **Pantothenic acid deficiency:** 100 to 200 mg daily
[+] **Riboflavin deficiency:** 5 to 10 mg daily
[+] **Thiamine deficiency:** 50 mg daily orally or intramuscularly
[+] **Vitamin B$_6$ deficiency:** 50 to 100 mg daily
[+] **Vitamin C deficiency:** 500 mg twice daily
[+] **Vitamin E deficiency:** D,L-alpha-tocopheryl acetate 200 to 2000 mg or IU daily for 6 weeks
[+] **Copper deficiency:** 2 mg twice daily for up to 6 weeks along with 50 mg zinc daily
[+] **Magnesium deficiency:** Usual oral dosage ≈ 400 mg daily (Consider IM or IV administration.)

Other Factors
* **Hydrochloric acid deficiency:** Betaine or glutamic hydrochloride 10 to 50 gr following meals (Beware of gastric irritation.)

[+] rule out **gluten sensitivity**
[+] rule out **milk sensitivity** (infants with iron-deficiency anemia)

Source: Werbach & Moss, 1999.

A child with megaloblastic anemia failed to respond to vitamin B$_{12}$ or folic acid but responded to supplementation with oral thiamine 20 mg daily. When, on two occasions, the thiamine supplement was stopped, anemia recurred (Rogers, 1964).

Vitamin B$_6$ deficiency may be associated with both a microcytic anemia (Bernat, 1983a) and a megaloblastic anemia (Hines & Harrison, 1964); both respond to supplementation. When the vitamin is deficient, sickle cell anemia may also show a response to vitamin supplements (Natta & Reynolds, 1984). Furthermore, if a sideroblastic anemia is unresponsive to pyridoxine, supplementation with pyridoxal-5'-phosphate may be effective, as the anemia may be due to defective phosphorylation of pyridoxine to its active form (Hines & Love, 1975).

Table 10–2 Nutrient Deficiencies in Anemias

	Anemia (general)	Beta-Thalassemia	Sickle Cell	Sideroblastic
Copper	X		X	
Folic Acid	X		X	
Iron	X		X	
Magnesium	X	X	X	
Riboflavin	X		X	
Thiamine	X			
Vitamin A	X		X	
Vitamin B_6	X		X	X
Vitamin B_{12}	X		X	
Vitamin C	X	X		
Vitamin E	X	X	X	
Zinc		X	X	

Source: Werbach & Moss, 1999.

A patient with primary acquired sideroblastic anemia was unresponsive to pyridoxine 100 mg daily, but showed a prompt reticulocytosis when given pyridoxal-5-phosphate 20 mg daily (Hines, 1970).

Of course, *vitamin B_{12}* deficiency is a well-known cause of pernicious anemia, a megaloblastic anemia, and supplementation may be able to reverse the neurologic damage (Berk et al., 1998). Moreover, a B_{12} deficiency may be associated with sickle cell anemia, which can respond to intramuscular supplementation (al-Momen, 1995).

Vitamin C Deficiency

Vitamin C deficiency is occasionally associated with a normochromic, normocytic, or macrocytic anemia (Sauberlich, 1984). Furthermore, the nutrient may be reduced in beta-thalassemia (Giuberti, 1987). Vitamin C enhances non-heme iron absorption, which can aid in the prevention and treatment of iron-deficiency anemia (Monsen, 1982) and may stimulate hematopoiesis (Ajayi & Nnaji, 1980).

Vitamin E Deficiency

When a nonspecific anemia is found to be associated with vitamin E deficiency, it may respond to supplementation (Drake & Fitch, 1980). In addition, there are a number of specific forms of anemia that are associated with deficiency, all of which may also respond to repletion. These include sickle cell anemia (Sindel et al., 1990; Natta et al., 1980), beta-thalassemia (Giuberti et al., 1987; Osoylu & Gurgey, 1991), and the anemias associated with cystic fibrosis (Farrell et al., 1977) and Mediterranean G_6PD deficiency (Corash et al., 1980).

MINERAL DEFICIENCIES

Copper Deficiency

Copper deficiency, which can be instigated by a high level of zinc supplementation, is associated with a hypochromic, microcytic anemia (Williams, 1983). In addition, due to its effects on ceruloplasmin, copper deficiency may cause an iron deficiency anemia due to impaired iron absorption and reduced heme synthesis while iron accumulates in storage tissues. When induced by a copper deficiency, iron deficiency anemia can only be corrected with copper supplementation (Watts, 1989). Serum copper levels may also be reduced in sickle cell anemia (Ishir et al., 1995).

A 35-year-old Caucasian woman ingested 110 to 165 mg elemental zinc as zinc sulfate for 10 months. She developed a slowly worsening microcytic, hypochromic anemia found to be due to copper deficiency. Zinc supplementation was eliminated and she was supplemented with 2 mg copper daily. After 2 months, her anemia was unchanged. She received 10 mg copper chloride intravenously over a period of 5 days, and responded (Hoffman, 1988).

Iron Deficiency and Overload

Iron deficiency is likely to be the most frequent cause of anemia. It responds well to iron supplementation (Bernat, 1983b). In addition, iron is often deficient in pernicious anemia (Carmel et al., 1987) as well as in sickle cell anemia (Reed et al., 1987). (See Hydrochloric Acid Deficiency and Food Sensitivities sections later in the chapter, and Copper Deficiency described earlier.)

By contrast, beta-thalassemia major (Cooley's anemia), an inherited microcytic anemia, may be associated with iron overload; and levels of ferritin, an iron storage protein, may be positively correlated with lipid peroxidation product concentrations in this disorder (Livrea et al., 1996). Iron supplementation is therefore contraindicated in the treatment of a microcytic anemia unless there is evidence of iron deficiency.

Magnesium Deficiency

Magnesium nutriture may be reduced in a number of anemias, including sickle cell anemia (Ishir et al., 1995), beta-thalassemia (Hyman et al., 1980) and sideropenic anemia (Abbasciano et al., 1991). In sickle cell anemia, magnesium depletion appears to be at least partly due to excessive urinary excretion (Olukoga et al., 1993). Supplementation may increase the absolute reticulocyte count and the number of immature reticulocytes, while reducing the number of dense sickle erythrocytes (De Franceschi et al., 1997a).

In regard to beta-thalassemia, results of a study in mice suggest that dietary magnesium supplementation may improve the anemia (De Franceschi et al.,1997b); the results of human trials have yet to be reported.

Zinc Deficiency

Plasma levels of *zinc* may be low in sickle cell anemia (Ishir et al., 1995) which may be corrected by supplementation (Sindel et al., 1990). Pharmacologic doses of zinc (100–300 mg daily) for several months can, however, produce a severe copper deficiency causing a sideroblastic anemia with hypocupremia, anemia, leukopenia, and neutropenia (Broun et al., 1990).

COMBINED NUTRIENT DEFICIENCIES

A handicapped child initially presented with iron-deficiency anemia. Despite treatment with iron supplements, after 5 weeks the anemia had worsened and symptoms of bruising and joint pain appeared.

When biochemical tests indicated deficiencies of vitamin C and folic acid, the child was then given vitamin C and folic acid supplementation to which he responded. The initial lack of response to iron suggests that vitamin C deficiency may have been the primary cause for the decreased utilization of iron. Alternatively, iron supplementation could have precipitated scurvy by increasing the oxidation of ascorbic acid. Because of a lack of bone marrow response, it is unlikely that iron supplementation precipitated folic acid deficiency, but ascorbic acid deficiency may have further depleted the patient's low folate stores (Clark, 1992).

In beta-thalassemia, chronic hemolysis causing hyperzincuria appears to be the cause of zinc deficiency (Vatanavicharn et al., 1992).

OTHER RELATED FACTORS

Hydrochloric Acid Deficiency

A deficiency of hydrochloric acid may impair iron absorption, leading to an iron-deficiency anemia (Jacobs et al., 1966). Conversely, hydrochloric acid output may improve following iron supplementation (Shearman et al., 1966), although atrophic gastritis does not appear to be causally related to the anemia (Cater, 1992). Adequate supplementation with glutamic or betaine hydrochloride should normalize iron nutriture and correct the anemia (Jacobs et al., 1964).

Also, patients with sickle cell anemia may have intestinal bacterial overgrowth which can be associated with nutritional deficiencies (Heyman et al., 1989). This overgrowth, in turn, could be secondary to hydrochloric acid deficiency causing increased survival of ingested bacteria (Giannella et al., 1973).

Food Sensitivities

In infants, milk sensitivity may cause intestinal bleeding. This can lead to the development of iron deficiency anemia (Oski, 1983). Also, anemia is a characteristic sign of celiac disease due to gluten sensitivity, although it is rarely the only sign (Kaiser, 1991).

For approximately 2 years, a 23-year-old asymptomatic, normal-weight woman had been known to have an iron-deficiency anemia. Radiography of the small intestine revealed a coarse rugal pattern of the duodenum. Endoscopically-obtained duodenal biopsy demonstrated villous atrophy. Elevated anti-gliadin antibody titers, as well as her response to a gluten-free diet, confirmed the diagnosis of celiac disease (Kaiser, 1991).

REFERENCES

Abbasciano V, et al. Serum and erythrocyte levels of magnesium in microcytosis: Comparison between heterozygous beta-thalassemia and sideropenic anemia. *Haematologica.* 1991;76(4):339–341.

Ajayi OA, Nnaji UR. Effect of ascorbic acid supplementation on haematological response and ascorbic acid status of young female adults. *Ann Nutr Metab.* 1990;34:32–36.

al-Momen AK. Diminished vitamin B_{12} levels in patients with severe sickle cell disease. *J Intern Med.* 1995;23796:551–555.

Berk L, et al. Effectiveness of vitamin B_{12} in combined system disease. *N Engl J Med.* 1948;239:328.

Bernat I. Pyridoxine responsive anemias. *Iron Metabolism.* New York, NY: Plenum Press; 1983a:313–314.

Bernat I. Iron deficiency. *Iron Metabolism.* New York, NY: Plenum Press; 1983b: 215–274.

Branda RF, et al. Folate-induced remission in aplastic anemia with familial defect of cellular folate uptake. *N Engl J Med.* 1978;298(9):469–475.

Broun RE, et al. Excessive zinc ingestion: A reversible cause of sideroblastic anemia and bone marrow depression. *JAMA.* 1990;264:1441–1443.

Carmel R, et al. Iron deficiency occurs frequently in patients with pernicious anemia. *JAMA.* 1987;257(8): 1081–1083.

Cater RE II. The clinical importance of hypochlorhydria. (A consequence of chronic helicobacter infection): its possible etiological role in mineral and amino acid malabsorption, depression, and other syndromes. *Med Hypotheses.* 1992;39:375–383.

Clark NG, et al. Treatment of iron-deficient anemia complicated by scurvy and folic acid deficiency. *Nutr Rev.* 1992;50(5):134–137.

Corash L, et al. Reduced chronic hemolysis during high-dose vitamin E administration in Mediterranean type glucose-6-phosphate dehydrogenase deficiency. *N Engl J Med.* 1980;303:416–420.

De Franceschi L, et al. Oral magnesium supplements reduce erythrocyte dehydration in patients with sickle cell disease. *J Clin Invest.* 1997a;100(7):1847–1852.

De Franceschi L, et al. Dietary magnesium supplementation ameliorates anemia in a mouse model of beta-thalassemia. *Blood.* 1997b;90(3):1283–1290.

Drake JR, Fitch CD. Status of vitamin E as an erythropoietic factor. *Am J Clin Nutr.* 1980;33:2386–2393.

Farrell PM, et al. The occurrence and effects of human vitamin E deficiency. A study in patients with cystic fibrosis. *J Clin Invest.* 1977;60:233–241.

Giannella RA, et al. Influence of gastric acidity on bacterial and parasitic enteric infections. *Ann Intern Med.* 1973;78:271–276.

Giuberti M, et al. Plasma vitamin E, platelet vitamin C and plasma ferritin levels in heterozygous beta-thalassemia. *Nutr Rep Int.* 1987;35(6):1141–1150.

Gothoni G, et al. High-dose folic acid treatment for red-cell aplasia. Letter. *Lancet.* 1995;345:1645–1646.

Heyman MB, et al. Elevated fasting breath hydrogen and abnormal hydrogen breath tests in children with sickle cell disease: a preliminary report. *Am J Clin Nutr.* 1989;49:654–657.

Hines JD, Grasso JA. The sideroblastic anemias. *Semin Hematol.* 1970;7(1):86–106.

Hines JD, Harris JW. Pyridoxine-responsive anemia: description of three patients with megaloblastic erythropoiesis. *Am J Clin Nutr.* 1964;14:137–146.

Hines JD, Love D. Abnormal vitamin B_6 metabolism in sideroblastic anemia: effect of pyridoxal phosphate therapy. *Clin Res.* 1975;23:403A.

Hodges RE, et al. Hematopoietic studies in vitamin A deficiency. *Am J Clin Nutr.* 1978;31:876–885.

Hoffman HN, et al. Zinc-induced copper deficiency. *Gastroenterology.* 1988;94:508–512.

Hyman CB, et al. The clinical significance of magnesium depletion in thalassemia. *Ann N Y Acad Sci.* 1980;344:436–443.

Ishir T, et al. Zinc, copper, magnesium and sickle cell anemia. *Trace Elem Electrolytes.* 1995;12(3):161.

Jacobs A, et al. Gastric acidity and iron absorption. *Br J Haematol.* 1966;12:728–736.

Jacobs A, et al. Role of hydrochloric acid in iron absorption. *J Appl Physiol.* 1964;19(2):187–188.

Kaiser U. Monosymptomatic endemic sprue as a cause of iron-deficiency anemia. *Dtsch Med Wochenschr.* 1991;116(42):1588–1590.

Lane M, Alfrey CP Jr. The anemia of human riboflavin deficiency. *Blood.* 1965;25(4):432–442.

Livrea MA, et al. Oxidative stress and antioxidant status in b-thalassemia major: Iron overload and depletion of lipid-soluble antioxidants. *Blood.* 1996; 88(9):3608–3614.

Mangel H, et al. Thiamine-dependent beriberi in the "thiamine-responsive anemia syndrome." *N Engl J Med.* 1984;311:836–838.

McCurdy PR. Is there an anemia responsive to pantothenic acid? *J Am Geriatr Soc.* 1973;21(2):88–91.

Monsen ER. Ascorbic acid: An enhancing factor in iron absorption. *Nutritional Bioavailability of Iron.* Washington, DC: American Chemical Society; 1982:85–95.

Natta CL, et al. A decrease in irreversibly sickled erythrocytes in sickle cell anemia patients given vitamin E. *Am J Clin Nutr* 1980;33:968–971.

Natta CL, Reynolds RD. Apparent vitamin B_6 deficiency in sickle cell anemia. *Am J Clin Nutr.* 1984; 40:235–239.

Olukoga AO, et al. Urinary magnesium excretion in steady-state sickle cell anaemia. *Acta Haematol.* 1993;90(3):136–138.

Oski FA. *Don't Drink Your Milk!* Syracuse, NY: Mollica Press; 1983.

Osoylu S, Gurgey A. Vitamin E treatment in triplicated alpha-globin gene-heterozygous beta-thalassemia. *Am J Hematol.* 1991;38:335–336.

Pierce LE, Rath, CE. Evidence for folic acid deficiency in the genesis of anemic sickle cell crisis. *Blood.* 1962;20:19.

Reed JD, et al. Nutrition in sickle cell disease. *Am J Hematol.* 1987;24(4):441–445.

Rogers LE et al. Thiamine-responsive megaloblastic anemia. *J Pediatr.* 1969;74(4):494–504.

Sauberlich HE. Ascorbic acid. *Nutrition Reviews' Present Knowledge in Nutrition,* 5th ed. Washington, DC: The Nutrition Foundation Inc; 1984.

Shearman DJC, et al. Gastric function and structure in iron deficiency. *Lancet.* 1966;i:845–848.

Sindel LJ, et al. Nutritional deficiencies associated with vitamin E deficiency in sickle cell patients: the effect of vitamin supplementation. *Nutr Res.* 1990; 10:267–273.

Vatanavicharn S, et al. Zinc and copper status in hemoglobin H disease and beta-thalassemia/hemoglo-
bin E disease. *Acta Haematol.* 1982;68(4):317–320.

Watts DL. The nutritional relationships of copper.
J Orthomol Med. 1989;4(2):99–108.

West CE, Roodenburg AJC. Role of vitamin A in iron
metabolism. *Voeding.* 1992;53:201–205.

Williams DM. Copper deficiency in humans. *Semin
Hematol.* 1983;20(2):118–28.

CHAPTER 11

Laboratory Testing for Food Allergies

Sidney MacDonald Baker, MD

To practice truly preventive medicine, we want to be able to identify that crucial period when health is beginning to slip away, before the damage has been done. We now have many of the pieces of the puzzle in our hands—the knowledge of the factors that lead to health and those that lead to greater likelihood of illness. A range of new laboratory tests are also available that clarify the meaning of various symptoms, testing based on the biochemical functions of the body that reflect interactions between the body and all aspects of the environment, including diet.

FOOD ALLERGY TESTING

When using nutritional medicine to treat illness, two simple questions are key in understanding related health problems: Is there a deficiency or unmet need for an essential nutrient? Could there be a toxin or allergen that should be avoided or eliminated?

"Avoid" is the key word in the second question. When the body is burdened by the metabolic costs of detoxification, it makes sense to lighten the burden on the system.

Sidney MacDonald Baker, MD, has served as director of the Gesell Institute of Human Development, and has taught at Yale Medical School and Southern Connecticut State University. A graduate of Yale University and Medical School, he is board certified in pediatrics. Dr. Baker is author of a number of books, including *Detoxification and Healing* and *The Circadian Prescription*.

Courtesy of Sidney MacDonald Baker, MD, Sag Harbor, New York. Portions of this chapter were adapted from Baker SM. Food allergy testing. In: Nichols TW, Faass, N, eds. *Optimal Digestive Health*. Rochester, VT: Healing Arts Press; 2005.

This involves basic preventive measures such as hand washing, minimizing exposure to chemicals, and eliminating allergens from the diet.

Elimination Diets

Using an elimination diet means avoiding offending substance(s) before they have a chance to become a burden to the body. One way to initiate an elimination diet is to advise patients to avoid suspected foods for at least 7 days. Foods that are common allergens include cereal grains and milk products, breads and fermented foods, oranges and other citrus fruits, spices, eggs, coconut, fish and shellfish, tea, and coffee.

In some cases patients may systematically eliminate suspected foods and still cannot determine the cause of their symptoms. In these situations, a test can be quite useful in evaluating the problem and providing a short list of possible causes. For example, allergens can cause delayed or intermittent allergic responses that are difficult to identify in an elimination diet. However, it is important to note that there is no perfect test. No test will identify all the foods that could trigger symptoms over the course of a patient's lifespan. Still, testing is available that can eliminate some of the guesswork.

One of the types of allergy tests used by many integrative physicians is ELISA (enzyme-linked immunosorbant assay) testing for IgG antibodies to foods. We know that antibodies are proteins produced by the body to combat bacteria or other pathogenic microbes, as well as offending foods or other threatening substances. IgE antibodies reflect immediate, acute reactivity; in the case of food allergies, these reactions can cause life-threatening anaphylaxis in certain individuals, in response to common foods such as peanuts or shrimp. IgM antibodies indicate a response to a currently active infection.

In contrast, IgG antibodies are associated with delayed sensitivities, rather than classic acute food allergy symptoms. A high level of IgG antibodies, measured through IgG ELISA testing, indicates that the immune system is responding abnormally and too aggressively to a particular food. We have found that this testing is valid when performed by a laboratory with reliable methodology. In certain medical situations, these evaluations can provide an important tool in the treatment of patients with complex chronic illness. Since food allergies can also be a factor that drives food cravings, allergy testing can also be useful in the treatment of weight gain and obesity.

Research on Laboratory Testing for Allergies

To study food intolerances, we explored the question of whether testing for IgG antibodies accurately reflects the reactions caused by particular foods. A series of double-blind, placebo-controlled studies were conducted. Reactivity was evaluated for each individual through blood tests, measuring the particular levels of IgG antibodies for that participant, for 115 commonly consumed foods. Patients were then randomized into two groups and assigned avoidance diets based on either their real scores or diets in which they avoided nonproblematic foods. In summary:

- Group A avoided foods associated with IgG reactivity on the ELISA testing.
- Group B avoided foods found to be nonreactive through the testing.

The study was blinded so that neither patients nor physicians knew which participants were on real allergy-avoidance diets. To learn which group did better, we asked study participants to track and report symptoms of any problems typically associated with food sensitivity, as well as all general health concerns, including fatigue, digestive discomfort, headaches, hyperactivity, respiratory symptoms such as wheezing or congestion, skin disorders including eczema or inflammation, and sleep problems.

As patients began to feel better, the scores that reflected their symptoms began to drop. The group that avoided the reactive foods indicated on the test improved by approximately 33%. For those who avoided nonreactive foods, symptoms dropped by approximately 20%.

All participants in the study did a little better. The intention to heal is powerful and accompanies any change we make. Because changing one's diet is one of the most significant lifestyle changes many people ever make, noticeable results can occur. However, the most significant results were those achieved by the patients who avoided allergenic foods confirmed by the antibody testing. They experienced a greater decrease in symptoms than those who avoided nonreactive foods.

It is understandable that the avoidance of nonreactive foods also had some powerful nonspecific effects in relieving symptoms. This reflects the placebo effect, which is always in play when patients have faith in the advice of their doctor. The results are also likely to reflect the effects of self-monitoring and "being on one's good behavior" for the test.

ELISA testing also identifies nonreactive foods, which can be especially important in the treatment of chronic conditions that involve excessive and inappropriate immune activation. In this type of disorder, it is important to know which foods trigger the least immune activity. Immune reactivity has been associated with disorders such as autoimmune disease, chronic fatigue syndrome, and hyperactivity. In summary, ELISA antibody testing can provide a great deal of information relevant to the needs of patients with food allergies, allergy-related symptoms, and chronic illness.

ADDITIONAL RESEARCH

Many integrative practitioners report improved clinical outcomes in the management of allergies and sensitivities using IgG immuno assays (Pizzorno et al., 2002). Yet reviewers in the field of allergy understandably complain about the paucity of research on IgG evaluations for food allergy. A search of the National Library of Medicine (NLM) database (fall 2004) yielded a total of 35 clinical trials on IgG and food allergy—only 14 of which were conducted in the last 10 years. In some of the research no correlation was found between allergic symptoms and IgG antibodies. However, four studies in particular found notable correlations between antibody levels and the presence of symptoms. These studies also reported measurable improvement in patient health status.

Irritable bowel syndrome (IBS) patients. One of the most interesting studies is a recent randomized, controlled trial from the UK which enlisted 150 patients with suspected allergies and IBS symptoms (Atkinson et al., 2004). Patients were evaluated for IgG levels with ELISA testing and then randomized to receive either a diet excluding all foods to which they had elevated IgG levels or a sham diet excluding foods with normal scores. Researchers found that "after 12 weeks, the true diet resulted in a 10% greater reduction in symptom score than the sham diet . . . with this value increasing to 26% in fully compliant patients. . . . All other outcomes showed trends favoring the true diet. Relaxing the diet led to a 25% greater deterioration in symptoms in those on the true diet" (Atkinson et al., 2004).

Asthmatic children. A study in Kuala Lumpur, Malaysia, tracked the symptoms, diet, and antibody levels of 22 children ages 3 to 14, with mild to moderate asthma (Yusoff et al., 2004). The children were evaluated by a pediatrician at the beginning and end of the study, an assessment of food intake was made periodically, blood samples were taken, and peak expiratory flow rate (PEFR) was measured. Children in the intervention group were placed on an egg- and milk-free diet. At the conclusion of the 8-week study period, testing indicated that children on the diet experienced a statistically significant decrease in serum IgG concentrations for anti-ovalbumin and anti-beta lactoglobin. "In contrast, the values for anti-ovalbumin IgG in the control group were significantly increased. . . . Over the study period, the PEFR of children in the experimental group able to perform the test was significantly increased, but no such change was noted in the children in the control group" (Yusoff et al., 2004).

Rheumatoid arthritis patients. The clinical effects of diet were studied in 66 patients in a study conducted at a university hospital in Stockholm (Hafstrom et al., 2001). Patients were randomized to a gluten-free vegan diet or a well-balanced nonvegan diet for 1 year. Results were analyzed at baseline and at 3, 6, and 12 months, using criteria of the American College of Rheumatology (ACR), antibody testing, and X-rays of their hands and feet. Forty-seven patients completed the study. Among "diet completers, 40.5% (nine patients) in the vegan group fulfilled the ACR 20 improvement criteria compared with 4% (one patient) in the nonvegan group. Antibody levels of IgG against gliadin and betalactoglobulin decreased in the vegan group but not in the control group" (Hafstrom et al., 2001).

Children with allergies. An Italian study of cow's milk allergy evaluated more than 500 children for serum values of IgG anti-betalactoglobulin (Iacono et al., 1995). The children were age 1 month to 6 years old, and the study included those who were healthy, those with symptoms of allergy to casein, and children who were symptomatic due to other types of disorders. "There was a marked difference in the distribution of IgG anti-betalactoglobulin values in the 3 study groups." In health controls, IgG values in the 90th percentile averaged 48%. In the children with cow's milk protein allergy, IgG values in the 90th percentile averaged 147%. Researchers indicated, "With a cut-off of over 58% we found only one false positive for diagnosis of cow's milk protein allergy" (Iacono et al., 1995).

The extensive use of ELISA evaluations in other areas of medicine suggests that there is value in further research on ELISA testing for allergies as well. Ideally future research would further describe the subset of patients for whom IgG phenomena apparently play a role in symptom development and potentially in symptom resolution.

REFERENCES

Atkinson WA, Sheldon TA, Shaath N, Whorwell PJ. Food elimination based on IgG antibodies in irritable bowel syndrome: a randomized controlled trial. *Gut.* 2004;53:1459–1464.

Hafstrom I, Ringertz B, Spangberg A, et al. A vegan diet free of gluten improves the signs and symptoms of rheumatoid arthritis: the effects on arthritis correlate with a reduction in antibodies to food antigens. *Rheumatology* (Oxford). 2001 Oct;40(10): 1175–1179.

Iacono G, Carroccio A, Cavataio F, et al. IgG anti-betalactoglobulin (betalactotest): its usefulness in the diagnosis of cow's milk allergy. *Ital J Gastroenterol.* 1995 Sep;27(7):355–360.

Pizzorno JE, Murray MT, Joiner-Bey H. *The Clinician's Handbook of Natural Medicine.* Edinburgh, Scotland: Churchill Livingston; 2002.

Wachholz PA, Durham SR. Mechanisms of immunotherapy: IgG revisited. *Curr Opin Allergy Clin Immunol.* 2004 Aug;4(4):313–318.

Yusoff NA, Hampton SM, Dickerson JW, Morgan JB. The effects of exclusion of dietary egg and milk in the management of asthmatic children: a pilot study. *J R Soc Health.* 2004 Mar;124(2):74–80.

RESOURCES

Medical Laboratories Offering ELISA Allergy Testing

ELISA/ACT Biotechnologies (Serammune Physicians Lab)
14 Pigeon Hill Drive, Suite 300
Sterling, VA 20165
Phone: (703) 450-2980
Fax: (703) 450-2981
Email: clientservices@elisaact.com
Web site: www.elisaact.com

Great Smokies Diagnostic Laboratory
63 Zillicoa Street
Asheville, NC 28801-1074
Phone: (800) 522-4762
Fax: (828) 232-1750
Email: customer service: cs@gsdl.com
Web site: www.gsdl.com

Immuno Laboratories
6801 Powerline Road
Fort Lauderdale, FL 33309
Phone: (800) 231-9197 or (954) 691-2500
Fax: (954) 691-2505
Web site: www.immunolabs.com

Immunosciences Lab, Inc.
8693 Wilshire Boulevard, Suite 200
Beverly Hills, CA 90211
Phone: (310) 657-1077
Fax: (310) 657-1053
Email: practitioner inquiries:
  DrAri@msn.com
Web site: www.immunoscienceslab.com

Meridian Valley Laboratory
801 SW 16th Suite 126
Renton, WA 98055
Phone: (425) 271-8689
Fax: (425) 271-8674
Email: meridian@meridianvalleylab.com
Web site: www.meridianvalleylab.com

CHAPTER 12

Testing for Nutritional and Digestive Status

Patrick Hanaway, MD

EVALUATING DIGESTIVE STATUS

Digestion is one of the keys to health and wellbeing. Yet in the United States alone, 35 million people have irritable bowel syndrome (IBS). Another 35 million people take some type of medication for reflux. Aggregated data from the National Institutes of Health suggests that as many as 90 million Americans may have some type of digestive disorder.

A related concern focuses on the nutritional needs of our patients. How do we begin to individualize our recommendations for each client or patient? In the practice of medicine, there is a tendency to discuss nutrition with patients from a global perspective—often we recommend a high-fiber, low-fat diet, with fewer simple sugars and junk foods. How can we move beyond these generalized dietary recommendations using an evidence-based approach? What is the most efficient manner to determine the nutritional needs of specific patients? How can we further assist patients who have IBS, reflux, or heartburn?

Patrick Hanaway, MD, is board certified in family medicine with a medical degree from Washington University, residency training at the University of New Mexico, and a bachelor's in molecular biology from the University of Wisconsin. He is also board certified in holistic medicine and is treasurer of the American Board of Holistic Medicine. Dr. Hanaway is founder and medical director of the Family to Family Clinic in Asheville, North Carolina, and medical director for Great Smokies Diagnostic Laboratory.

Courtesy of Patrick Hanaway, MD, and Great Smokies Diagnostic Laboratory, Asheville, North Carolina.

These are common symptoms that primary care physicians across the country must address in their practices every day. Unfortunately, it is not cost-effective for physicians to coach their patients in the details of dietary change—economic factors generally limit the role of physicians with regard to diet and lifestyle counseling.

One way to help patients is to begin with an evaluation of their digestive function. This is initiated with a dietary history and a list of the supplements they are taking. The next determination is how well they are digesting and assimilating what they consume.

How do we know whether our patients have good digestion? How do we evaluate digestion in a coherent, thoughtful, and scientific way? To objectively assess digestive competence, it is important to consider:

- Overall digestive function
- Absorption
- Levels of gastrointestinal flora
- The presence of inflammation
- Possible infection or bacterial overgrowth

Assessing digestion. This information is relatively simple to obtain. If we are what we eat, then our stool will provide important clues as to what we are taking in and how our body is assimilating it. Consequently, stool testing becomes a useful construct for being able to assess digestion and digestive function.

The first step is to assure that digestion is occurring properly. Is there adequate acid in the stomach to initiate the breakdown of food? Are adequate pancreatic enzymes being secreted to further break down fats and proteins into more refined phospholipids and amino acids? After being processed in the gut and the liver, are these foods metabolized sufficiently to be incorporated into the cells of the body?

Absorption and flora. The next step is to evaluate absorption. Certain imbalances can interfere with the ability to assimilate food, which will have a significant impact on nutrient intake, as well as the potential for inflammation due to increased intestinal permeability. Those factors also have an impact on the balance of bacteria living in the large and small intestine. The balance of the microflora can be evaluated by measuring by-products of normal bacterial activity—for example, the level of short-chain fatty acids. The fatty acids are energy factors that provide nutrients for repair. These bacteria-generated fuels are essential components for the proper function of the lining of the gastrointestinal tract (which is renewed every five to six days).

The barrier function. This type of lab analysis also considers the integrity of the gut barrier function. Are there sufficient nutrients to sustain the health of the gastrointestinal tract lining and maintain the barrier function to exclude pathogenic organisms? If this barrier function is impaired, the body will be unable to repel pathogens, which can stimulate a degree of inflammation. When the barrier is compromised, food proteins and other molecules can cross the gut lining into the system, due to increased intestinal permeability. These dynamics can impinge on health, with symptoms that seem apparently

unrelated to digestion, evident for example in cases of celiac disease and associated neurological sequelae.

In summary, critical factors in digestive health include maximizing appropriate absorption, maintaining the intestinal barrier function, and supporting beneficial bacteria. Compromise in any of these functions increases vulnerability to infection and inflammation.

COMPREHENSIVE DIGESTIVE ANALYSIS

Overview

The comprehensive digestive analysis is an evaluation of stool that provides some 20 different measures of digestive function. It assesses the absorption of fats, levels of digestive enzymes, markers of inflammation, and indicators of allergic activity in the digestive tract. This laboratory test evaluates levels of bacteria and yeast in the GI tract, the presence (or absence) of parasites, and important by-products in the colon (both beneficial and toxic).

This analysis also provides indications of whether symptoms are likely to be due to inflammatory conditions such as infection or post-infectious IBS, inflammatory bowel disease (IBD), or triggered by food allergies. A comprehensive evaluation assesses pancreatic function and markers for risk of colon cancer. The test results can be used as the basis for individualizing the patient's diet and supplement plan to enhance digestion, which can avoid unnecessary guesswork.

Key Markers of Digestion and Absorption

Pancreatic elastase 1—Pancreatic elastase is an enzyme that serves as an indicator of exocrine pancreatic output of key enzymes such as chymotripsin and lipase. The information provided by this test can contribute to a prompt and reliable diagnosis in suspected cases of pancreatic insufficiency. Reduced levels of pancreatic elastase have been found in patients with diabetes, cholelithiasis, and osteoporosis. This enzyme has been shown to decline with age. Test results can be used to monitor or adjust the dosage of pancreatic enzyme supplementation required.

Valerate, isovalerate, and isobutyrate— Elevated levels of these particular short-chain fatty acids result from putrified anaerobic bacterial fermentation of peptides, which suggests inadequate protein digestion due to low levels of hydrochloric acid (hypochlorhydria), pancreatic insufficiency, bacterial overgrowth of the small intestine, or malabsorption.

Total short-chain fatty acids (butyrate, acetate, and propionate)—These beneficial short-chain fatty acids are produced by anaerobic bacterial fermentation of nonabsorbed dietary fiber. Low levels of these particular fatty acids typically reflect insufficient dietary fiber, decreased colonic flora, and/or constipation.

n-Butyrate—Among the short-chain fatty acids, n-butyrate is the preferred substrate that serves as fuel for colonocytes, assisting in the maintenance of colonic integrity and cellular differentiation. Low levels of this fatty acid imply that the cells lining the colon are lacking the necessary nutrients for proper maintenance. Such low levels have also been associated with increased risk of colon cancer.

Key Markers of Gut Immunology

Calprotectin—Fecal calprotectin is a direct measure of inflammation in the gut and has been correlated with disease activity in inflammatory bowel disease (IBD). Elevations of calprotectin can also indicate possible infection, the development of neoplastic tissue, the presence of polyps, or post-infectious IBS. Abnormal levels warrant further investigation.

Eosinophil protein X (EPX)—This is one of a number of proteins found in eosinophils that indicate increased immune activity. Therefore, these proteins serve as markers for evaluating disease activity and can be seen in cases of chronic diarrhea, parasitic infection, food allergies, IBD, and GI cancer.

Metabolic Factors

The markers in the following tests are a measure of the metabolic function of the gut. Results that fall outside the reference range may be an indication of increased risk of colon cancer.

pH—An excessively alkaline stool can result when there is excessive protein consumption, inadequate dietary fiber, slow transit time, and/or constipation. (If stool is too alkaline, this is an indication that the body is too acidic.) Conversely, excessive acidity of the stool is often related to small bowel bacterial overgrowth, carbohydrate maldigestion, fat malabsorption, diarrhea, and/or rapid transit time.

Beta-glucuronidase—Beta-glucuronidase is an anaerobic bacterial enzyme that can deconjugate and release potential toxins, thus increasing the formation of local carcinogens in the bowel as well as the recirculation of toxins, hormones, and various drugs normally detoxified by the liver. Increased beta-glucuronidase activity has been associated with colon cancer.

Bile acids. An elevated secondary bile acid ratio is associated with an increased risk of breast and colorectal cancer. Elevated levels may occur with formation of gallbladder stones (cholelithiasis) in patients following gallbladder removal (cholecystectomy), and in patients with altered fat absorption.

Digestion and absorption are principle interfaces with our environment, that have major implications in the development of health and disease. Consequently, using these tools can help us promote better health in our patients.

RESOURCES

Laboratories That Offer Comprehensive Digestive Analysis

Great Smokies Diagnostic Laboratory
63 Zillicoa Street
Asheville, NC 28801-1074
Phone: (800) 522-4762
Fax: (828) 232-1750
Customer service email: cs@gsdl.com
Web site: www.gsdl.com

Doctor's Data, Inc.
P.O. Box 111
West Chicago, IL 60186
Phone: (800) 323-2784 or (630) 377-8139
Fax: (630) 587-7860
E-mail: inquiries@doctorsdata.com
Web site: www.doctorsdata.com

Meridian Valley Laboratory
801 SW 16th, Suite 126
Renton, WA 98055
Phone: (425) 271-8689
Fax: (425) 271-8674
Email: meridian@meridianvalleylab.com
Web site: www.meridianvalleylab.com

CHAPTER 13

Nutrition from a Functional Perspective

Institute for Functional Medicine

WHAT IS FUNCTIONAL MEDICINE?

Functional medicine is a science-based field of health care that is grounded in the following principles:

- Biochemical individuality
- Patient-centered care
- Dynamic balance of internal and external factors
- Web-like interconnections of physiological factors
- Health as positive vitality
- Promotion of organ reserve

Functional medicine involves examining the core clinical imbalances that underlie a disease or condition—looking beyond physical signs and symptoms to a deeper understanding of functionality. These imbalances arise as environmental inputs, such as diet and nutrients (including water), exercise, and trauma are processed by a patient's body, through his or her unique metabolism. (We also keep in mind that literally everything about a patient is also affected by his or her mind, spirit, attitudes, and beliefs.) The principles of functional medicine present a different context for identifying and understanding these imbalances.

Fundamental physiological processes that support healthy balance and optimal functioning include:

- Communication (intra- and inter-cellular)
- Bioenergetics, or the transformation of food into energy
- Replication and maintenance of structural integrity, from the cellular to the whole-body level
- Waste elimination and defense
- Circulation and transport of nutrients in the body

From a functional medicine standpoint, imbalances in these processes can lead to changes in many different physiological systems that then become precursors to the signs and symptoms that we diagnose as organ system disease. Figure 13–1 provides a simplified model of the system described briefly in this chapter.

Approaching clinical nutrition from a functional medicine perspective also means identifying the core metabolic imbalances that most often result from system breakdowns at any point. The main categories of metabolic imbalances include:

The Institute for Functional Medicine provides continuing medical education for physicians and other health care professionals through seminars and an annual symposium. They also publish books; a monthly audio subscription series, *Functional Medicine Updates*; and other educational materials on emerging research and clinical applications. The mission of the institute is to improve patient outcomes through the prevention, early assessment, and comprehensive management of complex chronic diseases.

Courtesy of the Institute for Functional Medicine. Nutrition from a functional perspective. In: *Clinical Nutrition: A Functional Approach.* 2nd ed. Gig Harbor, WA: IFM; 2004.

- Digestive, absorptive, and microbiological imbalances
- Detoxification and biotransformation imbalances
- Oxidation-reduction imbalances and mitochondropathies
- Hormonal and neurotransmitter imbalances
- Immune and inflammatory imbalances
- Structural imbalances, from cellular membrane function to musculoskeletal system

Data are continuing to accumulate showing that dietary influences have repercussions on the development of many diseases. Research is now focusing on how to assess these imbalances earlier in life, and then readjust the metabolic balance to decrease the risk those conditions and diseases pose to the well-being and quality of life for our patients.

Consider just one example of how the complex system we have briefly described can be influenced by nutrition. We now recognize that several factors affect the amount of estrogen

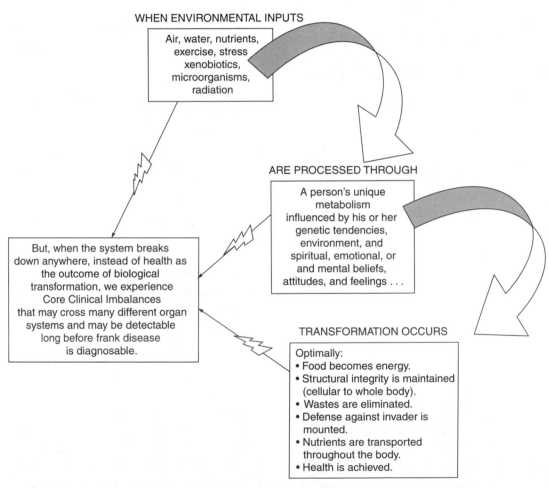

Figure 13–1 Nutrition and Functional Medicine—a Simplified Model

Source: Institute for Functional Medicine, Gig Harbor, WA.

that is produced in and flows through a woman's body at any given time. In particular, in the postmenopausal years, estrogen is no longer produced by the ovaries, but is still produced in other cells in the body (Gruber et al., 2002). The production of estrogen by adipose tissue in postmenopausal women is now understood to be one of the mechanisms linking obesity and the increased risk of post-menopausal, hormone-dependent cancers (Bray, 2002). Diet and lifestyle choices that affect adiposity can, therefore, influence the amount of estrogen produced in a post-menopausal woman's body. Excess estrogen, in turn, can create imbalances that influence the development of many problematic conditions. However, we need to know more than this to be effective with the patient.

Science has also recognized that "estrogen" is more than just estrone, estriol, and estradiol—it is a whole class of molecules that includes many metabolites of estrone and estradiol (Zhu & Conney, 1998). Some of these metabolites are extremely active and have been linked to increased risk of post-menopausal, hormone-dependent cancers. On the other hand, some of these metabolites appear to be protective of the body and are linked to a lower incidence of postmeno-pausal, hormone-dependent cancers (Liehr, 2000). We know that dietary substances, including vitamin and non-vitamin components, can modify how much of these estrogenic metabolites are made in the body, and which ones predominate. Therefore, diet can influence health in more ways than just the amount of adipose tissue; it can also affect the balance of metabolites in the body, and thus we believe it has a key role to play in hormone-dependent breast cancer prevention (Lord et al., 2002).

As this brief example demonstrates, nutrition is one of the key environmental inputs that can be reviewed with a patient and mod-ified to support optimal health and function. The following section describes each of the principles of functional medicine from the perspective of nutrition.

BIOCHEMICAL INDIVIDUALITY IN NUTRITION

A core principle in functional medicine is biochemical individuality. As children, we were told that all snowflakes are a little different and no two are exactly alike. As clinical scientists, we learn about the role of individuality in our voluntary activities— how we make decisions, how we develop our personalities, how we evolve our style of doing things. But, what about our everyday bodily processes?

We tend to think that our bodily processes are "all in our genes," particularly such involuntary activities as metabolism, cellular information processing, and internal communication systems. That is, they are all pre-determined, static, defined by our DNA, and out of our control. At some point, clinical science lost the inclination to distinguish how individuality can impact everyday involuntary physical functions as well as voluntary ones.

A functional perspective includes an awareness of the relationship between voluntary and involuntary processes, and between psychological and biological uniqueness. From a functional perspective, the concept of uniqueness extends to our physiological and biochemical life as much as it does to our psychological life. Biochemical individuality means that your way of digesting food is different than my way of digesting food; the bile synthesized in your liver is different than the bile synthesized in my liver; the food that nourishes you may not be the same food that nourishes me. The following examples illustrate how biochemically diverse we are.

Individuality in Metabolism of B Vitamins

In 1993, a study was published showing the levels of vitamins B_{12}, B_6, and folic acid in 64 healthy older adults (20 male, 44 female; mean age 76) (Joosten et al., 1992). Of these subjects, 94% had "normal" serum levels of vitamin B_6, vitamin B_{12}, and folate. Yet, when these researchers measured serum levels of three metabolites known to accumulate in the blood when vitamins B_6, B_{12}, and folate are deficient—methylmalonic acid (MMA), 2-methylcitric acid (2-MCA), and homocysteine (HCys)—they found that over 63% of the subjects had elevated serum metabolites, indicating intracellular deficiency of at least one of these vitamins.

Even more striking was the interindividual variability in the serum metabolites. Subjects showing normal serum levels of vitamins B_6, B_{12}, and folate frequently differed radically in their serum homocysteine levels (between 10 and 50 mu M/L). Subjects differed dramatically in their methylmalonic acid levels as well. This study gives us just one example of how metabolically different healthy individuals can be, given a strikingly similar and normal snapshot glance at their vitamin status. Science is continuing to document that many of these differences relate to the interaction between a person's genetics and environment, and that each of us is "wired" to express a different need for these crucial B vitamins, depending on our unique biochemistry, which is influenced by lifelong behaviors and exposures.

Individuality in Metabolism of Vitamin C

The B vitamins are by no means the only examples of our biochemical differences.

Vitamin E requirements have been reported to show, at minimum, a five-fold variance in normal, healthy adults, and an even greater interindividual variability when dietary intake of polyunsaturated fatty acids is substantially different (Blumberg, 1999). Plasma ascorbate (vitamin C) levels regularly vary in healthy individuals by 25% to 30% but disease states like diabetes, inflammatory conditions, and the presence of infections can lead to a substantially increased need for this vitamin. Most organizations now indicate a minimum requirement and a maximum amount between 100 and 1000 milligrams per day as the levels to consider (Levine et al., 1999).

Levine and colleagues have reported that the level of vitamin C within the neutrophil increases by as much as 10-fold over normal levels depending upon the activation state of the cell (Washko et al., 1993). This means, for example, that a cell in an inflammatory state will accept as much as 10 times the amount of vitamin C as a cell in a noninflammatory state. The environment affects how much vitamin C the body's cells need at any particular time.

The first and foremost guiding principle of a functional approach, namely the principle of biochemical individuality, tells us that we are as different at the biochemical level—at the level of our everyday involuntary processes—as we are psychologically.

PATIENT-CENTERED NUTRITION

The functional focus on biochemical individuality may leave you thinking: "If everyone is so different, where do I begin?" Clinical nutrition works hand in hand with patient-centered medicine. One focus is eliciting and analyzing the patient's whole story. As developed by Leo Galland, MD, in the mid-1990s, key components of the patient's story are:

- Antecedents—What preceded the patient's illness?
- Triggers—What factors, given the patient's antecedent history, tipped the patient's health into a dysfunctional state?
- Mediators—Given the initial disease or condition, what has kept the process going, so that health is still out of reach?

This kind of analysis explicitly recognizes that each person's path to disease (or health) is unique. We need to understand that individual's particular path in order to modify it and change the momentum away from disease and toward health. Learning the patient's full story is the best place to start.

The term "personalized nutrition" is beginning to be used in relation to how the information from the human genome project can become directly beneficial to the public (Grimaldi et al., 2003). Individualized information—specific genetic patterns and anomalies—can be detected in "single nucleotide polymorphisms," or "SNPs." Many SNPs are being actively investigated now to find ways to personalize drug dosages and dietary recommendations (Collins & Guttmacher, 2001; Ames et al., 2002). For example, one of the best understood SNPs is coded for an enzyme necessary in the folate pathway. The majority of the population does not contain this SNP. But 20% to 30% of the population does carry at least one copy of this SNP (called the MTHFR C-T), and it appears that these individuals may need more than the RDA level of 400 mcg per day of folate.

DYNAMIC BALANCE AND NUTRITION

A functional medicine approach to health care means examining core clinical imbalances that underlie a disease or condition. The concept of homeostasis was first detailed

in the seminal 1865 work by Claude Bernard, a contemporary of Pasteur, entitled: *An Introduction to the Study of Experimental Medicine.* In this work, Bernard described "homeostasis" and the "milieu intérieure" — the interior environment whose stability serves as the "primary condition for freedom and independence of existence." Bernard viewed maintaining constancy in this interior environment as the foremost goal of an organism, toward which all vital mechanisms in the body are oriented.

Modern textbooks of medicine define homeostasis as: "the relatively stable physical and chemical composition of the internal environment of the body which results from the actions of compensating regulatory systems." Homeostatic systems, then, are systems that function to keep the physical or chemical internal environment relatively constant.

Dynamic Balance and Body Temperature

Perhaps the most commonly used example of homeostasis is the body's thermoregulatory system, which keeps our temperature so constant it is the reason we humans are referred to as "homeotherms."

This system is designed to maintain our body temperature at around $98.2° \pm 0.6°$. Most people experience convulsions at body temperatures near or above 106° Fahrenheit and cannot survive temperatures much greater than 109°. At the other end of the spectrum, heat-producing mechanisms (including vasoconstriction, increased thyroxine production, increased metabolic rate, and shivering) occur with increasing exposure to cold. Our thermoregulatory system maintains a relatively narrow temperature range throughout healthy life. Only with the loss of vitality (for example, in the loss of health that can accompany aging) does this thermoregulatory function become less sensitive. So, we conclude that body temperature is characterized by homeostasis—a constant, fixed parameter of life.

Body temperature in a clinical context, however, is not a fixed parameter. When we take a temperature, we get a single, fixed number, but that number is not a constant in the body. Body temperature actually fluctuates within about 3° Fahrenheit (from 97° to 100°) throughout the day. It is different at the extremities than at internal sites, where it is a bit higher on average. Body temperature is also lower in the mornings and after rest than it is after exertion or intake of food, when the body is more active metabolically. Therefore, body temperature is not static, but rather dynamic. It is in dynamic balance, maintained around 98.2° Fahrenheit, not always right on the dot, but constantly fluctuating to adjust to the environment and the needs of the body at each moment in time.

Dynamic Balance and pH

This same perspective could be applied to the subtle control of blood pH (which is maintained between 7.35 and 7.45) or the subtle differences between alveolar and atmospheric pressure of 760 and 758 mm Hg. The metabolic pathways in our bodies are the same, fluctuating up and down in activity around an average point. Although there is a tendency to focus on the average number and not on the range, it is the ability to adjust that keeps us connected and interacting in a healthy way with the world around us.

One way in which this discussion relates to nutrition, and more importantly to functional medicine, is in how we view a single number from a laboratory or physical test. Is that number telling the whole story? Or is that number just one point that needs to be put into the context of the whole individual? Identifying imbalance means understanding that we are not looking at fixed points, but at a dynamic process that fluctuates, and the range of fluctuation needs our attention so we can look at the whole person within the context of his or her environment.

WEB-LIKE INTERCONNECTIONS AND NUTRITION

Dynamic balance helps us think more completely about the range of changes a person's body goes through every single day, realizing that nothing is entirely "fixed." Looking at interconnections moves us out of the "single-agent—single-outcome" mode of thinking. Instead, we see the body as a fully interconnected organism, within which everything affects everything else and nothing is truly isolated.

From another perspective, we now know a fair amount about the diverse effects that stress has on health (it increases cortisol levels, for example). But that connection goes both ways—not only does stress increase your need for certain nutrients, but the use of certain nutrients can palliate not only the physical symptoms (blood pressure and cortisol) but the subjective response to acute psychological stress as well (Brody et al., 2002). The whole system is interconnected and multidirectional, from the mind to the body and back again.

Restoring balance to underlying metabolic patterns is a process that makes demands upon the body. The classic macro- and micronutrients that act to restore and maintain balance must be accompanied by other necessary nutritional factors that also have important parts to play in this orchestration of life. An objective of nutritional therapy is to make sure the appropriate complementary relationships or companionships are in place. For example, the companion presence of different molecules has a dramatic effect on nutrient absorption:

- Certain minerals in an inorganic delivery form require adequate secretion of hydrochloric acid (HCl) by the stomach for proper digestion and absorption.
- Many nutrients must attach to organic acids or amino acids for proper absorption.
- The presence of flavonoids along with vitamin C alters and enhances vitamin C absorption.

These are examples of how nutrients and other food factors work in concert and synergistically. The functional approach to nutrition looks not just at providing all the basic nutrients, but also at supporting these critical relationships as part of nutritional therapy.

Interrelationships of Copper and Zinc

Another example of this web-like interconnectivity is seen with Wilson's disease, a disorder of excess copper absorption and deposition. In this progressive disorder, which leads to cirrhosis of the liver and degeneration of brain tissue, zinc therapy can lower excessively high levels of copper in the blood (Chandra, 1994). This approach recognizes the natural balance (or antagonism) that can occur in the body between copper and zinc. In other words, what is important is not just what is there that should not be, or what is not there that should be, but also the balance and connection of these different factors with each other.

Interrelationships in Bone Health

The body's web of interconnections is very complex. For example, look at the issue of maintaining healthy bone. Historically, when nutrition researchers observed resorption of bone calcium, they perceived absolute quantitative calcium deficiency and recommended calcium supplements. However, "calcium deficiency" is not an isolated deficiency but a problem of balance among nutritional and other parameters. We cannot achieve bone remineralization with supplemental calcium alone. Other nutrients—such as magnesium, manganese, zinc, copper, boron, and phosphorus—are equally important for formation of hydroxyapatite and a healthy bone matrix. These other nutrients must also be present in certain ratios.

Bone restoration involves more than just the presence of the right nutrients in the right amounts. In space, when astronauts are in a zero-gravity environment, minerals leach from their bones because load-bearing movement is difficult without gravity. Similarly, the bones of people who are bedridden lose minerals because those individuals are not upright, engaging in load-bearing activity. From much other research, we now know that building and maintaining healthy bone requires load-bearing on a regular basis. That is, adequate nutrients are necessary, but physical activity is also required for the nutrition to "work" and the bones to mineralize properly.

This web of interactions is even more complex than just minerals and physical exercise. We also know that many other factors affect bones. Systemic inflammation, such as seen with rheumatoid arthritis, can cause bone resorption; hormonal changes influence bone resorption; and certain drugs also influence bone resorption (Richette et al., 2003; Haugeberg et al., 2003).

In addition, bone health can influence other body functions. For example, lead is a toxic metal that, in its ionic form (as it occurs in things like lead pipe found in old plumbing fixtures), can mimic calcium in the body. Small amounts of lead can even affect gene expression by its ability to replace calcium in key regulatory control proteins (Bouton & Pevsner, 2000). A person with a significant exposure to lead will have bones in which some of the calcium has been replaced by lead. Lead can stay in the body for a long time—years, or even decades—sequestered in the bones (Olmstead, 2000). Studies suggest that the majority of the body's lead burden resides in the bone and during times of increased bone turnover, such as seen with calcium deficiency, osteoporosis, repair of broken bones, and pregnancy and lactation, this lead will be released (Vig & Hu, 2000; Sowers et al., 2002). If a person has a history of high lead exposure, the newly liberated lead can create functional brain problems that do not seem directly related to the bone, such as learning disabilities, seizures, and even comas.

HOW NUTRITION SUPPORTS HEALTH AS POSITIVE VITALITY

The historical focus on deficiency and negative outcomes is still apparent in many clinical nutrition textbooks where problem avoidance is the exclusive intervention. Examples of this type of intervention include: elimination of high oxalate foods to avoid recurrence of calcium oxalate nephrolithiasis, reduction of dietary fat to avoid exacerbation of intestinal malabsorption, and decreased simple-sugar intake in the management of dysglycemia. Although the problem-avoidance intervention might be critical in the symptomatic management of a health condition, it does not address functionality or the reestablishment of a positive balance in underlying metabolic patterns.

Negative outcomes such as vitamin deficiency have been the traditional focus of clinical nutrition. Therefore, most nutritional interventions have been designed to remedy deficiency states. The formula has been fairly simple, involving three basic steps:

- First, the presence of clinical deficiency symptoms is determined—usually by examining some visible, morphological change occurring at an end-stage clinical level. Examples of such observations include rachitic rosary (vitamin D), angular stomatitis or cheilosis (vitamin B_2), koilonychias (iron), glossitis (folate), and gingival enlargement or gingivitis (vitamin C).
- Second, a dietary or laboratory confirmation (or both) is obtained. For example, a diet diary could be entered into a computer software program and could confirm a deficiency in vitamin D intake, or a laboratory panel could help verify an iron-deficiency anemia.
- Third, the necessary nutrient(s) are provided (often through supplementation) to treat the deficiency.

A functional perspective certainly acknowledges the importance of this basic approach to nutrient deficiency and recognizes such deficiencies as a reason for intervention. However, a functional approach also seeks to enhance the effectiveness of clinical nutrition by bringing "function" more directly into the intervention process. The integration of functional thinking occurs at each step of the process, and might radically alter the final components of the intervention by bringing different considerations into the process at an earlier stage.

Subclinical Deficiencies

What would happen if we could go back in time prior to the appearance of the end-stage, morphological change, or frank deficiency? We would likely find that many "invisible" biochemical and physiological changes were occurring for some time prior to the appearance of the deficiency or disease. In other words, subclinical changes were going on long before the patient arrived in our office. Using such knowledge to prevent or treat disease has been called "upstream medicine"— which is what functional medicine at its best can deliver.

A clear example of this issue of "subclinical" effects can be seen in the development of metabolic syndrome, a condition that has been linked to further development of Type 2 diabetes mellitus, and one that is prevalent in our current society. Metabolic syndrome is called the "deadly quartet" and is characterized by high triglycerides, insulin resistance, low HDL cholesterol, and high blood pressure (Kelley, 2000; Ford et al., 2002). Much research has shown that metabolic syndrome does not occur overnight, but involves many changes in how the body handles glucose and insulin, and is influenced by many other factors over time. We can look at fasting glucose and insulin in an individual and find healthy levels, but if we do a challenge test (i.e., give a glucose dose, and then look at blood glucose and insulin in a 2-hour postprandial assessment), we may see something quite different. A significantly elevated insulin level may indicate that the body is beginning to have problems adjusting to a glucose challenge. Having this information, we can intervene before things become worse, giving us a much better opportunity to fully restore normal function.

As clinicians, we become versed in the signs and symptoms that signal the presence of a disease or condition. How do we become versed in observing—or noting the absence of—the signs of optimal balance in our patients? How do we evaluate "positive vitality," not just diagnose disease? Understanding key subclinical imbalances and their potential effects on an individual is one way to begin seeing health as the presence of positive vitality, not just the absence of disease.

PROMOTION OF ORGAN RESERVE

Underlying all balance, all homeostasis, is proper nutriture. Optimal health is more than the ability of the body to operate adequately in a particular moment; it also means the ability of the body to withstand the challenges of everyday life. These challenges may arise from communicable diseases (like flu and colds), increased stress, increased physical activity, a more toxic environment, or dietary changes. A functional approach to health means supporting the body in such a way that it can thrive (and not just survive), despite the challenges of living. The body, therefore, needs reserves, some storehouse upon which it can draw when it is challenged. Functional medicine looks at these reserves as part of overall health.

Conventional approaches to nutriture have placed all nutrients within one of two categories: essential or nonessential. "Essential nutrients" have been defined as nutrients that the body cannot synthesize and that must, therefore, be supplied through the diet. "Nonessential nutrients" have been defined as nutrients that the body can synthesize and, therefore, need not be obtained through dietary intake. A functional perspective argues that many nutrients cannot be placed accurately within a single category. In many cases, nutrients that have been conventionally described as "nonessential" may be required in the diet, at specific times or in a specific individual. Therefore, a functional understanding of clinical nutrition involves a new classification for nutrients within a third category, described as "conditionally essential."

Conditionally Essential Nutrients

Nutrients can become conditionally essential for a variety of reasons. A human body may have a constitutional genetic "defect" which prevents an ordinary level of synthesis of the nutrient. In other cases, the body may have an induced defect, in which the nutrient-synthesizing enzyme has been inhibited by a toxic substance, resulting in a lower production of the nutrient. The body might have an atypically high need for the nutrient and, although the body synthesizes that nutrient in an amount considered adequate for a typical human body, the nutrient needs would still not be met. In each of these cases, the nutrient in question would conventionally be classified as "nonessential" but would, in fact, need to be supplied exogenously through the diet or through supplementation.

To avoid the dilemma of a "nonessential" nutrient needing to be supplied exogenously, the functional perspective has adopted the term "conditionally essential" to apply to nutrients that can be synthesized by the body but need to be obtained from the diet or supplementation in a specific person at a specific time.

Whether the average human body *can* synthesize a nutrient and whether a specific human body *is* actually synthesizing a nutrient are two distinctly different issues. Only the latter issue relates directly to what is going on in a unique individual at a particular moment.

SUMMARY

A functional approach to nutrition means analyzing the multiple roles of various nutrients and other necessary food factors (including "non-nutrients"). A functional approach to nutrition means knowing what these key life-sustaining substances are really doing in the body and asking the question: Are these nutrients truly supporting health in this particular person's body the way they should?

Please remember that no book can substitute for an individualized, thoughtful decision-making process by patients and providers. Clinically-related material is not presented as a prescription for care, but rather as an indicator of the kind of information clinicians may want to consider in making treatment decisions for their patients.

REFERENCES

Ames, BN, Elson-Schwab I, Silver EA. High-dose vitamin therapy stimulates variant enzymes with decreased coenzyme binding affinity (increased Km): relevance to genetic disease and polymorphisms. *Am J Clin Nutr.* 2002;75:616–658.

Bernard C. *An Introduction to the Study of Experimental Medicine.* Henry Copley Greene, trans. New York, NY: The MacMillan Co; 1865.

Blumberg JB. Dietary reference intakes for vitamin E. *Nutr.* 1999;15:797–798.

Bouton CM, Pevsner J. Effects of lead on gene expression. *Neurotoxicology.* 2000;21:1045–1055.

Bray GA. The underlying basis for obesity: relationship to cancer. *J Nutr.* 2002;132(suppl 11): S3451–S3455.

Brody S, Preut R, Schommer K, Schurmeyer TH. A randomized controlled trial of high dose ascorbic acid for reduction of blood pressure, cortisol, and subjective responses to psychological stress. *Psychopharmacology.* 2002;159:319–324.

Chandra RK. Zinc and immunity. *Nutr.* 1994;10:79–80.

Collins FS, Guttmacher AE. Genetics moves into the medical mainstream. *JAMA.* 2001;286:2322–2323.

Ford ES, Giles WH, Dietz WH. Prevalence of the metabolic syndrome among US adults. *JAMA*. 2002; 287:356–359.

Grimaldi K, Gill-Garrison R, Roberts G. Personalized nutrition: an early win from the human genome project. *Integrative Med*. 2003;2:34–45.

Gruber CJ, Tschugguel W, Schneeberger C, Huber JC. Production and actions of estrogens. *N Eng J Med*. 2002;346:340–350.

Haugeberg G, Orstavik R, Kvien T. Effects of rheumatoid arthritis on bone. *Curr Opin Rheumatol*. 2003; 15:469–475.

Institute for Functional Medicine. *Clinical Nutrition: A Function Approach*. 2nd ed. Gig Harbor, WA: IFM; 2004.

Joosten E, van den Berg A, Riezler R, et al. Metabolic evidence that deficiencies of vitamin B_{12} (cobalamin), folate, and vitamin B_6 occur commonly in older people. *Am J Clin Nutr*. 1992;58:468–476.

Kelley DE. Overview: what is insulin resistance? *Nutr Rev*. 2000;58(Suppl II):S2–S3.

Levine M, Rumsey SC, Daruwala R, Park JB, Wang Y. Criteria and recommendations for vitamin C intake. *JAMA*. 1999;281:1415–1423.

Liehr JG. Is estradiol a genotoxic mutagenic carcinogen? *Endocrine Rev*. 2000;21(1):40–54.

Lord RS, Bongiovanni B, Bralley JA. Estrogen metabolism and the diet-cancer connection: rationale for assessing the ratio of urinary hydroxylated estrogen metabolites. *Altern Med Rev*. 2002;7: 112–129.

Olmstead MJ. Heavy metal sources, effects, and detoxification. *Altern Complementary Med*. 2000: 347–354.

Richette P, Corvol M, Bardin T. Estrogens, cartilage, and osteoarthritis. *J Bone Spine*. 2003;70:257–262.

Sowers MR, Scholl TO, Hall G, et al. Lead in breast milk and maternal bone turnover. *Am J Obstet Gynecol*. 2002;187:770–776.

Vig EK, Hu H. Lead toxicity in older adults. *J Am Geriatr Soc*. 2000;48:1501–1506.

Washko PW, Wang Y, Levine M. Ascorbic acid recycling in human neutrophils. *J Biol Chem*. 1993; 268:15531–15535.

Zhu BT, Conney AH. Functional role of estrogen metabolism in target cells: review and perspectives. *Carcinogenesis*. 1998;19:1–27.

CHAPTER 14

Behavioral Nutrition Coaching

Joy Kettler Gurgevich

Behavioral nutrition is an emerging area within the field of nutrition that involves the use of behavioral techniques to support patients in adopting healthy eating patterns. This is an experiential approach that engages clients in the pleasurable aspects of tasting new foods, dining out, shopping, and cooking with wholesome and nourishing foods. The following are five suggestions that will help your patients achieve healthier eating habits.

1. ***Focus on change in one area at a time.*** For example, in working with patients who have diabetes, one place to start could be a focus on making better selections in their choice of sweeteners. They can begin by shopping for new products, incorporating them into their diet, and generally becoming more conscious about how, when, and why they use sweeteners. By focusing on just one aspect of their eating patterns, they are less likely to become overwhelmed and more likely to stay motivated. In some cases, the physician may set clear priorities for diet recommendations. In other situations, the change is less urgent and practitioner and patient can work collaboratively to select the area of focus.

2. ***Help clients find their place on the continuum.*** At one end of the spectrum is a junk-food lifestyle and at the other, a diet of 100% organically grown, unprocessed foods. Where does your client fit on that continuum? Where is their comfort level? What are their time constraints, and which changes can they make with a reasonable degree of comfort?

3. ***Encourage clients to experience healthy eating.*** The educational aspect of nutrition is extremely important. However, as a nutritionist, I have found that the most effective means of influencing clients' eating habits and diet is first-hand experience. Many clients tend to be more motivated when they have the opportunity to actually taste and experience delicious natural foods that they can substitute for less healthy options. For example, once they have tasted quality extra-virgin olive oil, well-prepared hearty grains, or fresh-roasted nuts and seeds, they are more likely to take the initiative to incorporate those foods into their diet. At that point, the new food is no longer unfamiliar, and they are more motivated to actually purchase and prepare the food.

There are a number of behavioral approaches that can be used to help clients create a new lifestyle. As a nutritionist, I sometimes shop with clients, cook with them, or help them reorganize and restock their kitchens. This approach can demys-

---

Joy Kettler Gurgevich is a preceptor for Dr. Andrew Weil's Program in Integrative Medicine, the behavioral nutrition expert on Dr.Weil.com, and is in private practice in Tucson, Arizona.

tify nutrition, make it more practical, and providing the basis for change. Many nutritionists, however, do not have the opportunity to spend this much time with clients.

However, a number of venues are now available that can provide some of these experiences for your clients. In most cities there are now large health food stores that have hot food delis, marketing displays, and other venues for sampling their products. Although some of these activities are clearly promotional, the experience is also extremely educational for people interested in expanding their diets to include new and healthier foods. Shopping in these environments allows clients to experience the pleasures of natural foods first hand.

4. ***Provide information on easy, healthy meals and snacks.*** We have to be realistic. Most people do not have the time to prepare gourmet meals, but healthy meals need not be complicated. There are a surprising number of meals that require no cooking at all, and many others that can be prepared quickly. Consider developing a handout with suggestions for practical, healthy snacks, menu plans, or recipes. Another approach is to focus on resources that provide this information, including the best of the cookbooks and Web sites.

5. ***Provide resources on dining out and healthy restaurants.*** Currently, most major cities have restaurants that feature local produce and products, and in some cases organically grown food. Their style of preparation tends to focus on natural flavors, featuring local produce in season, fresh seafood, and grains. In some cities, guidebooks that list natural food restaurants are available. Information can also be found on the Internet.

When resource guides are not available, consider developing a resource list for your clients. Include health food stores, farmers' markets, supermarkets that feature organic produce (and also those that provide home delivery), as well as services that provide weekly delivery of locally grown organic fruits and vegetables. Additional resources might include cooking classes, cable TV shows, and other types of venues in your area.

These simple, practical experiences can have a major impact by promoting healthier nutrition. One small change provides the opportunity for more change. Over time, clients can enhance both their health and quality of life.

CHAPTER 15

Research on Clinical Nutrition

Nancy Faass, MSW, MPH

Extensive data from longitudinal studies and research on large populations are providing the basis for a new level of sophistication in the science of nutrition. These data make possible more precise and targeted efforts in the prevention and treatment of chronic, degenerative diseases. Emerging data are expanding the range of therapies available in the field of clinical nutrition.

Insulin resistance, blood lipids, and coronary disease. The Framingham study, one of the most extensive longitudinal studies in history, has involved two generations of residents in the town of Framingham, Massachusetts. The study was initiated in 1948 using a prospective epidemiological approach to investigate what was then an epidemic of coronary disease in the United States (Kannel, 1986, 2000). The findings have provided insight into the prevalence, incidence, spectrum, predisposing factors, and major risk factors for coronary disease, stroke, peripheral artery disease, and heart failure. This research has served to dispel clinical misconceptions regarding hypertension, dyslipidemia, atrial fibrillation, and glucose intolerance.

Results: Through this work, seminal understandings regarding cholesterol and cholesterol fractions were established, including the role of triglycerides, LDL (low-density lipoprotein), and HDL (high-density lipoprotein) (Kannel, 2000).

High triglycerides were found to be associated with reduced HDL, indicating insulin resistance. All the risk factors tended to cluster—and were shown to be promoted by insulin resistance and induced by weight gain. These factors have also been associated with higher incidence of coronary disease.

For the past decade, the Framingham Study has been engaged in quantifying the effects of homocysteine, lipoprotein (A), insulin resistance, small dense LDL, C-reactive protein, clotting factors, and genetic determinants of cardiovascular disease. It is now possible to estimate the lifetime risk of all atherosclerotic cardiovascular disease outcomes (Kannel, 2000).

Homocysteine and dementia. Framingham data have been utilized to evaluate the impact of homocysteine levels on a range of conditions including mental function and dementia. This raises the question of whether elevated homocysteine precedes the onset of dementia or results from dementia-related nutritional and vitamin deficiencies. A sample of 1092 subjects without dementia (667 women and 425 men; mean age, 76 years) were evaluated. Homocysteine was measured at diagnosis, and homocysteine levels measured 8 years earlier and found to be elevated, were reviewed (Seshadri et al., 2002). The goal of the analysis was to identify possible correlations between plasma homocysteine levels and dementia risk.

Results: Over the follow-up period of 8 years, dementia developed in 111 subjects, including 83 with a diagnosis of Alzheimer's disease. When plasma homocysteine levels exceeded 14 mM/L, the risk of Alzheimer's disease nearly doubled (relative risk 1.8) (Seshadri et al., 2002).

A brief biography of Ms. Faass appears in Chapter 2.

Homocysteine and atherosclerosis. Increased plasma homocysteine has also been associated with atherosclerotic vascular disease in elderly persons. A team of researchers from New York Medical College (Storey et al., 2003) investigated the association of plasma homocysteine with atherosclerotic vascular disease and dementia in 200 patients of an academic nursing home. Four groups were evaluated for mean plasma homocysteine with the following findings:

1. Atherosclerotic vascular disease and dementia: homocysteine 15.3 mM/L
2. Atherosclerotic vascular disease with no dementia: homocysteine 15.1 mM/L
3. Dementia with no atherosclerotic vascular disease: homocysteine 14.4 mM/L
4. No dementia or atherosclerotic vascular disease: homocysteine 10.6 mM/L

Results: Mean plasma homocysteine level was significantly higher in elderly patients with atherosclerotic vascular disease and/or dementia compared with patients who had no dementia or atherosclerotic vascular disease (Storey et al., 2003).

Homocysteine, insulin resistance, and endothelial dysfunction. The Framingham study examined relationships between homocysteine levels and features of insulin-resistance syndrome in participants who were offspring of those in the original study (Meigs et al., 2001). Subjects were evaluated for plasma levels of fasting homocysteine, folate, B vitamins, creatinine, insulin, and glucose (fasting and 2-hour levels, after a 75-g oral glucose tolerance test). Subjects who met the study criteria (N = 2011, mean age 54 years, range 28–82; 55% women) were categorized as having none, one, two, or all three of the phenotypes of insulin-resistance syndrome: impaired glucose tolerance, hypertension, and/or a central metabolic syndrome (two or more traits: obesity, dyslipidemia, or hyperinsulinemia). Urine albumin/creatinine ratios were also measured in 1592 subjects participating in the sixth examination (1995–1998).

Results: Among study participants, 12.3% had hyperinsulinemia, and 15.9% had two or more insulin-resistance syndrome phenotypes. Adjusted mean homocysteine levels were higher among those with hyperinsulinemia (9.8 mM/L) compared with those without (9.4 mM/L). Homocysteine levels were also higher among subjects with two or more insulin-resistance phenotypes (9.9 mM/L) compared with those with one or none (9.3 mM/L). Mean urine albumin/creatinine ratio levels were higher among subjects with two or more insulin-resistance phenotypes (7.2 mg/g) compared with those with one or none (5.5 mg/g).

Researchers concluded, "Hyperhomocysteinemia and abnormal urinary albumin excretion are both associated with hyperinsulinemia and may partially account for increased risk of cardiovascular disease associated with insulin resistance. Because hyperhomocysteinemia and microalbuminuria also reflect endothelial injury, these observations also support the hypothesis that endothelial dysfunction is associated with expression of insulin resistance syndrome" (Meigs et al., 2001).

The role of carbohydrates in obesity and heart disease. In another study population, a team of Harvard researchers tracked the effect of carbohydrates in the diet on weight gain and coronary heart disease over a 10-year period, monitoring the diet and health of more than 75,000 women, 38 to 63 years of age. The participants had no prior history of heart disease, stroke, or diabetes. Dietary evaluation included rating carbohydrates on the Glycemic Index. Carbohydrates high on the Index tend to trigger greater release of insulin. Foods low on the Glycemic Index are metabolized more slowly and tend to be insulin sparing.

Results: The risk of heart disease was found to be "directly associated" with a diet high in carbohydrate content. Over the course of the study, 761 cases of heart disease developed. Consumption of a diet high in carbohydrates was found to double the risk of heart attack in the top 40% of participants, with even greater risk among the top 20%. Researchers reported associations between high glycemic load, obesity, insulin resistance, and coronary heart disease (Liu et al., 2000).

Inverse relationship between Mediterranean diet and obesity. This study, conducted at the Medical Research Institute of Barcelona, assessed the relationship between body mass index (BMI), obesity, and the level of adherence to the traditional Mediterranean diet (Schroder et al., 2004). In a population-based cross-sectional study, Spanish men (N = 1547) and women (N = 1615) from northeastern Spain, aged 25–74, were evaluated from 1999–2000. A food frequency questionnaire was used to assess dietary intake. A Mediterranean diet score was developed to identify consumption of foods considered to be characteristic of the traditional Mediterranean diet (vegetables, fruits, legumes, nuts, fish, meat, cereals, olive oil, and wine).

Results: Decreased risk of obesity correlated in both men and women with increased adherence to the traditional Mediterranean dietary pattern. The top one third of participants of both genders with this adherence score were 40% less likely to be obese (odds ratio of 0.61). "These data suggest that the traditional Mediterranean dietary pattern is inversely associated with body mass index and obesity" (Schroder et al., 2004).

Mediterranean diet and reduction in markers of heart disease. Researchers from the University of Athens School of Medicine evaluated potential mechanisms by which the Mediterranean diet reduces cardiovascular risk. The effects of this diet were evaluated in relation to plasma levels of C-reactive protein (CRP), white blood cell counts, interleukin-6 (IL-6), tumor necrosis factor-alpha, amyloid-A, fibrinogen, and homocysteine. The study randomly enrolled and then tracked the health of 1514 men (18 to 87 years old) and 1528 women (18 to 89 years old) from the Attica region of Greece (2000–2001). Adherence to the Mediterranean diet was assessed by a diet score, with higher score values indicating closer adherence to the diet.

Results: Participants in the top one third of the diet score had, on average, 20% lower C-reactive protein levels, 17% lower IL-6 levels, 15% lower homocysteine levels, 14% lower white blood cell counts, and 6% lower fibrinogen levels as compared with those in the lowest 33%. Conclusions: This research found that "adherence to the traditional Mediterranean diet was associated with a reduction in the concentrations of inflammation and coagulation markers. This may partly explain the beneficial actions of this diet on the cardiovascular system" (Chrysohoou et al., 2004a).

Mediterranean diet and markers for hypertension. A second population-based evaluation in Attica by the University of Athens School of Medicine examined the association between prehypertension status and inflammatory markers (C-reactive protein, white blood cells, IL-6, tumor necrosis factor-alpha, amyloid-A, homocysteine, and fibrinogen) in a random sample of cardiovascular disease-free adults. The evaluation included a detailed interview, blood samples collected after 12 hours of fasting, and a range of clinical measurements, including blood pressure levels.

Results: The prehypertensive population included 653 men and 535 women. Compared to normotensives, prehypertensive men and women had 31% higher C-reactive protein, 32% higher tumor necrosis factor-alpha, 9% higher amyloid-A, 6% higher homocysteine levels, and 10% higher white blood cell counts. Researchers concluded: "Studying a large sample of cardiovascular disease-free adults . . . an association between prehypertension and inflammatory markers [was] linked to the atherosclerotic process, independently of other coexisting risk factors or unhealthy lifestyle behaviors. Our findings may be of clinical importance, as they suggest that prehypertension might be a pro-inflammatory condition" (Chrysohoou, 2004b).

Animal protein and cancer. A team of researchers at the Harvard School of Public Health that included Walter Willett, MD, studied possible associations between dietary animal products and prostate cancer. Researchers commented that this association has been noted in observational studies. This research evaluated detailed dietary data on 51,529 men who were participants in the Health Professionals Follow-Up Study (1986, 1990, and 1994). From 1986 to 1996, 1897 total cases of prostate cancer (excluding stage A1) and 249 metastatic cancers were identified. Data on these cases were analyzed using pooled logistic regression.

Results: Researchers reported that the intake of total meat, red meat, and dairy products was not associated with the risk of total or advanced prostate cancer. However, an elevated risk for metastatic prostate cancer was observed with intake of red meat (relative risk 1.6 for highest vs. lowest quintile). Processed meats, bacon, beef, pork, or lamb as a main dish, and dairy products each contributed to an elevated risk of metastatic prostate cancer. (Michaud et al., 2001). Although nutrients such as fatty acids and excessive calcium intake may explain most of the dairy association observed, a portion of the risk of metastatic prostate cancer associated with red meat intake remains unexplained.

Antioxidant protective effects against radiation exposure. Another large population study conducted in Japan evaluated the protective effects of green and yellow vegetables among more than 38,000 radiation-exposed atomic bomb survivors. Consuming green-yellow vegetables two to four times a week was found to cut the risk of bladder cancer by almost 40%, compared with the risk of those consuming vegetables once a week or less. A diet that also included fruit decreased risk as much as 40% to 50%. Chicken in the diet was associated with decreased risk to some degree. The consumption of other dietary items, including meat and green tea, was not found to be related to risk. "The findings add to evidence that high consumption of vegetables and fruit are protective against bladder cancer" (Nagano et al., 2000).

Diabetes and breast cancer. The Nurses' Health Study was a multicentered study conducted at the Harvard Medical School that included a prospective evaluation of the association between Type 2 diabetes and invasive breast cancer. The research followed the health of 116,488 female nurses (30 to 55 years old, free of cancer at baseline) from 1976 through 1996 for the occurrence of Type 2 diabetes, and through 1998 for the incidence of invasive breast cancer.

Results: During 2.3 million person-years of follow-up, researchers identified 6220 women with Type 2 diabetes and 5189 cases of invasive breast cancer. Diagnoses were verified through medical records and pathology reports. Researchers indicated, "Women with Type 2 diabetes had a modestly elevated incidence of breast cancer (hazard ratio 1.17, indicating their risk increased by approximately 17%) compared with women without diabetes. This finding was independent of age, obesity, family history of breast cancer, history of benign breast disease, reproductive factors, physical activity, or alcohol consumption" (Michels et al., 2003). The association was apparent among postmenopausal women (risk ratio 1.16) but not premenopausal women (risk ratio 0.83). The association was predominant among women with estrogen receptor-positive breast cancer (risk ratio 1.22).

Physicians' Health Study: antioxidants and heart disease. Researchers at Harvard Medical School prospectively evaluated the relationship between vegetable intake and coronary heart disease risk in the Physicians' Health Study, a randomized trial of aspirin and beta-carotene among 22,071 US male physicians aged 40–84 years conducted in 1982. This component of the study evaluated 15,220 men without heart disease, stroke, or cancer at baseline. Information on vegetable intake was obtained through a food frequency ques-

tionnaire that included eight vegetables; participants utilized the questionnaire at baseline, and in the 2nd, 4th, and 6th years of follow-up.

Results: During the 12 years of follow-up, 1148 incident cases of coronary heart disease were confirmed: 387 cases of myocardial infarction and 761 cases of coronary artery bypass grafting or percutaneous transluminal coronary angioplasty. After adjusting for other risk factors, including age, randomized treatment, body mass index (BMI), smoking, alcohol intake, physical activity, multivitamin intake, and history of diabetes, hypertension, and high cholesterol, it was found that men who consumed at least 2.5 servings/day of vegetables had a relative risk of 0.77 for coronary heart disease, compared with men in the lowest category ($<$ 1 serving/day). The inverse relationship between vegetable intake and coronary heart disease risk was more evident among men with a body mass index $\geq$ 25 and among current smokers. Researchers concluded, "These prospective data support current dietary guidelines to increase vegetable intake for the prevention of coronary heart disease" (Liu et al., 2001).

REFERENCES

Chrysohoou C, Panagiotakos DB, Pitsavos C, Das UN, Stefanadis C. Adherence to the Mediterranean diet attenuates inflammation and coagulation process in healthy adults: the ATTICA Study. *J Am Coll Cardiol.* 2004a;44(1):152–158.

Chrysohoou C, Pitsavos C, Panagiotakos DB, Skoumas J, Stefanadis C. Association between prehypertension status and inflammatory markers related to atherosclerotic disease: the ATTICA Study. *Am J Hypertens.* 2004b;17(7):568–573.

Kannel WB. The Framingham Study: its 50-year legacy and future promise. *J Atheroscler Thromb.* 2000;6(2):60–66.

Kannel WB. Nutritional contributors to cardiovascular disease in the elderly. *J Am Geriatr Soc.* 1986:34(1):27–36.

Liu S, Lee IM, Ajani U, Cole SR, Buring JE, Manson JE, Physicians' Health Study. Intake of vegetables rich in carotenoids and risk of coronary heart disease in men: the Physicians' Health Study. *Int J Epidemiol.* 2001;30(1):130–135.

Liu S, Willett WC, Stamfer MJ, et al. A prospective study of dietary glycemic load, carbohydrate intake, and risk of coronary heart disease in women. *Am J Clin Nutr.* 2000;71(6):1455–1461.

Meigs JB, Jacques PF, Selhub J, et al. Fasting plasma homocysteine levels in the insulin resistance syndrome: the Framingham offspring study. *Diabetes Care.* 2001;24(8):1403–1410.

Michaud DS, Augustsson K, Rimm EB, Stampfer MJ, Willett WC, Giovannucci E. A prospective study on intake of animal products and risk of prostate cancer. *Cancer Causes Control*. 2001; 12(6):557–567.

Michels KB, Solomon CG, Hu FB, et al. Type 2 diabetes and subsequent incidence of breast cancer in the Nurses' Health Study. *Diabetes Care*. 2003; 26(6):1752–1758.

Nagano J, Kono S, Preston DL, et al. Bladder-cancer incidence in relation to vegetable and fruit consumption: a prospective study of atomic-bomb survivors. *Int J Cancer*. 2000;86(1):132–138.

Schroder H, Marrugat J, Vila J, Covas MI, Elosua R. Adherence to the traditional Mediterranean diet is inversely associated with body mass index and obesity in a Spanish population. *J Nutr*. 2004;134(12): 3355–3361.

Seshadri S, Beiser A, Selhub J, et al. Plasma homocysteine as a risk factor for dementia and Alzheimer's disease. *N Engl J Med*. 2002;346(7):476–483.

Storey SG, Suryadevara V, Aronow WS, Ahn C. Association of plasma homocysteine in elderly persons with atherosclerotic vascular disease and dementia, atherosclerotic vascular disease without dementia, dementia without atherosclerotic vascular disease, and no dementia or atherosclerotic vascular disease. *J Gerontol A Biol Sci Med Sci*. 2003; 58(12):M1135–1136.

CHAPTER 16

Resources in Clinical Nutrition

Nancy Faass, MSW, MPH

The field of clinical nutrition encompasses an enormous amount of information. To some degree, access to this information is being streamlined through a growing number of resources designed specifically for health practitioners. For those who want to deepen their knowledge in this area, a seminar can be a good place to begin. This initial foundation can be expanded through reading and the use of Web sites, databases, and software, accessed by computer or personal digital assistant (PDA). Once a greater knowledge base has been established, learning can be kept current through workshops and/or a monthly publication or audio series. The range of resources includes:

- Books, software, and videos
- Training, workshops, and conferences
- PDA resources, databases, and Web sites

BOOKS, SOFTWARE, AND VIDEOS

Reviews of the Research: Melvyn Werbach, MD

These books review and abstract the peer-reviewed clinical literature on nutrition, organizing clinical data by both disease category and nutrient or botanical. Each volume contains hundreds of abstracts and a complete bibliography. Publications include:

Werbach MR. *Foundations of Nutritional Medicine. A Sourcebook of Clinical Research*. Tarzana, CA: Third Line Press, Inc; 1997.

A brief biography of Ms. Faass appears in Chapter 2.

Werbach MR. *Nutritional Influences on Illness*. 2nd ed. Tarzana, CA: Third Line Press, Inc; 1996.

Werbach, MR. *Nutritional Influences on Illness*. (CD-ROM). Tarzana, CA: Third Line Press, Inc; 1999. This CD, which includes both *Nutritional Influences on Illness* (2nd ed., 1996) and *Nutritional Influences on Mental Illness* (2nd ed., 1999), can be searched by key word.

Werbach MR. *Nutritional Influences on Mental Illness: A Sourcebook of Clinical Research*. 2nd ed. Tarzana, CA: Third Line Press, Inc; 1999.

Werbach MR, Moss J. *Textbook of Nutritional Medicine*. Tarzana, CA: Third Line Press, Inc; 1999.

Werbach MR, Murray MT. *Botanical Influences on Illness: A Sourcebook of Clinical Research*. 2nd ed. Tarzana, CA: Third Line Press, Inc; 2000.

These publications are available from:
Third Line Press
4751 Viviana Drive
Tarzana, CA 91356
Phone: (818) 996-0076
Fax: (818) 774-1575
Email: tlp@www.third-line.com
Web site: www.third-line.com

Software and Videos: Leo Galland, MD

The Drug Nutrient Workshop Software. Intended for use by health professionals as a clinical management tool, this software includes a questionnaire that can be filled out by the patient or by office staff to provide an analysis and a report for individual patients of potential interactions between drugs, nutrients, supplements, and foods they are consuming. This database includes:

- Approximately 900 medications, cross-referenced
- Approximately 600 nutritional and herbal supplements
- More than 2000 documented interactions, both potentially hazardous and beneficial

The software can also serve as an electronic reference system on the applied pharmacology of natural products. The entire database can be browsed as if it were an electronic book or searched for content by key words, drug names, nutritional supplement names, or pharmacological classes. References can also be copied and pasted into Google Scholar through a direct link, for further research. A reference-only version of the Drug-Nutrient Workshop is also available, intended for professional training programs, health libraries, and users not engaged in clinical practice.

The Nutrition Workshop Software. This is a dietary analysis tool in a software format, designed to provide health practitioners with quantitative and descriptive information about their patients' diets. The food frequency questionnaire has been adapted for clinical use from a database originally developed at the NIH. The patient's answers to the questionnaire can be transferred to the health practitioner via Internet, office intranet, or on disk or CD. The analysis software generates a report that includes:

- A dietary analysis of estimated daily intake of calories, protein, carbohydrates, fat, fiber, vitamins, minerals, and carotenoids.

- Significant characteristics of the patient's diet that have been shown in scientific studies to influence health and longevity.
- To assess weight management, the patient's activity level is also addressed, providing an estimate of the total daily caloric expenditure, compared with estimated caloric intake.

Integrative Medicine Video. A 6-hour educational workshop on the principles and practices of integrative and nutritional medicine. Topics include (1) the mediators, antecedents, and triggers of illness; (2) nutritional influences on cell function and the effects of antioxidant nutrients; and (3) intestinal toxicity, dysbiosis, and leaky gut syndrome, focusing on causes, consequences, diagnosis, and treatment.

Information on the Drug-Nutrient Workshop, the Nutrition Workshop, and videotapes by Leo Galland, MD, can be obtained through:

Applied Nutrition, Inc.
133 East 73 Street
NY, New York 10021
Fax: (212) 794-0170
Email: drgalland@NutritionWorkshop.com
Web site: www.NutritionWorkshop.com

Recent Publications of the Institute for Functional Medicine (IFM) and Jeffrey Bland, PhD

Bland JS. *Genetic Nutritioneering*. New Canaan, CT: McGraw-Hill/Keats Publishing; 1999. For consumers and professionals.

Bland J. *Improving Health Outcomes Through Nutritional Support for Metabolic Biotransformation.* Gig Harbor, WA: IFM; 2003.

Bland J. *New Approach to Anti-Aging: Nutritional Neuroendocrinology.* Gig Harbor, WA: IFM; 2001.

Bland J. *Nutrigenomic Modulation of Inflammatory Disorders.* Gig Harbor, WA: IFM; 2004.

Bland J. *Nutritional Endocrinology: Breakthrough Approaches for Improving Adrenal and Thyroid Function.* Gig Harbor, WA: IFM; 2002.

Bland J. *Nutritional Management of the Underlying Causes of Chronic Disease.* Gig Harbor, WA: IFM; 2004.

Institute for Functional Medicine. *Clinical Nutrition: A Functional Approach.* 2nd ed. Gig Harbor, WA: IFM; 2004. (See Chapter 12 for an excerpt from this work.)

Institute for Functional Medicine. *Textbook of Functional Medicine.* Gig Harbor, WA: IFM; 2005.

Audio series: Functional Medicine Updates. This is a monthly audio subscription series features reports and analysis by Jeffrey Bland, PhD, on emerging research. The series is available on audiocassette, audio CD, or as a quarterly data CD containing searchable text, indexed back to 1997.

For publication orders and course registrations, contact:

Institute for Functional Medicine
4411 Pt. Fosdick Drive NW, Suite 305
PO Box 1697
Gig Harbor, WA 98335
Phone: (800) 228-0622
Fax: (253) 853-6766
Email: client_services@fxmed.com
Web site: www.functionalmedicine.org

Further Reading and References

Agatston A. *The South Beach Diet.* New York, NY: Rodale Books; 2003. Written by a cardiologist, this book is a practical resource for glycemic and cholesterol management, relevant to both consumers and health care professionals.

Atkins RA. *Atkins for Life.* New York, NY: St. Martin's Griffin; 2003.

Murray MT. *Encyclopedia of Nutritional Supplements.* New York, NY: Three Rivers Press; 1996.

Murray MT, Pizzorno JE. *Encyclopedia of Natural Medicine.* Revised 2nd ed. New York, NY: Prima Lifestyles; 1997.

Pizzorno J, Murray M, eds. *Textbook of Natural Medicine.* (2 vol. set) 2nd ed. Edinburgh, Scotland: Churchill Livingstone; 1999. This is a comprehensive, definitive text on naturopathic medicine.

Pizzorno JE, Murray MT, Joiner-Bey H. *The Clinician's Handbook of Natural Medicine.* Edinburgh, Scotland: Churchill Livingstone; 2002. A practical, insightful clinical text on nutritional medicine, referenced to the *Textbook of Natural Medicine* for in-depth explanations.

PDR Physicians' Desk Reference for Nutritional Supplements. Montvale, NJ: Medical Economics Data; 2001. This resource can be ordered from www.pdrbookstore.com.

Schwarzbein D, Brown M. *The Schwarzbein Principle II.* Deerfield Beach, FL: Health Communications, Inc.; 2002. Written by an endocrinologist, this book addresses both management of the stress response and glycemic control.

Shils ME, Olson JA, Shike M, Ross AC, eds. *Modern Nutrition in Health and Disease.* 9th ed. Philadelphia, PA: Lippincott Williams & Wilkins; 1998. Written for health care professionals, this is an outstanding reference on nutrition in two volumes.

TRAINING, WORKSHOPS, AND CONFERENCES

Course: Food as Medicine, James Gordon, MD, and the Center for Mind-Body Medicine

This practical course is designed to help physicians and other health professionals deepen their knowledge of nutrition. Content includes assessing the nutritional status of patients, recommending individualized diets, answering questions about food and supplements, and supporting the psychological needs of patients in changing their diets. It is intended for physicians, medical staff, medical school faculty, nurses and nurse practitioners, dietitians and nutritionists, chiropractors, and other health practitioners. The course provides information on clinical management of common health problems, including allergies, arthritis, asthma, cancer, diabetes, digestive disorders, heart disease, neurological conditions, obesity, and women's health issues. For additional information, contact:

Center for Mind-Body Medicine
5225 Connecticut Ave., NW, Suite 414
Washington, DC 20015
Phone: (202) 966-7338
Web site: www.cmbm.org

Online Courses: University of Arizona, Program in Integrative Medicine

A series of 3-month online courses in *Nutrition and Health* and *Botanical Studies* has been developed by the Program in Integrative Medicine. The first of these modules, Nutrition and Cardiovascular Health, is available via the Internet to all health care professionals. The course covers the fundamentals of diet and nutrition for heart health, including: macro- and micronutrients, fad diets, supplements, phytonutrients, motivating patient change, the state of the research in this field, and more. Virtual case histories are included as learning tools. Continuing education credits of 16.5 hours are provided to physicians, nurses, and registered dieticians. For additional information, contact:

Program in Integrative Medicine
University of Arizona Medical School
PO Box 245153
Tucson, AZ 85724-5153
Email: piminfo@ahsc.arizona.edu
Phone: (520) 626-5662
Web site: www.integrativemedicine.arizona.edu

Training and Conferences: Institute for Functional Medicine

Foundational Course. This 6-day course, *Applying Functional Medicine in Clinical Practice*, is designed to teach practitioners how to apply the principles and science of functional medicine to enhance patient outcomes. Grounded in emerging science, and directed at clinicians who want to improve their management of complex, chronic diseases, this educational forum provides lectures, case-based small group breakouts, and exceptional faculty. Two sessions are taught each year: usually one in the western United States and one in the east. The course provides 41.5 CME (continuing medical education credits).

Clinical Modules. These 1- to 3-day courses are designed to expand and deepen the knowledge base established in the Institute's 6-day intensive. The modules are offered in a convenient weekend format and provide approximately 20 hours CME credit.

Conferences. The IFM hosts an annual multiday symposium, the *International Symposium on Functional Medicine,* which presents a comprehensive exploration of emerging research and clinical perspectives on a specific, focal health care topic. Recent symposium themes have included: The Immune System under Siege (2005), Diabetes and Metabolic Syndrome (2004), The Heart on Fire: Modifiable Factors Beyond Cholesterol (2003), and

Emerging Therapies in Complex Neurological and Psychiatric Conditions (2002). Up to 28 CME credits are provided.

PDA RESOURCES, DATABASES, AND WEB SITES

Personal Digital Assistant Resources

Databases are becoming more widely utilized in clinical practice with the increasing availability of handheld computers—personal digital assistants. Clinicians can now tap major databases and Web sites for diagnostic information, research, full-text articles, drug formularies, botanical and nutritional resources, and information on interactions and contraindications. Some databases are available without charge, such as PubMed, while others are accessible only by subscription. The following Web sites represent a small fraction of the vast information resources now available in electronic form on the Internet:

PubMed, a database of the National Library of Medicine, NIH
Web site: www.ncbi.nih.nlm.gov/PubMed

Natural Standard Research Collaboration
Web site: www.naturalstandard.com

Natural Medicines Comprehensive Database
Web site: www.naturaldatabase.com

InfoRetriever and InfoPoems: evidence-based resources
Web site: www.infopoems.com

MDConsult, a publication of Elsevier Science
Web site: www.MDConsult.com

*Web*MD Sites:
www.Medscape.com
www.*Web*MD.com

Major Databases and Links

Abstracted Research: Medline/PubMed

The Medline database of the National Library of Medicine is the largest biomedical database in the world, encompassing more than 12 million references. Over 6000 journals from more than 70 countries are indexed, with entries dating from 1966 to the present. To search topics in nutrition, it is important to use the specific scientific or chemical term. For example, journal articles on vitamin C may be listed under "ascorbic acid." When a search is unsuccessful, check terminology by clicking on "MeSH headings" on the vertical toolbar, and entering the common name to check other terms used in Medline.
Web site: www.ncbi.nlm.nih.gov/PubMed

Directory of Databases: Rosenthal Center for Complementary and Alternative Medicine

This directory of the Rosenthal Center, Columbia University, includes databases specific to CAM, herbology, and disciplines such as traditional Chinese medicine. A second database of botanical resources is also featured on the Rosenthal site.

Directory of Databases
Web site: www.rosenthal.hs.columbia.edu/Databases/html#2

Botanical Medicine Information Resources
Web site: www.rosenthal.hs.columbia.edu/Botanicals.html

Google Scholar

Google Scholar supports Web searches for scholarly and research literature, including peer-reviewed articles, papers, theses, books, abstracts, and technical reports. This interface can be used to find articles from academic publishers, professional societies, preprint repositories, and universities, as well as across the Web.

Web site: www.scholar.google.com

Cochrane Collaboration

This international consortium seeks to meet the growing need for evidence-based documentation in medicine, including the field of complementary medicine. The Cochrane Collaboration is involved in the creation and maintenance of an international registry of completed and ongoing randomized, controlled clinical trials, and in the development of guidelines and software to systematize and facilitate the preparation and updating of these systematic reviews. More information can be obtained from:

Cochrane Complementary Medicine Field Trial Registry Coordinator
Complementary Medicine Program
University of Maryland School of Medicine
2200 Kernan Drive
Baltimore, MD 21207-6697
Phone: (410) 448-6997
Fax: (410) 448-6875
Web site: www.compmed.umm.edu/cochrane

Clinical Nutrition Database: Clinical Pearls Online

This open-source database contains a decade of peer-reviewed research in nutrition and integrative medicine with weekly research updates. The database includes more than 500 archived interviews of expert researchers in the field; it is available to health care professionals and the public at no charge. Click on Clinical Pearls Online Subscribers, and log in: username: "clinical"; password: "pearls" (all lowercase). For further information, contact:

Clinical Pearls Publications, Inc.
Phone: (916) 483-1085
Email: service@clinicalpearls.com
Web site: www.clinicalpearls.com

Literature Reviews: Current Contents

Monthly reviews of the scientific literature, including clinical nutrition, by Current Contents Clinical Medicine and Current Contents Life Sciences are available through university and public libraries, and can be purchased in print and on disc from:

The Institute for Scientific Information
350 Market Street
Philadelphia, PA 19104
Phone: (800) 523-1850
Fax: (215) 386-2915
Web site: www.isinet.com

Database: Embase

Produced by Elsevier Science, the Netherlands, Embase provides extensive coverage of pharmacological and biomedical research. The database, which includes publications from 1975 onward, encompasses more than 9 million references from more than 4,000 journals, as well as selected Medline records. Access to the database is available by subscription.
www.embase.com

Databases: Healthnotes

This content provider develops databases on nutrition and health for use by doctors, pharmacists, hospitals, schools, and medical libraries throughout the world. Healthnotes offers a subscription-based resource for health care practitioners that includes science-based information on self-care options, vitamins and minerals, herbs, homeopathic remedies, diet, and drug-nutrient interactions. These databases are available from:

Healthnotes
1505 SE Gideon, Suite 200
Portland, OR 97202
Phone: (800) 659-6330 or (503) 234-4092
Web site: www.healthnotes.com

Health and Nutrition Web Sites

Harvard School of Public Health, Nutrition
  Source
Web site: www.hsph.harvard.edu/nutrition
  source

Web sites that provide diagrams of metabolic
  pathways:
www.unisanet.unisa.edu.au/08366/h&p2carb.
  htm
www.genome.ad.jp/kegg/metabolism.html
www.gwu.edu/~mpb

Organic Trade Association (with links to
  products)
Web site: http://www.ota.com/index.html

Preventive Medicine Research Institute of
  Dean Ornish, MD
Web site: www.pmri.org

Software for assessment of nutrition and of
  interactions:
www.epocrates.com
www.hightechnutrition.com
www.nutrition-toolbox.com
www.NutritionWorkshop.com

Tufts University Nutrition Navigator (with
  links)
Web site: www.navigator.tufts.edu

Government-Sponsored Web Sites

Centers for Disease Control and Prevention
Web site: www.cdc.gov

Center for Food Safety and Applied Nutrition
FDA Food Information Line
Phone: (888) SAFEFOOD (24 hours a day)
Web site: www.cfsan.fda.gov

Food and Drug Administration (FDA)
Web site: www.fda.gov

Government directory of clinical trials
Web site: www.clinicaltrials.gov

National Center for Complementary and
  Alternative Medicine (NCCAM)
Web site: www.nccam.gov

National Institutes of Health, Office of
  Dietary Supplements
Web site: http://dietary-supplements.info.
nih.gov

US Department of Agriculture (USDA) Food
  Safety
USDA Meat and Poultry Hotline
Phone: (800) 535-4555 or TTY (800) 256-
  7072
Web site: www.fsis.usda.gov

USDA Nutrient Data Laboratory
Web site: www.nal.usda.gov/fnic/foodcomp

United States Pharmacopeia Convention,
  Inc.
Web site: www.usp.org

PART III

Exercise and Fitness

CHAPTER 17

Exercise Therapy in Medicine

Neil Sol, PhD

MEDICAL FITNESS

Evidence from mounting research suggests that exercise may be one of the most universal forms of therapy. We know that exercise provides benefits in maintaining health and in preventing conditions such as cardiovascular disease. As a treatment modality, *medical exercise* is a therapeutic intervention usually provided in a facility that integrates medicine and fitness. Medical exercise can be prescribed for rehabilitation to restore health, for example, following a cardiovascular episode.

When exercise is provided by a medical team, it can be adapted to improve almost any type of health condition including cancer, diabetes, hypertension, low back pain, lung disease, lupus, obesity, orthopedic injuries, or renal disease. For example, in diabetes, prescribed exercise can lower or eliminate the need for supplemental insulin. Although almost everyone in the clinical world has heard this at one time or another, there is a tendency to undervalue such a basic approach.

Medical fitness is a new and rapidly expanding field. Exercise specialists or physiologists are essentially personal trainers with

Neil Sol, PhD, has been a leader in the fields of health enhancement and fitness for the past two decades. He has extensive experience in creating, managing, and marketing health-related products and services in academic environments, the commercial fitness industry, and hospital health systems. Currently, he is vice president of Outpatient Services at ValleyCare Health System in Pleasanton, California.

Courtesy of Neil Sol, PhD, Pleasanton, California.

expertise in medical fitness. Having access to a knowledgeable exercise specialist enables the physician to refer patients with confidence. Just as physicians and health care providers need a referral list of capable specialists, patients are also well served if referrals include a good exercise specialist and a medical fitness facility. We anticipate the day when access to these services will be considered essential resources by most health care professionals.

PRIMARY AND SECONDARY REHABILITATION

A good medical fitness professional can develop individualized exercise programs for primary prevention to prevent the initial occurrence of disease, and for secondary prevention to prevent a second occurrence. Primary rehabilitation refers to health maintenance, health promotion, health enhancement, wellness, and performance enhancement. Secondary rehabilitation is provided as a therapeutic intervention in response to disease or disability. In these cases, exercise is prescribed for the needs and requirements of the individual, specifying the correct amount of exercise necessary to prevent a second occurrence of disease and to enhance quality of life.

Exercise as a clinical treatment modality can have a substantial positive impact on the health of patients. Medical fitness can be adapted to address a broad range of needs— from those of children and adolescents in sports who are not utilizing the right form of conditioning to those of adults who want to avoid diabetes or its sequelae.

Primary and secondary prevention are now being applied with greater frequency in clinical care. As a health care practitioner, medical fitness programs provide a resource to which you can refer patients. This obviates the necessity for physicians and health care practitioners to become experts in medical fitness. Just as you do not need to know everything there is to know when you make a referral to an allergist, a physical therapist, or a surgeon, you do not need to be an expert in medical fitness to make an intelligent referral.

WEIGHT LOSS

Consider the situation of patients who are struggling with their weight. Typically, long before they see a physician, they have made some effort at weight loss on their own. They may seek information from magazine articles, books, Web sites, videos, or infomercials. Many people do their own research and then come to their physician with questions relative to a particular exercise program, device, or nutritional product.

Physicians and health care providers are in a better position if they have a range of alternatives and referrals to offer the patient. In the context of specific health conditions, the availability of a hospital-based medical fitness center expands the options. When providers can refer patients to such a facility, staffed by skilled professionals, then that is frequently at the top of their referral list. Having these resources available, health care practitioners are no longer required to be totally knowledgeable about the credibility or the details of every resource on the Internet.

With regard to weight loss, there are essentially two levels of need: people who want to lose a little weight and those who are morbidly obese. When patients have a high body mass index (BMI), it is important that they receive timely referral. Guidelines indicate that these conditions need to be addressed when there is a BMI of 35 or above (accompanied by comorbidities) or a BMI of 40 or above (whether or not there are comorbidities). The multidisciplinary approach utilized in medical fitness centers applies various types of expertise to the needs of patients. This approach is consistent with that used by physicians and other health professionals, who typically recommend a combination of diet counseling, exercise, and possibly medication.

In assessing programs, the important criteria include:

- Sponsorship by a health care organization
- Credentialed staff
- A program tailored to each individual's capacity
- Nutritional counseling
- Guidance on regular physical activity
- An approach that helps participants avoid injury or disappointment
- Client encouragement, communication, and feedback
- Convenient location in the community of the health care provider or the patient

At ValleyCare Health System in Northern California, for example, we offer a program called LifeStyleRx in a medically integrated facility that provides weight management programs and a broad range of other fitness and medical exercise programs. We serve people from childhood through every phase of adulthood. For the person who simply wants to lose a few pounds, we provide dietary consultation and exercise programs to control the intake and utilization of calories.

Conditions involving morbid obesity frequently require bariatric surgery, which is performed at ValleyCare for patients who qualify. Typically these patients are case managed by bariatric physicians. We provide a screening process that involves dietary counseling and intervention, as well as psychological and medical evaluation to determine if surgery is the right option for the patient. When this surgery is elected, it is important that patients take some initiative. To maximize their success, we provide presurgical exercise and a dietary program to help them lose a few pounds (typically 10 or 15 pounds). This also enables patients to explore their level of commitment and whether they are ready to change their lifestyle. Following the surgery, we offer a program that helps them maintain their weight loss through correct eating, exercise, and the effects of the surgery. We also provide postsurgery support groups to help people adhere to their new regimen and make a successful adjustment.

PRESCRIPTION FOR FITNESS

When medical fitness expertise is available, physicians no longer have to become experts in exercise or exercise physiology. They simply need to make informed referrals to skilled exercise professionals or to a reputable medical fitness facility. This presents a few questions:

1. How do health care professionals determine their patients' needs in terms of therapeutic exercise?
2. How can providers educate themselves in this field so they can write good exercise prescriptions, describing the limitations or special requirements of their patients?

3. How do they find skilled exercise professionals and medical fitness centers in their community or region?

Training and licensure. Exercise physiologists are trained through programs on both a bachelor's and a master's level. Currently there is no formal licensure. However, there are many quality certification programs for exercise providers. In the future, we anticipate that fitness professionals will be licensed, and physicians will write prescriptions to these professionals and regard them as essential members of the clinical team, much as they now view other allied health professionals.

Referral Sources

- Referrals to medical fitness professionals: This information can be obtained through national certification boards, such as the American College of Sports Medicine and the Aerobic and Fitness Association of America, as well as many others.
- Referrals to personal fitness trainers: Contact information on trainers can be obtained through national associations such as the Aerobic and Fitness Council of America and the National Federation of Professional Trainers.
- Referrals to hospital fitness centers: Many hospitals across the country are now building medical fitness centers, and it is anticipated that in the near future a greater number of resources will be in place. The majority of the professionals in these centers are likely to be credentialed.
- Networking within the professional community: Currently the onus is on both physicians and exercise providers to build professional relationships and establish mutual referral lists.

RESOURCES

Publications

American College of Sports Medicine. *ACSM's Exercise Management for Persons with Disease and Disabilities.* 2nd ed. Champaign, IL: Human Kinetics Publishers; 2002.

American College of Sports Medicine. *ACSM's Resource Manual for Guidelines for Exercise Testing and Prescription.* 7th ed. Philadelphia, PA: Lippincott Williams & Wilkins; 2005.

Rippe JM. *Lifestyle Medicine.* Boston, MA: Blackwell Publishing; 1999.

United States Department of Health and Human Services (USHHS). *Physical Activity and Health: A Report of the Surgeon General.* Atlanta, GA: Centers for Disease Control and Prevention, National Center for Chronic Disease Prevention and Health Promotion; 1996.

Associations and Agencies

American College of Sport Medicine (ACSM)
PO Box 1440
Indianapolis, IN 46206-1440
Phone, national center: (317) 637-9200
Phone, regional chapters: (317) 637-9200, ext. 138
Fax: (317) 634-7817
Web site: www.acsm.org

Centers for Disease Control and Prevention
National Center for Chronic Disease Prevention and Health Promotion
Division of Nutrition and Physical Activity, MS K-46
4770 Buford Highway, NE
Atlanta, GA 30341-3724
Phone: (888) 232-4674
Web site: www.cdc.gov

National Academy of Sports Medicine (NASM)
26632 Agoura Road
Calabasas, CA 91302
Phone: (800) 460-6276 or (818) 595-1200
Fax: (818) 878-9511
Web site: www.nasm.org

Associations of Fitness Trainers and Facilities

Aerobic and Fitness Association of America (AFAA)
15250 Ventura Blvd., Suite 200
Sherman Oaks, CA 91403
Phone: (877) 968-7263
Web site: www.afaa.com

American Council on Exercise (ACE)
4851 Paramount Drive
San Diego, CA 92123
Phone: (800) 825-3636 or (858) 279-8227
Fax: (858) 279-8064
Web site: www.acefitness.org

International Health, Racquet and Sportsclub Association (IHRSA)
263 Summer Street
Boston, MA 02210
Phone: (800) 228-4772 or (617) 951-0055
Fax: (617) 951-0056
Email: info@ihrsa.org.
Web site: www.ihrsa.org

National Federation of Professional Trainers/ NFPT, Inc.
PO Box 4579
Lafayette, IN 47903
Phone: (800) 729-6378 or (765) 471-4514
Fax: (765) 471-7369
Email: info@nfpt.com
Web site: www.nfpt.com

National Strength and Conditioning Association
1885 Bob Johnson Drive
Colorado Springs, CO 80906
Phone: (800) 815-6826 or (719) 632-6722
Fax: (719) 632-6367

Email, national headquarters: nsca@nsca-lift.org
Email, certification: commission@nsca-cc.org
Web site: www.nsca-lift.org or www.nsca.com

CHAPTER 18

Exercise Is Medicine

Cedric X. Bryant, PhD, FACSM, and James A. Peterson, PhD, FACSM

The beneficial effects of exercising on a regular basis are well documented. Not only has exercise been shown to enhance a person's ability to perform daily activities without undue fatigue or injury, it has also been found to help decrease the risk of developing a number of chronic medical conditions, including coronary heart disease, hypertension, diabetes, and obesity. In fact, over the last 20 years, an overwhelming body of research evidence has emerged supporting the notion that being physically active improves overall health and well-being.

Two of the most widely publicized research efforts to investigate the possible relationship between exercise and disease were longitudinal studies, each of which involved more than 10,000 subjects. In a renowned study of 17,000 Harvard graduates, Ralph Paffenbarger, MD, found that men who expended approximately 300 calories a day—the equivalent of walking briskly for 45 minutes—delayed mortality from all causes by an extraordinary 28% and lived an average of more than two years longer than their sedentary former classmates. The other study, conducted in the mid-1990s by Steven Blair, PED, of the Institute of Aerobics Research in Dallas, documented the fact that a relatively modest amount of exercise can have a significant effect on the longevity of both men and women. This study found that the higher the fitness level, the greater the longevity (after the data was adjusted for age differences between subjects in this 8-year investigation of 13,344 individuals). An analysis of the extensive data yielded by both studies suggests one inescapable conclusion—*exercise is medicine*.

Cedric X. Bryant, PhD, FACSM, serves as the chief exercise physiologist and vice president of educational services for the American Council on Exercise. Dr. Bryant has served on the faculty of the United States Military Academy at West Point, Pennsylvania State University, and Arizona State University, and has been senior vice president for StairMaster Health and Fitness Products Inc. where he was responsible for research, development, and design. He also lectures internationally and has authored or coauthored more than 200 journal articles and 18 books.

James A. Peterson, PhD, FACSM, is a sports medicine consultant who resides in Monterey, California. Dr. Peterson is a prolific writer, having authored 63 books and over 200 published articles on a variety of topics in sports medicine, fitness, and management. An active member and fellow of the American College of Sports Medicine, Dr. Peterson was the coeditor of the 2nd edition of *ACSM's Standards and Guidelines for Health/Fitness Facilities* and currently serves as the associate editor-in-chief for *ACSM's Health and Fitness Journal*.

REDUCING CARDIOVASCULAR RISK WITH EXERCISE

The number one cause of death of men and women in the United States is cardiovascular disease (CVD). Each year, more than 930,000 deaths can be directly attributed to CVD. Unfortunately, even though this condition has been found to begin relatively early in life (sometimes as early as the teenage years for males), the symptoms of this disorder do not typically manifest until the disease is far advanced in an individual. Approximately 25% of the US population suffers from CVD. Prevention is, without question, the most appropriate approach to this pandemic medical problem. Exercise can moderate a number of risk factors for CVD.

HDL cholesterol. Exercise helps to prevent CVD by positively affecting blood lipid levels. For example, exercising on a regular basis has been found to raise levels of beneficial high-density lipoprotein (HDL). HDL cholesterol is important from a health-risk standpoint because of its ability to help protect against CVD through its efforts to collect cholesterol, transport it to the liver, and safely dispose of it as bile acids in the stool. By transferring cholesterol to the liver, HDL helps prevent the accumulation of lipids on the walls of the arteries in atherosclerosis. Exercise also facilitates the formation of HDL and helps slow the eventual breakdown of HDL, enabling individuals to maintain higher levels of this cardioprotective lipoprotein.

Hypertension. Exercise also helps to prevent CVD by enabling individuals to more effectively control blood pressure/hypertension. Research shows that low-intensity aerobic exercise (40%–70% of VO_2 max) can lower systolic blood pressure by approximately 11 mm Hg and diastolic blood pressure by approximately 9 mm Hg in mild-to-moderate hypertensive patients. Not surprisingly, individuals who already suffer from high blood pressure can significantly lower their mortality risk by exercising on a regular basis.

Smoking cessation. Exercise has also been observed to help prevent CVD by aiding some people (though not all) in their attempts to quit smoking. Evidence suggests that physically active individuals reduce their craving for cigarettes with exercise participation. Other studies have shown that many individuals who had previously smoked voluntarily gave up this habit once they became involved in a program of regular physical activity. Unfortunately, the addictive qualities of nicotine (nicotine is a drug that is six to eight times more addictive than alcohol) in many instances override a smoker's capacity to adequately consider the beneficial consequences of exercise. At the present time, statistics indicate that more than 45 million Americans still smoke (approximately 22.5% of the adult population).

Obesity. Exercise has also been found to play a major role in lowering body fat. Obesity is a significant risk factor for CVD—particularly when body fat is accumulated around the waist. Regular exercise helps to improve body composition in two primary ways. One way is by increasing caloric expenditure, thereby creating a caloric deficit. If a previously sedentary individual walks two miles a day at a speed of 4 mph, five days a week, that person can expect to lose 9.5 to 11.0 pounds over a 1-year period of time—provided their caloric intake remains stable. These calculations are based on individuals of average size: women weighing approximately 130 pounds (60 kg) and men weighing approximately 155 pounds (70 kg). Exercise helps to improve body composition by ensuring that the majority of weight loss is from fat rather than lean body tissue. Exercise also helps to counteract high blood pressure, glucose intolerance, and low self-esteem.

EXERCISE IN DISEASE MANAGEMENT

Over the last decade, many health experts have concluded that medical science has (for many chronic health problems) achieved about as much as can be expected in the battle against sickness and death. Furthermore, based on increasing evidence, many experts have surmised that additional expenditures for health care are not likely to produce the financial benefits that could be achieved if every American adopted better health practices—particularly a physically active lifestyle. In the past three decades, several major epidemiological studies have demonstrated that regular physical activity is associated with an improved quality of life and longevity.

In numerous instances, exercise can be an extremely effective adjunctive treatment modality for individuals suffering from a diverse array of chronic medical problems. As a result, properly prescribed exercise programs can lower health care costs, not only by reducing the incidence or severity of health problems in many cases, but also by diminishing an individual's reliance on medications and limited medical resources when illness does occur.

The range of medical problems and health-related conditions that can be at least partially treated and controlled by exercise is extensive. In addition to cardiovascular disease, three of the most significant health concerns in this regard are hypertension, diabetes, and obesity.

Hypertension

An estimated 60 million American adults have high blood pressure. Individuals are classified as hypertensive when their blood pressure level exceeds 140 mm Hg systolic and/or 90 mm Hg diastolic on two or more consecutive measurements. Hypertension adds to the workload of the heart and arteries and contributes to CVD and arteriosclerosis. As a result, the heart may become enlarged (left ventricular hypertrophy) and less efficient; the artery walls may also become damaged. Fatty plaque may be deposited on the walls, increasing the possibility that these vessels may be scarred and hardened. Such damage can reduce the flow of blood and oxygen to the kidneys, heart, brain, or eyes. Even

more serious, it can lead to blood clot formation with the potential for stroke.

Although drug therapy is traditionally considered to be the most effective form of treatment for high blood pressure, exercising on a regular basis has been found to be a beneficial and safe adjunctive therapy for many hypertensive individuals. In fact, a sound exercise program may serve as an effective nondrug alternative for some people. Exercise is thought to lower resting blood pressure by decreasing the activity of the sympathetic nervous system. A reduction in sympathetic nerve activity could lower one or both of the two principal determinants of blood pressure, since mean arterial blood pressure equals the product of cardiac output and total peripheral resistance.

Given the aforementioned, hypertensive patients should be encouraged to make a firm commitment to exercise, because even a small amount of regular activity (and the subsequent reduction in blood pressure) can go a long way toward diminishing the long-term consequences of hypertension. For example, lowering systolic blood pressure by a mere 2 millimeters of mercury has been shown to reduce deaths from stroke by 6%, heart disease by 4%, and from all causes by 3%.

Diabetes

Approximately 90% of the more than 16 million Americans suffering from diabetes have Type 2, noninsulin dependent diabetes, the more easily controlled form of the disease. Formerly referred to as adult-onset diabetes, it is typically diagnosed after an individual reaches age 40 and is usually the result of insulin resistance. In some Type 2 diabetics, the malady results because the pancreas simply does not produce enough insulin. Obesity, family history, and a sedentary lifestyle appear to be the most significant risk factors for Type 2 diabetes. It is also important to note that the number of children who are being diagnosed with Type 2 diabetes has made the term "adult-onset diabetes" obsolete.

In Type 1 or juvenile-onset diabetes, insulin injections are required. Although a family history of Type 1 diabetes affects an individual's risk of developing the disease, a genetic predisposition for this condition is not nearly as common as in Type 2 diabetes.

As every physician knows, hyperglycemia (high blood sugar) can cause fatigue, dehydration, and blurred vision, and unchecked can result in loss of consciousness, coma, or even death. Over an extended period, moderately elevated blood sugar levels can affect the blood vessels that feed the brain, eyes, heart, and kidneys, can cause damage to those vital organs, and can lead to nerve damage. Fortunately, exercise can help diabetics control their condition and reduce their risk of life-threatening complications.

Prevention. Research shows that regular exercise can reduce an individual's likelihood of developing diabetes by more than half—even in those who are obese or are genetically predisposed to the disease. In a major study conducted at the University of California, Berkeley, researchers found that for every extra 500 calories (kcal) a week that an individual expends during exercise, the risk of developing diabetes is reduced by 6%. The expenditure of 500 calories per week can be accomplished by engaging in the following activities:

- Walking one mile 4 to 5 times per week
- Bicycling 5 miles 3 to 4 times per week
- Circuit strength training for 30 minutes two times per week

The beneficial aspects of exercise that are either directly or indirectly related to diabetes include the following:

- Regulation of blood sugar levels. Exercise encourages the body to use more glucose—its primary fuel source. As a result, exercise has the effect of lowering elevated blood sugar levels by helping transport glucose out of the bloodstream and into the cells where it can be expended rather than stored as fat. In fact, exercising on a regular basis can enable some diabetics who require medication to control their blood sugar levels, which reduces the amount of insulin they require. Some Type 2 diabetics who exercise regularly find they can eventually discontinue glucose-regulating medications. When individuals stop working out for just three days in a row, however, the beneficial effects of exercise are almost completely lost. Of the various types of conditioning regimens, aerobic exercise appears to provide the greatest benefit in terms of blood sugar control. Strength training has also been shown to have a positive impact on blood sugar levels.

- Minimizing the health risk of diabetes. In diabetics, the most common causes of illness and death are coronary heart disease (CHD), stroke, and various cardiovascular complications due to atherosclerosis. With regard to minimizing the likelihood of atherosclerosis, regular exercise improves blood lipid profiles. Exercise also helps lower heart rate, blood pressure, and blood platelet adhesiveness levels, making the blood less likely to clot.

- Reduction of body weight and fat stores. Exercise helps reduce excess weight and body fat—each of which is a major contributing factor to the development of Type 2 diabetes in many individuals as they age. Insulin sensitivity (i.e., the responsiveness of cells to insulin) is significantly enhanced following exercise-induced reductions in weight and body fat levels. As a result, the diabetic's need for insulin is reduced. The lower the insulin dosage, the closer the body's metabolic system functions to its normal physiological level. As a result, there is a substantial reduction in the metabolic roller coaster that diabetics tend to suffer, allowing for more consistent blood sugar regulation.

- Enhancing psychological well-being. Although the physiological effects of exercise are most frequently examined, exercise also can have a positive psychological impact on diabetics. For example, regular exercise may effectively reduce emotional stress, increase feelings of well-being, and improve overall quality of life. Although these psychological effects are more difficult to quantify, they are well supported anecdotally and represent important benefits for those with diabetes.

The role of exercise in treating diabetes involves a carefully considered balance. When properly combined with a sensible diet and appropriate medications, exercise can have a positive impact on the lives of diabetics. The challenge is to strike the proper balance among the critical elements of an effective treatment program. Note that any major change in one of these primary treatment factors usually requires a concurrent adjustment in the other two elements as well. An increase in the level of physical activity by a diabetic often necessitates an increase in food intake and/or an alteration in the dosage or timing of that individual's medication.

Obesity

Obesity, defined as weighing 20% more than recommended for a given body height, affects approximately 60 million adults, with the highest rates found among minority groups and the poor. The proportion of adults in the United States who are classified as obese, when defined by a body mass index (BMI) greater than or equal to 30 kg/m^2, rose 49% over the last decade. (BMI is calculated by dividing weight in pounds by height in inches.) The greatest increases in BMI occurred among young adults, college-educated people, and those of Hispanic ethnicity. During this time period, obesity increased in every state, in both sexes, and across all age groups, races, and educational levels, both smokers and nonsmokers. The latest figures show that more than half of all Americans are overweight or obese. Perhaps most startling is the fact that one out of five children and adolescents ages 5 to 17 is obese.

The dramatic rise in the prevalence of overweight individuals and obesity in the United States has created a serious public health concern for a large percentage of the population. Being overweight has been directly or indirectly linked to insulin resistance and Type 2 diabetes, coronary heart disease, certain types of cancer, hypertension, osteoarthritis, and gallbladder disease. In 1998, in response to an emerging body of scientific evidence, the American Heart Association reclassified obesity as a major modifiable risk factor for coronary heart disease. Consequently, weight reduction is often prescribed in the prevention and treatment of many chronic diseases and medical conditions.

For successful lifelong weight management, sensible eating and regular exercise go hand in hand. The optimal approach to weight loss combines mild caloric restriction (energy intake not lower than 1200 kcal/day), a negative caloric balance (not to exceed 500 to 1000 kcal/day), and an exercise program that promotes a daily caloric expenditure of more than 300 kcal. Note that multiple short bouts of exercise have been shown to be as effective (or even more effective in some instances) than longer continuous sessions in promoting reductions in body weight and fat stores, if the total caloric expenditure is comparable.

In addition, strength-training exercise can help to maintain or build muscle tissue or, at a minimum, counter the tendency for a calorie-restricted diet to cause a significant loss of lean muscle mass. With regard to strength training, a minimum of one set involving each of the major muscle groups of the body, performed at least two times per week, is recommended. Such a regimen should include 8 to 10 different exercises, performed at a load that permits 8 to 12 repetitions per set for healthy, sedentary adults, or 8 or more repetitions per set for persons older than 50 years of age.

Exercise can improve physical appearance, even if a significant amount of weight is not lost. Because muscle is denser than fat, individuals can look more fit and trim without changing their total body weight. Although a personally enjoyable physical activity will help to promote some degree of weight loss, an exercise program that combines aerobic conditioning, increased physical activity in daily living, and sensible strength training represents the best approach for using exercise to control body composition. The goal should be a gradual weight loss (i.e., not more than approximately 2.5 pounds or 1 kg/week) without inducing metabolic derangements such as ketosis.

EXERCISE: THE RIGHT R_X

Considerable evidence confirms that the United States is in the midst of a serious epidemic of physical inactivity. The human and health care costs of that epidemic are enormous. The available scientific evidence is irrefutable, indicating that most Americans desperately need to experience the many health and medical benefits of a physically active lifestyle.

One of the most compelling insights that patients can acquire is an understanding of the relationship between lack of regular exercise and major health concerns. Exercise can provide an excellent R_X for effective health care. In the near future this may become the standard prescription—not the exception—for those interested in achieving and maintaining a full, healthy lifestyle.

GENERAL REFERENCES

American College of Sports Medicine. *ACSM's Resource Manual for Exercise Testing and Exercise Prescription.* 4th ed. Philadelphia, PA: Lippincott Williams & Wilkins; 2001.

American College of Sports Medicine. *ACSM's Guidelines for Exercise Testing and Exercise Prescription.* 6th ed. Philadelphia, PA: Lippincott Williams & Wilkins; 2000.

American Council on Exercise. *ACE Personal Trainer Manual.* San Diego, CA: American Council on Exercise; 2003.

American Council on Exercise. *ACE Clinical Exercise Specialist Manual.* San Diego, CA: American Council on Exercise; 1999.

Blair SN, Kohl HW 3rd, Barlow CE, Paffenbarger RS Jr, Gibbons LW, Macera CA. Changes in physical fitness and all-cause mortality: a prospective study of healthy and unhealthy men. *JAMA.* 1995;273: 1093–1098.

Bryant CX, Franklin BA, Conviser JM. *Exercise Testing and Program Design.* Monterrey, CA: Healthy Learning; 2002.

Nieman DC. *The Exercise-Health Connection.* Champaign, IL: Human Kinetics Publishers; 1998.

United States Department of Health and Human Services. *Physical Activity and Health: A Report of the Surgeon General.* Atlanta, GA: Centers for Disease Control and Prevention, National Center for Chronic Disease Prevention and Health Promotion; 1996.

CHAPTER 19

Medically Supervised Exercise

Donna Manning, MS

Hospitals frequently offer programs in cardiac rehabilitation that include Phase 3 outpatient exercise classes. In some hospitals, these Phase 3 programs are no longer restricted to patients with cardiac conditions. Services have been broadened to include a population of patients who have a risk factor or special condition and would benefit from an exercise program. Some of these programs are also open to people in the community.

Patient reports indicate that many of those who are at risk want supervision with regard to exercise. These programs provide them an opportunity to begin exercising under medical supervision. Phase 3 classes are intended for patients who are not currently being treated for a life-threatening health condition. These programs also serve patients who have recovered from a cardiac episode and have graduated from more intensively supervised exercise.

Currently, Phase 3 services are not usually covered by insurance and are paid for out-of-pocket in the majority of cases. In California, for example, these programs are available on a self-pay basis through community hospitals for approximately $8 to $9 per class. Classes are typically held 2 or 3 times a week; thus a 1-month program would cost approximately $90 to $110. In some cases, 1 to 2 months of Phase 3 monitoring is sufficient to get a patient started with a home exercise program.

Physicians in the community have the option of recommending their patients to these programs. An initial stress test may be performed in the doctor's office before the patient joins the program. The physician may also write an exercise prescription defining any limitations on exercise necessitated by the patient's condition. Services of a Phase 3 program can include:

- Health education
- The development of an exercise program
- Monitoring for a health condition
- A health resource

Health education. Participation in a Phase 3 program often provides access to health education services in conjunction with supervised exercise. A comprehensive Phase 3 program may provide some of the following services:

- Review of patients' medical history
- Review of medications and answers to any related questions
- Health education regarding a specific condition and steps the patient can take to prevent its progression
- Discussion of the role of lifestyle, including diet, exercise, and stress management

Donna Manning, MS, holds a Master of Science degree from the University of Florida in Exercise Physiology and Athletic Training, and her experience includes community college teaching. She is certified in advanced cardiac life support (ACLS) and has been employed as an exercise physiologist in cardiac rehabilitation programs of several major hospitals. Ms. Manning currently serves in the cardiac rehabilitation unit of ValleyCare Health System, in Livermore, California.

- An explanation of the various tests the patient has been prescribed
- Monitoring of vital signs as a preliminary to exercise: blood pressure, heart rate readings, ausculatation, and checking for edema

Working with an exercise physiologist. Patients typically participate in these programs for 4 to 10 weeks on average. The exercise physiologist works with the patient to develop an individualized exercise program that will be beneficial without putting him/her at risk of injury or health complications. Once that program is developed, the physiologist monitors the patient's exercise and performance until both are comfortable with the new program. Steps in setting up a program can include:

- Baseline body composition measurements
- Determination of the appropriate level of exercise and development of an exercise prescription
- Review of guidelines regarding appropriate exercise intensity levels for any given individual and how to monitor the intensity of exercise
- How to monitor one's own pulse and perceived rate of exertion
- Increased awareness of how one should feel when exercising, including signs and symptoms of overexertion
- How to use the exercise equipment
- Monitoring during a 6-minute supervised walk
- Development of an exercise or walking program the patient can do at home

Monitoring a specific health condition, such as diabetes. Patients who have diabetes, for example, are coached in managing their blood sugar with regard to exercise. The physiologist or nurse will:

- Provide guidelines on optimal blood sugar levels before, during, and after exercise.
- Have patients check their blood sugar before they exercise.
- If the blood sugar level is initially too low, they are encouraged to have a snack before they begin and provided with information on healthy snacking both before and after exercise.

Health resources. These programs often serve patients as an available resource to which they can turn for information and guidance. When they graduate, they know they can return if they have a question about their medication, want a blood pressure check, or have questions about their exercise program.

Once patients have been educated with regard to the intensity and self-management of their exercise, they can become more independent and are more likely to exercise on their own. Many are fearful of exercising when they have a medical condition or have been prescribed new medication. A Phase 3 cardiac rehabilitation program is a valuable resource to help educate and inform patients about their condition, to make healthy lifestyle changes and learn safe exercise habits.

CHAPTER 20

Physiology of Qigong, Tai Chi, and Yoga

Roger Jahnke, OMD

Qigong and tai chi (a form of Qigong) from China and yoga from India are ancient methodologies developed and refined over thousands of years for sustaining and enhancing the natural healing systems of the human body. The traditional rationale for the effectiveness and benefits of such practices was ascribed to their maximization of natural healing energies in the body—*Chi* or *Qi* in China, and *prana* in India. A growing body of research indicates that Qigong and yoga promote a range of beneficial physiological effects through breath practice, relaxed patterns of movement, and focused awareness. These effects involve mechanisms that are currently well understood in Western biomedicine (Oschman, 2000; Jahnke, 2002).

For mobilizing healing capacity or reducing health risk, the research suggests that moderate exercise is often preferable to vigorous exercise (Blair et al., 1995). This type of finding has triggered a surge of interest in the traditional systems of healing exercise and mind-body practices from ancient cultures. Reviews of clinical studies on Qigong and tai chi have reported a range of physiological and health benefits, including pain management; enhanced cardiovascular, respiratory, musculoskeletal, and immune function; and improved muscular strength, stamina, posture, flexibility, balance, and mood (Li et al., 2001; Klein & Adams, 2004; Wang et al., 2004).

Three important aspects of physiology and the body's natural system of self-repair are supported by these therapeutic mind-body practices:

1. Oxygen delivery
2. Lymph generation and propulsion
3. Neurological and brain activity

In addition to these mechanisms, the physiological functions enhanced by meditative, therapeutic exercise include many less understood mechanisms such as the production and delivery of co-enzymes and antioxidants, connective tissue repair, and the enhancement of stem cell development. Ongoing research promises to further clarify these benefits.

OXYGEN

To contrast meditative exercise such as Qigong with more vigorous aerobic exercise such as running, swimming, or cycling, it is useful to trace the oxidation and energy cycle. In both vigorous and moderate

Roger Jahnke, OMD, with nearly 25 years clinical practice of traditional Chinese medicine, has been to China eight times to research the health enhancement methods of meditative and therapeutic exercise. Author of *The Healer Within* (HarperCollins, 1999) and *The Healing Promise of Qi* (McGraw-Hill, 2002), he teaches Qigong in venues that include the Esalen Institute, Omega Institute, and Kripalu Center. He is a diplomate in acupuncture and classical Chinese medicine, director and research coordinator of the Institute of Integral Qigong and Tai Chi, a founding board member of the National Qigong Association, and CEO of Health Action, a consulting firm in Santa Barbara, California.

Courtesy of Roger Jahnke, OMD, Santa Barbara, CA © 2005.

exercise the body naturally produces a powerful mix of metabolic resources. In vigorous exercise this energy production provides endogenous fuel to support muscle activity. In the less intense fitness systems of ancient cultures, this inner resource has historically been considered therapeutic or medicinal. In therapeutic exercise such as Qigong and yoga, the metabolic energy produced is conserved so it can be circulated throughout the body as an internal healing resource— referred to in ancient China as "the inner medicine" or "the healer within."

In vigorous exercise this fuel or inner resource is spent to feed hungry muscles. In milder forms of exercise this resource is not completely expended, but is circulated internally and utilized as a reserve of self-repair factors to sustain and heal tissues, organs, and glands. At advanced levels of Qigong, these endogenous healing factors are intended to support optimal function of the body and brain, as well as longevity.

Increased oxygen availability from the practice of therapeutic exercise has at least three potential benefits:

• Support for energy production
• Cellular and intercellular hydration, as a by-product of energy metabolism
• Enhanced immune function

Energy production. The energy necessary to fuel cellular processes and regulate body heat is supplied through the interaction of oxygen and glucose. This metabolic reaction occurs in the presence of ATP (adenosine triphosphate), which serves as a catalyst. Oxygen from the air and glucose from food are catalyzed by ATP to release the biochemical energy (ergs) that accomplishes cellular processes throughout the body. The efficiency of this process is a critical factor in the ability of the human organism to sustain a high level of vitality. In Chinese research it has been observed that blood levels of ATP increase with therapeutic practices such as tai chi and Qigong (Wang et al., 1988). These types of therapeutic exercise efficiently activate the body's energy metabolism cycle (the Krebs cycle). The term Chi or Qi means "essential energy" in traditional Chinese medicine.

In the West, ancient medicine is generally characterized as unscientific. From this perspective, the Chinese "formula" for the transformation of energy (Qi) seems overly simplified. However, it can be equated with the metabolic formula for energy generation used in modern physiologic chemistry (see Table 20–1).

Hydration. A second critical benefit of increased oxygen metabolism is linked to the cellular production of water as a by-product of the energy production (Krebs) cycle (Shields, 1990). Through this process, water is incorporated into various types of fluids throughout the body including lymph, blood serum, cerebrospinal fluid, synovial fluid, tears, and perspiration. This internal hydration supports a range of immune and repair functions, particularly those associated with the lymph system. Both the production and circulation of this fluid are increased in therapeutic mind-body exercises.

Oxygen and immune function. The scientific evidence indicates that immune function is dependent on oxygen availability for the production of white blood cells, lymphocytes, T-cells, and killer cells. Mild to moderate exercise (including breathing exercise) is known to increase immune function. For example, mind-body exercise mobilizes the effect of natural killer (NK) cells (Pedersen et al., 1988), the production of white blood cells and lymphocytes (Lee et al., 2003a), and favorable T-cell ratios (Yao, 1989), and increase production of interleukin-4 (Carlson et al., 2003).

Table 20–1 Conceptualization of Energy Generation

Gu Qi (grain) energy derived from food	+ Kong Qi energy derived from air	<catalyst> Qigong, tai chi, massage, or acupuncture	= Zhen Qi life energy or vital force	
$C_6H_{12}O_6$ glucose	+ $6O_2$ air	<ATP> adenosine-triphosphate	= Ergs biological energy	+ $6CO_2$ + H_2O carbon dioxide and water

Source: Roger Jahnke, OMD, Santa Barbara, CA, © 2005.

Conversely, oxygen deficiency has been found to decrease immune function. In individuals who exercise so vigorously that they exceed the aerobic level and cross the anaerobic threshold, immune function is actually decreased (Brahmi et al., 1985).

Oxygen deficiency has also been associated with a range of disorders including cancer cell proliferation, confirmed in the research of Nobel Prize recipient Otto Warburg (1966). Numerous studies have associated reduced lung volume and oxygen exchange capacity with less resistance to disease and increased risk of mortality (Gordon & Kannel, 1970; Cullen et al., 1983). In studies of elderly patients, reduced oxygen metabolism was associated with immunodeficiency (Saltzman & Peterson, 1987). More recent clinical research has found that relaxation and breathing exercises, as in yoga, can be beneficial for patients with lung cancer (Corner et al., 1996).

LYMPH SYSTEM FUNCTION

The lymphatic system supports a range of immune and eliminative functions. We now know that physical activity and deepened breathing enhance circulation of the lymph and overall function of the lymphatic system. The practice of mild therapeutic exercise has

been found to activate a number of self-healing mechanisms:

- Lymph generation
- Lymph propulsion
- Support for immune function
- Circulation of cerebrospinal fluid
- The transport of nutrients

Lymph generation. A significant portion of the water in the body's fluids is produced by the same physiological process that generates the body's biological energy (Shields, 1980). Respiration is inherent in the function of every cell. For each gram of glucose metabolized, in excess of a gram of water is produced. In a moderately active human weighing about 155 pounds (70 kg), between 2100 cc and 2800 cc (454 kg) of lymph enters the blood stream daily at the subclavian vein through the thoracic duct (Shields, 1972). In a person engaging in moderate exercise, such as Qigong, yoga, or walking, up to 1400 cc of additional aerobically generated water can be produced daily. When an individual is participating in moderate physical activity, as much as one half of the water propelled through the lymph system is actually a by-product of cellular metabolism. Increased lymph flow accelerates the elimination of metabolic by-products and bacterial toxins, and increases the circulation of immune factors.

Lymph propulsion. The lymph has no distinct heart in humans; however, research has revealed that birds and reptiles have specific lymph hearts (Shields, 1980). In humans the lymph is propelled by a *composite lymph heart*, which involves a number of physiological functions working in coordination. The circulation of lymph against gravity is accomplished through contractions of skeletal muscles that propel the lymph through the lymphatic vessels, which contain one-way valves, in a unidirectional system. "Spontaneous, intrinsic pulsatory contraction of the peripheral lymphatic vessels" has been demonstrated in humans (Smith, 1949; Reimenschneider & Shields, 1981). Propulsion of lymph, initiated by breath and movement, occurs through several mechanisms including aerobic production of water and mechanical pumping of the lungs and diaphragm:

1. *Aerobic propulsion*—The aerobic production of water as a by-product of metabolism contributes to lymph propulsion mechanically. The fluid volume and holding capacity of the interstitial spaces between the cells throughout the body are naturally limited. As that limit is reached, the discharge and overflow of additional fluid due to oxygen metabolism drives the excess fluid into the terminal lymphatic vessels, the initial vascular openings of the lymphatic system (Yoffey & Courtice, 1970; Shields, 1980; Adair & Guyton, 1985; Olszewski, 1985). Like a cup that is running over, the interstitial space fills, building volume and pressure, and then flows over into the lymphatic system.

2. *Intrinsic smooth muscle contraction*—Within the lymphatic vessels and the peripheral lymphatic capillaries, the autonomic response of the smooth muscle tissue is to contract when filled and stretched to a certain tolerance (Olszewski, 1985).

This contraction moves the lymph forward through the lymphatic vessels with the assistance of one-way valves located throughout the system. This mechanism functions as a systemic pump which act in a manner somewhat similar to the contractions of the heart as it pumps the blood through the arteries (Bradbury & Cserr, 1985).

3. *Striated skeletal muscle contraction*—The effect of muscle contraction on lymph is one of the classic explanations for propulsion of the lymph (Adair & Guyton, 1985; Bradbury & Cserr, 1985). Even slight contractions of the skeletal muscles propel the lymph through this unidirectional system. In more dynamic aerobic exercise practices, the pumping of the skeletal muscles and compression of the tissues increases interstitial fluid flow. In Qigong and yoga this mechanism is triggered by relaxation and contraction of striated muscles through various patterns of movement entailed in these practices.

4. *Gravitational propulsion*—Any inversion of the limbs or lying in the prone position allows for a freer flow of lymph, due to the reduced force of gravity. This is one of the reasons elevation of the limbs is frequently prescribed for health problems characterized by a pooling of interstitial fluids (edema). In therapeutic exercise practices, many postures and movements create this mechanical dynamic in which the lymph is actually propelled by gravity. For example, in certain walking forms of Qigong (tai chi and Guo Lin Qigong are the most well-known), the individual moves all the limbs in beautiful circular motions, slowly and continuously, to activate this inversion mechanism. In yoga a number of the postures (asanas) invert the limbs; for example, in the head and shoulder stands the entire body is inverted.

5. *Mechanical lymph propulsion through the process of breathing*—One of the most powerful aspects of the lymph heart mechanism is the action of the lungs and diaphragm (Shields, 1980). Located below the diaphragm is a substantial and expanded portion of the lymphoid tissue known as the cisterna chyli. This cistern-like structure collects lymph from multiple incoming lymphatic vessels in an expanded balloonlike area of the vessel, which functions as a holding chamber. This large chamber holds the most substantial accumulation of lymph fluid anywhere in the body.

Another major repository of lymph fluid is concentrated in spongelike webs of lymphoid tissue located throughout the abdominal organs. With the downward movement of the diaphragm, particularly in deeper breathing, a wave of lymphatic fluid is compressed from the cisterna chyli and the spongelike webs of tissue. This lymph is moved forward in the system through the one-way valves in the lymphatic vessels, and propelled upward into the thoracic duct (Adair & Guyton, 1985).

The size of the thoracic duct is many times that of peripheral lymphatic vessels. Above the diaphragm, the thoracic duct collects lymph from the organs within the rib cage and also transfers lymph upward from lymph-rich areas in the abdominal cavity.

Through the activity of the lymph heart, lymphatic fluid is transported from all areas of the body. This fluid accumulates centrally and is then propelled by the diaphragm and the action of breathing in a final rush through the thoracic lymph duct into the blood at the subclavian vein. There it merges with blood to become a component of blood serum (Shields, 1980). The lymph-borne by-products of metabolism are then detoxified in the liver, filtered through the kidneys, and discharged from the body in bile and urine.

Lymph and immune function. The role of the lymphatic system in immune activity is well documented in the scientific literature (Drinker & Yoffey, 1941; Bradbury & Cserr, 1985; Olszewski, 1985; Van Rooijen, 1987). Lymph is an important medium for the transport and delivery of immune cells. Bone marrow, thymus, spleen, and lymph nodes are all involved in the interaction of the lymph and the immune system. Immune cells in the lymph originate from a number of sources:

- Transported to the lymph from the immunogenic tissues and organs (spleen, thymus, and bone marrow)
- Exchanged from blood circulating through the lymph nodes
- Formed within lymph nodes themselves (Bradbury & Cserr, 1985)

Greater numbers of these cells are diffused into the system when lymph flow or volume is increased (Adair & Guyton, 1985).

Lymph fluid contains a number of active immune agents including lymphocytes, antibodies, and macrophages (Olszewski, 1985). Both Qigong (Lee et al., 2004) and yoga (Lee et al., 2003a) have been found to increase levels of these immune components.

- Lymphocytes—The concentration and functionality of lymphocytes, monocytes, and neutrophils have been found to increase following Qigong training (Lee et al., 2003b, 2004). We also know that neurotransmitter receptor sites on lymphocytes interface with the neuropeptides that drive immune function (Smith et al., 1985). This reflects an important link between lymphatic function, neurochemistry, and neuroimmunity.

- Antibodies—The development of antibody-generating cells in lymph nodes has been delineated, localized, and quantified in the research (Van Rooijen, 1987). Research indicates that mind-body practices, such as meditation, can increase antibody titers (Davidson et al., 2003).

Circulation of cerebrospinal fluid. Historically, cerebrospinal fluid was perceived as a closed system. However, it has been acknowledged for several decades that cerebrospinal fluid (CSF) travels along the cranial and spinal nerves and into the perineural lymphatics (Kimber & Kimber, 1977; Bradbury & Cserr, 1985). The effects of pressure and posture on this flow suggest that certain types of movement, postural adjustment, and deep breathing activate the CSF/lymphatic interaction (Bradbury & Cserr, 1985).

Nutritive function. The importance of a broad availability of nutritional factors to the tissues is now widely accepted. However, the role of the lymphatic system in the delivery of nutrients was little known before 1972 (Shields, 1972). More recent findings indicate that the lacteals (specialized lymphatic vessels in the small intestine), have been found to mediate this nutritive mechanism (Adair & Guyton, 1985). *Chyle* is the milky fluid of nutrients absorbed from *chyme* in the small intestine; chyle is then passed into the circulating blood, as previously described. The effect of diaphragmatic movement during deep inspiration on the cysterna chyli, small intestine, and abdominal organs appears to significantly enhance nutrient absorption.

In traditional Asian systems of medicine and self-care, breath practice, deep breathing, and mild exercise are considered therapeutic. These techniques are enlisted to improve circulation and the absorption of micronutrients from therapeutic diet and medicinal herbal formulas. Therapeutic exercise maximizes the nutrifying potential of the lymphatic fluid by increasing volume and flow rates of the lymph. In individuals whose health is compromised, these functions can be enhanced through therapeutic exercise such as Qigong (Lee et al., 2003b, 2004).

BRAIN AND NERVOUS SYSTEM FUNCTION

Another of the goals of traditional healing systems is the restoration of *homeostasis*. In Chinese medicine the balance of forces or energies (yin and yang) serve as a metaphor for the equilibrium between the sympathetic and parasympathetic nervous systems. Much of the research on mind-body practice suggests that this equilibrium enhances nervous system function through a number of mechanisms, including:

- Initiation of the relaxation response
- Shift to a more beneficial neurotransmitter profile
- Increased microcirculation
- Support for neurological aspects of immune function
- Promotion of alpha/theta brain wave activity

Initiation of the relaxation response. When the autonomic nervous system is primarily in the sympathetic, adrenergic mode, the system is expending rather than conserving energy. In the extreme, this is the *fight or flight response* with increased heart rate and blood pressure, and more rapid breathing. Catabolic activity may also occur in this mode, associated with elevated cortisol levels (Girod & Brotman, 2004). The stress response, if protracted, can lead to adrenal exhaustion (Selye, 1978). Biological stress can also be a precursor to a number of functional disorders including depression, hypertension, arrthymias, immune deficiency, and inflammation (Benson, 1975).

Balancing sympathetic autonomic activity is the parasympathetic (cholinergic) phase of rest and repair, which is also described as the *relaxation response* (Benson, 1975). This conservative, anabolic repair phase of metabolism is characterized by decreased blood pressure and heart and breath rate. Activation of the parasympathetic mode can neutralize the potentially harmful effects of fight or flight overactivity.

The parasympathetic profile can be engaged consciously, initiated through deep, slow breathing coupled with the intention to relax (Benson, 1975). These are also the initiating steps for Qigong and yoga, which have been practiced for millennia in the East. It is well documented that traditional Asian health maintenance practices provide effective techniques for generating the relaxation response (Benson, 1975; Chang et al., 2004) and the biofeedback response (Green & Green, 1977), normalizing blood pressure and heart rate (Lee et al., 2003b).

Improved neurotransmitter profile. Certain characteristic profiles of neurotransmitter dominance are typically associated with mood states such as pain, anxiety, or depression (Lechin et al., 1996); other profiles are associated with positive emotions such as joy or comfort (Ornstein & Sobel, 1987; Rein et al., 1995). In patients suffering from chronic pain, profiles of increased norepinephrine, reduced cholinesterase, and depressed beta endorphins have been found to be characteristic (Lechin et al, 1996).

Research indicates that therapeutic mind-body exercise can moderate sympathetic function through the hypothalamus, promoting a more favorable neurotransmitter profile characterized by decreased norepinephrine, elevated cholinesterase and beta endorphins

(Brown et al., 1995), and elevated melatonin (Coker, 1999). The neurotransmitter profile of the predominantly parasympathetic and more anabolic environment has been documented to support several aspects of positive mental and physiological functioning:

- Research indicates that a parasympathetic profile tends to reduce depression (Lechin et al., 1996) and cravings for addictive substances (Kovacs & Telegdy, 1988).
- The relaxation response has been found to improve postoperative distress (Levin et al., 1987).
- Breathing and progressive muscle relaxation have been shown to have the potential to enhance control of acute pain (Heffline, 1990).
- The effects of Qigong have been found to increase norepinephrine and dopamine levels and to support pain management in conditions such as fibromyalgia (Creamer et al., 2000).

Increased microcirculation. During the stress response/fight or flight, the arterioles in the skin, muscles, and certain organs constrict. The systematic deactivation of sympathetic function in the relaxation response, typical in Qigong and yoga, promotes vasodilation with accompanying warmth of the surface of the skin and enhanced microcirculation (Wang et al., 2001). This can result in a significant increase in oxygen, nourishment, immune components, and self-healing factors. Biofeedback research has further confirmed an association between elevated skin temperature and the relaxation response (Green & Green, 1977). A number of studies from China have explored this microcirculatory mechanism and concluded that this effect can be promoted through Qigong and other health improvement practices (Wei et al., 1988; Xiu et al., 1988; Zhao et al., 1988).

Clinical research in China has further confirmed this effect (Zhao et al., 1988; Wang & Xu, 1991; Wang et al., 2001; Liu et al., 2003).

Neurological aspects of immune function. Research in the field of psychoneuroimmunology has demonstrated that mental and emotional states alter resistance to disease and infection (Ornstein & Sobel, 1987; Pert, 1997). Lymphocytes and macrophages have receptors for neurochemicals produced by the endocrine and nervous systems, the brain and the gut, including catecholamines, serotonin, and endorphins, as well as prostaglandins (Roszman et al., 1985; Ornstein & Sobel, 1987). These findings reflect the interface among brain function, the nervous system, and immune capability.

The hypothalamus appears to be a nexus for these various interrelated influences, since it contains 40 times more receptor sites than any other area of the brain or nervous system (Pert et al., 1985; Pert, 1986). A number of studies have confirmed the effects of the hypothalamus on immune function (Ornstein & Sobel, 1987). The practice of Qigong and yoga influences these relationships via the hypothalamus, by down-regulating sympathetic activity (Green & Green, 1977; Benson, 1975). Clinical research has corroborated the positive effect of therapeutic mind-body exercise on immune function (Shannahoff-Khalsa, 1988; Xiu et al., 1988).

Induction of alpha/theta brain wave activity. The intention to relax and the deepening of the breath are classic initiating actions that trigger the relaxation response. Research conducted on practitioners of yoga (Green & Green, 1977) and Qigong (Beijing College of Traditional Chinese Medicine, 1988) has shown that these practices elicit the relaxation response, with brain wave frequency toward the alpha range and in certain cases theta frequency. Alpha brain wave function is a result of relaxation and is conducive to healing. Common physiological effects of the alpha state include slowing the heart rate, reducing blood pressure, and increasing skin temperature and circulation.

In Qigong and yoga the goal is to achieve the lowest possible frequency of brain wave activity through the practice. In standing Qigong (which involves no movement), the quiescent meditative state has been found to promote the theta range of brain activity in EEG studies from China (Pan et al., 1994). However, the dynamic or moving methods of Qigong can also be effective in promoting alpha or theta states. In general, mind-body practices tend to promote favorable neurological activity.

CONCLUSION

Qigong, tai chi, yoga, and various other mind-body methods such as the Feldenkrais and Alexander methods have demonstrated viable potential for immune support, circulatory efficiency of blood and lymph, improved neurotransmitter profiles, and overall health enhancement. The efficacy of these techniques can be explained through our scientific understanding of the body's basic self-regulatory mechanisms. Each of the mechanisms discussed here produces internal resources historically referred to in Asia as inner medicine (the healer within). They also serve to balance body energy (Qi and prana). In Western terms we would describe this dynamic as up-regulating immune function and supporting neurotransmitter production. Now that we have ample physiological and clinical evidence to confirm the value of these practices, it is apparent that Qigong, yoga, and other forms of therapeutic exercise are practical, timely, and inexpensive tools for improving health and enhancing healing.

REFERENCES

Adair TJ, Guyton AC. Introduction to the lymphatic system. In: Johnston MG, ed. *Experimental Biology of the Lymphatic Circulation*. Amsterdam, Netherlands: Elsevier Science Publishers; 1985.

Beijing College of Traditional Chinese Medicine. *Proceedings of the First World Conference for Academic Exchange of Medical Qigong*. Beijing, China: Beijing College of Traditional Chinese Medicine; 1988.

Benson HR. *The Relaxation Response*. New York, NY: William Morrow and Company; 1975.

Blair SN, Kohl HW, Barlow CE III, Paffenbarger RS Jr, Gibbons LW, Macera CA. Changes in physical fitness and all-cause mortality. A prospective study of healthy and unhealthy men. *JAMA*. 1995;273: 1093–1098.

Bradbury MWB, Cserr HF. Drainage of cerebral interstitial fluid and of cerebral spinal fluid into lymphatics. In: Johnston MG, ed. *Experimental Biology of the Lymphatic Circulation*. Amsterdam, Netherlands: Elsevier Science Publishers; 1985.

Brahmi Z, Thomas JE, Park M, Park M, Dowdeswell IR. Effect of acute exercise on natural killer cell activity in trained and sedentary human subjects. *J Clin Immunol*. 1985;5:321–328.

Brown DR, Wang Y, Ward A, et al. Chronic psychological effects of exercise and exercise plus cognitive strategies. *Med Sci Sports Exerc*. 1995;27:765–775.

Carlson LE, Speca M, Patel KD, Goodey E. Mindfulness-based stress reduction in relation to quality of life, mood, symptoms of stress, and immune parameters in breast and prostate cancer outpatients. *Psychosom Med*. 2003;65:571–581.

Chang BH, Jones D, Hendricks A, Boehmer U, Locastro JS, Slawsky M. Relaxation response for Veterans Affairs patients with congestive heart failure: results from a qualitative study within a clinical trial. *Prev Cardiol*. 2004;7:64–70.

Coker KH. Meditation and prostate cancer: integrating a mind-body intervention with traditional therapies. *Semin Urol Oncol*. 1999;17:111–118.

Corner J, Plant H, A'Hern R, Bailey C. Nonpharmacological intervention for breathlessness in lung cancer. *Palliat Med*. 1996;10:299–305.

Creamer P, Singh BB, Hochberg MC, Berman BM. Sustained improvement produced by nonpharmacologic intervention in fibromyalgia: results of a pilot study. *Arthritis Care Res*. 2000;13:198–204.

Cullen K, Stenhouse NS, Wearne KL, Welborn TA. Multiple regression analysis of risk factors for cardiovascular disease and cancer mortality in Busselton, West Australia: a 13 year study. *J Chronic Dis*. 1983;36:371–377.

Davidson RJ, Kabat-Zinn J, Schumacher J. Alterations in brain and immune function produced by mindfulness meditation. *Psychosom Med*. 2003;65: 564–570.

Drinker CK, Yoffey JM. *Lymphatics, Lymph and Lymphoid Tissue*. Cambridge, MA: Harvard University Press; 1941.

Girod JP, Brotman DJ. Does altered glucocorticoid homeostasis increase cardiovascular risk? *Cardiovasc Res*. 2004;64:217–226.

Gordon T, Kannel WB. *The Framingham Study. An Epidemiological Investigation of Cardiovascular Disease*. Sections 1–26. Bethesda, MD: National Heart and Lung Institute; 1970.

Green E, Green A. *Beyond Biofeedback*. New York, NY: Delacorte Press; 1977.

Heffline MS. Exploring nursing interventions for acute pain in the postanesthesia care unit. *J Post Anesth Nurs*. 1990;5:321–328.

Jahnke, R. *The Healing Promise of Qi*. New York, NY: Contemporary Books/McGraw-Hill; 2002: chap 16.

Kimber DC, Kimber G. *Stackpole's Anatomy and Physiology*. 17th ed. New York, NY: Macmillan Publishing Co; 1977.

Klein PJ, Adams WD. Comprehensive therapeutic benefits of Taiji: a critical review. *Am J Phys Med Rehabil*. 2004;83:735–745.

Kovacs GL, Telegdy G. Hypothalamo-neurohypophyseal neuropeptides and experimental drug addiction. *Brain Res Bull*. 1988;20:893–895.

Lechin F, Van der Dijs B, Benaim M. Stress versus depression. *Prog Neuropsychopharmacol Biol Psychiatry*. 1996;20(6):899–950.

Lee MS, Huh HJ, Jeong SM. Effects of Qigong on immune cells. *Am J Chin Med*. 2003a;31:327–335.

Lee MS, Jeong SM, Kim YK. Qi-training enhances respiratory burst function and adhesive capacity of neutrophils in young adults: a preliminary study. *Am J Chin Med*. 2003b;31:141–148.

Lee MS, Kang CW, Ryu H, Moon SR. Endocrine and immune effects of Qi-training. *Int J Neurosci*. 2004;114(4):529–537.

Levin RF, Malloy GB, Hyman RB. Nursing management of postoperative pain: use of relaxation techniques with female cholecystectomy patients. *J Adv Nurs*. 1987;12(4):463–472.

Li JX, Hong Y, Chan KM. Tai chi: physiological characteristics and beneficial effects on health. *Br J Sports Med.* 2001;35:148–156.

Liu Y, Mimura K, Wang L, Ikuda K. Physiological benefits of 24-style Taijiquan exercise in middle-aged women. *J Physiol Anthropol Appl Human Sci.* 2003;22:219–225.

Olszewski WL. *Peripheral Lymph: Formation and Immune Function.* Boca Raton, FL: CRC Press; 1985.

Ornstein R, Sobel D. *The Healing Brain.* New York, NY: Simon and Schuster; 1987.

Oschman, James. *Energy Medicine.* New York, NY: Churchill Livingstone; 2000.

Pan W, Zhang L, Xia Y. The difference in EEG theta waves between concentrative and non-concentrative qigong states—a power spectrum and topographic mapping study. *J Tradit Chin Med.* 1994;14(3): 212–218.

Pedersen BK, Jackson JC, Cross RJ, Titus MJ, Markesbery WR, Brooks WH. Modulation of natural killer cell activity in the peripheral blood by physical exercise. *Scand J Immunol.* 1988;27: 673–678.

Pert CB. *Molecules of Emotion.* New York, NY: Scribner; 1997.

Pert CB. The wisdom of the receptors: neuropeptides, the emotions and the bodymind. *Advances.* 1986; 3:8–16.

Pert CB, Ruff MR, Weber RJ, Herkenham M. Neuropeptides and their receptors: a psychosomatic network. *J Immunol.* 1985;135:820–826.

Reimenschneider PA, Shields JW. Human central lymph propulsion. *JAMA.* 1981;246:2066–2067.

Rein G, Atkinson M, McCraty R. The physiological and psychological effects of compassion and anger. *J Advancement Med.* 1995;8(2):87–105.

Roszman TL, Jackson JC, Cross RJ, Titus MJ, Markesbery WR, Brooks WH. Neuroanatomic and neurotransmitter influences on immune function. *J Immunol.* 1985;135(suppl 2):769s–772s.

Saltzman RL, Peterson PK. Immunodeficiency of the elderly. *Rev Infect Dis.* 1987;9(suppl 2): 1127s–1139s.

Selye H. *The Stress of Life.* New York, NY: McGraw-Hill Book Co; 1978.

Shannahoff-Khalsa D. A contemporary view of life force biology: the merging of Kundalini Yoga and the neurosciences. In: Srinivasan TM, ed. *Energy Medicine Around the World.* Phoenix, AZ: Gabriel Press; 1988.

Shields JW. The aerobic production and central propulsion of lymph. In: Nishi M, ed. *Progress in Lymph-ology XII: Proceedings of the XIIth International Congress of Lymphology. Tokyo, Japan; September 1989.* Amsterdam, Netherlands: Elsevier Science, Ltd; 1990.

Shields JW. Central lymph propulsion. *J Int Soc Lymphol.* 1980;13:9–17.

Shields JW. *The Trophic Function of the Lymphoid Elements.* Springfield, IL: Thomas; 1972.

Smith EM, Harbour-McMenarnin D, Blalock JE. Lymphocyte production of endorphins and endorphin-mediated immunoregulatory activity. *J Immunol.* 1985;135:779–782.

Smith RO. Lymphatic contractility: a possible intrinsic mechanism of the lymph vessels for transport of lymph. *J Exp Med.* 1949;90:497.

Van Rooijen N. The "in situ" immune response in the lymph nodes: a review. *Anat Rec.* 1987;218: 359–364.

Wang C, Collet JP, Lau J. The effect of Tai Chi on health outcomes in patients with chronic conditions: a systematic review. *Arch Intern Med.* 2004;164: 493–501.

Wang CX, Xu DH. The beneficial effect of qigong on the ventricular function and microcirculation in deficiency of heart-energy hypertensive patients. *Zhong Xi Yi Jie He Za Zhi.* 1991;11:659–660, 644.

Wang JS, Lan C, Wong MK. Tai Chi Chuan training to enhance microcirculatory function in healthy elderly men. *Arch Phys Med Rehabil.* 2001;82:1176–1180.

Wang Z, et al. A preliminary study of the relationship between Qigong and energy metabolism: the changes of blood ATP content in Qigong masters in the Qigong state. In: *Proceedings of the First World Conference for Academic Exchange of Medical Qigong.* Beijing, China: Beijing College of Traditional Chinese Medicine; 1988.

Warburg O. *The prime cause and prevention of cancer.* Lindau Lecture. Wurzburg, Germany: Triltsch K; 1966.

Wei S, et al. An experimental research on the changes of blood volume in the brain and the changes of the heart rate in the Qigong and PSI state. In: *Proceedings of the First World Conference for Academic Exchange of Medical Qigong.* Beijing, China: Beijing College of Traditional Chinese Medicine; 1988.

Xiu R, et al. Studies of Qigong effect on the human body by the computerized synchronous system for macro and microcirculatory parameters measurement. In: *Proceedings of the First World Conference for Academic Exchange of Medical Qigong.* Beijing, China: Beijing College of Traditional Chinese Medicine; 1988.

Yao BS. A preliminary study on the changes of T-cell subsets in patients with aplastic anemia treated with qigong. *Zhong Xi Yi Jie He Za Zhi.* 1989;9:341–342, 324.

Yoffey JM, Courtice FC. *Lymphatics, Lymph and the Lymphomyeloid Complex.* London, UK: Academic Press; 1970.

Zhao B, et al. Effects of Qigong on cerebral blood flow (CBF) and extremitic blood flow (EBF). In: *Proceedings of the First World Conference for Academic Exchange of Medical Qigong.* Beijing, China: Beijing College of Traditional Chinese Medicine; 1988.

Part IV

Mind-Body Medicine

CHAPTER 21

Mind-Body Medicine

James S. Gordon, MD

OVERVIEW

The term "mind-body medicine" emphasizes not only the deep interconnection between mind and body, but also our capacity to have a positive influence on mental function, emotions, and physiology. In addition, mind-body medicine emphasizes a variety of psychological, mental, and physical techniques and approaches we can consciously use to effect change. This perspective acknowledges that what we do mentally and psychologically affects the body. It also affirms the reciprocal effects of physiology on the mind. Consequently, it is just as reasonable to consider physical activity such as yoga or jogging as mind-body techniques as it is to think of more traditional psychospiritual approaches such as meditation or relaxation.

Mind-body medicine now encompasses a wide range of techniques, some very ancient, such as meditation, guided imagery, hatha yoga, Qigong, and tai chi. Others are quite modern; for example, biofeedback, which depends on the use of technology and instrumentation to feed back information about the effects of our thoughts and emotions on aspects of our physical functioning, such as heart rate or blood pressure.

Traditional approaches to healing. Most mind-body techniques have been used in one form or another for thousands of years and are an integral aspect of the healing systems of many cultures. Guided imagery, for instance, is sometimes viewed as a modern technique that began with Jung, when in fact the use of imagery is an intrinsic aspect of the most ancient shamanic traditions. In this context, imagery techniques were applied to bring about a shift in the subject's consciousness or to promote healing.

Evidence-based techniques. We now have solid scientific evidence regarding the benefits of mind-body approaches from research performed over the last 40 years. The initial studies on biofeedback, performed by Neil Miller at Yale University and the Rockefeller Institute, were the first to document the fact that animals could exercise significant control over autonomic nervous system functions, which until then were believed to have been beyond conscious control—not only of animals but also of humans. Elmer and Alyce Green of the Menninger Institute were pioneers in the exploration of biofeedback with human beings. They began their work with the observation of yogis in India, whom

James S. Gordon, MD, is the founder and director of the Center for Mind-Body Medicine in Washington, DC, and is a clinical professor in the Departments of Psychiatry and Family Medicine at the Georgetown University School of Medicine. Dr. Gordon has served as chairman of the White House Commission on Complementary and Alternative Medicine Policy, as first chair of the Program Advisory Council of the NIH Office of Alternative Medicine, and as a research psychiatrist at the National Institute of Mental Health. A Harvard Medical School graduate and author/editor of 11 books and 120 articles, his recent work has focused on the development of comprehensive mind-body programs for health care professionals, for people with chronic health conditions, for traumatized children and families, and for those who serve them in war-torn areas such as Bosnia, Kosovo, Israel, and Gaza.

they discovered could exercise significant control over autonomic nervous functions such as heart rate and pain perception. The Greens documented this in India and then became involved in the development of biofeedback. Their research showed that people in the West (including people with very little or no training in this area) could begin to exercise some of the same control over the autonomic nervous system by using biofeedback equipment.

Psychoneuroimmunology. Since that time, there has been a great deal of research on guided imagery and various meditation and relaxation techniques, as well as yoga, tai chi, Qigong, and other approaches. The research has shown that these techniques can have direct effects not only on the autonomic nervous system, but also on endocrine and immune function. Some of the most interesting and challenging work performed in the last three decades has focused on the intimate connections among these three systems. These fields of investigation, known as psychoneuroimmunology and psychoneuroendocrinology, have been extremely important in revealing the therapeutic possibilities of mind-body techniques and have also served as catalysts for a fundamental reassessment of how the human body works.

In the West for much of the 20th century it was assumed that immune function operated with complete independence from other systems in the body and beyond the control of the central nervous system. The initial research on psychoneuroimmunology clearly demonstrated interaction between the central nervous system and immune system function. The work of Robert Ader at the University of Rochester also provided indications that the immune system can be conditioned, just as behavior can be conditioned. Solomon Snyder and Candace Pert at Johns Hopkins and the National Institute of Mental Health demonstrated that the same neurotransmitters that send messages to the central nervous system also send information to the immune and endocrine systems. Ader's work focused on the influence of patterns of thoughts and emotions on immune function while Solomon and Pert's established our biochemical understanding of communication between these systems.

This research makes it apparent that mind-body medicine makes very clear anatomic and physiologic sense. We now know that the cerebral cortex is intimately connected to the brain's limbic system, the seat of our most basic emotions, which is closely connected with parts of the brain concerned with imagery. These areas are also closely connected with the hypothalamus—the central switching and control station for the autonomic nervous system, as well as the immune and endocrine systems. The research on psychoneuroimmunology shows that these connections are not only reciprocal but multidirectional, and that they are hard wired into the body. They can be influenced and utilized with surprising ease.

Optimal self-care. One of the most important aspects of mind-body medicine is that it relies upon what individuals can do for themselves. This is one of the reasons it is so central to the creation of truly integrative health care. Mind-body medicine is fundamentally a form of self-care that can be taught to almost anyone of any educational level. These approaches and techniques can make profound changes in physiological functioning; for example, decreasing blood pressure, decreasing intensity and frequency of asthma attacks, supporting immune function, and improving mood. The use of mind-body techniques can also profoundly change the attitude people have towards their illness.

Instead of feeling like a victim of cancer, heart disease, or asthma, people have the opportunity to influence their thought patterns and emotions, their immune response, and their sense of well-being.

This empowerment represents one of the most significant trends in health care today. Complementary therapies are important, but a more fundamental aspect of integrative medicine is its emphasis on the shift from health care dependent on professionals to one in which people are partners with these providers and learn approaches that are central to their own healing.

In considering the range of techniques within mind-body medicine, it is important to look at each technique individually, matching that approach with the psychology of a specific patient. For example, some people enjoy working with imagery—using the imagination as a means of influencing the function of the autonomic or endocrine system. Imagery can also be an effective tool for problem solving or rehearsing one's response to a medical procedure. Other people are more attracted to techniques that involve technology or the use of biofeedback, which can also aid people in moderating the effects of stress.

Mind-body medicine in medical education. At present there are efforts underway to bring mind-body medicine into medical education. For example, the Center for Mind-Body Medicine is currently training faculty from more than a dozen medical schools in the United States to integrate this approach into the education of students. Our hope is that eventually all medical students will have the opportunity to learn this approach and experience its benefits. One of the most effective ways of teaching these techniques is through mind-body skills groups, which offer participants the practical experience of mind-body approaches and the opportunity to review the scientific support for them.

Learning about mind-body medicine is fundamentally experiential as well as intellectual. If one wants to become skilled in using these approaches, the techniques need to be experienced and practiced over a period of time. This is the only way to gain a sense of their potential effectiveness, the difficulties in using them, the range of situations in which they can be helpful, and how different approaches may be individualized for different people.

CHAPTER 22

Group Support

James Gordon, MD

OVERVIEW

In traditional societies, whenever someone is seriously ill, a family or an entire group is summoned to contribute to the healing. This is one of the most fundamental ways human beings have historically dealt with illness. It is understood that serious illness represents an imbalance between the individual and the community and that the participation of the whole community is required to restore balance. In contemporary society, we focus on disease and abnormalities within the individual, and have lost sight of the context of illness and the healing power of the group. However, in the past 50 years in the West, we have begun to recover that understanding.

One of the major influences on group work has been the success, beginning in the 1930s, of Alcoholics Anonymous and all the associated programs in which group support is of central importance. In the 1960s in psychiatry and mental health we also began to rediscover the power of group therapy, often based on psychodynamic principles, and support groups. As these two very different models have developed and been studied, it has become increasingly clear to large numbers of professionals and lay people that groups can play an important role in helping and healing people with various different types of conditions (Gordon, 1996).

Extensive research has been conducted over the last 30 years on the efficacy of group support in the healing process. These studies have focused on people with disorders that have included cancer, heart disease, HIV, chronic pain, and post-traumatic stress disorder. A variety of studies have shown that group support involving some form of self-expression, education, and basic mind/body techniques can significantly improve quality of life, enhance immune function, and lower levels of stress hormones (Gordon & Curtin, 2000).

The research of David Spiegel and colleagues, first published in *Lancet* (1989), is very important in our understanding of the effect of group theory in this area. He found that women with metastatic breast cancer who were in a supportive, expressive group not only felt better but actually lived longer. Both support group participants and those in the control group also received conventional state-of-the-art cancer therapy. Participants in these support groups lived on average 15 months longer than those in a control group. That study's methodology was replicated by Pam Goodwin et al. (2001) in Canada and published in the *New England Journal of Medicine*. Although she showed the same types of improvement in quality of life, there was no life extension.

It is not clear that this kind of supportive and expressive group support extends life, but it is clear that for the majority of participants, it improves psychological and physiological functioning (Targ & Levine, 2002). These studies also help us to identify some of the elements that distinguish the most successful groups (Deckro et al., 2002; Nakao et al., 2001).

A brief biography of Mr. Gordon appears in Chapter 21.

Additional research has been performed that may explain the discrepancy in life extension in Spiegel and Goodwin's studies. Alistair Cunningham in Canada uses a model very similar to the one we use at the Center for Mind-Body Medicine. It provides people in the group with a variety of approaches to self-awareness and self-care and encourages them to support their health independently of the group (Cunningham & Watson, 2004). Cunningham emphasizes the need to practice a variety of different techniques on one's own, such as journaling, meditation, guided imagery, movement, and exercise. These groups also emphasize the spiritual dimension of healing and the fact that life-threatening illness can be a catalyst for life transformations.

Cunningham's studies show that although average lifespan is not always extended, there is a subgroup of people in the groups who do live longer. These are people who literally take the group to heart—who get the message that their illness can be transformative. They actively engage in all aspects of group work and apply these approaches in their daily lives. It is apparent from Cunningham's work that benefits from group membership are far greater for those who commit themselves to the group and to practices that are rich with therapeutic and spiritual possibilities.

Other benefits of group support reported in the research include improved immune function in HIV positive people (Antoni, 1991), as well as decreased pain and improved mood in people with chronic pain (Davidson et al., 2003). Group support is also one of the central elements in Dean Ornish's programs for people with significant heart disease (Ornish et al., 1990). Ornish combines a low-fat, plant-based diet with exercise, yoga, and meditation. The small group format is the medium that makes it far easier for people to learn and successfully continue the diet, the meditation practice, and the exercise program.

At the Center for Mind-Body Medicine (CMBM), our training also emphasizes the importance of the group, the necessity for commitment to the group's work, and transformative opportunities that participation offers. The essential elements of CMBM's mind-body skills group have remained constant since we created this model more than a decade ago. We have offered these groups to patients with chronic and life-threatening illnesses, inner city high school teachers and students, and medical school faculty and students. These groups have also been provided to those traumatized by war and terrorism in the United States (New York City firefighters post 9/11), in the Balkans, and in the Middle East (Gordon et al., 2004).

ESSENTIAL ELEMENTS OF GROUP WORK

We have identified a number of basic elements associated with effective group process.

1. Ours is a meditative group. It is not a psychotherapy group, so it is not appropriate to analyze, interpret, or discuss the group process. Participants come into the group to learn specific techniques (meditation, guided imagery, and self-expression), but most importantly to learn to be present in the group—to be relaxed and aware, and become a witness to their moment-to-moment experience.

2. The group is a safe place. In the context of these groups, whatever you have to say, whoever you are, is accepted. For example, in working with people who have a health condition, such as cancer

or post-traumatic stress disorder, we do not push them to talk about their "presenting problem." They are allowed to be themselves and talk about whatever is important to them, as it comes up.

3. Respect is fundamental. Everyone has the full respect of the group leader, and everyone in the group is expected to respect one another. Sometimes in other groups, particular group members are allowed to dominate the conversation, set the emotional tone, or present themselves as more knowledgeable. The principle here is that everyone is equally worthy of respect and of being heard. It is the leader's function to make sure this occurs.

4. The groups are educational. In each group, we teach members new techniques they can apply in problem solving in their own lives (such as guided imagery and biofeedback techniques). In each 12-session series, there is also a balance between education and self-expression. Every didactic experience is followed by an opportunity to share that experience.

5. The groups are focused in the moment. The issue is not what happened to someone 20 years ago or even the roots of one's present problem, but what is occurring right now. We are always calling participants back to the present moment. How are you feeling now about what happened to you then, or about what someone else in the group just said?

6. The leader is both teacher and participant. He or she is the one who is teaching the techniques, making sure that group members respect one another, and assuring that the process of the group is respected. At the same time the leader is a real person, and is on the same journey as the members, toward greater self-awareness and better self-care. Consequently, when group members check in, so does the leader. If everyone is drawing, the leader does so as well and shares his or her own drawing and experience.

7. Everyone has the capacity to know themselves. We have observed that this is true even with very young children, as well as with adults who have little or no formal education. In essence, if people are willing to use their intuition and to participate in the exercises, they will learn what they need to know about themselves. In order to tap each person's intuitive wisdom, we use a variety of techniques including guided imagery, meditation, art, verbal exercises, and movement.

8. Everyone has the capacity to care for themselves. Although we hope there is compassion and love in the group, this is not a place where people are regarded or treated as helpless, no matter how troubled or ill they are. We believe that although they may need assistance from others at times, everyone can learn a great deal about taking care of and loving themselves.

9. The group is mutual. We are all mirrors for each other and everything that comes up for one person in the group can teach everyone else. If a participant is talking to the group about something she is experiencing (anxiety, for example), the task of other participants is not to help the speaker with her anxiety. Rather, their task is to look inside themselves and see what the other member's words are evoking in them—to learn from one another.

10. The group grows and changes. Some groups come together quickly, while others require more time. Certain people take on different roles within the group. People learn things in different phases, and the group keeps changing. Over time we find that people in the groups tend to develop a deep sense of compassion for each other. As a result, the quality of the group can change significantly over the course of time.

The group ideally balances flexibility and structure. Although we have a clear structure for each group, which includes the specific exercises and techniques that are taught, there is also room to respond to pressing concerns. If something distressing, poignant, or exciting emerges, it is important that the leader be open and flexible enough to create a space for that awareness to be experienced and then expressed.

RESEARCH AT THE CENTER FOR MIND-BODY MEDICINE

Group Work with Health Care Professionals

We now have research data on the effectiveness of our training programs for health care and mental health professionals in the United States. What we have found is that professionals who go through our training experience improvement in mood, in their sense of direction, and in their motivation for their work. They report decreased levels of stress and enhanced capacity to help themselves and others.

These findings also hold true for medical students with whom we have worked. For the past six years, we have trained medical school faculty from around the country. At Georgetown Medical School, which is our model program, we have now trained 18 faculty members to lead mind-body skills groups using the prototype developed at the Center for Mind-Body Medicine. The initial research on the effects of these groups on medical students is currently being prepared for publication. The findings indicate the same types of benefits reported by other health professionals and also show that the students feel less stressed about medical school and more enthusiastic about becoming physicians. They do better academically, with less effort, and feel more compassionate toward their classmates.

Group Work in Kosovo

In postwar Kosovo we have trained more than 900 health care practitioners and other professionals. In evaluations following the trainings, these professionals reported significant decreases in their levels of anxiety and rage, and improvements in mood and energy. The research (using standardized measures) also indicates decreases in levels of stress and increased optimism. Following their training, these professionals provide groups in their own community. Consequently, their experience and the training they have been given become available throughout the population.

In Kosovo we have been able to train not only health care professionals, but also teachers, leaders of women's groups, and religious leaders who work with children and families. What we have found is that people who are intelligent and willing to be open, self-critical, and thoughtful about themselves are able to do very good work as leaders of mind-body skills groups, with the support of some psychiatric or psychological consultation.

In the Suhareka region of Kosovo, we have carefully studied the work of high school teachers who received the training and subsequently provided group work to children who have post-traumatic stress disorder (Gordon et al., 2004). During the war in Kosovo, 90% of the homes in Suhareka were burned or bombed, and 20% of the high school students lost one or both parents. After the war, the high school teachers we trained offered our model to young people in their school, combining large-group instruction and small-group experiential work. In a pilot study, mind-body groups were provided for a period of 6 weeks to 139 students. Groups were conducted for 3 hours, once a week, and included 1-hour presentations on mind-body techniques and 2 hours of small group work. Levels of post-traumatic stress disorder in participating students decreased from approximately 85% to an average of 35% in only 6 weeks. Data from 250 more students are being analyzed and the results will be submitted for publication. A randomized, controlled trial of our method in Kosovo is also currently underway.

The program of training and clinical practice using our model is now central to the entire Kosovo community mental health system. It has also prompted major nongovernmental Israeli and Palestinian organizations (NGOs) to contact us. Trainings are currently underway and are being planned in the Middle East in collaboration with both Israeli and Palestinian governments as well as with NGOs.

Clinical Applications

Based on our experience in the United States, Kosovo, and elsewhere, we have come to believe that this type of group work can be of central importance to people with many kinds of debilitating disorders and for those affected by war and terrorism. Group work can also provide effective support for those who want to prevent illness and enhance their health. Our work at the Center for Mind-Body Medicine is to train as many professionals as possible to make these mind-body skills groups widely available in medical practices, health care institutions, and community-based programs. A major focus of our training is work with faculty of medical and other professional schools, so these skills can be incorporated into the training and clinical work of all health professionals. Our work is to make this training available to all those who are interested, and to publish research conducted on the training, and on the clinical and educational use of these groups.

Types of group structure. The group model can be structured to serve people with a particular condition, or those with a variety of illnesses and issues. It has proved useful with children and adults of all ages and a wide variety of diseases, disorders, and concerns. In some cases we have chosen to offer groups serving participants with a specific condition, whether it is cancer, HIV, depression, or post-traumatic stress. At other times we have provided groups focused on a range of conditions or issues—mixed groups in which there may be one person with cancer, another with heart disease, a medical student who has anxiety, a stressed-out executive, and an older person who is concerned about depression. The mixed groups serve people from all walks of life, with different needs, all participating in the same group.

Each approach has certain advantages. When we are working with patients who all have the same condition, they share common experiences and bond quickly. On the other hand, working with people who have different types of conditions and are of different ages gives everyone a new perspective. This kind of group seems to help participants shift the focus from their illnesses to their lives as a whole, from common response to illness to the common humanity of all participants. Both kinds of mind-body skills groups work extremely well.

Training. The Center for Mind-Body Medicine has trained more than 1100 health professionals in the United States. Currently, approximately a dozen medical schools are using this work. In Kosovo, everyone who works in the nationwide community mental health system has been trained in this approach. We are hoping to make this training available over the next two years to hundreds of leaders in the mental health field in Israel, Gaza, and the West Bank.

Reimbursement. Mind-body groups are reimbursed as group therapy. In some cases, physicians are able to include group work as a component of the treatment plan for individual patients with specific medical conditions.

Certification and referrals. The Center for Mind-Body Medicine offers a professional certification program that includes 124 hours of individual and group supervision and training. Approximately 100 people in the United States and abroad are currently certified. Information about these certified trainers, and referrals to them are available on the Center's Web site (www.cmbm.org).

The Center for Mind-Body Medicine offers the following training programs:

MindBodySpirit Medicine: This program is designed to guide health professionals in the integration of MindBodySpirit medicine in the clinical practice of medicine, psychology, social work, nursing, and all other healing professions.

Healing the Wounds of War: This is our international version of the *MindBodySpirit Medicine* program in which mental health professionals, teachers, and community leaders in war-torn areas are taught MindBodySpirit approaches in order to deal with the stress and trauma of the people in their communities. Our previous programs have been provided in South Africa, Mozambique, Bosnia, New York City (to firefighters), Kosovo, and presently, in Israel and Gaza.

For more information, see the Center's Web site: www.cmbm.org
Center for Mind-Body Medicine
5225 Connecticut Ave. NW, Suite 414
Washington, DC 20015
Phone: (202) 966-7338
Fax: (202) 363-7247

REFERENCES

Antoni MH. Psychosocial stressors and behavioral interactions in gay men with HIV infection. *Int Rev Psychiatry*. 1991;3:383–399.

Cunningham AJ, Watson K. How psychological therapy may prolong survival in cancer patients: new evidence and a simple theory. *Integr Cancer Ther*. 2004;3(3):214–229.

Davidson RJ, Kabat-Zinn J, Schumacher J, et al. Alterations in brain and immune function produced by mindfulness meditation. *Psychosom Med*. 2003;65(4):564–570.

Deckro GR, Ballinger KM, Hoyt M, et al. The evaluation of a mind/body intervention to reduce psychological distress and perceived stress in college students. *J Am Coll Health*. 2002;50(6):281–287.

Goodwin PJ, Leszcz M, Ennis M, et al. The effect of group psychosocial support on survival in metastatic breast cancer. *N Engl J Med*. 2001;345(24):1719–1726.

Gordon JS. *Manifesto for a New Medicine: Your Guide to Healing Partnerships and the Wise Use of Alternative Therapies*. Reading, MA: Addison-Wesley Publishing; 1996.

Gordon JS, Curtin S. *Comprehensive Cancer Care: Integrating Alternative, Complementary and Conventional Therapies*. Cambridge, MA: Perseus; 2000.

Gordon JS, Staples JK, Blyta A, Bytyqi M. Treatment of posttraumatic stress disorder in postwar Kosovo high school students using mind-body skills groups: a pilot study. *J Trauma Stress*. 2004;17(2):143–147.

Nakao M, Fricchione G, Myers P, et al. Anxiety is a good indicator for somatic symptom reduction through behavioral medicine intervention in a mind/body medicine clinic. *Psychother Psychosom*. 2001;70(1):50–57.

Ornish D, Brown SE, Scherwitz LW, et al. Can lifestyle changes reverse coronary heart disease? The Lifestyle Heart Trial. *Lancet*. 1990;336(8708):129–133.

Spiegel D, Bloom JR, Kraemer HC, Gottheil E. Effect of psychosocial treatment on survival of patients with metastatic breast cancer. *Lancet*. 1989;2(8668):888–891.

Targ EF, Levine EG. The efficacy of a mind-body-spirit group for women with breast cancer: a randomized controlled trial. *Gen Hosp Psychiatry*. 2002;24(4):238–248.

CHAPTER 23

Biofeedback Applications

Patricia Norris, PhD

INTRODUCTION

The term "biofeedback" was coined in 1969, when a group of psychologists and psychophysiologists formed the Biofeedback Research Society to study parameters of self-regulation with feedback produced by electronic instrumentation. Biofeedback provides objective information on the effects of thoughts and emotions on any internal physiologic process being monitored, such as brain wave patterns, activity of muscle neurons, or hand temperature.

Through instrumentation, the effects of conscious intentions are instantly available to conscious awareness. Physiological changes that can be enhanced through biofeedback include deep relaxation, reduced muscle tension, lowered heart rate, and improved circulation. Consequently, biofeedback can be utilized to promote greater control over physiological function in the management of conditions such as chronic pain, headaches, high blood pressure, anxiety, and numerous other disorders. Self-regulation acquired through biofeedback can play an important role in moderating illnesses such as asthma and chronic obstructive pulmonary disease, cancer, diabetes, and heart disease. This approach can also enhance the ability to establish peak performance and has been used with success in the training of everyone from Olympic athletes and NASA pilots to opera stars and concert pianists.

Self-regulation and voluntary control have a history that goes back thousands of years, with roots in both the East and the West. In contemporary applications, the use of electronic instrumentation, with the capacity to provide moment-by-moment biological feedback, enables us to examine the relationships between conscious and unconscious, voluntary and involuntary, and cortical and subcortical processes in our physiologic responses.

PRACTICAL IMPLICATIONS OF BIOFEEDBACK

In essence, biofeedback involves visualizing the desired outcome in tandem with any type of feedback that provides information on physiologic function such as muscle tension or heart rate, provided through instrumentation. Biofeedback demonstrates the potential to exert greater control over oneself, including functions normally thought to be beyond conscious control.

An example of the application of this approach is evident from research on the train-

Patricia Norris, PhD, has served as clinical director of the Menninger Center for Applied Psychophysiology and Biofeedback (1980–1994) and is currently clinical director at Life Sciences Institute of Mind-Body Health. Dr. Norris has been using biofeedback and psychophysiologic psychotherapy in her therapeutic work since 1970, in which she emphasizes integrating body, emotions, mind, and spirit; visualization and imagery; psychosynthesis; and psychoneuroimmunology. She has been president of the Biofeedback Society of America, now the Association for Applied Psychophysiology and Biofeedback (AAPB), president of the International Society for the Study of Subtle Energies and Energy Medicine, a faculty member of the Karl Menninger School of Psychiatry, and is currently an Associate Professor of Holos University Graduate Seminary, and an Adjunct Professor at Union Graduate School.

Courtesy of Patricia Norris, PhD, Topeka, Kansas.

ing of Russian Olympic athletes two decades ago. This particular study focused on the use of visualization in preparation for competition. (Visualization plays a role in many biofeedback therapeutic processes. In this study, visualization was used without biofeedback equipment. The feedback was ultimately the effectiveness of the method, reflected in athletic achievement.)

Researchers tracked the efficacy of various types of training in speed skating and other sports using a regimen that included a visualization component. For some of the athletes, preparation for competition included time spent *mentally* practicing their sport, while others focused solely on physical training. (In general, visualization for peak performance involves mentally seeing and feeling the activity being performed flawlessly, experiencing in the mind's eye every aspect of the performance step-by-step, minute-by-minute, in real time.)

One group participated in physical training 100% of the time, another spent 25% of its time on mental training and 75% on physical training, a third group spent 50% of its time on each type of training, and the fourth group spent 75% of its time on mental training and only 25% on physical training.

At the next Olympic trials, athletes in the fourth group, who spent 75% of their time on visualization, scored highest in performance and showed the greatest improvement. The next best was the group that spent half the time visualizing their performance, and the least successful group was the one that spent all the time in physical training. As a result of this type of research, the power of imagery is now acknowledged and applied in many professional sports (for example, *The Zen of Golf* and *The Inner Game of Tennis*).

To date, there have been thousands of studies on biofeedback, with a broad range of applications. One interesting example is work done at NASA over the past two decades with these techniques. Biofeedback is utilized to help astronauts overcome free-fall sickness that occurs due to lack of gravity. NASA also applies biofeedback in training to aid pilots in remaining mentally alert during flights. Researchers have developed a helmet with sensors that detect brain wave frequencies. If brain waves begin to slow, indicating distraction or lack of alertness, the pilot immediately receives this feedback. Pilots who fly at extremely high speeds must learn to remain exceptionally responsive and this device provides an effective form of biofeedback to achieve that.

CLINICAL APPLICATIONS

Safety and contraindications. Biofeedback is not generally contraindicated; in fact it can be an effective form of treatment for conditions such as hypertension or diabetes (see Table 23–1). However, for disorders of this type that require medication, it is essential that patients carefully monitor their physiological responses. That monitoring process is always a component of our training. In cases of hypertension, for example, we recommend that clients take their blood pressure daily, before and after their biofeedback session. When people practice biofeedback effectively, physiology such as blood pressure, blood sugar, or thyroid function may begin to normalize. As that occurs, the dosage of medication must be adjusted and gradually decreased in response to the improvement.

If an individual with hypertension was practicing biofeedback and not paying attention to his blood pressure, there would be the risk of overmedication. The same is true to some extent with diabetes; most diabetics who are practicing stress manage-

Table 23–1 Clinical Biofeedback Applications

Brain wave biofeedback, using the EEG (electroencephalogram) to measure and feed back brain wave frequencies

• ADD, ADHD (attention deficit disorder, attention deficit/hyperactivity disorder)	• Pain management
• Alcoholism	• Performance enhancement and personal growth
• Bipolar disorders	• Seizure management
• Closed head injury	• Sleep disorders
• Drug addiction	

Muscle biofeedback, using the EMG (electromyogram) to measure muscle activation, tension, and relaxation

• Bladder and bowel training and incontinence problems (using a pubococcygeal probe)	• Recovery from the effects of immobilization (e.g., being in a cast, extended bed rest)
• Muscle tension	• Spinal cord injuries
• Pain management	• Sports applications
• Partial paralysis	• Stroke
• Physical therapy applications	• Tension headaches

Heart rate using the EKG (electrocardiogram) and HeartMath (heart rate variability)

• Anger management	• Headaches
• Anxiety attacks	• Mood disorders
• Breath control	• Pain management

Temperature biofeedback, measuring skin temperature (hand temperature reflects sympathetic nervous system arousal/stress response)

• Anxiety	• IBS (irritable bowel syndrome)
• Cancer and immune system disorders such as ALS (amyotrophic lateral sclerosis), multiple sclerosis, and rheumatoid arthritis	• Migraine headaches
	• Pain management
	• Panic attacks
• Circulatory problems	• Performance enhancement
• Diabetic skin ulcers, neuropathy, and retinopathy	• Respiratory disorders
	• Sleep disorders
• Hypertension	• Stress disorders

ment need to closely monitor their blood sugar because their requirement for insulin could be reduced. Again, this monitoring is important in order to avoid the risk of overmedication.

Brainwave biofeedback with the EEG (electroencephalograph). This process involves learning to produce desired brainwave patterns to improve functioning. We have had very encouraging results working with clients in the management of addictions and alcoholism, attention deficit disorder and learning disabilities, bipolar disorders, chronic pain, head injuries, and other neurological conditions.

Some disorders are associated with a particular pattern of EEG brain waves. For example, people with attention deficit disorder usually display one of two patterns—either excessive slow wave activity associated with daydreaming, creativity, and poor focus of attention, or a pattern of low-amplitude waves in all frequencies associated with vigilance and distractibility. Both these brain wave patterns lead to difficulty with concentration.

In cases of attention deficit disorder and hyperactivity, behavior and learning patterns can be normalized by reducing excessive slow wave or low-amplitude activity. Each particular wave frequency is picked up through a sensor in an electrode, typically placed at the crown of the head. Feedback to the participant is provided through a computer with a display of an image or a graph (for example, an airplane that ascends when concentration is greater and descends as concentration is lost). This process tends to promote alertness and focus.

On the other hand, many clinical applications require increasing slow wave activity to quiet the mind. This approach is relevant to the management of pain conditions, drug addictions, and alcoholism, as well as psychotherapeutic applications. This is accomplished using alpha-theta brainwave training in which the participant reclines quietly, eyes closed, and focuses inward. Over time, he learns to increase the abundance of alpha and theta freqencies. Every time his brain produces the desired frequency, he simultaneously hears a tone that signifies that particular brain wave. For each individual certain internal sensations accompany the various brain wave frequencies. Biofeedback training enables one to recognize and reproduce those internal sensations of consciousness created by the specific frequencies. This approach can

be invaluable in the treatment of many pain disorders and a number of other conditions.

We have also used alpha-theta brain wave biofeedback in two pilot programs in the prison system with prisoners incarcerated for addictions, in an effort to reduce their recidivism after parole. The success rate in those programs after two years included no recidivism in 50% of participants (compared with a typical success rate of 10% to 20%) and no further use of addictive substances.

EMG (electromyogram) measuring muscle tension and relaxation. This training enables the participant to gain greater muscular control by providing feedback on the activation and relaxation of specific muscles. For example, EMG feedback can be useful for people who have been in a cast and developed excessive muscle tension and weakness due to immobilization. The process can train them to both relax and reactivate those muscles.

This type of biofeedback can also be used to teach relaxation. People who carry excessive physical tension can learn to relax tense muscles by experiencing what it feels like to become deeply relaxed. There is a general tendency to confuse immobilization with relaxation. For some individuals this may be the first time they have ever experienced genuine relaxation after a lifetime of fighting their bodies.

Continence training using the EMG. This method involves the use of a small device (a pubococcygeal probe) with a sensor that can pick up feedback from the pubococcygeal muscles (the muscles used in Kagel exercises). The feedback indicates the level of tension in those muscles, enabling the participant to increase or decrease muscle tension. In individuals with bowel or bladder incontinence due to neurological damage, the process can help restore normal control.

For example, one of our clients was a 6-year-old boy with spina bifida who experienced frequent episodes of fecal incontinence. He had just begun school and would often have to leave early because of these problems. He came to treatment with his father, who helped him become comfortable using the equipment (which is quite simple and minimally intrusive). As he became aware of that muscle through the feedback, and as his level of voluntary control over the muscle increased, he was able to resolve the incontinence. Within a few weeks, he had gained complete bowel control and had no further problems. He was proud of what he had accomplished and happy about being able to stay in school and lead a normal life.

Incontinence can be a major life issue and is frequently one of the primary reasons people are placed in nursing homes. The research suggests that perhaps 50% of these cases could be resolved with this type of biofeedback training; clinically we see that as many as 70% of these cases are resolved.

Heart-rate variability. There are several types of equipment that provide feedback on heart rate, including EKG (electrocardiogram) instrumentation and HeartMath software. We have used these applications for general stress reduction and anxiety, as well as arrythmias, hypertension, and PVC (premature ventricular contractions). When rapid heart rate is problematic, EKG biofeedback can be used to help clients learn to reduce their resting heart rate.

We also work with heart rate to improve breathing, using HeartMath computer software. Ideally, the heart accelerates when we inhale and slows as we exhale. During periods in which we are sitting quietly, breathing slowly and deeply, the pattern of a healthy heart will alternately accelerate and slow. Using the feedback from heart rate patterns, we can teach clients to retrain their breathing patterns.

Heart rate feedback can also be used to teach techniques for coping with stress. As we all know, heart rate changes significantly in response to negative or positive mental thoughts and imagery. Participants can use this feedback to identify the effects of their thoughts on their physiology. In general, visualization and imagery are very effective techniques for stress management. The use of imagery and biofeedback in tandem can play an important role in healing, since stress tends to exacerbate any condition. Biofeedback is a perfect vehicle for this training, because it measures and feeds back the effects of various types of visualization, thoughts, and emotions.

Temperature control. Temperature training through hand warming is probably the most important and widely used biofeedback tool in our work. We utilize this technique with almost all new clients to introduce the process of biofeedback and to provide them with an effective tool for stress reduction. This is a good initial step whether they are being seen for physiological or psychological disorders, post accident, or for cancer. Whenever anyone learns the self-mastery of biofeedback, they develop a different relationship with their body. They gain a greater sense of confidence, empowerment, and physiological competence that can help with healing or enhanced performance. Any physiological function that can be measured and indicated through feedback instrumentation can be applied in a process of learning to gain greater influence over one's physiology.

SELF-CARE: HAND WARMING AND STRESS REDUCTION

The hand-warming technique is an excellent method of self-care that can be learned by essentially anyone to manage stress, reduce anxiety, and promote relaxation. This is a very practical approach, since the only instrument required is a digital indoor–outdoor thermometer available at some hardware stores and on the Internet for $10 to $20. The technique is particularly relevant in times of stress or crisis situations. As mentioned, biofeedback is also useful to those with health disorders since stress can make any condition worse.

The following dialogue is the type of coaching we usually provide to teach the process of hand warming.

DIALOGUE FOR HAND-WARMING EXERCISE

The body is highly responsive to the focus of our attention. For example, if you think about your salivary glands and what it feels like when they release saliva under your tongue, almost inevitably that will occur. You do not even need to use any type of imagery such as thinking of the taste of lemon juice. The mental contact alone is sufficient.

To experience hand warming, place your hands together and focus on the sensation. As your hands become warmer, that lowers arousal and the stress response—the sympathetic mode—increasing your sense of calm and well-being. To begin the process, cup your fingers over your palms and then slip one set of fingers into the other, so they are crossed, the backs of the fingers of one hand touching the palm of the other. Let them curl gently together, becoming totally aware of the sensation. Experience your fingers and the way they feel—sense each finger—your little fingers and then your thumbs in terms of their vol-

ume and how they are bent. Then put your awareness on just the fingernail, first the full fingernail bed and then the area under the tip of your nail, where it meets the finger. Then hold your focus on the sensation of the fingertip for a moment.

Now move your attention gradually, placing your attention on one finger at a time. Let your awareness move down your little finger to the space between that finger and your ring finger. Then become very aware of the volume of the ring finger and the joints. Now shift your attention to the end of that finger and out to the fingertip and then to the space between the ring finger and the next finger. During this time one's temperature will almost always begin to rise. Work your way through this exercise quite slowly, spending perhaps five minutes or more.

Clinical Aspects of Hand Warming. During this mental exercise, using a digital thermometer as a feedback device, most people observe that their temperature begins to increase almost immediately. Temperature is conveyed through a small thermal sensor taped to their little finger, attached by wire to the thermometer, which has a digital display.

Indoor-outdoor thermometers can be adapted very nicely to this application. These thermometers include two thermal sensors—the outdoor sensor is at the end of a wire a number of feet long. The participant tapes the outdoor sensor onto a little finger and sets the thermometer to "outside." With that sensor in place one can go use the hand-warming exercise or monitor temperature in response to various emotions and thought processes.

The great value of this exercise is that it tends to lower arousal, shifting the autonomic nervous system out of the stress response. Once someone becomes skilled at this form of stress reduction, they have a resource they can draw on in times of crisis. For example, this method has applications in reducing anxiety and aborting panic attacks. People who are fearful of airplane travel can use hand warming during takeoff or when the plane encounters turbulence. We have had clients with panic disorder who can now freely travel by air without anxiety using this technique.

Thermal training can be used to moderate migraine headaches, high blood pressure, and irritable bowel syndrome. It is useful as a first step in becoming familiar with biofeedback before embarking on a more complex process such as brain wave biofeedback. This technique is also good for people who have circulation problems. The process of hand warming tends to increase circulation as the blood vessels relax: this phenomenon can occur in any area of the body by directing one's attention and applying this same process of awareness. Due to this effect, thermal feedback can be used by diabetics, for example, to improve circulation in their legs and feet, or for conditions such as diabetic ulcers or neuropathy.

The process is exceptionally easy to learn and apply. In fact, the longer one uses this technique, the easier it becomes. Those who have been using this method for some time find that when the need arises they are able to apply it with exceptional effectiveness. Yet even patients who have only been using the hand-warming technique for a week or two find it very helpful. Biofeedback training increases access to our greatest strengths and capacities—by coordinating the conscious mind with the unconscious.

RESOURCES

Training and licensure. There are two perspectives on the use of biofeedback by health care practitioners. One philosophy is

THEORY: THE PROCESS OF LEARNING

All our physical activity is initiated by mental imagery, although it is not always conscious or deliberate. Learning a skill consists of image, action, and feedback. Practicing a skill consists of repeating a performance until the feedback shows us that the action matches our mental image. This is obvious, for example, in developing skills in a sport such as basketball. When shooting baskets, the feedback is the visual information about where the ball goes.

Clearly, whether we are learning to walk, serve a tennis ball, balance a bike, or decrease tension headaches, we are not really training our body, we are training the brain. We are learning to gain cortical control over subcortical processes, to exert conscious control over the unconscious. Although this may seem obvious, in biofeedback this same process of learning is applied to physiologic functions normally thought of as beyond conscious control, such as heart rate or circulation. It is becoming clear that control of many internal body processes is just as easy to learn as riding a bike or shooting baskets.

Traditionally, the nervous system has been separated into the voluntary and involuntary nervous systems—the voluntary system operating the striate muscles in the arms, legs, and other areas, and the involuntary system operating smooth muscles such as those in the stomach, intestines, and blood vessels. We have long known that the smooth muscles of the heart, stomach, and intestines (functioning unconsciously) respond to thoughts and emotions such as fear. Biofeedback indicates that these same smooth muscles also respond to volition and images. The technology of biofeedback makes this knowledge and these abilities accessible to anyone interested in increasing voluntary control, to influence their physiological functioning in a measurable, verifiable evidence-based approach.

Source: Adapted from Norris P. Biofeedback, voluntary control, and human potential. *Biofeedback and Self-Regulation.* 1986;14(1): 3,6. © Plenum Publishing/Springer.

that professionals simply incorporate it into their practices if they are already licensed. For example, physicians, nurses, and psychologists provide biofeedback under their respective licenses. Many physical therapists also utilize biofeedback in their work. The other philosophy is that biofeedback therapy should be a profession in its own right, as a degreed program taught in universities, encompassing all the psychophysiology, neurophysiology, and other medical knowledge related to biofeedback treatment.

Certification. The Association for Applied Psychophysiology and Biofeedback (AAPB) offers an entire course of study. Certification is currently awarded by AAPB to trained health care professionals, and an examination to certify practitioners is provided through their affiliate, the Biofeedback Certification Institute of America (BCIA). Certified practitioners must also meet continuing medical education requirements and be recertified every 4 years. Individuals who maintain certification over an extensive period of time and have contributed significantly to the field may qualify to become senior fellows in biofeedback.

Skill set. A good biofeedback practitioner is one who educates the client, explains the process clearly, and provides them with a good understanding of the method. We have found that even young children can learn and use biofeedback and respond well if they are given an understanding of how and why the feedback works. In general this approach is most effective when the practitioner is realistic, yet supportive. Since the purpose is to teach self-regulation, it is also important that the practitioner use a client-centered approach and accommodate the learning style of the client.

Insurance coverage and clinical availability. Some insurance plans cover biofeedback services; coverage varies from plan to plan.

Sources of practitioner referrals. The AAPB annually publishes a directory of all members that can be used to find biofeedback therapists by location or by category of service. Additionally, in many states there are biofeedback societies that list all state members and their specialties. This is useful since some practitioners belong to the state society and not to the national society. AAPB also maintains a list of the resource person for each state society.

Many hospitals now have a biofeedback group or a complementary medicine program that offers biofeedback as part of their service. In most, major cities the yellow pages of the phone book also include the category "biofeedback," and the organizations listed can lead one further.

Specific resources. The temperature instrument described earlier for the hand-warming exercise can be purchased at local hardware stores or ordered from a hardware supply house, Harbor Freight. This is an "indoor–outdoor" digital thermometer, item #33080, available at www.harborfreight. com. The device costs approximately $10, and is ideal for learning and teaching temperature control.

CONCLUSION

One of the major functions of biofeedback is to allow greater access to the unconscious mind. The unconscious is vast—for each of us, it contains the memory of every moment of our lives. The unconscious is also the repository of all our skills. Consider learning to play the piano, for example. Initially, one must learn the notes and keys, but eventually playing the piano occurs unconsciously. At that point, one can play effortlessly and may even be talking and playing simultaneously because the skills have become so automatic and unconscious. Over time, like learning to play the piano, the processes of self-regulation can be taught and become automatic.

CHAPTER 24

HeartMath

Douglas Mann, MD

OVERVIEW

Heart rate variability biofeedback is a new technology that has broad-based applications in health improvement, rehabilitation, and performance enhancement. There are now several decades of research on the physiology of heart rate variability (HRV), and the area is well established as a credible field of scientific investigation. HRV is a measure of the naturally occurring beat-to-beat changes in heart rate. The analysis of HRV, or heart rhythms, is a noninvasive measure of neurocardiac function that reflects heart-brain interactions.

HRV feedback also reflects the activity of the sympathetic and parasympathetic branches of the autonomic nervous system and the synchronization between them, providing a window into the dynamics of the system as a whole (McCraty et al., 1995). This form of biofeedback utilizes heart rhythm coherence feedback training, which has been proven to support improvement in a wide variety of clinical conditions. HRV can be used to facilitate the maintenance of a physiologically efficient and regenerative inner state, characterized by reduced nervous system chaos and increased synchronization. This psychophysiological mode, termed *physiological coherence*, is conducive to

Douglas Mann, MD is professor of neurology at the University of North Carolina School of Medicine, Chapel Hill, medical director of the UNC Program on Integrative Medicine and the UNC Neurology Clinics, and principal investigator on several NIH grants.

healing and rehabilitation, emotional stability, and optimal performance (Tiller et al., 1996; McCraty & Atkinson, 2003).

Clinical applications of HeartMath techniques and accompanying software include a range of therapeutic interventions:

• Pain management
• Oncology pain and symptom management
• Migraine headaches
• Hypertension
• Stress reduction and breath control
• Self-care

HRV can be derived either from the electrocardiogram (ECG), using electrodes placed on the chest, or from pulse wave recordings using a plethysmographic optical sensor placed at the fingertip or earlobe. ECG recordings have the advantage of producing fewer movement-related artifacts. However, pulse wave recording devices also provide data suitable for most biofeedback applications, and, as they require no electrode hookup, are adaptable for use with personal computers. Consequently, they have applications in a wide variety of settings.

The Freeze-Framer, a heart rhythm coherence biofeedback system that utilizes computer software, developed by D. Childre and the Institute of HeartMath, a nonprofit research center in Boulder Creek, California. The Institute has developed and tested a number of biofeedback techniques for positive emotional refocusing and repatterning.

The Freeze-Framer software and associated techniques have been tested and validated in a number of clinical studies. Clinical applications of HeartMath are taught through on-site training to appropriate health care professionals.

Research. There is now a significant body of research on heart rate variability. A bibliography is included in this chapter and additional bibliography is available on the Institute's Web site at www.heartmath.org. Outcomes research using this approach by the HeartMath Research Center suggests significant, measurable improvement in clients who use the software regularly.

Contraindications. The primary contraindications are psychological instability or major mental disorders, similar to the contraindications for hypnosis or guided imagery. Although little has been published on this topic, we know clinically that patients who are schizophrenic or who have boundary issues may encounter difficulties with mind-body approaches. Otherwise there are no reported side effects. For example, blood pressure is not lowered excessively by the use of this biofeedback technique, and there are no physiological changes with potential for harm.

APPLICATIONS

Pain management. I use this software in my work as a neurologist in the University Headache Clinic at the University of North Carolina Department of Neurology in Chapel Hill. My primary academic focus is pain management. In the headache clinic we specifically treat patients with chronic and recurrent headaches, providing diagnostic assessment and pharmacological consultation. I use HeartMath techniques and Freeze-Framer software in conjunction with this practice.

Oncology pain and symptom management. We also use Freeze-Framer software in work with patients referred by the Oncology Department to the UNC Program on Integrative Medicine for pain management and general care using complementary approaches. Cancer typically evokes a significant level of anxiety, and the HeartMath approach provides a set of tools patients can use to manage that anxiety and increase their sense of equanimity. I encourage patients to buy the software and practice with it at home. The most effective approach involves frequent practice.

Migraine headaches of moderate intensity. Patients report that many of their moderate to mid-level intensity headaches can be managed through regular use of these techniques to such an extent that they can reduce their use of medication significantly. Patients seem to develop better pain management skills if they have a technique that can help them relax, such as guided imagery. Utilizing the Freeze-Framer software in conjunction with the other skills I teach them enables them to identify the onset of pre-pain symptoms and pain itself much earlier. These patients have developed a greater awareness of the cues that indicate their pain levels are increasing, and they can begin using these pain management techniques earlier in the course of their headaches. We coach them to recognize their initial symptoms and then interrupt the progression of pain by focusing on positive feelings, along with their breathing.

Severe migraines. Intense migraine headaches are often difficult to manage with mind-body techniques. However, this approach does provide a means of deamplifying the pain. Although it does not necessarily cut down on patients' use of medication or the duration of the headaches, they report that their quality of life is improved with use of these techniques. In addition, this approach enables patients to sleep a little better.

Hypertension. HeartMath techniques have also been used to manage stress on the job. One study, for example, evaluated workplace stress, blood pressure, and emotional health in hypertensive employees. At 3 months postintervention, those in the treatment group who used the HeartMath techniques and Freeze-Framer software exhibited a mean reduction of 10 mm Hg in systolic blood pressure and 6 mm Hg diastolic blood pressure, which are significant improvements.

Stress management. Research indicates that HeartMath techniques are viable interventions to reduce stress. For example, an emotional self-management program for stress that utilized heart rate variability training found that measures of physiological and psychological health improved, including DHEA–cortisol ratios.

Self-care. More than half the patients with whom we work purchase the software. They can obtain it directly from the Institute of HeartMath. Patients like the idea of being in control of the process, and they like the user-friendly design of the software. The interface is easy to navigate and understand. The cost to the patient is approximately $290 for the complete system, including the software, which can be used on any computer or laptop and includes a finger cradle with a pulse detector. The software provides feedback that can motivate and indirectly coach users in managing their thoughts and emotions.

PHYSIOLOGICAL EFFECTS OF HEARTMATH BIOFEEDBACK

Research on HRV and emotion has identified a distinct mode of physiological functioning that is frequently associated with the experience of sustained positive emotion: *physiological coherence.* Coherence is used here as an umbrella term to describe a physiological mode that encompasses a range of distinct but related phenomena, including synchronization, entrainment, and resonance, all of which emerge from the harmonious interactions of the body's subsystems. Research (McCraty et al., 1995; Tiller et al., 1996; McCraty & Atkinson, 2003) indicates that correlates of physiological coherence include:

- Increased synchronization between the two branches of the autonomic nervous system
- A shift in autonomic balance toward increased parasympathetic activity
- Increased heart-brain synchronization (alpha rhythms become more synchronized to heartbeat)
- Increased vascular resonance
- Entrainment among diverse physiological oscillatory systems (i.e., heart rhythm patterns, respiratory, craniosacral, and blood pressure rhythms)

The coherent mode is reflected by a smooth, sine wavelike pattern in the heart rhythms (heart rhythm coherence) and a narrow-band, high-amplitude peak in the low frequency range of the HRV power spectrum, at a frequency of about 0.1 hertz (Tiller et al., 1996; McCraty & Atkinson, 2003).

In terms of physiological functioning, the coherent mode confers a number of benefits to the system. These include:

- Resetting of baroreceptor sensitivity, which is involved in short-term blood pressure control and has also been found to be related to increased respiratory efficiency (Lehrer et al., 2003)
- Increased vagal afferent traffic, which is involved in the inhibition of pain signals and sympathetic outflow (McCraty & Atkinson, 2003)

- Increased cardiac output in conjunction with increased efficiency in fluid exchange, filtration, and absorption between the capillaries and tissues
- Increased ability of the cardiovascular system to adapt to circulatory requirements
- Increased temporal synchronization of cells throughout the body (Langhorst et al., 1984)

Greater coherence results in increased systemwide energy efficiency and metabolic energy savings. The physiological coherence mode has also been associated with psychological benefits such as increased emotional stability and improved cognitive performance (McCraty et al., 1998; McCraty et al., 1999; McCraty, 2002).

Sustaining Benefits of Coherence

Although physiological coherence is a natural state that can occur spontaneously, sustained episodes are generally rare. Although specific rhythmic breathing methods can induce coherence and entrainment for brief periods, cognitively directed, paced breathing is difficult for many people to maintain for more than about 1 minute. On the other hand, our findings indicate that individuals can maintain extended periods of physiological coherence by actively self-generating and sustaining a positive emotional state, such as appreciation, care, or love. Using a positive emotion to drive the coherent mode appears to excite the system at its resonant frequency, and coherence emerges naturally, making it easy to sustain for long periods (McCraty & Childre, in press).

Individuals using HeartMath coherence-building techniques have demonstrated:

- Significant reductions in stress, anxiety, and depression (McCraty et al., 1998;

McCraty et al., 1999; Luskin et al., 2002; McCraty et al., 2003; Rozman et al., 1996; McCraty et al., 2000; Barrios-Choplin et al., 1997)
- Enhancement of humoral immunity (Rein et al., 1995; McCraty et al., 1996)
- Increases in positive affect and attitudes, and an increased DHEA/cortisol ratio (McCraty et al., 1998)

As discussed, these interventions have also been shown to produce significant improvements in health status in various clinical populations.

CLINICAL PRACTICE

Overview

The biofeedback Freeze-Framer software provides visual displays that show the pattern of heart rate variability in real time. The user places an index finger in a cradle with a pulse sensor (or a sensor is placed on the ear lobe), so the information on the computer screen reflects actual physiologic responses moment to moment. The computer display clearly indicates when the pattern is coherent or disrupted. There is also a visual that indicates autonomic nervous system activity—in both the sympathetic nervous system (stress response) and parasympathetic system (rest and repair).

The sensitivity of heart rate variability to changes in emotional state has been demonstrated in recent research conducted at the Institute of HeartMath. Both positive and negative emotions can be readily distinguished by changes in heart rhythm patterns that are independent of heart rate. Specifically, during the experience of negative emotions such as anger, frustration, or anxiety, heart rhythms become more erratic or disordered, indicating less synchronization in the reciprocal action between the parasympathetic and sympathetic branches of the autonomic nervous system. In contrast, sustained positive emotions, such as appreciation, love, or compassion, are associated with a highly ordered or coherent pattern in the heart rhythms, reflecting greater synchronization between the two branches of the autonomic nervous system (McCraty et al., 1995; Tiller et al., 1996).

Techniques. There are a number of guided scenarios that use imagery and invoked emotions, which the user can explore to improve heart rate variability including:

- Breathing techniques that are used to improve the client's pattern of breathing and consequently heart rate variability coherence
- Highly positive images, words, or feelings associated with a favorite pet or a loved one, to visibly demonstrate the effects of emotions on heart rate variability
- Highly charged or negative thoughts, images, or words such as job pressure, financial worries, or some recent catastrophe, to demonstrate the disruptive effects of those emotions on cardiac function

Using the software. In monitoring one's own responses on the computer screen, the effects of positive or negative emotions produce a visible change in heart rhythm pattern. Patients are encouraged to focus on feelings they experience in a positive relationship with a pet, a child, or a loved one. Pets can provide an especially effective example and we may encourage participants to mentally review pleasant interactions with a favorite pet in substantial detail, such as being greeted by their dog or playing ball with him. Positive emotions can also be elicited by feeling a sense of gratitude for some aspect of one's life or simply for being alive. In response to positive thoughts or emotions, the monitor usually reflects increased input from the parasympathetic system and improved heart rate coherence.

The effects of negative emotions such as frustration or anger are also examined. Those responses tend to be less consistent. In some cases, if the patient has a great deal of positive momentum, even negative thoughts will not have a major effect, which is equally useful to know.

Anchoring positive emotions. Another technique involves "anchoring" positive emotions, using a psychological marker or anchor such as a word, visual symbol, or even a body movement such as pinching two fingers together to remind oneself of that positive emotional state. The use of an anchor enables patients to return to those thoughts or images quickly and re-create the positive experience associated with good systemic coherence, even in times of stress. The goal is to be able to re-create those positive feelings in their own lives at will, using breathing techniques and positive thoughts and emotions. It is important that patients practice these techniques at home on a regular basis. Once they understand how the software works and are comfortable using it, we individualize the sessions according to their specific needs.

Changing patterns of thinking. Patients are also trained in techniques for interrupting negative thoughts. The Freeze-Framer software provides feedback that can motivate and indirectly coach the user. This feedback can support them in changing catastrophising, negative thoughts into positive emotions of appreciation, compassion, and love of others. Seeing the effect of one's thoughts reflected in cardiac physiology is essentially like cognitive behavioral therapy in action.

Customizing the application. These techniques can also be used in conjunction with mind-body meditation and other types of biofeedback, which can provide a powerful multidimensional approach to self-regulation.

HRV biofeedback is straightforward to learn and use compared to other forms of biofeedback. Consequently, the use of Freeze-Framer software can facilitate rapid improvement. Since the instrumentation utilizes only a simple pulse sensor requiring no electrode hookup, it is versatile and can be used easily and effectively not only in clinical settings, but also in the patient's home, in the workplace, in schools, or while traveling. Its cost-effectiveness also makes it accessible to a greater number of people and in a wide range of applications. In relation to other biofeedback modalities, heart rate variability feedback is also more reflective of changes in emotional or psychological state, and thus is particularly relevant in applications where reducing stress and increasing emotional stability are critical.

Training. The clinical applications of the HeartMath techniques are taught in on-site training sessions at the Institute of HeartMath to licensed health care professionals. This process involves an intensive 3-day course preceded by approximately 3 months of practice and reading. Completing the course successfully provides an in-depth understanding of HeartMath techniques and advanced biofeedback applications and enables the practitioner to become licensed in HeartMath providership. More than a thousand professionals have been licensed to date.

For health care professionals who simply want to use the Freeze-Framer software with patients or clients, other types of support are available. For example, a weekly teleconference is held for practitioners on the clinical applications of HeartMath. Currently, thousands of health professionals are successfully using the software with patients and clients. Additional information about the resources and training available through HeartMath,

LLC, can be obtained on the Web at www.heartmath.com or by contacting the Health Professional Program for inquiries or support at (800) 450-9111.

Skill set. Health care professionals who are interested in communication tend to have a personal skill set that lends itself to this approach. The practitioner takes on a teaching or coaching role to assist patients in learning to use the software. This process involves observing and monitoring their interaction with the feedback system, educating them about stress and its effects on the body, and coaching them to be able to elicit positive responses in terms of mood.

Insurance coverage and reimbursement. Some insurance plans that cover biofeedback will cover HeartMath if it is identified as a biofeedback training technique. It is very similar to other types of biofeedback, with specific endpoints reflected in changes in the functioning of the heart.

Nonprofit research institute. HeartMath Institute can be contacted for information on the research or to discuss potential collaboration on a research study, The Institute is also a resource for educational programs and materials for teachers and students, K through 20. These programs are designed for children and young adults with ADD, impulse control, and emotional and anger management issues. Further information can be obtained from:

Institute of HeartMath and HeartMath
   Research Center
14700 West Park Avenue
Boulder Creek, CA 95006
Phone: (800) 450-9111 or (831) 338-8500
Fax: (831) 338-8504
Email: info@heartmath.org

The research Web site, which includes downloadable .pdf copies of research studies is available at: www.heartmath.org

RESOURCES

The Freeze-Framer software and related training materials can be purchased through HeartMath, LLC. This resource center also provides information on training and licensure for health care professionals in HeartMath stress reduction, as well as practitioner referrals and books and audio learning programs:

HeartMath, LLC
14700 West Park Avenue
Boulder Creek, CA 95006
Phone—Health Professional Program and practitioner referrals: (800) 450-9111 or (831) 338-8700
Fax: (831) 338-9861
Email: info@heartmath.com
Web site—information on providership and practitioner referrals: www.heartmath.com

HeartMath store, online. Both HeartMath Web sites serve as resources for software, CDs, and learning programs for software users, as well as books for consumers and health care professionals:
Web sites: heartmath.com and heartmath.org

Books. Publications of the Institute of HeartMath are available directly from the Institute and on the Web, for example, through Amazon.com.

Childre D, Cryer B. *From Chaos to Coherence*. Boulder Creek, CA: HeartMath Institute; 2000.

Childre D, Martin H. *The HeartMath Solution*. New York, NY: HarperSanFrancisco; 2000.

Childre D, Rozman D. *Overcoming Emotional Chaos*. San Diego, CA: Jodere Group; 2002.

Childre D, Rozman D, McKay M. *Transforming Anger*. Oakland, CA: New Harbinger Publications; 2003.

REFERENCES

Barrios-Choplin B, McCraty R, Cryer B. An inner quality approach to reducing stress and improving physical and emotional wellbeing at work. *Stress Med.* 1997;13(3):193–201.

Langhorst P, Schulz G, Lambertz M. Oscillating neuronal network of the "common brainstem system." In: Miyakawa K, Koepchen HP, Polosa C, eds. *Mechanisms of Blood Pressure Waves*. Tokyo, Japan: Scientific Societies Press; 1984: 257–275.

Lehrer PM, Vaschillo E, Vaschillo B, et al. Heart rate variability biofeedback increases baro-reflex gain and peak expiratory flow. *Psychosomatic Med.* 2003;65(5):796–805.

Luskin F, Reitz M, Newell K, Quinn TG, Haskell W. A controlled pilot study of stress management training of elderly patients with congestive heart failure. *Prev Cardiol.* 2002;5(4):168–172, 176.

McCraty R. Influence of cardiac afferent input on heart-brain synchronization and cognitive performance. *Int J Psychophysiol.* 2002;45(1–2):72–73.

McCraty R, Atkinson M. *Psychophysiological coherence*. Boulder Creek, CA: HeartMath Research Center, Institute of HeartMath. Publication 03-016; 2003.

McCraty R, Atkinson M, Lipsenthal L. *Emotional self-regulation program enhances psychological health and quality of life in patients with diabetes*. Boulder Creek, CA: HeartMath Research Center, Institute of HeartMath. Publication 00-006; 2000.

McCraty R, Atkinson M, Rein G, Watkins AD. Music enhances the effect of positive emotional states on salivary IgA. *Stress Med.* 1996;12(3):167–175.

McCraty R, Atkinson M, Tiller WA, Rein G, Watkins AD. The effects of emotions on short term heart rate variability using power spectrum analysis. *Am J Cardiol.* 1995;76(14):1089–1093.

McCraty R, Atkinson M, Tomasino D. Impact of a workplace stress reduction program on blood pressure and emotional health in hypertensive employees. *J Altern Complement Med.* 2003;9(3):355–369.

McCraty R, Atkinson M, Tomasino D, Goelitz J, Mayrovitz HN. The impact of an emotional self-management skills course on psychosocial functioning and autonomic recovery to stress in middle school children. *Integr Physiol Behav Sci.* 1999; 34(4):246–268.

McCraty R, Barrios-Choplin B, Rozman D, Atkinson M, Watkins AD. The impact of a new emotional self-management program on stress, emotions, heart rate variability, DHEA and cortisol. *Integr Physiol Behav Sci.* 1998;33(2):151–170.

McCraty R, Childre D. The grateful heart: the psychophysiology of appreciation. In: Emmons RA, McCullough ME, eds. *The Psychology of Gratitude.* New York, NY: Oxford University Press; in press.

McCraty R, Singer D. Heart rate variability: a measure of autonomic balance and physiological coherence. In: Watkins A, Childre D, eds. *HeartMath: The Science of Emotional Sovereignty.* Amsterdam, the Netherlands: Harwood Academic Publishers; in press.

Rein G, Atkinson M, McCraty R. The physiological and psychological effects of compassion and anger. *J Advancement Med.* 1995;8(2):87–105.

Rozman D, Whitaker R, Beckman R, Jones D. A pilot intervention program which reduces psychological symptomatology in individuals with human immunodeficiency virus. *Complement Ther Med.* 1996;4(4):226–232.

Tiller WA, McCraty R, Atkinson M. Cardiac coherence: a new, noninvasive measure of autonomic nervous system order. *Altern Ther Health Med.* 1996;2(1):52–65.

CHAPTER 25

Health Coaching

Debra Harris, RN, BSN, and Rebecca McLean

OVERVIEW

Health coaching is one of the more effective advances today in preventive medicine and disease management. Analogous to the personal trainer or life coach, the health coach supports clients in achieving specific health goals. This approach may also incorporate life coaching, health education, risk management, or support for the management of chronic illness.

Coaching occurs initially in weekly sessions that provide a behavioral framework for lifestyle change or medical compliance. The process may involve one-on-one coaching or group support to assist clients in setting goals and working toward them. Change is defined in achievable steps taken by the client, tracked and reinforced through weekly meetings in person or by phone.

Role of the health coach. The health coach can serve as a mentor to the client in situations in which behavioral change is important. Physicians usually do not have the time to see their patients on a weekly basis for the behavioral support and structure often necessary to achieve medical compliance. Many patients realize that they need a new approach, but may not know where to begin. Coaching can provide support change in a number of areas:

- Behavioral/lifestyle change
- Risk reduction (diet and exercise programs, smoking cessation)
- Addressing addictive behaviors
- Medical management or compliance
- Behavioral management of disease and chronic conditions

The health coach fills a unique niche within health care that can be complementary to both case management and counseling. The function of case management has historically been to coordinate referrals made by the physician and to follow up on care. However, case managers do not typically intervene in terms of lifestyle changes. In a counseling model, the goal is to help the client gain greater understanding and insight. In contrast to both these approaches, the

Debra Harris and Rebecca McLean are among the initial developers of the health coaching concept in the United States.

Debra Harris, RN, has 20 years of experience in clinical nursing as both staff nurse and in various management positions. For the past decade, Ms. Harris has served as program coordinator for patient-care projects at St. Charles Medical Center, and as program director of the Center for Health and Learning, developing hospital-based educational programs for physicians, staff, and the community. She also has extensive experience as a health coach and facilitator and as cofounder of Harris 2 Consulting provides coaching, training, and consulting.

Rebecca McLean is national director of the Circle of Life Coaches Training and Certification, which prepares health coaches for one-on-one coaching, and facilitators for wellness support groups in hospitals, clinics, parishes, agencies, and businesses. In 1983, she cofounded Health Action Clinic and Consulting, an interdisciplinary health care organization. Over the past two decades, Ms. McLean has facilitated thousands of people with heart disease, cancer, diabetes, HIV, and other chronic disorders in both group sessions and individual coaching.

Courtesy of Debra Harris, RN, Bend, Oregon, and Rebecca McLean, Santa Barbara, California.

health coach works within a structured format to support behavioral change.

Interfacing with Practitioners

Referrals from physicians. In the context of hospital-based work, a health coach's caseload may be as much as 90% physician-referred. For a private health coach, 80% to 100% of clients may be self-referred. Orders from the physician may be in the form of a prescription, written orders, or a verbal request. Typically, the referral is broadly worded within the context of a particular health issue, for example, "needs exercise and diet" or "needs stress reduction."

The role of the coach varies depending on his or her training and the setting. Coaches with broad training and experience in group work may facilitate support groups. Coaches trained as nurses are qualified to provide medical and case management. Sessions focus on the client's most critical health risk factor (for example, exercise to prevent diabetes).

Readiness for change. The initial assessment process involves identifying the client's level of motivation and readiness for change. Frequently, clients believe they are ready to change until they begin to fully understand what is required. The challenges include breaking old habits, trying new behaviors, fear of the unknown, and taking risks. The most effective coaches are those who begin the process by helping clients discover their own strengths. The most effective clients are those who want to take an active role in their own life and are willing to put effort into improving their health.

Contraindications. Patients who are not proactive on their own behalf tend to have the least success in a coaching program. On the other hand, it is always important to create the opportunity for success. In some cases, clients may have been in a particular circumstance for so long they no longer remember that there is another way. These people are most likely to benefit from a process in which they gain a vision of the potential for change and how their situation could be different. Ultimately, successful coaching requires that the client be both motivated to make changes and supported in creating appropriate action steps.

THE COACHING PROCESS

The Initial Session

The first meeting is typically for an hour and a half and involves a process of assessment and goal setting. Meetings are initially held in person because personal contact can establish greater rapport between coach and client and tends to be more supportive. In the first or second session, the client identifies one to three goals on which they want to begin work. Subsequent meetings typically occur weekly, in person or on the phone, either one-on-one or in a group setting, depending on the needs and desires of the client. After the initial assessment, sessions are usually 30 to 60 minutes long and involve check-ins on the goals of the preceding week and goal setting for the coming week. Typically, the coaching process includes:

1. Assessment to affirm strengths and identify challenges
2. Developing a realistic action plan
3. Implementing the plan
4. Assessing progress and modifying the plan
5. Reinforcing success

1. Assessment

Affirming the client's strengths. Coaching typically begins by identifying the clients' strengths to build their confidence, empower them, and support their efforts toward change. Clients who have experienced a life crisis or chronic illness tend to forget their strengths. Over time, they may come to identify with their problems and lose their sense of self. One of the most important aspects of this work is to reconnect the individual with their inner strength and motivation. The encouragement of the coach provides an additional source of substance, that can enable the client to make positive changes. Drawing on this emotional sustenance, clients frequently expand their own personal support systems.

Coaching also involves asking good questions—the better the question, the better the response. That process places the coach in a more neutral position, lessening the degree to which they are directive. It enables them to refer the process and the decision making back to the client. The goal of these questions is to open new paradigms of thinking and provide a subtle form of feedback.

Identifying challenges. Once the assessment is complete and the client has gained a better sense of their strengths, the next step is to identify habits or other barriers that may be impeding their progress. The core work of coaching helps the client gain an increased understanding of the emotional drivers of his or her behavior. Although lifestyle is certainly an issue, there is often an emotional component that contributes to lifestyle choices.

The process of identifying the challenges or barriers to change is usually where the most important health coaching work occurs. Progressing toward the goal is relatively easy once this step has been taken. A variety of personal awareness exercises are used to help the client identify barriers and how they get in the way of making healthy choices. For example, the Event Perception Model can be used to expand the client's awareness of how frequently they overreact to stress, out of habit. Those negative reactions lead to habits

of behavior that can remain long after the initial trigger event. One of the coach's primary roles is to help the client recognize obsolete perceptions which tend to get in the way of more positive behavior.

Coaching or group support always involves a greater understanding of day-to-day habits and thought patterns—and the impact of these habits on health. Most of us tend to run on automatic a surprising amount of the time. Although this provides a certain degree of efficiency, it can also be a major deterrent to making healthy choices. Once a client gains a clearer understanding of how and why their situation has developed, they realize they can do something about it. Behaviors that are maintained simply by force of habit *can* be modified. This focus on the role of habits tends to relieve a great deal of guilt and provides clients with an enhanced sense of control and confidence. Once current habit patterns are recognized, coach and client can begin mapping out incremental steps for change, enabling the client to create healthier new patterns of positive thinking, new habits, and self-enhancing behaviors.

2. Developing a Realistic Action Plan

Clarifying goals. The first step in goal setting is to help the client identify what he or she wishes to accomplish. Clients who are referred by a physician or health care practitioner work within goals that may already be predefined to some degree. Even within this framework, the client always has the opportunity to choose how they want to approach the goal.

The health coach asks defining questions. The task is to identify or refine the goals more specifically and individualize them to the client. What do they want or need to do differently? What part of their life calls for attention? Restoring balance may involve not only physical health, but also mental, emotional, and spiritual aspects of life. Although the focus is on health, the process could involve anything from changing eating or working habits to changing relationships.

Creating an action plan. When the goals have been identified, the client and health coach develop a personal action plan consisting of the steps the client will take to achieve these goals. Based on insights gained in the assessment process, the client then develops short-term objectives, working with the coach to create a practical, realistic plan. These objectives focus on incremental, achievable action steps to move the client toward his goal and build his confidence. By defining the goal in achievable steps, the chance of failure is minimized and success is more attainable.

3. Implementing the Plan

Tracking progress. Once clients begin their program, coaching involves tracking progress and rethinking strategies that are not working. At these sessions, the coach asks questions such as:

- Was there an opportunity to take the action step?
- If the step was taken, what was successful?
- What worked and why?
- What did the client learn?
- At this point, the coach reinforces those successes—both the achievements and the learning.
- The next question is, What does the client want to do now—what is the next step?

Identifying critical success factors. This review process focuses on what was most effective:

- What enabled the client to accomplish the goal?

- What creates success for that particular client? This information begins to clarify critical success factors for clients, providing greater insight into their process.
- What challenges did the client overcome?
- Were there frustrations or disappointments and how were they handled?
- What were the key factors that supported success: for example, structure, support, energy, resources, or mindset?
- How can this knowledge be applied to the next step?

4. Assessing Progress and Modifying the Plan

When a specific objective is not met, the coach and client work collaboratively to identify key issues and develop new strategies for success:

- If the client did not take the next step, what got in the way? This phase involves exploring what was learned and acknowledging that learning as a form of progress.
- Should the action steps be smaller?
- Is there need for additional resources?
- Should the goal be changed?
- If the client took the step and it did not work, why?
- In either case, what was learned? Again, the increased understanding is acknowledged as a form of progress.
- Should the goal be redefined or is this the wrong goal?
- What type of support would have been helpful and what does the client want for the coming week?

Through this process, the client can continue to move toward the goal. One step at a time, a track record of successes is built and confidence is gained. Coaching provides a continuous improvement process: the system is designed to be fail-safe.

5. Reinforcing Success

From the very first session, we focus on strengths—this reinforces clients' belief in themselves, so they will be more motivated to continue the process of change:

- We affirm strengths at every opportunity, naming the qualities that enabled the client to take the next step, for example, the courage to break an old habit or implement a new behavior.
- We note and affirm all victories, even the small ones. This also teaches clients to reinforce their *own* successes.
- We acknowledge all learning as progress.

Positive self-talk is another important component of this work. An exploration of self-talk and inner dialogue provides an opportunity for clients to get in touch with the kind of messages they are giving themselves. Is there inner support for positive change? What can the client do to move forward to the next step? An evaluation of self-talk provides an opportunity to minimize negativity and self-defeating messages.

THE BASIS FOR LONG-TERM CHANGE

The coaching process also extends beyond immediate change—it addresses not only how to create change, but also how to sustain it. Coaching supports people in achieving clarity about what they value and how to live a life that is in greater alignment with those values. Clients gain insight into the effects of various habits and behaviors on their health. This increased awareness frequently evolves into a commitment to greater quality of life and health, which could involve exercising more, managing stress, or improving their relationships.

MAINTAINING A NEW LIFESTYLE

When the client is ready to transition into the next phase, coach and client develop a long-term plan for maintaining the changes that have been made and continuing the process. The coach provides support and structure for change, using behavioral approaches confirmed in the research literature and through clinical experience. A long-term program may also include periodic work with the health coach, other health professionals, a support group, a personal trainer, or peer counseling.

Ongoing progress and change are supported by:

- Continued use of the tools and resources from coaching
- Utilizing a personal tracking system
- Rewarding and reinforcing accomplishments
- Identifying the need for support and knowing how to enlist it
- Sharing the process with an accountability partner
- Participating in a support group
- Understanding relapse and how to manage it
- Engaging other support as needed or desired

RESOURCES

Self-care. Coaches frequently encourage clients to use support groups because they are an inexpensive venue for support, community, and access to resources. Many clients also opt to remain in one-on-one coaching. The combination of group work and coaching means that clients can have individual support and the opportunity to participate in a group. For many, this enables them to stay in the process longer because there is less expense. In one model of group work, developed at Stanford

University, clients participate in a facilitated group that transitions into a peer-support group without a leader. Participants continue to draw on support in the group in lieu of individual coaching sessions. Some clients also choose to use a one-on-one peer-facilitated model, working on an ongoing basis with one other person as a source of accountability and ongoing support.

Training and licensure. Instruction on health coaching is currently available through private training venues (see Health Coaching Resources). Life coaching is offered through a number of private training institutes. There is currently no national association for health coaching.

Skill set. It is vital that the coach encourage participants to make the personal improvement process their own. The goal is always empowerment. Facilitators who see themselves as catalysts of change rather than as experts are likely to be more effective in enabling people to grow and heal.

Insurance coverage and reimbursement. In the hospital environment, services may be covered by insurance when they are associated with a specific clinical service such as a symptom-reduction program. However, when a coach is not working under the direct supervision of a physician or a health care facility, these services are not typically reimbursed by insurance. Clients who are self-referred pay out-of-pocket. Private-pay services limit access based on income. However, the positive aspect of private pay is that clients are highly motivated.

HEALTH COACHING RESOURCES

Health Action

Circle of Life Coaches Training and Certification
Rebecca McLean, Director

243 Pebble Beach Drive
Santa Barbara, CA 93117
Phone: (805) 685-4670
Fax: (805) 685-4710
Email: rmclean@west.net
Web site: www.circleoflife.net

Services include training of one-to-one coaches and group facilitators; providing the Circle of Life experience for conferences and retreats for groups, departments, and boards; and consulting to design complementary and integrative medicine programs. Referrals are available at http:www.circleoflife.net for nationally certified Circle of Life wellness coaches with their location, specialty, and credentials. See the Health Action Client List at http://www.HealthAction.net.

Circle of Life Publications

McLean R, Annich L, Jahnke, R. *The Circle of Life Facilitator Training Manual.* 5th ed. Santa Barbara, CA: Health Action; 2005. This manual provides the knowledge base and skills training for Circle of Life coaching and group support.

McLean R, Jahnke R. *The Circle of Life, Personal Health Assessment & Self Energizing System, Participants Guide.* 5th ed. Santa Barbara, CA: Health Action; 2005. This guide provides the participant's tool set and guide book for Circle of Life coaching and group support.

McLean R. *Circle of Life Coaching/Facilitator Training CDs* (2 CDs). Santa Barbara, CA: Health Action; 2004. These CDs offer guidance on facilitating and coaching others in the Circle of Life health and life coaching process.

McLean R. *Circle of Life Tools for Health and Wellness CDs* (3 CDs). Santa Barbara, CA: Health Action; 2004. Five processes and exercises for coaches, facilitators, and participants are described in these three CDs.

Harris 2 Consulting

Debra Harris, RN
Michael Harris, MD
86 SW Century Drive, MB # 169
Bend, OR 97702

Phone: (541) 480-7498
Email: mndrharris@bendcable.com
Web site: www.harris2consulting.com

Harris 2 Consulting provides individual health coaching and resources for individuals and businesses. Services include on-site executive coaching in leadership and communication skills, corporate/workplace health presentations, health screening, integrative program development, and executive wellness retreats. Personal health coaching is designed to serve clients with needs that range from performance enhancement to chronic illness.

GENERAL COACHING RESOURCES

Training

International Coach Federation
1444 "I" Street NW, Suite 700
Washington, DC 20005
Phone: (888) 423-3131 or (202) 712-9039
Fax: (888) 329-2423 or (202) 216-9646
Web site: www.coachfederation.org
Email: icfoffice@coachfederation.org

The International Coach Federation is the largest nonprofit professional association of personal and business coaches worldwide with more than 7000 members and over 132 chapters in 30 countries. The ICF provides credentialing for coaches and referrals to training institutions.

The Coaches Training Institute
1879 Second Street
San Rafael, CA 94901
Phone: (800) 691-6008 or (415) 451-6000
Fax: (415) 460-6878
Email: CTIinfo@thecoaches.com
Web site: www.thecoaches.com

The Coaches Training Institute (CTI) is the largest nonprofit educational institution devoted exclusively to the training of coaches. In the United States, CTI currently offers coaches training for personal/life coaching, and executive/corporate coaching in six major American cities. International affiliates are located in the United Kingdom, Norway, Japan, Australia, and New Zealand.

Leadership Institute of Seattle
14506 Juanita Drive NE
Kenmore, WA 98028-4966
Phone: (800) 789-LIOS or (425) 939-8100
Fax: (425) 939-8110
Web site: www.lios.org

The Leadership Institute of Seattle (LIOS) provides training in leadership skills and personal growth for leaders, consultants, and counselors. The mission of LIOS is to teach people how to lead with integrity, use power ethically, collaborate successfully, and use personal awareness to affect change in others. This type of training is useful in helping coaches identify their own process and become more effective.

Books

Amazon.com currently lists numerous books on personal/life coaching and professional/business coaching but none on health coaching.

Whitworth L, Sandahl P, Kimsey-House H. *Co-Active Coaching: New Skills for Coaching People Toward Success in Work and Life*. Mountain View, CA: Davies-Black Publishing; 1998. This best-selling book is written for coaching professionals by the cofounders of the Coaches Training Institute; their coactive model encompasses specific skill sets and key principles of coaching.

CHAPTER 26

Imagery

Martin L. Rossman, MD

INTRODUCTION TO IMAGERY

Imagery is best thought of as a way of working with the patient, rather than a way of treating particular disease entities. As an adjunctive therapy, imagery has applications in a wide variety of medical and surgical conditions. It is almost always useful, although rarely as a sole therapy. Since imagery is a natural language of the unconscious and the human nervous system, its potential uses in health care are extensive. The following are some of the major applications in the healing professions:

- Stress reduction and relaxation
- Stimulation of psychophysiologic effects, including altered blood flow, muscle relaxation, and immune stimulation
- Enhanced attunement to symptoms and increased mind-body awareness
- Preparing and supporting patients to make healthy lifestyle changes
- Pain management
- Reduction of anxiety and complications in conjunction with surgery, difficult medical procedures, or childbirth
- Provision of skills for coping with chronic illness
- Treatment of depression, post-traumatic stress disorder, and traumatic abuse
- Counseling, life coaching, and performance enhancement

A brief biography of Martin Rossman appears in Chapter 3. Courtesy of Martin L. Rossman, MD, Mill Valley, California.

Precautions and Contraindications

Imagery should not be substituted for necessary medical or surgical interventions, or in lieu of appropriate medical diagnosis and/or treatment. Mental health practitioners will want to ascertain the medical status or diagnosis of patients to make certain they are also aware of their medical options. Conversely, while imagery is generally quite safe, it can be harmful if used inappropriately with patients who have experienced significant trauma or who have psychopathology, such as those who are psychotic or on the verge of a psychotic break, those with dissociative disorders, or those with borderline personality disorders. Patients should be referred to mental health practitioners if the work becomes psychologically complex. Imagery can be quite helpful to people with these conditions if it is used by health professionals with expertise in these diagnostic categories and in imagery work.

OVERVIEW

Definitions

- *Guided imagery* is a term variously used to describe a range of techniques from simple visualization and direct imagery-based suggestion, through metaphor and story telling. Guided imagery is used to help teach psychophysiologic relaxation (Walker et al., 1999), to relieve symptoms (NIH, 1996), to stimulate healing responses in the body (Hall et al., 1993), to support lifestyle change (Richardson et al., 1997), and to help people tolerate procedures and treatments more easily (Blankfield, 1991).

• *Interactive Guided Imagery* is a service-marked term coined by the Academy for Guided Imagery to represent a process in which imagery is used in a highly interactive format to evoke patient autonomy. This approach provides patients with ways to draw on their own inner resources to support healing and to make appropriate adaptations to changes in their health.

Development

Historically, most healing rituals have involved imagery, either overtly or covertly. In this sense, imagery can be considered one of the oldest and most ubiquitous forms of medicine. The healing rituals of various cultures all have a certain level of efficacy or they would not have persisted. Although we may attribute these therapeutic benefits to placebo responses, they do stimulate real and measurable effects with important implications for our understanding of the healing process (Frank, 1974).

Carl Jung, the eminent Swiss psychiatrist, believed that imagery may be a reflection of the unconscious mind revealing itself (Meissner et al., 1975). Jung employed a method he called active imagination as a means of gaining insight into his clients' unconscious processes. He would invite his patients to relax and focus their attention on their symptoms, and then have them describe the images that came to mind. He found that the images conveyed relevant information, directly related to his patients' individual development, growth, and healing.

Imagery again came to light in medicine in the late 1960s. Startling research by radiation oncologist O. Carl Simonton and psychologist Stephanie Simonton reported unexpected longevity in cancer patients following the use of imagery and visualization to stimulate immune response (Simonton et al., 1980; Simonton & Matthews–Simonton, 1981). The Simontons taught their patients simple relaxation and imagery techniques for enhancing performance, relaxation, memory, and healing (Simonton et al., 1978). Although the Simonton's work stirred great interest and controversy, very little clinical research was done in this area until the late 1980s.

Psychologists Jeanne Achterberg (1985) and Frank Lawlis, working with the Simontons, helped to formulate some of the earliest research in this area, developing the *Image CA*, a rating scale of imagery drawings by cancer patients. They found that certain aspects of imagery work may predict clinical outcome; they have subsequently developed similar scales and imagery interventions in the areas of chronic pain, diabetes, and spinal injuries.

Psychoneuroimmunology. The development of psychoneuroimmunology as a field of study (Pert, 1997) has encouraged researchers to cross disciplinary boundaries, to study the effects of the mind on physiology and healing in earnest. Many studies have already validated the Simontons' early hypothesis that people can stimulate their immune response through imagery (Watson et al., 1999). Studies also indicate that psychosocial interventions may extend the life or quality of life of cancer patients (Cunningham, 2000). Although additional research still needs to be done to clarify the roles of imagery in cancer survival, a robust body of literature now supports its uses—for reducing anxiety and depression associated with cancer and its treatment, reducing the adverse effects of chemotherapy and radiation, relieving pain, and improving quality of life in cancer patients (Richardson et al., 1997).

Clinical applications. Imagery is becoming widely accepted as a safe, efficacious, and cost-effective means of helping patients prepare for surgery and other invasive medical procedures (Bennett et al., 1986). For example, a number of studies have reported reduced presurgical anxiety, fewer surgical complications, and shorter postsurgical hospital stays (Hathaway 1986; Jamison, 1987). Evidence also supports the use of imagery in the management of conditions such as arthritis and asthma (Smyth et al., 1999), allergies and hypertension, and for helping patients with chronic illnesses such as diabetes and coronary artery disease. Imagery has been shown to help people change potentially harmful lifestyle habits such as smoking or overeating and thus has ubiquitous applications in medical practice.

Theory

Images encode our beliefs about healing. Mental images, formed long before we learn to understand and use words, lie at the core of who we think we are, what we believe the world is like, what we feel we deserve, and how motivated we are to take care of ourselves. These images strongly influence our beliefs and attitudes about how we fall ill, what will help us get better, and whether or not medical and/or psychological interventions will be effective. Imagery also has powerful physiological consequences that are directly related to the healing systems of the body.

The power of placebo. Research on the placebo effect, the standard to which we compare all other modalities (and find relatively few more powerful), has provided some of the strongest evidence for the power of the imagination in healing. It is well documented that from 30% to 55% of all patients given inactive placebos respond as well as or better than those given active treatments or agents.

Engaging the placebo response. Extensive research has confirmed that people can derive not only symptomatic relief, but actual physiologic healing in response to treatments that primarily work through beliefs and attitudes. Consequently, learning to better mobilize this phenomenon in a purposeful, conscious way becomes an important, if not critical, area of investigation for modern medicine. Although all responses to imagery are not placebo responses, imagery offers an entrance into this important arena. The existance of placebo effect is one of the strangest pieces of evidence for the power of the imagination. The only reason we go to the trouble and expense of randomized, double-blind placebo controlled trials is that it is so difficult to eliminate the power of people's expectations.

Principal Concepts

Imagery has physiologic consequences. Imagery is essentially a way of thinking that involves sensory attributes. In the absence of competing sensory cues, the body tends to respond to imagery as it would to a genuine external experience. The most common and familiar example of this phenomenon is sexual fantasy and its attendant physiologic responses. Imagery has been shown to potentially affect almost all major physiologic control systems of the body, including respiration, heart rate, blood pressure, metabolic rates in cellular function, gastrointestinal mobility and secretion, sexual function, and even immune responsiveness.

Imagery is a primary encoding language of the nervous system. Imagery can be thought of as one of the brain's two higher-order encoding systems. The system we are most familiar with is the *sequential information processing system*, which underlies linear, analytic, and conscious verbal thinking (predominately "left-brain" functions). Most health professionals are highly educated and highly rewarded for their abilities using this mode of information processing.

- Imagery utilizes a *simultaneous information processing* mode that underlies holistic, more integrative patterns of thinking that engage the right brain and the unconscious mind.
- Many of us learn to give the majority of our attention to the conscious, verbal part of our mind that narrates a linear, logical, rational, analytic monologue describing its perspective of the world and how we think about it.
- However, we all have other ways of experiencing ourselves that are more connected to our emotional and psychophysiologic status: the richness of intuitions, emotions, feelings, memories, drives, goals, appetites, aspirations, ambitions, values, beliefs, and sensations. Any or all of these aspects of ourselves may require and even demand attention, finding ways to intrude on everyday consciousness through physical, emotional, or behavioral symptoms.
- These symptoms can serve as reflections of underlying dynamics or stressors. Focusing attention on these symptoms in a relaxed state of mind, and inviting imagery to arise that represents those underlying needs, provides the opportunity to identify unmet needs or unresolved problems, to reconnect with these important issues, and to improve the quality of one's life.
- The use of imagery enables health care professionals to coach patients through this process of insight, to reduce stress, and to remove barriers to healing.

Applying imagery to promote insight or change. Imagery is a powerful tool in healing in part because of its close relationship to the emotions—imagery is the language of the emotional self. Emotions show us what is important to us and can be either potent motivators or barriers to changing lifestyle.

Imagery is also the language of visioning and planning. When one identifies a lifestyle pattern or habit to be changed, imagery can be used to envision and plan in detail how that change will become integrated into daily life. Imagery rehearsal of successful change can provide motivation and energy to support this process.

Once we have identified a change we want to make, such as a lifestyle pattern or habit, we can begin to envision and plan in detail how we will make it a part of our daily lives. Imagery rehearsal of successfully making a change can provide motivation and energy that can help us actually accomplish it.

CLINICAL PRACTICE

Setting goals for treatment. In interactive imagery, the health care practitioner or psychologist serves as a guide, working with the client to establish the desired goals and objectives for their work together. The goals can be defined in physical, emotional or behavioral terms, and a reasonable trial period of exploration is then agreed upon. We often ask patients to participate in three exploratory sessions and then decide whether this approach seems useful to them. At that point they can decide whether they would like to use it as a form of self-care or elect to participate in a series of 10 to 15 sessions. They also have the option of using this approach in longer-term work. At the end of each session, and at the end of the agreed upon time period, the goals of the work are reviewed and progress assessed.

Treatment options. Since imagery is a natural way we think, and since it can almost always be helpful, there are virtually an unlimited number of situations for which it can be used in health care settings. For simplicity, it may be helpful to consider some of the major applications of imagery:

1. Relaxation and stress reduction, which are easy to teach, easy to learn, and almost universally helpful.
2. Visualization, or directed imagery, in which the client or patient is encouraged to imagine desired outcomes in a relaxed state of mind. This affords the patient a sense of participation and control in their own healing, which in itself is of significant value. In addition, research suggests that it may relieve or reduce symptoms, stimulate healing responses in the body or healthy behaviors, and/or provide effective motivation for making positive life changes.
3. Receptive, or insight-oriented imagery, which involves the use of imagery to gather information about a symptom, illness, mood, situation, or solution.

The patient experience. If the client has no prior experience with relaxation or imagery, the guide typically invites them to relax while being guided through a brief relaxation technique. The client is then encouraged to imagine being in a beautiful, safe, and peaceful place and to describe what they see, hear, smell, and feel there. The guide may suggest that this "special place" has other qualities that might also be helpful to the client. For example, a fearful client might be encouraged to imagine being in "a powerful place," "a sanctuary," or "a place where you are completely safe and beyond harm." A client who feels too exhausted to deal with a situation might be encouraged to imagine a place of "great energy and vitality" or "a place of rest, renewal, and refreshment." A patient primarily concerned with recovering from a serious illness may be invited to imagine a "healing place" and to notice and emphasize the qualities of the place that make it particularly healing for them.

Case History

A brief clinical example may serve to suggest the power of interactive guided imagery. A 57-year-old executive with diabetes mellitus was recalcitrant and noncompliant with the medical regimen for his illness, despite good diabetes education and the urging of his physician, family, and friends. When asked to allow an image to emerge for his disease, he imagined it as a ball and chain around his ankle. When prompted to express his thoughts and feelings about it, he replied that he hated it because it was weighing him down, preventing him from leading a normal life.

We encouraged him to express his feelings toward the image, and then to let it communicate back to him in a way he could understand. The ball took on a sad face and said that it was sorry, it didn't want to hurt him, but it was exhausted and needed some special care. The patient began to feel some empathy for it, and as he expressed this empathic feeling, the ball and chain turned into a small dog on a leash. In his imaginary dialogues, the little dog told him that if he fed it well, and let it both rest and exercise appropriately, it would become a friend to him and would walk by his side rather than drag him down.

The patient realized that this was clearly in his own interest. As he began taking better care of his "little dog," he became more physically active, changed his diet, lost weight, and within months reported feeling "better than I have in years!" The imagery helped him gain a different perspective on his problem, and to access and express his emotions. This enabled him to find a better way of relating to his illness and led him to make the changes that brought about good control of his disease. Although disease remission does not always occur, this type of imagery experience almost always leads to better self-understanding and enhanced coping skills for dealing with a chronic illness or health condition.

Self-care vs. professional care. Another set of options to consider is whether the client will benefit from the use of imagery as a self-care technique, in a group or class, or in the context of an individual counseling or therapy relationship. Self-help books, tapes, and CDs are inexpensive resources for many clients who are effective in utilizing these techniques on their own. In practice, most patients and practitioners will explore all of the above options and utilize those that suit the client best, given the unique nature of the issue, their coping responses, their approach to life, and the amount of time, energy, and funds they are willing or able to invest in the process.

Insurance reimbursement. Practitioners typically use imagery as one component of psychotherapy, counseling, stress reduction training, or medical hypnosis. Consequently, work with imagery is usually billed and reimbursed in the context of other professional services. When applied for medical purposes, medical practitioners may ethically bill for medical services, although insurance companies may challenge this if services are lengthy and repetitive. There are currently no separate billing codes for guided imagery or Interactive Guided Imagery, although ABC codes have been developed for these services.

Sources of practitioner referrals. Studies have recently shown that as many as 60% of physicians refer patients to complementary mind-body approaches. The most prevalent utilization of mind-body therapies involves meditation, relaxation techniques, imagery, hypnosis, and biofeedback (Barnes et al., 2004). Research also shows that a substantial number of physicians utilize these services for themselves and their families (Berman et al., 1998).

Professional training, certification, and scope of practice. Health professionals utilize imagery within their practice, based on the scope of their licensure, education, experience, and competence. Using guided imagery does not turn a physician or nurse into a psychotherapist, or a psychotherapist into a physician or nurse. Instead, it gives each a greater range of skills in working with issues that involve both mind and body, emotions, and behavioral change.

The Academy for Guided Imagery provides a 150-hour certification program for health care and mental health professionals. Certification through the Academy for Guided Imagery is restricted to professionals licensed in their states of residence in medicine, nursing, psychology, or other health care profession, or in a counseling or health services field. For professionals in states that have no licensing for therapists, training and certification are evaluated on a case-by-case basis. Within these guidelines, the use of imagery provides professionals with additional tools to be even more effective at what they already do.

RESOURCES

Self-care instructional materials using guided imagery are available for patients, including books, tapes, and CDs from the following sources:

Martin L. Rossman, MD
Phone: 415-389-8941
Web site: www.guidedimageryhealing.com

Belleruth Naparstek, LCSW
Web site: www.healthjourneys.com

Emmett Miller, MD
Web site: www.drmiller.com

Professional training and certification:
The Academy for Guided Imagery
30765 Pacific Coast Highway, Suite 369
Malibu, CA 90265
Phone: (800) 726-2070
Fax: (800) 727-2070
Email for enrollment information: train@
AcademyforGuidedImagery.com
Web site: www.AcademyforGuidedImagery.
com

REFERENCES

Achterberg J. *Imagery in Healing.* Boston, MA: Shambala; 1985.

Barnes PM, Powell-Griner E, McFann K, Nahin R. Complementary and alternative medicine use among adults: United States, 2002. *Adv Data.* 2004;(343):1–16.

Bennett HL, Benson DR, Kuiken DA. Preoperative instructions for decreased bleeding during spine surgery. *Anesthesiology.* 1986;65:A245.

Berman BM, Singh BB, Hartnol SM, et al. Primary care physicians and complementary-alternative medicine: training, attitudes, and practice patterns. *J Am Board Fam Pract.* 1998;11:272–281.

Blankfield RP. Suggestion, relaxation, and hypnosis as adjuncts in the care of surgery patients: a review of the literature. *Am J Clin Hypnosis.* 1991;33(3):172–186.

Cunningham AJ, Edmonds CV, Phillips C, Soots KI, Hedley D, Lockwood GA. A prospective, longitudinal study of the relationship of psychosocial work to duration of survival in patients with metastic cancer. *Psychooncology.* 2000;9(4):323–339.

Frank J. *Persuasion and Healing.* New York, NY: Schocken Books; 1974

Hall H, Minnes L, Olness K. The psychophysiology of voluntary immunomodulation. *Intl J Neurosci.* 1993;69(1–4):221–234.

Hathaway D. Effects of preoperative instructions on postoperative outcomes: a meta-analysis. *Nursing Research.* 1986;35:269–275.

Jamison RN, Parris WC, Maxson WS. Psychological factors influencing recovery from outpatient surgery. *Behavior Research Therapy.* 1987;25:31–37.

Meissner WW, Mack JE, Semrad EV. In: Freedman AM, Kaplan HI, Sadock BJ, eds. *Comprehensive Textbook of Psychiatry II,* Vol. I. 2nd ed. Philadelphia, PA: Williams & Wilkins; 1975:486–487.

NIH Technology Assessment Panel. Integration of behavioral and relaxation approaches into the treatment of chronic pain and insomnia. *JAMA.* 1996;276(4):313–318

Pert CB. *Molecules of Emotion.* New York, NY: Scribner; 1997.

Richardson MA, Post-White J, Grimm EA, Moye LA, Singletary SE, Justice B. Coping, life attitudes, and immune responses to imagery and group support after breast cancer treatment. *Altern Therapies Health Med.* 1997;3(5):62–70.

Simonton OC, Matthews-Simonton S. Cancer and stress: counseling the cancer patient. *Med J Aust.* 1981;1(13):679, 682–683.

Simonton OC, Matthews-Simonton S, Sparks TF. Psychological intervention in the treatment of cancer. *Psychosomatics.* 1980;21(3):226–227, 231–233.

Simonton OC, Simonton SM, Creighton J. *Getting Well Again.* Los Angeles, CA: Tarcher; 1978.

Smyth JM, Stone AA, Hurewitz A, Kaell A. Effects of writing about stressful experiences on symptom reduction in patients with asthma or rheumatoid arthritis: a randomized trial. *JAMA.* 1999;281(14):1304–1309.

Spiegel D. Mind matters: coping and cancer progression. *J Psychosomatic Research.* 2001;50(5):287–290.

Walker LG, Walker MB, Ogston K, et al. Psychological, clinical, and pathological effects of relaxation training and guided imagery during primary chemotherapy. *British J Cancer.* 1999;80(1–2):262–268.

Watson M, Haviland JS, Greer S, Davidson J, Bliss JM. Influence of psychological response on survival in breast cancer: a population-based cohort study. *Lancet.* 1999;354(9187):1331–1336.

CHAPTER 27

Hypnosis

Steven Gurgevich, PhD

THERAPEUTIC APPLICATIONS

Clinical hypnosis, as an adjunct to the management of pain disorders or chronic conditions, can support highly positive health outcomes. In the author's clinical practice, approximately 95% of patients respond well to hypnosis, in part because of their high level of motivation. Smoking-cessation patients in the practice experience a quit rate of approximately 80%. This is a safe, cost-effective, and empowering approach that can be taught to patients for proactive self-care.

We use the terms *focused daydream* or *trance* to describe a state in which one is absorbed in his own thoughts and lessens his attention on his surroundings. When we work with children in pain management, for example, we simply ask them to pretend. Daydream (focused) and trance are basically identical in nature. However, what distinguishes hypnotherapy from a daydream state is that it involves a deliberate choice to enter this state of consciousness and utilize it to promote healing.

Steven Gurgevich, PhD, is a licensed psychologist specializing in behavioral and mind-body medicine who serves as faculty member and clinician within Dr. Andrew Weil's Program in Integrative Medicine, and as a core consultant to the Pediatric Complementary and Alternative Medicine Center at the University of Arizona Health Sciences Center. He is section chief at the Tucson Medical Center, Psychiatry Executive Committee (since 1980), and has taught at the University of Arizona in a number of capacities. He also teaches professionals through the American Society of Clinical Hypnosis and maintains a private practice at Behavioral Medicine, Ltd., and Sabine Canyon Integrative Medicine, LLC, in Tucson, Arizona.

Hypnosis or trance has been described as a psychophysiological state of altered consciousness consisting of narrowed awareness, restricted and focused attentiveness, selected wakefulness, and heightened suggestibility (Marmer, 1959). Others define it as a state of arousal—attentive, receptive, focused, and concentrative, with a corresponding diminution in peripheral awareness. These states include daydreaming, intense concentration, distraction, and selective perception (Spiegel & Spiegel, 2004).

This aspect of selective perception is one of the key features that differentiates hypnosis from other states of mind. In this state of internally focused concentration, there is selective awareness of incoming stimuli. However, in pain control, the subject is taught to become detached not only from external stimuli, but also from internal stimuli. As a result, the individual does not experience discomfort in situations that would normally be quite painful, such as dental or surgical procedures.

Interestingly, EEG evaluations of patients in trance show that it is a waking state, with brain activity different than that of sleep. Participants are awake, but more internally focused. Hypnosis is described as a state in which both conscious and unconscious processes are available simultaneously. Consequently, it is one of the primary techniques for accessing the mind-body connection

In the author's practice, typically half of patients are referred for chronic pain disorders.

The other half of the practice serves clients with a variety of medical concerns such as sleep, digestive, and skin disorders; rheumatological conditions; asthma; and other functional disorders. Hypnosis can also be beneficial in preparing patients for surgery, or helping them manage the discomfort of chemotherapy or cancer treatment. Behavioral issues can be addressed with hypnosis to overcome habitual behaviors such as smoking, nail biting, thumb sucking, or hair pulling. Clinical hypnosis can also be used to address the problems underlying such behaviors. Table 27–1 reflects the range of applications for hypnosis in medicine and psychotherapy.

DISPELLING THE MYTHS OF HYPNOSIS

One of the first steps with a new client is to dispel the patient's myths and misconceptions. For example, no one can actually hypnotize another person. The clinician can facilitate the process of entering that focused daydream state, but they cannot actually hypnotize or exercise control over another person.

Another common misconception is that while in a hypnotic state subjects can be motivated to act against their will. In reality, no one can override the best intentions, ideals, or values of another. What we can do is offer hypnotic suggestions, statements designed to influence the mind-body connection in a therapeutic manner.

There is no loss of consciousness, no "going out" or "going under." The individual remains aware of where they are and what they are doing at all times. There is no relinquishing of control, action, or activity that would embarrass the subject or reflect an action taken against their will.

Another myth is that one must be naïve or "feeble-minded" to be hypnotizable. Quite the contrary, the better the intellect, the better the subject. There is also the fear that one may not be able to be dehypnotized, that they might be unable to exit that trancelike state. In reality, the worst thing that can happen is that occasionally a subject falls asleep. Realizing that the hypnotic state is essentially identical to a daydream quickly alleviates these fears.

Table 27–1 Clinical Applications of Hypnosis

- Burns—reduction of pain and inflammation
- Childbirth—analgesic for labor and general ease of delivery
- Chronic jaw pain and bruxism
- Dental anesthesia
- Dental anxiety
- Dermatologic disorders—eczema, herpes, neurodermatitis, pruritus, psoriasis, warts
- Gastrointestinal disorders—ulcers, irritable bowel syndrome, colitis, Crohn's disease
- Hemophilia—self-hypnosis to control vascular flow and minimize transfusions
- Nausea and vomiting—associated with chemotherapy, pregnancy/morning sickness
- Pain—arthritis or rheumatism, back pain, cancer pain, dental anesthesia, headaches and migraines
- Post-traumatic stress—utilized for victims of abuse and various other traumatic situations
- Surgery/anesthesia—useful to lessen the need for chemical anesthesia, reduce post-operative pain, and speed recovery and wound healing

CLINICAL METHODOLOGY

Clinical hypnosis involves two key strategies. One is symptomatic, which means focusing on the symptoms. For example, in the case of a skin disorder such as hives, itching, or warts, we address the symptoms by providing an affirmation: Your skin is clear, and beneath your skin there is a wonderful blood supply. Your body is doing an excellent job of healing your skin. These positive messages are all symptom directed.

The other strategy is a psychodynamic approach. In this approach, we ask the individual about the underlying source of their problem using very metaphorical questions. In the case of a skin disorder, I might ask: What's getting under your skin? What's rubbing you the wrong way? or, What are you itching to do? Those types of metaphors use the literal language of the unconscious mind. The unconscious can only process language literally. If someone says, I want to lose weight so badly, the body only understands that literally. Badly? When the weight loss program goes "badly," the subject wonders why.

In cases of cardiac pain with no cardiac organicity, I ask questions such as: What do you need to get off your chest? What is breaking your heart? or, Who is breaking your heart? In the case of digestive disorders, I might say: What's burning you up inside? What's got you tied in knots? or, What's your gut reaction? With asthma patients we ask: Who or what is suffocating or smothering you?

In terms of diagnosis, hypnosis works best in cases of functional disorders—disorders that are not due to infectious process such as bacterial, fungal, or viral infection. It is most often used to address conditions that involve healthy tissue behaving in an inappropriate fashion in conditions such as reflux, irritable bowel syndrome, or skin disorders, as well

RESEARCH ON HYPNOSIS IN THE OPERATING ROOM

A recent meta-analysis of 20 published controlled studies on hypnosis in surgical applications found that patients in the hypnosis treatment groups experienced better outcomes than 89% of those in control groups (Montgomery et al., 2002). The analysis compared outcomes across six clinical categories: amount of pain medication used, degree of pain, negative affect, physiological indicators, recovery time, and treatment time.

One randomized, controlled clinical trial involved 241 patients undergoing percutaneous vascular and renal procedures. Patients received standard care or hypnosis; in addition, all patients were provided with access to analgesia (Lang et al., 2000). Investigators found that those in standard care used twice as much pain medication as those in the hypnosis group. Those using hypnosis also had significantly shorter procedure times, decreased anxiety, and greater hemodynamic stability.

A study of 60 patients undergoing hand surgery found lower pain intensity and anxiety, higher progress ratings, and fewer postoperative complications (Mauer et al., 1999). A retrospective study that reviewed 197 thyroidectomies found less pain, less analgesic use, shorter hospital stays, and improved postoperative convalescence (Defechereux et al., 1999).

A review panel appointed by the NIH (1996) found "strong evidence" for the use of hypnosis in alleviating pain associated with cancer.

Source: Gurgerich S, 2003.

as autoimmune conditions. Hypnosis can also be used as an adjunctive therapy to promote healing and support healthy immune function. It can be applied to promote behavioral change, healthy lifestyle, and stress reduction. Hypnosis can be used to address self-esteem issues, poor self-care, and compliance, which can be underlying causal factors in disease processes.

The Client Evaluation

As the first step in treatment, I perform a comprehensive psychological evaluation of all patients. The evaluation can provide insight into the history of their disorder, its origins, and the obstacles that are impeding healing. The effect of their lifestyle and mind-set on their illness is also considered. The goal of this evaluation is to identify the beliefs that may be contributing to their symptoms or illness. As part of this process, I may also talk with them about life experiences that could have contributed to their condition. Ultimately, they may be unaware of the role of their beliefs in their development of symptoms.

Once we understand the origin of their condition, we must determine how we can create a bridge into the subconscious, so that they can change those beliefs. We want them to change enough to experience the effects of their new beliefs. We can influence them by asking relevant questions and listening carefully to what they say and how they say it. Once we have determined their negative beliefs, more positive beliefs can be created, offering them alternatives that move them in a positive direction.

In any type of mind-body intervention, including hypnosis, a common obstacle we encounter is resistance. Resistance is normal and to be expected. This resistance may occur consciously or unconsciously—it reflects the critical inner voice within that says, "I can't" or "I won't." The client may have a negative self-image based on beliefs established in childhood. For many people, this inner critical voice is always present, evaluating every-

thing. In some cases these messages from the past can short-circuit a person's life.

Our work involves undoing or erasing those negative beliefs. Since the unconscious mind tends to be more receptive to new ideas, access to the unconscious through hypnosis can provide a point of leverage. One of the most challenging aspects of this type of psychological dynamic is helping clients change their conception of what is possible and what they can achieve.

Teaching the Process of Hypnosis

The next step is to teach them how to go into a trance or daydream state, to deliberately become absorbed inside themselves in a mind-set comparable to deep meditation. Their response is monitored by observing changes in respiration, muscle relaxation, or slight involuntary twitching movements (similar to the types of responses that occur when people fall asleep). Once they have achieved a trancelike state, I offer positive suggestions that relate to their particular health issue and suggest positive imagery, for example, imagining their skin clearing or picturing their entire digestive tract becoming relaxed. I may use various metaphors or images. For a patient with reflux, I may compare the digestive tract to a river that flows smoothly in one direction and remind the subject that they can slow down or speed up that flow in a way that enhances their comfort and nourishment. The suggestions are written with a symptomatic approach in mind. Applying hypnosis on a regular basis, patients come to realize they can influence their bodies and their health.

Near the end of the session, I suggest that they will feel refreshed, alert, and comfortable and will be able to use this approach for themselves whenever they would like. Usually I record the session and make them a CD of it before they leave, with instructions on practicing every day for at least three weeks.

How well they do depends on how well they practice or rehearse what they are learning with hypnosis—and how consistently they practice. In essence, all hypnosis is self-hypnosis, which patients must learn and then practice for themselves. Although there may be wide differences in hypnotizability among individuals, almost everyone can learn this skill and achieve results with instruction and practice. The real skill in hypnosis involves understanding the language of the unconscious mind. The unconscious interprets everything on a literal level, so learning the language of the unconscious is one of the skills the therapist conveys to the patient. However, it may take years for the therapist to become adept at understanding and utilizing this language.

Even a stage hypnotist applies some understanding of the language of hypnosis. Although much of their act is illusion, they are using some of the same principles of persuasion and suggestibility that are applied in clinical hypnosis. For example, they may have the subject clasp their hands together and imagine that they are glued tight. At that point, the stage hypnotist suggests: "*Try* to pull your hands apart." The key here is the word "try." The hypnotist did not literally say: "Pull your hands apart." He said "Try." From the perspective of the unconscious mind, the concept "try" is only an idea. (It implies an attempt, but not something that is accomplished.) For example, when anyone tries to fall asleep (an unconscious process), the harder they "try," the more wide awake they become. As the sage said in *Star Wars*, "There is no try—there is only do or not do." An increased understanding of the innuendos of language and self-talk is important in the effective use of hypnosis.

Self-Care and Professional Intervention

Typically in my practice I see people from one to four times overall, and it is rare that I have seen anyone more than four times. My role is basically instructional in nature. I introduce patients to hypnosis and teach them how to do this process themselves. Providing them with a CD of our session gives them a script they can use to practice on their own.

There are three key elements that make hypnosis effective.

- Motivation—If someone really wants to improve his or her condition, motivation is vital. It is vital they have the desire to achieve and experience a therapeutic outcome. If they do not *really want it*, it will not happen.

- Belief—What are their beliefs about their possibilities with hypnosis? How do they envision this improvement occurring—and what do they believe will be the result?

- Expectation—What do they expect will be the result? It is important for them to define what they want and expect to experience.

Most of the people I see are highly motivated. They may have been through several years of treatment for a debilitating condition such as asthma, IBS, or chronic pain. They want to be well again, and they want their life back. They are motivated to find a new approach, and they are especially interested in using an approach in which they can participate. They are willing to invest their time, energy, and money to achieve a therapeutic outcome. If they do not possess this level of motivation, the results will reflect it.

Safety. There are two dangers to hypnosis. When hypnosis is administered by someone who is not trained and the subject has a strong underlying unconscious conflict or history of trauma, they might not be able to handle a dramatic unbinding of emotion—abreaction. An *abreaction* is the term we use to describe the spontaneous release or unbinding of emotion associated with trauma that has been repressed. These emotions can be very distressing for the patient, as they may involve events that were repressed many years ago. Therapeutically, an abreaction will allow the clinician to address and treat the underlying problem very effectively. However, in untrained hands, it can be very distressing for a patient and often cannot be competently helped by an unqualified practitioner.

The other concern is that hypnosis might be used to eliminate pain that is serving as a warning that pathology is present. I have seen cases in which the patient sought assistance from lay practitioners to diminish pain using hypnosis—only to learn later that the pain was a warning signal associated with a tumor or some other disorder requiring medical attention. My rule of thumb is that practitioners should not use hypnosis to treat a condition unless they are also trained to treat it without hypnosis.

Research. There have been many articles reporting research using clinical hypnosis over the past 50 years. This literature is well summarized in professional journals, particularly those published by the two major societies for medical hypnosis: the American Society of Clinical Hypnosis, www.ASCH. net, and the Society for Clinical and Experimental Hypnosis, http://ijceh.educ.wsu.edu/ijcehframes.htm. In addition, a great many studies on hypnosis have been published in other medical journals.

Clinical outcomes. Hypnosis can be highly effective and the results are usually dramatic. These benefits often occur quite rapidly. For example, we see skin conditions clear in a matter of days or weeks. Consider the example of patients who are experiencing vomiting due to chemotherapy. Dramatic changes occur when they realize they can use their mind to increase their appetite and overcome nausea. What we believe and what we put our faith in has a major influence on what we experience. It is possible the average person does not realize the tremendous power of their unconscious beliefs as they play out in their lives.

I follow up with patients to obtain feedback on our work and determine if any obstacles are present. I might see them in the clinic or communicate on the telephone or through email to determine how they are doing. In some ways I liken my work to that of a music teacher. People come for a lesson, I show them how to use the instrument, and if I can motivate them and help them experience enough of a reward from that interaction, they will practice it on their own with dedication. In most cases, it is their motivated and compliant practice that produces the beneficial effects.

CLINICAL RESOURCES

Training and licensure. Health care and counseling professionals who use hypnosis in their work include physicians, dentists, social workers, marriage and family counselors, and some members of the clergy. However, hypnosis is not a therapy in and of itself, so the term hypnotherapist is actually a misnomer.

People who do not have a professional education can become a certified hypnotherapist (CHT). However, without the broader context of a professional background, that training has limited scope. I compare that training to the education of a phlebotomist: they learn how to set up IVs, provide subcutaneous or intravenous injections, and meet sterilization requirements, but they have little training beyond those procedures. For health care and counseling professionals, hypnosis is a useful tool with a range of applications when applied in the context of clinical practice.

Training is provided by the two major professional societies, their regional component associations, and certified members. Both societies offer a certification process that requires approximately 60 to 80 hours of approved supervised training. Two years of independent practice utilizing clinical hypnosis are required to receive certification from the American Society of Clinical Hypnosis.

Insurance. Some insurance plans pay for sessions of medical hypnosis, which has a procedure code in the diagnostic manuals. Reimbursement for hypnosis services varies from one insurance company to the next. Many patients have received reimbursement or partial reimbursement.

Sources of referrals. In my own practice, I only see patients by physician referral. I view this as the best way I can provide physi-

cians the opportunity to see firsthand the clinical benefits of hypnosis. After 30 years in practice, I still receive most of my referrals from doctors, through word of mouth, and through media such as books, television, newsletters, or the Internet. I also see people from other parts of the country who ask to come in for a few sessions to be helped with a particular chronic disorder or issue.

Skilled and competent clinicians can be located through the Web site of the American Society of Clinical Hypnosis at www.ASCH.net through the link, *Finding Certified Practitioners*. The practitioner database can be searched by city or state and provides a list of all the physicians and psychologists who have been certified in a given geographic area. Additional resources for referral are posted on my Web site, www.tranceformation.com.

REFERENCES

Defechcreux T, et al. Hypnoanesthesia for endocrine cervical surgery: a statement of practice. *J Altern Complement Med*. 1999;5:509–520.

Gurgerich S. Clinical hypnosis and surgery. *Alt Med Alert*. 2003;6(10):115.

Lang EV, et al. Adjunctive non-pharmacological analgesia for invasive medical procedures: a randomised trial. *Lancet*. 2000;355:1486–1490.

Marmer J. *Hypnosis in Anesthesiology*. Springfield, IL: Charles C. Thomas; 1959.

Mauer MG, et al. Medical hypnosis and orthopedic hand surgery: pain perception, postoperative recovery, and therapeutic comfort. *Int J Clin Exp Hypn*. 1999;47:144–161.

Montgomery GH, et al. The effectiveness of adjunctive hypnosis with surgical patients: a meta-analysis. *Anesth Analg*. 2002;94:1639–1645.

NIH Technology Assessment Panel. Integration of behavioral and relaxation approaches into the treatment of chronic pain and insomnia. *JAMA*. 1996;276:313–318.

Spiegel H, Spiegel D. *Trance and Treatment: Clinical Uses of Hypnosis*. 2nd ed. Washington, DC: American Psychiatric Press; 2004.

RESOURCES

Books for Patients

Temes, Roberta. *The Complete Idiot's Guide to Hypnosis*. Indianapolis, IN: Alpha Books; 1999. This is a comprehensive, user-friendly book that can be recommended to patients.

Burns, David D. *Feeling Good*. New York, NY: Avon; 1999. This classic has advanced our understanding of the dynamics of self-

talk. Burns has created a psychotherapeutic structure enabling counselors and therapists to help patients learn these skills. His book is also an accessible self-help guide for consumers.

Rosen, Sid. *My Voice Will Go With You: The Teaching Tales of Milton H. Erickson, MD*. New York, NY: W.W. Norton & Company, 1991. This classic, still a best-seller, focuses on the work of Milton Erickson and provides insight on unconscious interactions and the language of the subconscious.

Books for Professionals

Barber J. *Hypnosis and Suggestion in the Treatment of Pain*. New York, NY: W.W. Norton & Co; 1996.

Brown DP, Fromm E. *Hypnosis and Behavioral Medicine*. Mahwah, NJ: Lawrence Erlbaum Associates; 1987.

Crasilneck HB, Hall JA. *Clinical Hypnosis*: *Principles and Applications*. 2nd ed. New York, NY: Grunke & Stratton; 1985.

Hammond DC. *Handbook of Hypnotic Suggestions and Metaphors*. New York, NY: W.W. Norton & Co; 1990.

Kroger W. *Clinical and Experimental Hypnosis*. Philadelphia, PA: JB Lippincott; 1963.

Meyer RG. *Practical Clinical Hypnosis*. New York, NY: Lexington Books; 1992.

Olness K, Kohen DP. *Hypnosis and Hypnotherapy with Children*. 3rd ed. New York, NY: Guilford Press; 1996.

Rossi EL, Cheek DB. *Mind-Body Therapy*: *Methods of Ideodynamic Healing in Hypnosis*. New York, NY: W.W. Norton & Co; 1988.

Spiegel H, Spiegel D. *Trance and Treatment*: *Clinical Uses of Hypnosis*. 2nd ed. Washington, DC: American Psychiatric Press; 2004.

Zeig J. *Ericksonian Approaches to Hypnosis and Psychotherapy*. New York, NY: Brunner/Mazel; 1982.

Journals

The American Journal of Hypnosis, published by:

American Society of Clinical Hypnosis
140 N. Bloomingdale Road
Bloomingdale, IL 60108-1017
Phone: (630) 980-4740
Fax: (630) 351-8490
Email: info@asch.net
Web site: www.asch.net

The International Journal of Clinical Hypnosis is published by:

Society for Clinical and Experimental Hypnosis
Massachusetts School of Professional Psychology
221 Rivermoor Street
Boston, MA 02132
Phone: (617) 469-1981
Fax: (617) 469-1889
Email: sceh@mspp.edu
Web site: http://ijceh.educ.wsu.edu/

Both are good peer-reviewed journals, written on a professional level for members of these societies. Membership is open to people with a doctorate or a master's degree.

Audio CDs and Tapes

About seventy titles are available on my Web site, www.tranceformation.com, which we distribute throughout the country and the world. Of these, my favorites are:

- *Healing Mind. Healing Body*
- *Sleepy Time Hypnosis*
- *Private Healing Island*. This tape involves a great deal of imagery.
- *The Smoking Cessation Program*. I worked on this program for 12 years until the effectiveness rate was equivalent to that I achieve in my office with patients, which is approximately 80%.

CHAPTER 28

Spiritual Counseling

Mary Elizabeth O'Brien, PhD, MTS, RN, FAAN

Even though an acutely ill person may be facing a potentially life-threatening situation, the concept of spiritual health is not only possible, but may be the key factor in his or her coping successfully with the physiological deficit. In discussing the spiritual health of the acutely ill patient, Peterson and Potter (1997) suggested that "the strength of a client's spirituality influences how he or she copes with sudden illness, and how quickly he or she can move to recovery."

SPIRITUAL WELL-BEING DEFINED

The term spiritual well-being is described historically as having emerged following a 1971 White House Conference on Aging. Sociologist of religion David Moberg (1979) identified spiritual well-being as relating to the "wellness or health of the totality of the inner resources of people, the ultimate concerns around which all other values are focused, the central philosophy of life that guides conduct, and the meaning-giving center of human life which influences all individual and social behavior." The concept of

hope is central to a number of definitions of spiritual well-being. In a discussion of holistic nursing care, spiritual well-being is described as "an integrating aspect of human wholeness, characterized by meaning and hope" (Clark et al., 1991). Lindberg, Hunter, and Kruszewski (1994) included "the need to feel hopeful about one's destiny" in a litany of patient needs related to spiritual well-being.

Most notions of spiritual well-being also contain some reference to philosophy of life and transcendence. Blaikie and Kelson (1979) described spiritual well-being as "that type of existential well being which incorporates some reference to the supernatural, the sacred, or the transcendental"; and Barker observed that spiritual well-being is "to be in communication, in communion with that which goes beyond oneself in order to be whole in oneself" (1979). For the Christian, spiritual well-being is identified as "a right relationship of the person to God, and, following that, a right relationship to neighbor and self" (Christy & Lyon, 1979).

Spirituality is generally identified as being related to issues of transcendence and ultimate life goals. Nurse theorist Barbara Dossey (1989) explained spirituality as encompassing "values, meanings, and purpose" in life; it includes belief in the existence of a "higher authority"; and it may or may not involve "organized religion." O'Brien (1989), in reporting on research with the chronically ill, suggested that spirituality is a broad concept relating to transcendence (God); to the

Sister Mary Elizabeth O'Brien, PhD, MTS, RN, FAAN is a Professor of Nursing at The Catholic University of America School of Nursing and a Spiritual Advisor in the school. She holds a master's degree in theological studies and has been commissioned as a parish nurse. Sister Mary Elizabeth is author of 11 books, 6 of which are on the topic of spirituality and care of the sick.

Source: Courtesy of Mary Elizabeth O'Brien, SFCC, PhD, MTS, RN, FAAN, and Jones and Bartlett Publishers. Adapted from: O'Brien ME. *Spirituality in Nursing.* 2nd ed. Sudbury, MA: Jones and Bartlett; 2003.

"non-material forces or elements within man (or woman); spirituality is that which inspires in one the desire to transcend the realm of the material."

Religiousness, or "religiosity," as it is sometimes identified in sociological literature, refers to religious affiliation and/or practice. Kaufman (1979) described religiousness as "the degree to which religious beliefs, attitudes, and behaviors permeate the life of an individual." In their classic work of 1968, Stark and Glock identified five primary elements of religiousness: belief, religious practice (ritual, devotional), religious experience, religious knowledge, and consequence of religious practice on day-to-day living.

The "spirituality" dimension of spiritual well-being is measured in terms of the concepts of personal faith and spiritual contentment; the "religiousness" element of the construct is reflected in the concept of religious practice.

Personal faith. Personal faith, as a component concept of the spiritual well-being construct, has been described as a "personal relationship with God on whose strength and sureness one can literally stake one's life" (Fatula & Faith, 1993). Personal faith is a reflection of an individual's transcendent values and philosophy of life.

Religious practice. Religious practice is primarily operationalized in terms of religious rituals such as attendance at formal group worship services, private prayer and meditation, reading of spiritual books and articles, and/or the carrying out of such activities as volunteer work or charity.

Spiritual contentment. Spiritual contentment, the opposite of spiritual distress, is likened to spiritual peace (Johnson, 1992), a concept whose correlates include "living in the now of God's love," "accepting the ulti-

mate strength of God," knowledge that all are "children of God," knowing that "God is in control," and "finding peace in God's love and forgiveness." When an individual reports minimal to no notable spiritual distress, he or she may be considered to be in a state of "spiritual contentment."

SPIRITUAL NEEDS IN ILLNESS

Needs of patients with acute illness. Spiritual beliefs and, for some, religious practices may become more important during illness than at any other time in a person's life (Kozier et al., 1995). While an individual is enjoying good mental and physical health, spiritual or religious practices may be relegated, in terms of both time and energy, to a small portion of one's life activities. With the onset of acute illness, however, especially if associated with the exacerbation of a chronic condition, some significant life changes may occur both physically and emotionally. First, the ill person is usually forced to dramatically curtail physical activities, especially those associated with formal work or professional involvement. This may leave the individual with a great deal of uncommitted time to ponder the meaning of life and the illness experience. Such a time of forced physical "retreat" may effect considerable emotional change in one's assessment of past and future attitudes and behaviors.

The remarks of a 32-year-old male patient reflected such an experience during an episode of acute renal failure: "It enlightened me as to just how fast I was really going. It made me reevaluate my life. Now I can place my needs before my wants. It hasn't been so difficult in looking at the good advantages. This thing has made me think a lot about the way I used to live, and put different values on things." (O'Brien, 1983). A 47-year-old male renal-failure patient who had also suffered a serious bout of acute illness at the time of disease onset, commented in a similar vein: "This illness definitely made me think; get my mind together. I know all things happen for the good. It turned me around spiritually and mentally. Now I listen better. I try to be more patient, and I have more to learn from others" (O'Brien, 1983).

Despite a possible positive effect, however, the onset of a sudden and unanticipated acute illness may pose serious emotional and spiritual problems related to fear of possible death or disability. Psychological depression may occur as a result of severe physical symptoms such as acute pain and fatigue. Some patients question God's will and even express anger toward God for allowing the illness to occur. At this point, especially, the practitioner must be alert and astute in assessing the spiritual concerns and needs of an acutely ill patient. Although a diagnosis of spiritual distress may be masked by the physical and emotional symptoms of an illness, the patient's remarks can provide a hint as to the presence of spiritual symptoms in need of attention. For example, comments such as "God help me," or "I wonder where God is in all of this" can provide an opening for informal spiritual assessment.

The perioperative patient. In the model of perioperative nursing developed by Phippen, Wells, and Martinelli (1994), the spiritual dimension of the patient is influenced by underlying "religious and philosophical beliefs." The strategy suggested by Phippen et al. involves an exploration of the type of spiritual or religious practices to which the patient relates (for example, spiritual reading or a visit with a chaplain); the nurse may then intervene by providing materials or making appropriate referrals. Heiser, Chiles, Fudge, and Gray (1997) advocated, for example, that perioperative

nurses use music therapy in the immediate postoperative recovery period as a contemporary spiritual intervention strategy.

Patients in the intensive care unit. Critical care nurses comment on the need for the nursing practice of spiritual care in the ICU and its value: "My patients are all very sick, and communication is a key issue. When I talk to them about religious things, they often exhibit strengths related to how they are handling their illness. For some of these patients it's really tough, like with young bone marrow transplants in the ICU flunking the second transplant, and they're not going to live and they know it and the family knows it. They really need spiritual support . . . I'm trying to work on the nonpharmacologic approach to decreasing anxiety. Patients may be anxious because of unmet spiritual needs, so we're trying to use music, listening visitors, communication . . . just being open to whatever the patients' spiritual needs are, whether they're religious like associated with a church or just their own spirituality."

The patient in pain. Pain, whether acute, chronic, or related to a malignancy, is influenced by a multiplicity of physiological, psychological, sociocultural, and spiritual factors. Therapeutic interventions for the relief of pain include pharmacological (for example, analgesic drugs) and physiological (such as acupuncture, acupressure, cutaneous stimulation, surgery) measures, as well as nonpharmacoglogical measures such as biofeedback, meditation, relaxation, and guided imagery. For the nurse, in addition to recommending or participating in prayer (if acceptable to the patient in pain) and seeking counsel of a chaplain, another therapeutic spiritual care activity that the nurse may recommend and teach is the use of spiritual imagery (Ferszt & Taylor, 1988). Other spiritual care strategies for alleviating patients' pain include listening with a caring manner to the individual's fears and anxieties related to the pain experience, and facilitating the participation of family members and other significant persons who may be a primary source of support (Turk & Feldman, 1992; Warner, 1992).

Spiritual needs of the family. The family is an important resource in the provision of spiritual care, not only for the sick child but for the ill adult as well. There are a number of understandings of the term family in contemporary society. Friedmann (1992) defined *family* as "two or more persons who are joined together by bonds of sharing and emotional closeness, who identify themselves as being part of the family." Today, there is also a growing emergence of the single-parent family; for the single, unmarried individual, friends or associates belonging to a church or to friendship groups may also be loosely described as family.

Because healthy families generally function as units, it is important to minister to the spiritual needs of the entire family when one member is ill or in need of support (Clinebell, 1991). Families faced with serious short-term or chronic long-term illness of one of the members can benefit greatly from spiritual support provided by friends, church members, or pastoral care providers, both within and outside the health care system. The family's particular spiritual or religious tradition and experience will, of course, direct the kind and degree of spiritual care and support that will prove helpful during an illness. For the family not of religious tradition, spiritual care may consist simply of the presence and concern demonstrated by those providing the intervention.

The family in the intensive care unit. Clark and Heindenreich (1995) identified spiritual well-being for the acutely ill patient experiencing intensive care as encompassing the support of caregivers, family members and friends, and religion and faith beliefs. The family of an acutely ill patient hospitalized in an intensive care unit may spend long hours in waiting rooms, sometimes rarely leaving the hospital setting. This is a time when the arrival of a chaplain or nurse willing to provide spiritual care is generally welcomed unequivocally. Families need to verbalize their anxieties to someone with a caring heart as they attempt to face the severity of a loved one's illness (Niklas & Stefanics, 1975). Ultimately, spiritual support is reported to be a key dimension of family care in the ICU (Rukholm et al., 1991). For nursing staff some spiritual care interventions for the family might include giving information about the patient, environment, and staff, to the degree possible; encouraging the family to verbalize their anxieties and concerns; suggesting some coping strategies for attempting to keep up with physical needs such as nutrition and sleep; and reinforcing the fact that the family's anxiety is normal in such a situation, with the suggestion of some possible coping strategies to reduce stress (Gillman et al., 1996). The ICU nurse might also include patients' families in bedside discussions whenever acceptable and attempt to include family needs when developing a plan of care (Chesla & Stannard, 1997).

SPIRITUAL COUNSELING

In essence, meeting the spiritual needs of the acutely ill may encompass basic concepts of spiritual care such as listening, being present, and making a referral to a chaplain or other pastoral caregiver.

Pastoral care describes the interventions carried out by religious ministers in response to the spiritual or religious needs of others. The activities of the pastoral caregiver, "including sacramental and social ministries, can be as informal as conversational encounters and as formal as highly structured ritual events" (Studzinski, 1993). Howard Clinebell (1991) identified five specific pastoral care functions: "healing, sustaining, guiding, reconciling, and nurturing." Such spiritual care interventions may promote significant healing on the part of those who are ill.

Shelly and Fish (1988) noted the importance of the clergy as a resource in spiritual care of the ill; they asserted that spiritual care given by clergy and nurses should be complementary. For such complementarity to exist, three conditions are suggested: mutuality of goals in care giving, a delineation of role responsibilities, and communication. The activities of the minister or pastoral caregiver offer an important religious comfort dimension by providing the patient with familiar symbols and experiences (Atkinson & Fotunato, 1996). A pastoral advisor understands the patient's religious belief system and can plan care to be congruent with the individual's religious heritage (Krekeler & Yancey, 1993).

In making a pastoral care referral, the health care practitioner may contact a priest, minister, rabbi, imam, or other spiritual advisor of the patient's acquaintance and tradition, or refer the patient to a health care facility's department of pastoral care. Consider the influence of pastoral ministry in helping a patient cope with the acute onset of renal failure: "When I first went on dialysis and was in the hospital, I was sick as a dog. I had pneumonia plus kidney failure and I thought I might die. But the response that I got from my minister and the church was just fantastic. The minister prayed for me, and I had everybody wanting to know how's my dialysis going, and I got a list of 35 people from the church, especially the deacons, who were willing to drive me any place I needed to go."

Two aspects of faith are key in the provision of health care: spiritual sustenance and support for healing. The relationship between faith and illness is beautifully exemplified in the faith of Peter, a long-term survivor of HIV infection, who said, "God is the one reliable constant in my life." Spirituality is a resource that can be drawn upon to support the healing process, coping, and in some cases recovery, in response to the beliefs and needs of patients and their families.

REFERENCES

Atkinson LJ, Fortunato NM. *Berry & Kohn's Operating Room Technique*. St. Louis, MO: CV Mosby-Yearbook; 1996.

Barker E. Whose service is perfect freedom. In: Moberg DO, ed. *Spiritual Well-Being: Sociological Perspectives*. Washington, DC: University of America Press; 1979:154.

Blaikie NW, Kelson GP. Locating self and giving meaning to existence. In: Moberg DO, ed. *Spiritual Well-Being: Sociological Perspectives*. Washington, DC: University of America Press; 1979:137.

Chesla CA, Stannard D. Breakdown in the nursing care of families in the ICU. *Am J Crit Care*. 1997;6(1): 64–71.

Christy RD, Lyon D. Sociological perspectives on personhood. In: Moberg DO, ed. *Spiritual Well-Being: Sociological Perspectives*. Washington, DC: University of America Press; 1979:98.

Clark C, Heindenreich T. Spiritual care for the critically ill. *Am J Crit Care*. 1995;4(1):77–81.

Clark CC, Cross JR, Deane DM, Lowry LW. Spirituality: integral to quality care. *Holistic Nursing Process*. 1991;3(1):68.

Clinebell H. *Basic Types of Pastoral Care and Counseling*. Nashville, TN: Abington Press; 1991:430.

Dossey, BM. The transpersonal self and states of consciousness. In: Dossey BM, Keegan L, Kolkmeier LG, Guzzeta CE, eds. *Holistic Health Promotion*. Rockville, MD: Aspen; 1989:23–35.

Fatula MA. Faith. In: Downey M, ed. *The New Dictionary of Catholic Spirituality*. Collegeville, MN: The Liturgical Press; 1993:379.

Ferszt GG, Taylor PB. When your patient needs spiritual comfort. *Nursing '88*. 1988;18(4):48–49.

Friedmann MM. *Family Nursing: Theory and Practice*. 3rd ed. Norwalk, CT: Appleton & Lange; 1992:90.

Gillman J, Gable-Rodriguez J, Sutherland M, Whitacre JH. Pastoral care in a critical care setting. *Crit Care Nurs Q*. 1996;19(1):150.

Heiser R, Chiles K, Fudge M, Gray S. The use of music during the immediate postoperative recovery period. *AORN J*. 1997;65(4):66.

Johnson RP. *Body, Mind, Spirit: Trapping the Healing Power Within You*. Liguori, MO: Liguori;1992: 12–13.

Kaufman JH. Social correlates of spiritual maturity among North American Mennonites. In: Moberg DO, ed. *Spiritual Well-Being: Sociological Perspectives*. Washington, DC: University of America Press; 1979:237.

Kozier B, Erb G, Blais K, Wilkinson J. *Fundamentals of Nursing: Concepts, Process and Practice*. 5th ed. Menlo Park, CA: Addison-Wesley; 1995:314.

Krekeler K, Yancey V. Spiritual health. In: Potter PA, Perry AG, eds. *Fundamentals of Nursing: Concepts, Process and Practice*. 3rd ed. St. Louis, MO: Mosby; 1993:1000–1013.

Lindberg JB, Hunter ML, Kruszewski AZ. *Introduction to Nursing: Concepts, Issues and Opportunities*. Philadelphia, PA: JB Lippincott; 1994:110.

Moberg DO. The development of social indicators of spiritual well-being and quality of life. In: Moberg DO, ed. *Spiritual Well-Being: Sociological Perspectives*. Washington, DC: University of America Press; 1979:2.

Niklas GR, Stefanics C. *Ministry to the Hospitalized*. New York, NY: Paulist Press; 1975:81.

O'Brien ME. *The Courage to Survive: The Life Career of the Chronic Dialysis Patient*. New York, NY: Grune & Stratton; 1983:146.

O'Brien ME. *Anatomy of a Nursing Home: A New View of Resident Life*. Owings Mills, MD: National Health Publishing; 1989:24,88.

Peterson V, Potter PA. Spiritual health. In: Potter PS, Perry AG, eds. *Fundamentals of Nursing: Concepts, Process and Practice*. St. Louis, MO: CV Mosby; 1997:443.

Phippen ML, Wells MP, Martinelli AM. A conceptual model for perioperative nursing practice. In: Phippen ML, Wells MD, eds. *Perioperative Nursing Practice*. Philadelphia, PA: WB Saunders; 1994:4.

Rukholm EE, Bailey PH, Coutu-Wakulczyk G. Family needs and anxieties in the ICU. *Can J Nurs Res*. 1991;23(3):67–81.

Shelly JA, Fish S. *Spiritual Care: The Nurses' Role*. 3rd ed. Downer's Grove, IL: Intervarsity Press; 1988.

Stark R. Glock, C. *American Piety: The Nature of Religious Commitment*. Berkeley, CA: Univeristy of California Press; 1968.

Studzinski R. Pastoral care and counseling. In: Downey M, ed. *The New Dictionary of Catholic Spirituality*. Collegeville, MN: The Liturgical Press; 1993: 722–723.

Turk DC, Feldman CS. Facilitating the use of noninvasive pain management strategies with the terminally ill. *Hosp J*. 1992;8(1):193–214.

Warner JE. Involvement of families in pain control of terminally ill patients. *Hosp J*. 1992;8(1):155–170.

Self-Care

Chapter

CHAPTER 29

Patient Self-Care

M. Caroline Martin, RN, MHA

FOUR STEPS TO GOOD PATIENT SELF-CARE

1. Helping your patients know and understand their risk factors
2. Encouraging proactive self-care
3. Identifying the best resources available to patients in the community
4. Making your practice the place of choice for patient continuity of care

As the health care continuum expands, providers have greater opportunity to practice preventive medicine. If this is one of your goals, you may find that engaging patients in health promotion activities becomes as important as caring for them when they are ill. For preventive programs to be successful, your patients need the competence and confidence to practice good self-care. This approach is most successful when there is emphasis on collaboration with patients, health education, and healthy lifestyle choices. Even patients who require intensive health management can potentially benefit from lifestyle interventions.

1. HELPING PATIENTS UNDERSTAND THEIR RISK FACTORS

Health risk appraisals. One effective way to help your patients understand their risk factors is to provide health risk appraisals. A

A brief biography of M. Caroline Martin appears in Chapter 5.

health risk assessment or wellness profile is a questionnaire that can be used to capture information on general health issues, symptoms, and risk factors related to lifestyle. The assessment process can be integrated into day-to-day care delivery. Patients are asked to fill out a brief health assessment when they first come in for an office visit. Before the doctor sees the patient, the report can be scanned into the record and a printout provided to the physician.

The assessment is an additional source of information about the patient's health status that can be reviewed at the time of each appointment—information that can be captured without increasing time spent in the office visit. With the time constraints facing practitioners today, certain aspects of this process can and should be handled by educated trained paraprofessionals using good collateral materials for patient education. In some cases, the next step for patients may simply involve sitting down with a nurse after their appointment and reviewing the health assessment. It can also mean providing patients with a health manual or a handout specific to their needs.

Annual health risk appraisals. Health risk assessments can be repeated at the time of the annual physical, allowing year-to-year comparisons of lifestyle and behavioral risks. A copy of the assessment can also be given to the patient. This assessment provides a means of tracking the patient's progress and ascertaining whether their health risks are being minimized or exacerbated.

Capturing data electronically. The SF-36 (Short Form-36), SF-12, and SF-8 are widely utilized tools for health evaluation (one contains 36 questions, and the others 12 and 8 questions, respectively). These practical self-reports can be used to capture information on patient health status. The SF-36, for example, is a multipurpose, 36-item survey that measures patient perceptions in 8 domains of health: physical functioning, physical role, pain, energy/vitality, mental health, social functioning, emotional role, and general health. It yields scores for each of these 8 domains, and 2 summary measures of physical and mental health.

These questionnaires can also be used in conjunction with proprietary software, making it possible to scan the form and print out a report immediately. The self-assessments can be stored in digital form in patients' records, a decided advantage as more physicians move to the electronic medical record. Brief notes regarding observations, recommendations, or follow-up on progress can also be included.

Assessing readiness for change. Some self-assessment questionnaires, such as the *Healthwise Personal Wellness Profile*, also include questions to determine the patient's readiness for change. Results can be reviewed with patients to determine their level of motivation. The current theory of behavioral change suggests that it occurs in a process of identifiable stages. The type of feedback obtained from these assessment tools provides a snapshot of where patients are in the process of change. This information gives the physician greater ability to monitor progress and assist patients in making the changes necessary.

Opening the dialogue on risk factors. Many good assessment tools include recommendations which can be printed out and given to the patient. These printouts provide the basis for informal, yet focused discussions with patients. This is an opportunity to talk about interventions and options and to offer counseling and encouragement. These profiles are quite succinct, so the health care provider can gain a sense of the patient's current status in less than a minute and address the most critical issues reflected in the assessment at the time of the visit.

Targeting the intervention. Knowing the stage of readiness of your patients enables you to make individually tailored recommendations. Key information gleaned from the assessment will enable you to respond to patients' current interests and motivation. For example, if you discover that your patient is thinking about stopping smoking, having this information will allow you to target the intervention to his specific stage of readiness.

READINESS FOR CHANGE

Research suggests that approximately 5% to 10% of any given population are ready for change. For this receptive segment of the population, simply being provided with good information enables them to begin a process of change. Whether they buy a book or obtain information on the Internet, they will initiate the changes by themselves.

Another 5% to 10% of people on the other end of the spectrum are unlikely to make any change. Then there are the 80% in the middle; 40% are typically moving away from change, and 40% are moving toward change. Unless something dramatic happens, those moving away from change will probably not reverse their behavior. However, they may become motivated to change through a catastrophic life event; for example, learning that a family member has heart disease or discovering they have cardiovascular disease themselves.

Research from the Ornish program indicated that the most effective health interventions focus on the 40% of any population who are moving toward change. These are people who have tried various exercise programs and different diets without success; like most of us, they need a support structure to make major changes in their lives. Otherwise, they usually do not succeed on their own. People who are highly motivated tend to be more successful in achieving lifestyle changes. Those who are participating simply to please their family have a much harder time than those who are self-motivated.

Courtesy of Glenn Perelson, Ornish Preventive Medicine Research Institute, Sausalito, CA.

---

2. ENCOURAGING PROACTIVE PATIENT SELF-CARE

Supporting your patients in health promotion means increasing their level of understanding of good self-care—and their competence to achieve it. It also means providing the encouragement to build patients' confidence in their ability to create change in their own lives.

Prioritizing risk factors. The self-assessment provides cues to both the patient and the physician about increased risk. The next step is to correlate and prioritize risk factors to determine which are most urgent. For example, is the patient continuing to gain weight? The assessment provides a practical focus for opening this type of discussion and gently encouraging the patient to take action. This is an opportunity to explore new approaches with the patient that might be more effective. (Yet studies performed in physicians' offices find that many never mention good nutrition, obesity, smoking, or other lifestyle-related issues that underlie chronic health problems.) We now know that lifestyle can be a critical component of health and a powerful tool in both prevention and disease management.

This process enables the practitioner to make recommendations that are very specific to the needs of each patient. Generalized recommendations such as, "You need more exercise" may not be enough to bring about change. It is more likely to be motivating when the doctor suggests specific practical steps, such as, "I'm going to write you a prescription to the fitness center. If you take my prescription with you, you won't have to pay an initiation fee." Whenever physicians are able to determine patients' needs more clearly, they are in a better position to provide access to the most appropriate (and therefore cost-effective) services.

Prioritizing your recommendations will help patients understand that you consider lifestyle factors to be highly important. You can do this by being very purposeful in the questions you ask and the materials you provide. You also convey this emphasis on healthy lifestyle through the referrals and resources you encourage patients to use.

Reinforcing positive change. The health care practitioner can continue to track progress and provide encouragement at follow-up visits. Since the assessments (and a summary of the patient's goals) are stored in the medical record, they can be referred to during subsequent checkups. The practitioner can make note of any lifestyle change; for example, has the patient lost weight or begun a walking program? Lifestyle change can be encouraged through a positive comment or a question such as, "What helped you the most?" These periodic reviews also provide the opportunity to incorporate additional timely recommendations.

Tools for practice management. The process of reinforcing positive change not only enables you to focus your efforts in terms of each specific patient—it also supplies you with the data necessary to develop a profile of your practice. The brief assessments can be used to determine the most prevalent diagnoses and risk factors of your entire patient population. Once you have determined the key issues confronting the majority of your patients (and the prevalence of these issues), you can focus your own reading and research on those particular health conditions. Care pathways and resources can then be identified and targeted to the specific needs of the largest segments of your patient population. Clearly no practitioner can be knowledgeable about all the health resources available, but it is important to be aware of the selected resources most relevant to the needs of your patient population.

3. IDENTIFYING AVAILABLE RESOURCES

There are other steps to self-care that can be taught to patients so they do not require as much coaching on a one-on-one basis. Initially they may be able to utilize self-help books or the Internet before accessing the services of a nurse practitioner, other health care professionals—or you. Encourage patients to make good use of available resources:

- Health information such as wellness manuals
- Internet resources and telemedicine
- Community resources for health and wellness
- Support groups
- Services for those at risk but not yet symptomatic
- Disease management for patients with chronic illness

Health information such as wellness manuals. Our experience suggests that the use of resource manuals improves self-care and facilitates access to community resources. When you encourage patient self-care, this reflects the respect you have for your patients' ability to be participative in their own health.

If you choose to make a self-care manual available through your practice, information can be printed on the cover about your services so the manual becomes a marketing tool. Costs for this effort are a legitimate part of your practice expense and should be itemized as such, perhaps paid for out of the marketing budget. The manual could be given as a gift to new patients or provided at the time of the annual visit. If your practice participates in civic and community health events, these manuals are useful as indirect marketing. They serve not only to increase awareness of your services, but also to position your practice as one concerned about prevention and wellness.

The manual will be of most value if a brief patient coaching session is provided for the patient by a staff member to review its use. Follow-up calls by staff can be made 4 months after receipt of the manual to respond to questions your patients may have regarding the use of this resource. The follow-up can also inquire whether they used the manual, how it helped them, which tools and resources were the most beneficial, and the nature of their progress. If it is time and cost prohibitive to call all patients, a random sample of one in every five patients might allow your staff to ascertain the value of this resource. Another approach might be to implement an annual patient survey on service quality. This provides the opportunity to include questions about the usefulness of the manual and any self-care initiatives your patients may have begun. These efforts reflect your primary intention to benefit members of your patient community.

Internet resources and telemedicine. The problems with cyberspace—too much commercialism and some really bad advice—have raised concerns about whether this resource is actually of value. However, it also provides access to a wealth of good information and the opportunity for support through online forums. The following are some tips on how to get involved in providing online consumer health information.

Begin by putting your existing patient education materials on a Web site. Effective consumer health information is a must and should include the capability for two-way communication. If your site provides links to other sites, you have the opportunity to post only those sites you have reviewed and are comfortable in recommending. Your site can also include reading lists and community resources. This is another opportunity to cultivate smart patients. Take them seriously and encourage them to learn all they can about their own health.

Periodically review your site as if you were the patient. You will want to be very familiar with the content, links, usage, and value of your site. Physicians typically have one person on staff whose job it is to keep the Web site and printed materials up to date. This should be done on at least a semi-annual basis.

Have your staff determine if a call center or telephone health advisory service is available in your service area. Phone services can be used to improve continuity of care and timely treatment, and to monitor the condition of chronically ill patients. Many health information call services are operated as a community service.

Community resources for health and wellness. Some local health systems sponsor programs and support groups to meet a range of needs—from normal pregnancy and parenting to diabetes and heart disease.

These resources may include hospital-based fitness facilities or programs such as Phase 3 cardio exercise monitoring; classes in yoga, tai chi, or Qigong; and nutrition courses.

Support groups. Self-help groups are often consumer driven—examples range from Weight Watchers to Alcoholics Anonymous. These groups give patients the opportunity to share their experiences, trade resource information, and access psychosocial support. As a physician, if you recommend specific support groups, you or a staff member may want to attend a meeting initially to assure yourself of the expertise of the leader and the consistency with your own practice philosophy. When referring to disease management programs, you will also want to ensure that the group facilitators have the clinical expertise to deal with chronic conditions.

Services for those at risk (but not yet acutely ill). A different set of care management tools is required for those who are at risk but asymptomatic. Resources may be available in your community to help people reduce their health risks through programs described as well care management. This approach utilizes support groups, health management programs, and disease management processes. These programs usually focus on a targeted population, specific health condition (diabetes, for example), life stage (such as aging), or psychosocial need (such as families or teens at risk).

Most ideal are programs that use identified care guidelines and a broad range of resources to assist clients in managing their health conditions and individual needs. Well care management takes a very behavioral approach in which clients set specific goals and work toward tangible objectives and outcomes. Programs seek to provide resources or referrals that participants require to meet clinical and psychosocial needs, such as support, health care, and community services. This approach can be used for patients who are well, at risk, chronically ill, or acutely ill. The process is essentially the same for patients in each of these groups, although the tools and referral resources will vary. The point is to know what works best for your patients at each level of need, based on their clinical data, health-risk assessments, and level of readiness for change. With this information, you will be better prepared to link them with quality resources in your community.

Disease management for patients with chronic conditions. Additional resources are often needed for those who are symptomatic or who have chronic conditions. Check with your managed care provider or insurers to see if, as a participating physician, you can enroll your patients in their care management services. You will also want to determine how they link you into the program so that you can remain the coordinator of your patients' care. (The most highly developed care management currently available is that which occurs while the patient is within the hospital setting. However, out-patient care management tools and services are becoming increasingly more prevalent.)

Self-care is a critical component of disease management. Patients with chronic conditions will find that their efforts to live a healthy lifestyle are paramount in the effective management of their condition and in the reduction of complications.

For example, in the case of diabetic patients, support groups and self-care are exceptionally valuable, due to the chronicity of this condition, it's impact on quality of life, and the potential for severe complications. Third-party payers have begun to realize the benefit of knowledgeable and engaged patients, in terms of both cost reduction and the avoidance of medical complications. Insurance reimbursement is now available for individual and group diabetes education sessions when provided by certified diabetes educators within a physician's practice. This is an opportunity for doctors to expand their practice offerings while supporting the needs of their patients with chronic disorders. We have found that well care management is an important philosophy that can be utilized no matter where people are along the illness/wellness continuum.

Groups focused on diabetes management provide participants with information on the right foods to eat, exercise appropriate to their particular condition(s), and the management of insulin use. The practical goal in this population is to stabilize blood sugar, avoid a crisis lifestyle, and overcome the chronic side effects of poor disease management. Patient education also includes learning to self-manage specific risks associated with their condition, such as the need for good foot care and an annual retinal exam. In all disease management programs, the ultimate goals are enhanced health and quality of life.

4. MAKING YOUR PRACTICE THE PLACE OF CHOICE FOR PATIENTS

Today there are changes in the traditional patient-physician relationship—but with change comes opportunity. One aspect of this change is the transition from passive, dependent patients to active, healthy consumers, reflected in the growing interest in holistic health and consumer self-care. Empowered patients tend to be more compliant and more conscientious about their lifestyle and self-care.

Many patients are seeking a physician with whom they can partner in their own care. If you provide information to your patients that stresses the importance of working with a primary care provider, you will be speaking the same language as numerous consumers who are looking for a supportive patient-physician relationship. These relationships maximize continuity of care and minimize the use of the emergency room for nonemergent conditions.

It is important that patients know they have an established relationship with their physician. This involves two-way communication regarding their health in terms of what is working and what is not. Open communication tends to promote a greater level of trust. As your patients learn that you are supportive of them when they assume more responsibility for their own health, they will gain the realization that they have partnered with a physician who is committed to the practice of preventive medicine.

RESOURCES

SF-36 and SF-12
Medical Outcomes Trust
235 Wyman Street, Suite 130
Waltham, MA 02451
Phone: (781) 890-4884
Fax: (781) 890-0922
Email: info@outcomes-trust.org
Web site: www.outcomes-trust.org
Web site: www.sf36.com

SF-36 and SF-12
IQOLA Project
Health Assessment Lab
235 Wyman Street, Suite 130
Waltham, MA 02451 USA
Telephone: (781) 890-5544
Fax: (781) 890-0922
Email info@iqola.org
Web site: www.iqola.org

The Medical Outcomes Trust and the IQOLA Project provide research and product information on these assessment tools, which are now used worldwide and have been validated in 15 countries. A Google search on SF-36 or SF-12 also provides numerous links to sites with related products and information.

Healthwise Publications
PO Box 1989
Boise, Idaho 83701
Phone: (800) 706-9646
Web site: healthwise.org

Healthwise Publications provides a health manual and also an assessment form, the *Healthwise Personal Wellness Profile*, which includes an assessment of patient readiness for change.

CHAPTER 30

Prescribing Relaxation Techniques

David Rakel, MD

HISTORICAL PERSPECTIVE

In the early 20th century the physiologist, Walter Cannon, discovered that when subjects were exposed to a number of physically and mentally stressful events, they secreted a large amount of epinephrine that prepared them for action. He later coined the term "the fight or flight response" to describe this physical reaction to stress. On the other side of the coin was the Nobel Prize-winning Swiss physiologist, Walter Hess. In the 1930s, Hess found that by stimulating certain areas of the brain of laboratory animals, he was able to induce a physical reaction that was opposite to that seen with the fight or flight response. One area triggered signs of relaxation that included reduced muscle tone, breathing, and heart rate. Herbert Benson, working in the same laboratory as Cannon had years earlier, helped pioneer this field when he described the "relaxation response" and how meditation could be used to decrease the response of the sympathetic nervous system. Meditation was found to reduce heart rate, respiratory rate, plasma cortisol, and pulse rate, and to increase electroencephalogram alpha waves that are associated with relaxation (Shapiro, 1995). Evidence was accumulating supporting the fact that lifestyle practices can have a direct influence on disease and its prevention.

A brief biography of David Rakel appears in Chapter 1.

Courtesy of David Rakel, MD, and Elsevier Science. From: Rakel D. Prescribing relaxation techniques. In Rakel D, ed. *Integrative Medicine*. Philadelphia, PA: Saunders/Elsevier Science; 2003.

STRESS, RELAXATION, AND THEIR EFFECTS

It is now well established that stress has damaging effects on health and the immune system—through dysregulation of the autonomic nervous system and the hypothalamic-pituitary-adrenal axis (Stanford & Salmon, 1999). As can be seen in Figure 30–1, stress triggers emotions that release chemicals through these sites to stimulate somatic change that can lead to poor health. Chronic stress results in a continuous activation of cycle A, which helps explain the association between chronic stress and increased susceptibility to infection (Everly & Benson, 1989).

In this age of multitasking it is not uncommon to see someone driving a car while talking on a phone and jotting down a message. It takes time for our minds to change focus from one topic to another. The more we divert our attention, the less we are able to concentrate on any one task well. If we are constantly being distracted by multiple thoughts, our fight or flight response will be triggered due to fear of not being able to address them all. (I am sure many readers can relate.) Giving attention to lifestyle changes that reduce triggers and practicing techniques that will activate the relaxation response (cycle B) can have significant health benefits. It is important to remember that the relaxation response can be learned but takes practice for the body to benefit. Regular use results in long-term physiologic changes that last throughout the day, not only during the time that the relaxation technique is being practiced (Hoffman et al., 1982).

The evidence for relaxation. There are more than 3000 studies that show the benefi-

> *Relaxation techniques are tools that will help balance the effects of stress but are not substitutes for exploring problems that may be causing it.*

cial effects of relaxation on health. Table 30–1 lists common conditions in which relaxation has been found useful. Many studies docu-

ment the value of various relaxation exercises such as meditation, breathing, and progressive muscle relaxation. Beneficial effects have been shown in tension headaches (Blanchard et al., 1991), anxiety (Eppley et al., 1989), insomnia (Jacobs et al., 1996), psoriasis (Kabat-Zinn et al., 1998), blood pressure (Alexander et al., 1996; Stuart et al., 1987), cardiac ischemia and exercise tolerance (Zamarra et al., 1996), cardiac arrhythmia (Benson et al., 1975), premenstrual syndrome (Goodale et al., 1990), infertility (Domar et al., 1990), longevity and cognitive function in the elderly (Alexander et al., 1989), use of medical care (Orme-Johnson,

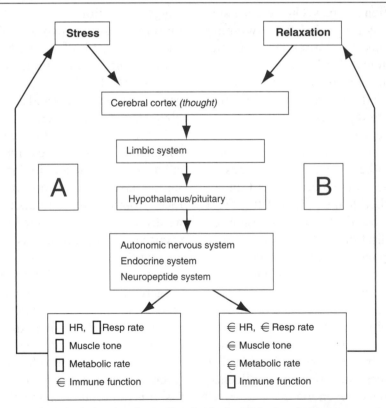

Figure 30–1 A simplified chart showing the cyclic mind-body and body-mind influences of stress (A) and relaxation (B) on health. As our body experiences the physical responses to stress and relaxation, our central nervous system remembers them causing a continuation of the cycle resulting in long-term positive or negative physical consequences.
Source: Rakel D. Prescribing relaxation techniques. In Rakel D, ed. *Integrative Medicine.* Philadelphia, PA: Saunders/Elsevier Science; 2003.

Table 30–1 Conditions That Benefit from Relaxation Exercises

- Anxiety, anger, and hostility
- Depression
- Infertility
- Pain, headaches
- Irritable bowel syndrome
- Essential hypertension
- Asthma
- Dermatologic conditions
- Raynaud's disease
- Rheumatoid arthritis
- Temporal mandibular joint disease
- Diabetes
- Chronic dyspepsia
- Premenstrual syndrome
- Cardiac arrhythmias
- Smoking cessation
- Cognitive function

Source: Rakel D. Prescribing relaxation techniques. In Rakel D, ed. *Integrative Medicine*. Philadelphia, PA: Saunders/Elsevier Science; 2003.

1987), medical costs in treating chronic pain (Caudill et al., 1991), smoking cessation (Royer-Bounour, 1989), and serum cholesterol (Cooper & Aygen, 1978). Recommending relaxation therapy is very important in the primary care setting since more than 60% of all doctor visits are stress related.

Relaxation and mental focus. It is our mind's thoughts that trigger the physiologic changes that can result in poor health. Efforts to "stop worrying," for example, involve focusing on something other than thoughts that cause stress. Mental focus is a common feature of all relaxation techniques. Meditation may focus on a mantra, yoga may focus on a body posture (asana) or the breath, guided imagery focuses on an image, and progressive muscle relaxation focuses on the muscles. Relaxation does not need to include these traditional mind-body therapies and may simply involve focusing on a hobby

such as painting, playing an instrument, or gardening. Whatever task is used, the mind will have a tendency to wander. If this happens, we can simply accept it and bring our attention back to the activity at hand. Using a more structured technique will help emphasize the importance of this. Focus frees the mind from its usual stressful thoughts, such as worry, planning, thinking, and reasoning, and dampens the production of adrenergic catecholamines that stimulate the limbic system, which in turn inhibit immune activity.

Relaxation and aerobic exercise. We usually do not associate relaxation with exercise but Herbert Benson and colleagues found that the relaxation response could also be elicited during aerobic exercise. Compared to a control group, volunteers who focused their thoughts on a word or phrase while riding a stationary bike reduced both their oxygen consumption and their metabolic rate, resulting in improved efficiency (Benson et al., 1978).

Few may have the time to meditate for 20 minutes twice a day, exercise for 30 minutes, spend quality time with their family, and make a living while getting 8 hours of sleep. Combining relaxation and exercise into one activity uses time more efficiently.

MATCHING THE TECHNIQUE TO THE INDIVIDUAL

Relaxation techniques are similar to ice cream flavors. Once someone finds a flavor they like, they think everyone should try it. The important thing is not to get everyone to meditate but to identify a technique that best suits that person's lifestyle. In fact, it has been shown that various relaxation techniques such as meditation, biofeedback, hypnosis, guided imagery, or progressive muscle relaxation induce the same physiologic response (Delmonte, 1984). There are many different ways to arrive at the desired outcome. Matching the technique to the individual will be more successful in inducing relaxation and it will be used more often. For example, a body vigilant woman with breast cancer might not respond well to progressive muscle relaxation since this requires focus on specific parts of the body. An anxious, type A individual may do better with a technique that gives an active mind something to focus on. A relaxation exercise should be as individualized as prescribing a medication for hypertension.

Relaxation exercises are a low-cost, well-tolerated therapy that can be recommended

> *The most important task is for the medical provider to match the relaxation technique to the patient's personality, beliefs, and lifestyle.*

for many problems seen in the primary care setting. Relaxation may be most useful in those suffering from anxiety, heart disease, recurring pain syndromes, and chronic illness, but will also be beneficial in helping patients find a balance in their lives—resulting in the best medicine of all, prevention. The following (Table 30–2) provides a brief summary of various relaxation exercises.

Table 30–2 Relaxation Techniques

Relaxation Technique	Summary	Further Resources
Breathing exercise (See Chapter 32, "Breathing Exercises")	The foundation of most relaxation techniques. Have the patient place one hand on the chest and the other on the abdomen. Instruct the patient to take a slow deep breath, as if sucking in all the air in the room. While doing this, the hand on the abdomen should rise higher than that on the chest. This promotes diaphragmatic breathing that increases alveolar expansion in the bases of the lungs. Have the patient hold the breath for a count of 7 and then exhale. Exhalation should take twice as long as inhalation. Repeat this for a total of 5 breaths, and encourage patients to do this three times a day.	*Conscious Breathing* by Gay Hendricks, PhD, is one of many good resources on using breathing for relaxation and health.
Transcendental meditation (TM)/The Relaxation Response (See Chapter 31, "Recommending Meditation")	To prevent distracting thoughts, the subject repeats a mantra (a word or sound) over and over again while sitting in a comfortable position. If a distracting thought comes to mind, it is accepted and let go	Visit www.mindbody. harvard.edu or read *The Relaxation Response* by Herbert Benson, MD. Visit

continues

Table 30–2 continued

Relaxation Technique	Summary	Further Resources
	with the mind focusing again on the mantra.	www.tm.org for information on transcendental meditation.
Mindful meditation (See Chapter 31)	Represents the philosophy of living in the present or the moment. The *body scan* is one technique in which the subject uses breathing to obtain a relaxed state while lying or sitting. The mind progressively focuses on different parts of the body where it feels any and all sensations intentionally but non-judgmentally before moving on to another part of the body. A patient with back pain may focus on the quality and characteristics of the pain as if to better understand it and bring it under control.	*Full Catastrophe Living* by Jon Kabat-Zinn, PhD, describes this technique in full and the program for stress reduction at the University of Massachusetts Medical Center.
Centering prayer	A form similar to TM that has a more religious foundation. The subject repeats a "sacred word" similar to a mantra. As thoughts come to mind they are accepted and let go, clearing the mind to become more centered on the spirit within, as if the mind's preoccupied thoughts are the layers of an onion that are pealed away allowing better understanding of the spirit at the core.	Visit www.centering prayer.com. Look under "method of centering prayer" for a nondenominational discussion.
Progressive muscle relaxation (PMR)	A form of relaxation in which the subject is attuned to the difference in feeling when the muscles are tensed and then relaxed. In a comfortable position, start by tensing the whole body from head to toe. While doing this, notice the feelings of tightness. Take a deep breath in and as you let it out, let the tension release and the muscles relax. This is then followed by progressive tension and relaxation throughout the body. Start by clenching the fists, then tensing	The Web site www.uaex.edu/Other_Areas/publications/HTML/FSHEI-28.asp offers a good review of PMR as well as other relaxation exercises. It is sponsored by the University of Arkansas. *You Must Relax* is a book by the developer of this technique, Edmund Jacobson.

continues

Table 30–2 continued

Relaxation Technique	Summary	Further Resources
	the arms, shoulders, chest, abdomen, hips, legs and so on, with each step followed by relaxation.	
Visualization/self-hypnosis (See Chapter 23 on imagery, as well as Chapters 24 through 26)	The subject uses visualization to recruit images that create a relaxed state. For example, if a person is anxious, visualizing images of a place and time that was peaceful and comforting would help induce relaxation. This is best used in conjunction with a breathing exercise.	There are many audio tapes that can guide people through a visualization "script" that can result in relaxation. Martin Rossman, MD, and Emmett Miller are well-known authors on this topic.
Autogenic training (See Chapter 23 on biofeedback)	Induces a physiologic response by using simple phrases. For example, "My legs are heavy and warm," is meant to increase the blood flow to this area resulting in relaxation. This is done progressively from head to toe with the use of deep breathing and repetition of the phrase. After completing this, focus attention on any body part that may still be tense, and then focus the breath and phrase to that area until the whole body is relaxed.	The British Autogenic Society Web site www.autogenictherapy. org.uk is a good resource for more information.
Aerobic exercise	While performing an aerobic exercise, focus attention on a phrase, sound, word, or prayer and passively disregard other thoughts that may enter the mind. Some may focus on their breathing, saying to themselves, "in" with inhalation and "out" with exhalation. Or repeating "one two, one two" with each step one may take with jogging. Doing this helps the mind focus, preventing other thoughts that may cause tension.	*Beyond the Relaxation Response* by Herbert Benson, MD, includes discussion of his research on inducing the relaxation response while exercising.
Yoga (See Chapter 33 on therapeutic exercise)	These techniques have been practiced for thousands of years in India. In America this system has	It is best to encourage your patients to take a class at a local commu-

continues

Table 30–2 continued

Relaxation Technique	Summary	Further Resources
	been divided into three aspects: breathing (pranayama yoga), bodily postures or asanas (hatha yoga), and meditation to maintain balance and health. Regular practice induces relaxation.	nity center or gym and to pick up an introductory book or video from a library or bookstore.
Tai chi (See Chapter 33)	An ancient Chinese martial art that uses slow, graceful movements combined with inner mindfulness and breathing techniques to help bring balance between the mind and body.	As above
Qigong (See Chapter 33)	A traditional Chinese practice that uses movement, meditation, and controlled breathing to balance the body's vital energy force, chi.	As above

Source: Rakel, DP, Shapiro DE. Mind-body medicine. In: Rakel RE et al. *Textbook of Family Practice.* 6th ed. Philadelphia, PA: Saunders; In press.

REFERENCES

Alexander C, Chandler HM, Langer EJ, et al. Transcendental meditation, mindfulness, and longevity: an experimental study with the elderly. *J Pers Soc Psychol.* 1989;57(6):950–964.

Alexander CN, Schneider RH, Staggers F, et al. Trial of stress reduction for hypertension in older African Americans. II. Sex and risk subgroup analysis. *Hypertension.* 1996;28:228–237.

Benson H, Alexander S, Feldman CL. Decreased premature ventricular contractions through use of the relaxation response in patients with stable ischemic heart-disease. *Lancet.* 1975;2:380–382.

Benson H, Dryer T, Hartley LH. Decreased VO2 consumption during exercise with elicitation of the relaxation response. *J Hum Stress.* 1978;4(2):38–42.

Blanchard EB, Nicholson NL, Taylor AE, Steffek BD, Radnitz CL, Appelbaum KA. *J Consult Clin Psychol.* 1991;59(3):467–470.

Caudill M, Schnable R, Zuttermeister P, et al. Decreased clinic use by chronic pain patients: response to behavioral medicine interventions. *Clin. J. Pain.* 1991; 7:305–310.

Cooper M, Aygen M. Effect of meditation on blood cholesterol and blood pressure. *Isr Med Assoc.* 1978;95:1–2.

Delmonte MM. Physiological concomitants of meditation practice. *Int J Psychosom.* 1984;31(4):23–36.

Domar AD, Seibel M, Benson H. The mind/body program for infertility: a new behavioral treatment approach for women with infertility. *Fertil Steril.* 1990;53:246–249.

Eppley KR, Abrams AL, Shear J. Differential effects of relaxation techniques on trait anxiety: a meta-analysis. *J Clin Psychol.* 1989;45(6):957–974

Everly GS, Benson H. Disorders of arousal and the relaxation response: speculations on the nature of treatment of stress-related diseases. *Int J Psychosom.* 1989;36:15–21.

Goodale IL, Domar AD, Benson H. Alleviation of premenstrual syndrome symptoms with the relaxation response. *Obstet Gynecol.* 1990;75:649–655.

Hoffman JW, Benson H, Arns PA, et al. Reduced sympathetic nervous system responsivity associated with the relaxation response. *Science,* 1982;215:190–192.

Jacobs GD, Benson H, Friedman R. Perceived benefits in a behavioral-medicine insomnia program: a clinical report. *Am J Med*. 1996;100:212–216.

Kabat-Zinn J, Wheeler E, Light T, et al. Influence of a mindfulness meditation-based stress reduction intervention on rates of skin clearing in patients with moderate to severe psoriasis undergoing phototherapy and photochemotherapy. *Psychosomatic Med*. 1998;60:625–632.

Orme-Johnson D. Medical care utilization and the transcendental meditation program. *Psychosom Med*. 1987;49:493–507.

Royer-Bounour P. The transcendental meditation technique: a new direction for smoking cessation programs. *Dissertation Abstr Int*. 1989;50(8):3428–B.

Shapiro D. Meditation. In: Strohecker J, Trivieri L, Lewis D, Florence M, eds. *Alternative Medicine: The Definitive Guide*. Fife, WA: Future Medicine Publishing; 1995:339–345

Stanford SC, Salmon P. *Stress: From Synapse to Syndrome*. London, UK: Academic Press; 1999.

Stuart E, Caudill M, Leserman, J, et al. Non-pharmacologic treatment of hypertension: a multiple-risk-factor approach. *J Cardiovasc Nurs*. 1987;1:1–14.

Zamarra J, Schneider RH, Bessighini I, et al. Usefulness of the transcendental meditation program in the treatment of patients with coronary artery disease. *Am J Cardiol*. 1996;77(10):867–870.

CHAPTER 31

Recommending Meditation

David Rakel, MD

OVERVIEW

What is it? "Meditation is simplicity itself. . . It's about stopping and being present . . . that is all." This quote by Jon Kabat-Zinn sums the process up nicely. In our culture, many of us are on autopilot, our thoughts focused on memories of the past or desires of the future. We may drive home from work a thousand times and not notice the objects that we pass because our minds are somewhere else. Meditation helps us quiet the mind of these distracting thoughts so we can live more in the present moment. It is here that we can explore our inner selves and bring peace, for the peace is already there once we stop disturbing it.

Meditation involves focusing the mind and paying attention. This attention may be directed toward a word, sound, picture, prayer, or the breath. This focus allows the mind to settle into the present moment, decreasing the many stressful thoughts that take us into the past or future. An analogy can be made with a radio. The static represents numerous thoughts of the day that preoccupy the mind, and meditation is a tool that allows fine tuning of the dial so the music and thoughts of the inner self can be heard more clearly.

There are many methods of meditating. When recommending meditation to patients the important thing is to encourage them to find an approach that best fits them.

What can it do? It has been well established that long-term stress has damaging effects on health and the immune system by creating an imbalance of the chemicals in the brain that control function (Stanford & Salmon, 1998). Herbert Benson, MD, pioneered this field when he described the "relaxation response" and how meditation could be used to decrease the response of the sympathetic nervous system, or what was termed the fight or flight response (Benson et al., 1977). Meditation was found to reduce heart rate, oxygen consumption, respiratory rate, plasma cortisol, and pulse rate, and to increase alpha brain waves that are associated with relaxation (Shapiro, 1995). Relaxation exercises such as meditation have shown beneficial effects on the severity of tension headaches (Blanchard et al., 1991), anxiety (Eppley et al., 1989), psoriasis (Kabat-Zinn et al., 1998), blood pressure (Alexander et al., 1996), cardiac ischemia and exercise tolerance (Zamarra et al., 1996), longevity and cognitive function in the elderly (Alexander et al., 1989), use of medical care (Orme-Johnson, 1987), medical costs in treating chronic pain (Caudill et al., 1991), smoking cessation (Royer-Bounour, 1989) and serum cholesterol (Cooper & Aygen, 1978).

Meditation not only results in health improvement and prevention of chronic disease, but also can lead to deeper spiritual understanding. Harvard's Herbert Benson found

A brief biography of David Rakel appears in Chapter 1.

Source: Courtesy of David Rakel, MD, and Elsevier Science. From: Rakel D. Learning to meditate. In Rakel D, ed. *Integrative Medicine*. Philadelphia, PA: Saunders/Elsevier Science; 2003.

that patients who were taught meditation for stress reduction often reported feeling more spiritual, more connected to all people and things. Meditation is an excellent tool that may open the door to infinite possibilities for exploring the spirit. Whether we know it or not, we are all on a spiritual journey. We are looking for a better, more meaningful way of life. Quieting the mind can be the first step to help us find that inner voice that rings true in this world of cluttered thought and expectations.

Many of the major religions would agree. Years ago, when practitioners of Christianity, Islam, Buddhism, Judaism, and Hinduism developed meditation techniques, their primary goal was not relaxation, but direct insight into the nature of God and the universe. Meditation was a means of letting go of the self or ego and of cultivating an understanding of love and compassion. Christian teachings claim, "The path leading to heaven is that of complete stillness." The Jewish Torah urges, "Be still and know that I am God." The Buddha teaches, "May you develop mental concentration . . . for whosoever is mentally concentrated sees things according to reality."

How is it done? The following are basic instructions that can be used by anyone interested in learning to meditate. Quieting the mind can be achieved successfully in many ways. For ease of demonstration we will focus on a mantra meditation which is similar to Transcendental Meditation (TM).

- First choose a word or phrase (mantra) that has meaning to you. This can be anything that brings you comfort. A neutral word may be peace, joy, one, or love. A religious example might include God, Shalom, or "the Lord is my shepherd."
- Find a quiet place to sit where there are few distractions.

- Commit to a set amount of time. Time yourself by periodically glancing at a clock, if needed, but don't set an alarm.
- Sit in a comfortable position that you can maintain with your back straight but not stiff.
- Close your eyes and relax.
- Allow yourself to notice your breath as you inhale and exhale. Breathe slowly and naturally. As you exhale, repeat your word or phrase. If you are using a long phrase, try focusing on half with inhalation and half with exhalation.
- When you notice your mind wandering, simply and gently return to your focus word. You will have thoughts of daydreams, tasks, worries, passions, etc., but simply say to yourself, "oh well" or "that's interesting" and return to the repetition.
- Assume a passive attitude and don't worry whether you are doing it right or wrong. Some find it helpful to use the analogy of swimming in the ocean. The idea is to drop 4 or 5 feet below the surface and observe the waves of thoughts as they go by. As you focus on your word or phrase, the sea will calm.
- At the end of your meditation, sit comfortably for a minute or two and then stand slowly when ready.

Tips

- Meditate on an empty stomach. Food has been found to inhibit the beneficial physiologic effects of meditation on the body.
- If you wish, meditate with a friend, spouse, or relative.

Expectations. The process of quieting the mind is unique for each individual and having a goal to reach contradicts the mission of the activity. With continued practice though, you may find it helpful to learn of the various experiences and benefits meditation may bring.

- The experienced practitioner will find it easier to quiet the mind. Although the beginner may have hundreds of thoughts during meditation, with time these will become less and less.
- Some may enter what is called "the gap," which is void of thought and mantra. This is a time for simply being present in the moment.
- Increased sense of control in the world instead of feeling like a passive "victim"
- Less focus on self or ego, which enhances a sense of love and compassion
- A deepening of spiritual life and/or religious experience
- A feeling of being more connected to all people and things

A simple Russian peasant who lived around the middle of the nineteenth century sums up the journey of a meditative practice nicely. "At first, spiritual practitioners feel that the mind is like a waterfall, bouncing from rock to rock, roaring and turbulent, impossible to tame or control. In midcourse, it is like a great river, calm and gentle, wide and deep. At the end, its boundaries expand beyond sight and its depth becomes unfathomable as it dissolves into the ocean, which is both its goal and Source" (Walsh, 1999).

Precautions. Meditation does not create unpleasant feelings. But quieting the mind may make you more aware of feelings that are already there. This can be a very important step in healing but often requires the help of a professional counselor to make sure that these thoughts and feelings are dealt with in a constructive and educational way. If you experience any strong or disturbing emotions, please discuss them with your medical care provider.

Quieting the mind can make one aware of preexisting stressors or memories that may require the aid of a counselor to deal with these emotions in a constructive way.

The dose. One to two times a day for 15 or 20 minutes is considered most effective. Meditating for shorter periods each day is better than one hour once a week.

FURTHER RESOURCES

- *Meditation: An Eight-Point Program* by Eknath Easwaran is a straightforward introduction to the subject.
- *How to Meditate: A Guide to Self Discovery* by Lawrence LeShan reviews different types of meditation and gives direction for practice.
- *The Miracle of Mindfulness: A Manual on Meditation* by Thich Nhat Hanh is an excellent, short, and practical guide.
- *Wherever You Go, There You Are* and *Full Catastrophe Living* by Jon Kabat-Zinn are excellent reviews on being mindful and mindfulness meditation.
- *Essential Spirituality* by Roger Walsh, MD, PhD, is an excellent review of how the great religions teach similar exercises for spiritual growth.
- www.centeringprayer.com is a form of meditation similar to TM but has a more religious foundation.
- The best way to learn is to find a class that is offered in your community. Check with a local hospital, community college, or the YMCA for classes.

REFERENCES

Alexander C, Chandler HM, Langer EJ, et al. Transcendental meditation, mindfulness, and longevity: an experimental study with the elderly. *J Pers Soc Psychol.* 1989;57(6):950–964.

Alexander CN, Schneider RH, Staggers F, et al. Trial of stress reduction for hypertension in older African Americans. II. Sex and risk subgroup analysis. *Hypertension.* 1996;28:228–237.

Benson H, Kotch JB, Crassweller KD. The relaxation response: a bridge between psychiatry and medicine. *Med Clin North Am.* 1977;61(4):929–938

Blanchard EB, Nicholson NL, Taylor AE, Steffek BD, Radnitz CL, Appelbaum KA. *J Consult Clin Psychol.* 1991;59(3):467–470.

Caudill M, Schnable R, Zuttermeister P, Benson H, Friedman R. Decreased clinic use by chronic pain patients: response to behavioral medicine intervention. *Clin J Pain.* 1991;7(4); 305–310.

Cooper M, Aygen M. Effect of meditation on blood cholesterol and blood pressure. *Isr Med Assoc.* 1978;95:1–2.

Eppley KR, Abrams AL, Shear J. Differential effects of relaxation techniques on trait anxiety: a meta-analysis. *J Clin Psychol.* 1989;45(6):957–974.

Kabat-Zinn J, Wheeler E, Light T, et al. Influence of a mindfulness meditation-based stress reduction intervention on rates of skin clearing in patients with moderate to severe psoriasis undergoing phototherapy and photochemotherapy. *Psychosom Med.* 1998;60:625–632.

Orme-Johnson D. Medical care utilization and the transcendental meditation program. *Psychosom Med.* 1987;49:493–507.

Royer-Bounour P. The transcendental meditation technique: a new direction for smoking cessation programs. *Dissertation Abstr Int.* 1989;50(8):3428–B.

Shapiro D. Meditation. In: Strohecker J, Trivieri L, Lewis D, Florence M, eds. *Alternative Medicine: The Definitive Guide.* Fife, WA: Future Medicine Publishing; 1995:339–345.

Stanford SC, Salmon P. *Stress: From Synapse to Syndrome.* London, UK: Academic Press; 1998.

Walsh, Roger. *Essential Spirituality.* New York, NY: John Wiley & Sons, Inc; 1999:170–171.

Zamarra J, Schneider RH, Bessighini I, et al. Usefulness of the transcendental meditation program in the treatment of patients with coronary artery disease. *Am J Cardiol.* 1996;77(10):867–870.

CHAPTER 32

Breathing Exercises

David Rakel, MD

BREATHING AS A BRIDGE

It is thought by many cultures that the process of breathing is the essence of being. A rhythmic process of expansion and contraction, breathing is one example of the consistent polarity we see in nature—night and day, wake and sleep, seasonal growth and decay, and ultimately life and death. In yoga, the breath is known as *prana*, a universal energy that can be used to find a balance between the body-mind, the conscious-unconscious, and the sympathetic-parasympathetic nervous systems.

Unlike other physiological functions, the breath is easily used to communicate between these systems, which gives us an excellent tool to help facilitate positive change. It is the only bodily function that we do both voluntarily and involuntarily. We can consciously use breathing to influence the involuntary (sympathetic nervous system) that regulates blood pressure, heart rate, circulation, digestion, and many other bodily functions. *Pranayama* is a yoga practice that literally means the control of life or energy. It uses breathing techniques to change subtle energies within the body for health and well-being. Breathing exercises can act as a bridge into those functions of the body of which we generally do not have conscious control.

A brief biography of David Rakel appears in Chapter 1.

Courtesy of David Rakel, MD, and Elsevier Science. From: Rakel D. Breathing exercises. In Rakel D, ed. *Integrative Medicine*. Philadelphia, PA: Saunders/Elsevier Science; 2003.

Our breathing provides an example of how life affects physiology. During times of emotional stress our sympathetic nervous system is stimulated and affects a number of physical responses. Our heart rate rises, we perspire, our muscles tense, and our breathing becomes rapid and shallow. If this process occurs frequently over a long period of time, the sympathetic nervous system becomes overstimulated, leading to an imbalance that can affect our physical health and result in a range of possible symptoms, including inflammation, high blood pressure, or muscle pain.

Consciously slowing our heart rate, decreasing perspiration, and relaxing muscles is more difficult than simply slowing and deepening breathing. The breath can be used to directly influence these stressful changes, causing a direct stimulation of the parasympathetic nervous system, resulting in relaxation and a reversal of the changes seen with the stimulation of the sympathetic nervous system. We can see how our bodies know to do this naturally when we take a deep breath or sigh when a stress is relieved.

BREATH TRAINING

Breathing can be trained for both positive and negative influences on health. Chronic stress can lead to a restriction of the connective and muscular tissue in the chest, resulting in a decreased range of motion of the chest wall. When breathing is rapid or shallow, the chest does not expand as much as it would with slower, deeper breaths, and much of the air exchange occurs at the top of the lung tissue towards the head. This results in "chest" breathing. You can see if you are a chest breather by placing your right hand on your chest and your left hand on your abdomen. As you breathe, see which hand rises more. If your right hand rises more, you are a chest breather. If your left hand rises more, you are an abdomen breather.

Chest breathing is inefficient because the greatest amount of blood flow occurs in the lower lobes of the lungs, areas that have limited air expansion in chest breathers. Rapid, shallow, chest breathing results in less oxygen transfer to the blood and subsequent poor delivery of nutrients to the tissues. The good news is that similar to learning to play an instrument or ride a bike, you can train the body to improve its breathing technique. With regular practice most people find that they breathe from the abdomen the majority of the time, even while asleep.

> *Using and learning proper breathing techniques is one of the most beneficial things that can be done for both short- and long-term physical and emotional health.*

THE BENEFITS OF ABDOMINAL BREATHING

Abdominal breathing is also known as *diaphragmatic breathing*. The diaphragm is a large muscle located between the chest and the abdomen. When it contracts it is forced downward causing the abdomen to expand. This causes a negative pressure within the chest, forcing air into the lungs. The negative pressure also pulls blood into the chest, improving the venous return to the heart. This leads to improved stamina in both disease resistance and athletic activity. The flow of

lymph, which is rich in immune cells, is also improved. By expanding the lungs' air pockets and improving the flow of blood and lymph, abdominal breathing also helps prevent infection of the lungs and other tissues. Most of all, it is an excellent tool to stimulate the relaxation response that results in less tension and an overall sense of well-being.

Abdominal Breathing Technique

Most patients find the following technique quite easy to learn. The instructions are relatively straight-forward:

Breathing exercises such as this one should be done twice a day or whenever you find your mind dwelling on upsetting thoughts or when you are experiencing pain.

- Place one hand on your chest and the other on your abdomen. When you take a deep breath in, the hand on the abdomen should rise higher than the one on the chest. This insures that the diaphragm is pulling air into the bases of the lungs.
- After exhaling through the mouth, take a slow deep breath in through your nose imagining that you are sucking in all the air in the room and hold it for a count of 7 (or as long as you are able, not exceeding 7).
- Slowly exhale through your mouth for a count of 8. As all the air is released with relaxation, gently contract your abdominal muscles to completely evacuate the remaining air from the lungs. It is important to remember that we deepen respirations not by inhaling more air but through completely exhaling it.
- Repeat the cycle four more times for a total of 5 deep breaths and try to breathe at a rate of one breath every 10 seconds (or 6 breaths per minute). At this rate our heart rate variability normalizes, which has a positive effect on cardiac health.

Once you feel comfortable with the above technique, you may want to incorporate words/thoughts that can enhance the exercise. Examples would be to say to yourself the word, "relaxation" (with inhalation), and "stress" or "anger" (with exhalation). The idea being to bring in the feelings or emotions you want with inhalation and release those you don't want with exhalation.

In general, exhalation should be twice as long as inhalation. The use of the hands on the chest and abdomen are only needed to help you train your breathing. Once you feel comfortable with your ability to breathe into the abdomen, they are no longer needed.

Abdominal breathing is just one of many breathing exercises, but it is the most important one to learn before exploring other techniques. The more it is practiced, the more natural it will become. Deeper breathing tends to improve the body's internal rhythm.

USING BREATHING EXERCISES TO INCREASE ENERGY

If practiced over time, the abdominal breathing exercise can result in improved energy throughout the day, but sometimes we are in need of a quick "pick-me-up." The Bellows breathing exercise (also called the stimulating breath) can be used during times of fatigue that may result from driving long distances or when you need to be revitalized at work. It should not be used in place of abdominal breathing but as an additional tool to increase energy when needed. This breathing exercise is opposite that of abdominal breathing. Short, fast, rhythmic breaths are used to increase energy, which are similar to the "chest" breathing we do when under stress. The bellows breath re-creates the adrenal stimulation that occurs with stress and results in the release of energizing chemicals such as epinephrine. Like most bodily functions, this serves an active purpose, but overuse results in the adverse effects discussed previously.

The Bellows Breathing Technique (the Stimulating Breath)

This yogic technique can be used to help stimulate energy when needed. It is a good approach to use before reaching for a cup of coffee.

- Sit in a comfortable upright position with your spine straight.
- With your mouth gently closed, breath in and out of your nose as fast as possible. To give an idea of how this is done, think of someone using a bicycle pump (a bellows) to quickly pump up a tire. The upstroke is inspiration, the downstroke is exhalation, and both are equal in length. The rate of breathing is rapid with as many as 2–3 cycles of inspiration/expiration per second.
- While doing the exercise, you should feel effort at the base of the neck, chest, and abdomen. The muscles in these areas will increase in strength the more this technique is practiced. This is truly a form of exercise.
- Do this for no longer than 15 seconds when first starting. With practice, slowly increase the length of the exercise by 5 seconds each time. Do it as long as you are comfortably able, not exceeding one full minute.
- There is a risk of hyperventilation that can result in loss of consciousness if this exercise is done too much in the beginning. For this reason, it should be practiced in a safe place such as a bed or chair.

This exercise can be used each morning upon awakening or when needed for an energy boost.

FURTHER RESOURCES

An excellent book to help explore more advanced breathing techniques is *Conscious Breathing* by Gay Hendricks (Bantam, 1995. ISBN# 0553374435).

An excellent audiotape/CD is *Breathing: The Master Key to Self Healing* by Andrew Weil. It discusses the health benefits of breathing and directs the listener through eight breathing exercises (Sounds True, 1999. ISBN# 156455726X).

The reader is encouraged to enroll in a yoga class through a local community or fitness center. Most well-trained instructors educate students on how the breath is used to enhance well-being with yoga practice.

PART VI

Therapeutic Massage

Chapter

CHAPTER 33

Referring Patients to Clinical Massage

Susan Rosen and Nancy Faass

OVERVIEW

Clinical massage implies therapeutic massage intended to treat specific medical conditions or injuries. This type of therapy is also described as manual therapy, orthopedic massage, or medical massage, and is included under the umbrella of manual medicine or rehabilitation therapy. The term *manual medicine* may also refer to physical therapy, occupational therapy, chiropractic, or osteopathic treatment.

Suggested Guidelines

At the time of this writing, the National Certification Board for Therapeutic Massage and Bodywork (NCBTMB) is in the process of developing advanced certification for clinical massage therapists, to differentiate practitioners trained to provide therapeutic, clinical interventions from those trained to provide massage for relaxation and stress reduction. The Board has performed an extensive job analysis and is finalizing eligibility criteria for this certification, as the first step in the development of an advanced national examination. An in-depth survey has been conducted by the Board to determine the knowledge, skills, training, and clinical experience most important for the advanced-level practitioner.

At the time of this writing, national guidelines are still in development. However, the eligibility criteria reviewed by the National Certification Board can provide useful guidelines when creating a referral list of clinical massage therapists. Minimum qualifications that have been discussed include:

Initial training. Entry-level massage education is widely considered a basic prerequisite (typically 500 to 1000 contact hours).

Questions to ask to identify a capable massage therapist:

1. Where did you receive your massage therapy training?
2. Are you a graduate of a training program accredited by the Commission on Massage Therapy Accreditation or that is a member of the AMTA Council of Schools?
3. Are you certified by the National Certification Board of Therapeutic Massage and Bodywork?
4. Do you have advanced training in any specific massage techniques?
5. Are you currently licensed as a massage therapist in this state?
6. Are you a member of a professional association?

Source: American Massage Therapy Association, www.amtamassage.org, 2004.

Susan Rosen is a founding member of the National Certification Board for Therapeutic Massage and Bodywork and has served as chair of the Washington State Massage Examining Board. She has practiced and taught massage professionally for more than 20 years. Owner of a group practice in a multidisciplinary health care clinic, Ms. Rosen is a leader in the integration of clinical and medical massage into mainstream health care.

Courtesy of Susan Rosen, Olympia, Washington.

In Washington State, for example, many massage schools provide training programs of 1400 contact hours.

Advanced Clinical Training. In addition to entry-level training, practitioners who work with medical conditions typically have 100 to 400 additional contact hours or more in advanced techniques in clinical or orthopedic massage. Many advanced practitioners have in-depth expertise gained through workshops, seminars, or preceptorships in therapeutic modalities, such as manual lymph drainage, Muscle Energy Technique, myofascial release, or Strain CounterStrain.

Clinical experience. Clinical experience is an important indicator of a practitioner's ability to apply advanced education in real life applications. Discussions among subject matter experts have suggested a minimum of 3 years in clinical/medical practice and an accumulation of at least 3000 session-hours of actual clinical practice. A session-hour is defined as a clock hour of clinical interaction with a patient(s). The hallmark of an advanced level practitioner is the direct application of educational experience to clinical practice, particularly under the supervision of a mentor.

Clinical experience is essential for a clinical therapist. For example, a massage practitioner who has worked in a spa setting for 3 or 4 years may still not have the requisite knowledge or skills necessary to work with medical referrals. Clinical practice provides the opportunity to apply specialized training and demonstrate increased competency. One should refrain from referring patients who require therapeutic clinical massage to practitioners with no clinical experience.

Certification. Certification is currently available to practitioners through two National Certification Examinations:

- National Certification Exam for Therapeutic Massage and Bodywork (which contains information on energy work as well as Asian-based models of bodywork)
- National Certification Exam for Therapeutic Massage (which does not contain the information on energy work and Asian-based models of bodywork, given for the first time in June 2005)

Licensure. Many states have licensure requirements. In a few states, licensure is unavailable and must be obtained through a local jurisdiction. Licensure recommendations are typically:

- A valid current state license to provide massage in the state of practice
- If no state licensure is available, documentation of practice within the legal parameters of the jurisdiction where massage is provided.

Additional Qualifications

Beyond the requirements of the National Board, qualifications to consider when selecting a clinical massage therapist include:

- Training and certification in massage or bodywork modalities with specific medical applications
- Clinical reasoning and decision-making skills; for example, when to refer clients to a physician to rule out more serious conditions, for diagnostic testing, or for follow-up
- Skills, training, and experience in client assessment, history taking, written communication, documentation, interpersonal communications, and medical ethics
- Ability to develop a treatment plan
- Advanced qualifications: supplemental learning experiences may also be reflected in academic hours or the equivalent, such as

an associate degree program, or publication of a book, research project, thesis, or dissertation. Practitioners coming to this work as a second career from other health care professions bring a wealth of knowledge and experience to their massage practice.

- Membership in a professional organization, as a reflection of their professionalism and their commitment to their work

INDICATIONS AND TECHNIQUES

Conditions Addressed

Clinical massage addresses a wide range of soft tissue and musculoskeletal disorders (acute and chronic), post-surgical conditions, injuries, and chronic pain disorders. Typically, indications for referral include pain, dysfunction, inflammation due to trauma, cumulative stress, or surgery, in conditions such as:

- Carpal tunnel syndrome
- Degeneration of a joint or disc
- Fibromyalgia
- Low back conditions, particularly those involving pain
- Muscle spasms
- Musculoskeletal misalignment (massage as an adjunctive therapy)
- Repetitive motion injuries
- Sciatica
- Scoliosis and kyphosis involving muscle imbalance
- Sprains and strains of various types
- Tendonitis or tendinosis
- Tension headaches
- Thoracic outlet syndrome
- Whiplash or other injuries due to an auto accident or a fall

For example, in cases of disc herniation or degeneration, patients who are not good candidates for surgery may be seen for pain management by a massage therapist. Massage, when provided by a practitioner trained in clinical practices, can be helpful in this regard. This would not typically involve palliative massage, but rather an emphasis on alignment work, balance of musculature, fascial release, decompression of the spine, and/or postural training.

Many of these conditions are also addressed by chiropractors, osteopaths, and physical therapists. Physicians and other practitioners can educate themselves about appropriate referral through reading or workshops. Useful resources for clinicians include an overview of the research, *A Physician's Guide to Therapeutic Massage* by Yates and an in-depth clinical guide, *Clinical Massage Therapy*, 2nd ed. by Rattray and Ludwig. There are a number of other comprehensive books and publications as well. (See Resources at the end of the chapter for a selected list.)

Therapeutic Modalities

The more extensive and varied the toolbox of therapeutic modalities that skilled massage practitioners have at their fingertips, the wider the range of conditions they can address effectively and successfully. Consequently, it is also useful to know the specific modalities in which practitioners are trained. Techniques most often utilized by advanced massage therapists include:

- Acupressure and shiatsu
- Craniosacral therapy
- Deep tissue massage (soft tissue mobilization)
- Manual lymph drainage
- Movement therapies, such as Feldenkrais and Alexander Technique

- Muscle Energy Technique, and other active and/or resisitive movement techniques
- Myofascial release
- Neuromuscular therapy
- Scar tissue mobilization
- Strain CounterStrain and other passive movement techniques
- Structural integration (Rolfing, Soma, Hellerwork)
- Trigger-point therapy
- Visceral massage

Adjunctive techniques utilized by advanced massage therapists include:

- Coaching in breathing exercises
- Hydrotherapy
- Self-care education

The choice of therapy will depend upon the patient's condition and the preference of the patient and physician. For example, specialized techniques are utilized for patients who are unable to handle much pressure, in conditions that involve chronic pain or sensitivity, such as cancer or rheumatoid arthritis. Ideally, the advanced practitioner should also be skilled in a range of techniques that can be adapted to the needs of the sensitive patient, such as:

- Craniosacral therapy, a technique developed by John Upledger and other osteopaths
- Manual lymph drainage techniques
- Reflexology, which involves the massage of pressure points on the hands and feet
- Strain CounterStrain/positional release
- Therapeutic Touch, developed by Dolores Krieger, PhD, which is used in hospitals; Reiki or Polarity therapy

CLINICAL PRACTICE

Scope of practice. In therapeutic massage, client referrals are frequently made by physicians or other health care practitioners. The referral is accompanied by a diagnosis and in some cases a prescription. The diagnosis is essential, since diagnostic evaluation is beyond the scope of practice of massage therapy. Massage therapists realize they do not have the knowledge base to serve as primary care providers. Rather, they see their contribution as appropriate once the client has been seen by a physician to rule out more serious conditions and to obtain a primary diagnosis.

Assessment. The ability to take a client history and perform a thorough clinical soft tissue assessment (such as palpation findings, postural observations, and movement tests) are important skills for the massage therapist. These are skills that the physician or practitioner will want to look for when identifying practitioners for potential referrals.

Although referrals are usually made in writing, the diagnosis may be brief or somewhat general, so a history and assessment are still necessary. Typically, the further assessment of diagnosed conditions such as soft tissue or joint injuries will involve skilled palpation and evaluation using a series of functional tests. These tests include passive and active range of motion and isometric tests to assess muscle-tendon injuries, such as the series of tests developed by the British orthopedic physician, James Cyriax.

Another purpose of the assessment is to identify symptoms that should be referred to a physician, particularly when clients are self-referred. This means that clinical massage therapists must be able to identify red flags or contraindications that suggest the need for medical evaluation and treatment, such as persistent headaches or severe chronic pain.

Reporting and communication. In the context of the referral process, good communication is vital. Therefore, massage therapists most ideal for referral are those who know how to communicate in writing, as well as verbally. This requires training in documentation and report writing, which are now included in many entry-level massage programs. In some organizations, such as Group Health, new reporting forms have been developed to streamline this process. Ongoing communication between the referring physician or their staff and the massage therapist is beneficial to both the patient and the health care team.

In certain situations, clinical massage therapists also provide documentation to insurance companies. For example, in Washington state massage is now covered by health insurance under some benefits programs, in cases of medical necessity. Consequently, providers in this state have become more experienced at interfacing with insurance providers. Documentation is usually required. Typically, reporting includes medical and functional goals for conditions that have an impact on the performance of activities of daily living (ADLs). Documentation also tracks changes in the patient's health status such as a decrease in pain.

DEVELOPING A REFERRAL LIST

Massage therapy is frequently offered through health plans as one of the services available in a network of credentialed providers. However, health care professionals may still want to develop their own referral list of practitioners. To screen for potential referrals, some providers have found it helpful to enlist a staff member to review brochures, resumes, or the Web sites of massage practitioners and then do phone interviews with the most appropriate candidates. Many massage therapists are willing to provide a massage *pro bono* to a staff member or give a presentation on clinical massage at a staff meeting. One of the best ways to learn of skilled massage therapists is through the recommendation of patients, who often report back on successful treatments and positive experiences. Ultimately, a massage therapist may have advanced training and provide thorough documentation, but the most important basis for future referrals is good results.

Effective therapeutic massage can contribute to positive clinical outcomes and patient satisfaction. A skilled clinical massage therapist can make a valuable contribution as a member of the clinical team or collaborative practitioner network.

RESOURCES

Andrade C, Clifford P. *Outcome-Based Massage*. Philadelphia, PA: Lippincott Williams & Wilkins; 2001.

Claire T. *Bodywork*. New York, NY: Harper Collins/Quill; 1996.

Hendrickson T. *Massage for Orthopedic Conditions*. Philadelphia, PA: Lippincott Williams & Wilkins; 2003.

Persad RS. *Massage Therapy and Medications*. Toronto, Canada: Curties-Overzet; 2001.

Rattray F, Ludwig L. *Clinical Massage Therapy*. Toronto, Canada: Talus, Inc.; 2000.

Thompson D. *Hands Heal: Communication, Documentation, and Insurance Billing for*

Manual Therapists. 2nd ed. Philadelphia, PA: Lippincott Williams & Wilkins; 2002.

Werner R. *A Massage Therapist's Guide to Pathology*. 2nd ed. Philadelphia, PA: Lippincott Williams & Wilkins; 2002.

Yates J, MD, PhD. *A Physician's Guide to Therapeutic Massage*. 3rd ed. Toronto, Canada: Curties-Overzet Publications; 2004.

(Also see Chapter 35. Definitions of Massage and Bodywork.)

CHAPTER 34

Overview of Clinical Massage

Karin Olsen and Linda Chrisman

THERAPEUTIC MECHANISMS OF CLINICAL MASSAGE

Massage therapy essentially involves hands-on manipulation of muscles and soft tissue. There are more than 150 variations of massage, bodywork, and somatic therapy disciplines (Associated Bodywork and Massage Professionals, 2004), involving thousands of techniques and variations. Therapeutic massage typically consists of a blend of Swedish massage, neuromuscular massage, and acupressure techniques (Field, 1999). The benefits of touch can enhance physiological function—particularly of the circulatory, lymphatic, muscular, and nervous systems. Consequently, massage may improve the rate at which the body recovers from injury and illness. Research indicates that massage can provide therapeutic benefit for conditions ranging from sports injuries to cancer pain.

Massage provides several basic therapeutic benefits. One of the primary areas of impact is improved circulation in muscles and soft tissues, which supports healing in conditions such as low back pain and injuries. Massage also has primary impact in stress reduction and pain management by stimulating the production of neurotransmitters such as serotonin and dopamine. Consequently, massage can be relevant to the needs of patients under stress—examples cited in the research include depression in hospitalized patients and in mothers of newborns. In some cases, manual therapies can provide almost immediate relief to patients by promoting measurable changes in physiology:

- Muscle relaxation (Field, 1999)
- Shift in the autonomic nervous system from sympathetic mode into the parasympathetic (Field et al., 1996)
- Release of endorphins, serotonin, and dopamine (Field, Hernandez-Reif, Taylor et al., 1997; Hernandez-Reif et al., 2001; Hernandez-Reif et al., 2004)
- Lower cortisol levels (Field, Schanberg, Kuhn et al., 1998; Hernandez-Reif et al., 2001)
- Deepened heart rate (Mok, 2004) and respiratory rate (Wang & Keck, 2004)
- Enhanced circulation (Agarwal et al., 2000; Mur et al., 2001)

Karin Olsen, BA, LMP, is an appointed board member of the Washington State Massage Examining Board and vice president of the Chamber of Commerce in her region. A graduate of Central Washington University, Ms. Olsen has developed and taught a range of courses in massage therapy. She holds professional certification in a number of massage disciplines and has practiced clinical massage since 1995; for the past decade, Ms. Olsen has been owner and manager of a group practice that provides clinical/medical massage therapy.

Linda Chrisman, MA, CMT, is an educator, writer, and practitioner with over 20 years of experience in the field of somatic bodywork. A graduate of Stanford University and the California Institute of Integral Studies, she has been certified in a number of disciplines, including Trager therapy and therapeutic massage. Ms. Chrisman practices and teaches in the San Francisco Bay area, where she specializes in Rosen Method, Continuum Movement, and Somatic Experiencing. She is a founding associate of the Health Medicine Institute, an integrative medicine center.

Table 34–1 Indications for Clinical Massage

Musculoskeletal Conditions (involving muscle and soft tissue)

Direct benefit	Secondary benefit
• Edema (Balzer et al., 1993) • Fibromyalgia (Sunshine et al., 1996) • Muscle and ligament strains and sprains (Hollis, 1987) • Muscle tension, stiffness, and spasms (AMTA, 2004) • Postural dysfunction (Paternostro-Sluga & Zoch, 2004) • Soft tissue rehabilitation (Mowen, 2000) • Thoracic outlet syndrome (Buonocore et al., 1998)	• Arthritis: osteoarthritis and rheumatoid arthritis (Field, Hernandez-Reif, Seligman et al., 1997) • Bursitis (Guler-Uysal & Kozanoglu, 2004) • Carpal tunnel syndrome (Sheon & the Goff Group, 1997) • Disc disease (Ulreich & Kullich, 1999) • Injuries due to biomechanical factors, such as back conditions (Ulreich & Kullich, 1999) • Injuries due to overuse (Sheon & the Goff Group, 1997; Lowe, 1999) • Injuries or trauma, including sports injuries (Chen & Wu, 1998; Lowe, 1999; Angus, 2001; van den Dolder & Roberts, 2003) • Joint conditions, restricted range of motion (AMTA, 2004) ***Secondary benefit*** • Scoliosis due to muscle imbalances (Tarola, 1994; Hawes & Brooks, 2002) • Temporomandibular joint (TMJ) dysfunction (Friedman, 1997) • Tendonitis (Gehlsen et al., 1999; Gimblett et al., 1999) • Whiplash (Ferrari & Russell, 2004)

Stress-Related, Mental-Emotional Conditions

Direct benefit	Secondary benefit
• Stress (Field et al., 1996; Birk et al., 2000) • Tension headache (Puustjarvi et al., 1990; Quinn et al., 2002)	• Anxiety (Field et al., 1996) • Depression (Field, Pickens, Prodromidis et al., 2000; Muller-Oerblinghausen, 2004) • Insomnia, stress-related (Richards, 2000; Chen et al., 1999) • Migraine headache (Wylie et al., 1997; Launso et al., 1999) • Stress associated with medical conditions or procedures (Richards, 1998)

continues

Table 34–1 Continued

Neurological and Pain Conditions

Direct benefit	Secondary benefit
• Pain conditions including cancer pain (Weinrich & Weinrich, 1990), chronic pain (Pope et al., 1994; Field, Hernandez-Reif, Seligman et al., 1997), and myofascial pain (Hollis, 1987)	• Cerebral palsy (Zhou et al., 1993) • Cervical spondylopathy (Colledge et al., 1996; Luo & Luo, 1997) • Hemiplegia [applying massage to increase circulation] (Chen & Wu, 1998) • Multiple sclerosis (Siev-Ner et al., 2003) • Parkinson's disease (Brefel-Courbon et al., 2003) • Spinal cord injury (Nayak et al., 2001; Diego et al., 2002; Warms et al., 2002)

Pregnancy, Labor, and Childbirth

Direct benefit	
• Pregnancy and labor (Field, Hernandez-Reif, Taylor et al., 1997; Osborne-Sheets, 1998) • Perineal massage [typically provided in hospitals by midwives] (Davidson et al., 2000; Stamp et al., 2001; Vendittelli et al., 2001) • Premature infant massage [typically provided in hospitals] (Field et al., 1986)	

Dermatological

Direct benefit	Secondary benefit
	• Burn treatment [typically provided in hospitals] (Field, Peck, Krugman et al., 1998; Field, Peck, Hernandez-Reif et al., 2000) • Scar tissue [including both hospital and outpatient therapy] (Rochet & Zaoui, 2002)] • Atopic dermatitis (Schachner et al., 1998)

Source: Karin Olsen and Nancy Faass, © 2005.

- Improved lymphatic circulation (Hollis, 1987; Balzer & Schonebeck, 1993)
- Increased production of immunoglobulins (Groer et al., 1994), natural killer cells, and lymphocytes (Hernandez-Rief et al., 2004), as well as cytotoxic T-cells (Ironson et al., 1996)

Major areas of function addressed by clinical massage include:

- Soft tissue injury—25 clinical trials have focused on the role of massage in addressing injury and massage is referenced in more than 500 journal articles listed under injury in the NLM database (for references to specific studies, see Table 34–1).
- Pain relief—More than 20 clinical trials have focused on the applications of massage in pain management, and massage is referenced in more than 100 journal articles on pain (at least 20 clinical trials have been conducted, including Chang et al., 2002; Kober et al., 2002; De Laat et al., 2003; Piotrowski et al., 2003; Walach et al., 2003; Yip & Tse, 2004; Bodhise et al., 2004; Wang & Keck, 2004).
- Stress reduction—35 clinical trials to date have focused on the potential of massage in moderating stress associated with medical conditions and hospitalization.

PHYSIOLOGICAL BENEFITS

Clinical or medical massage can be provided to support physiological function in a great many specific conditions. A growing body of research that includes more than 500 clinical trials provides an evidence basis for these indications (see Table 34–1). In addition, massage retains the human factor in the increasingly technologically oriented practice of medicine. Consequently, therapeutic massage can be a valuable, cost-effective primary or adjunctive therapy that is compatible with many other medical approaches to treatment (Greene, 2000). Research and clinical studies indicate improvement in a diverse range of conditions and diagnoses.

CONTRAINDICATIONS

Massage therapists warn of contraindications for massage (Hollis, 1987); yet, there is little research that identifies specific contraindications (Field, 1999). Each patient's needs should be considered on a case-by-case basis. However, there is general consensus on major contraindications (shown in Table 34–2).

Some situations involve a relative contraindication. For example, massage is not recommended for fragile healing tissue; however, massage of burn areas with cocoa butter can alleviate itching (Field, 1999). Massage therapy has also been used to reduce anxiety and indirectly reduce pain before and during the painful procedure of debridement (Field, Peck, Krugman et al., 1998). In addition, massage that focuses on intact tissue has been found to ameliorate the general perception of pain.

RESEARCH

The Medline database of the National Library of Medicine currently includes approximately 5000 citations on massage. This reflects major expansion in massage research over the past 20 years. Studies have also been conducted in Europe that have not yet been translated into English (Greene, 2000). Two additional sources of research on massage in the United States are the Touch Research Institutes (TRI) at the University of Miami School of Medicine and the National Center for Complementary and Alternative Medicine (NCCAM) at the NIH.

The NIH has funded 19 research projects at the time of this writing on both physio-

Table 34–2 Contraindications to Massage

Absolute Contraindications

Acute conditions requiring first aid or medical attention include: anaphylaxis, appendicitis, cerebrovascular accident, collapsed lung, diabetic coma or insulin shock, myocardial infarction, pneumothorax, severe asthmatic attack, acute seizure, or syncope (fainting)

- Atherosclerosis, severe
- Cancer, highly metastatic
- Cerebrovascular accident, postevent
- Diabetes with complications such as gangrene
- Eclampsia
- Fever ($> 101.5°F$; $> 38.5°C$)
- Headaches, severe, undiagnosed
- Hemophilia
- Hemorrhage
- Hypertension
- Infectious/contagious condition
- Organ failure (advanced heart, kidney, liver, or respiratory failure)
- Phlebitis
- Pneumonia, acute
- Shock

Absolute Contraindications to Local Conditions

Massage therapy is not appropriate locally for any of the following conditions: acute flare-up of inflammatory arthritis (rheumatoid arthritis, systemic lupus, or ankylosing spondylitis); acute neuritis, acute trigeminal neuralgia; life-threatening aneurisms, deep-vein thrombosis, phlebitis, or arteritis; ectopic pregnancy; esophageal varicosities; frostbite; localized infectious or irritable skin condition; malignancy, especially unstable conditions; open wounds, lesions, or decubitus ulcer; specific pain syndromes such as causalgia or reflex sympathetic dystrophy; radiation therapy, during therapy and several weeks posttreatment; recent burns (and new scar tissue); sepsis; tumors (and infected lymph nodes); varicosities

Source of content: Rattray F, Ludwig L. *Clinical Massage Therapy: Understanding, Assessing, and Treating Over 70 Conditions.* 2nd ed. Elora, Ontario, Canada: Talus, Incorporated; 2000; www.clinicalmassagetherapy.com.

logical mechanisms of massage and clinical outcomes. Topics of clinical studies have included various aspects of back pain, immune function, prostatitis, infant health, and depression in pregnant women, with findings of improved outcomes:

- Cortisol levels and blood pressure normalized more quickly in patients who received massage following abdominal surgery, compared with controls.
- Cancer patients who received massage therapy while undergoing bone marrow transplant were much less anxious and fatigued.
- HIV-exposed infants who received massage therapy fared better in terms of improved weight gain, neonatal performance, and decreased stress behaviors than those who did not receive massage.
- Medical and nursing students under stress who received massage therapy demonstrated increased immune response greater than that of controls, as measured by immunoglobulin levels.

The Touch Research Institute at the University of Miami Medical School supports the research of a multidisciplinary team of scientists, including Tiffany Field, PhD. TRI's earliest research focused on premature infants, finding that those who received massage treatments for three 15-minute periods per day for 10 days gained 47% more body weight than infants treated with standard therapy. Data indicated that massaged infants were hospitalized 6 days less than unmassaged infants for a cost savings of thousands of dollars per infant. Given that premature births accounted for 10% of total new births at University of Miami Hospital, the potential for cost savings is substantial. The massaged infants in the study maintained their weight advantage at 8-month follow-up and exhibited greater motor and mental skills than the babies who did not receive massage (Field et al., 1986; Dieter et al., 2003). (For additional information on studies by the Touch Research Institute, see Chapter 36.)

TRAINING AND LICENSURE

Clinical/medical massage therapy is a developing profession. Massage standards, training, and licensure vary from region to region. Certification is available through the National Board for Therapeutic Massage and Bodywork (NCBTMB), which sets standards for training and clinical experience. Standards for advanced practitioner status are in development at the time of this writing. (See Chapter 33 for more information.) The safety of this practice is reflected in the exceptionally low malpractice rates experienced by massage practitioners, which typically range from approximately $200 to $250 per year (ABMP, 2004; AMTA, 2004).

Certification. In most states, maintaining certification is voluntary. Certification is available through the National Certification Board for Therapeutic Massage and Bodywork, which administers a qualifying exam-

ination and certifies massage therapists who successfully pass the exam and maintain their status through continuing education.

Licensure. Standards for massage therapists, like those of most other health care professionals, are determined at the state level. At the time of this writing, massage is regulated in 33 states and the District of Columbia (AMTA, 2004). In 25 states, the NCBTMB exam is accepted as the state licensing examination (W. Lowe, written communication, December 1, 2004). In states where there are no specific requirements with regard to massage therapy, standards are determined by the local municipality. When developing credentialing guidelines, check with state and city governments to obtain the regulations relevant to your jurisdiction. For a summary of the licensure requirements of each state and links to the Web sites of the respective state boards, see www.amtamassage.org/about/state_boards.html.

Educational requirements. In at least 21 of the 33 states that offer massage therapy licensure, 500 hours of training are required. Three states require 1000 hours of training (Alabama, Nebraska, and New York) and a few others require training that ranges from 500 to 1000 hours. In sum, 500 hours of massage training is a good minimum standard. These hours represent time spent in the classroom and in clinical training. In Washington state, in massage institutes that are certified by the Department of Health, the vast majority of schools require 800 to 1400 hours of training for graduation.

Accredited training. Accreditation for schools of massage training is a rigorous process in some states and can involve months of effort to provide the required documentation (J. McKinnon, written communication, May 15, 2000). In states that regulate massage, standards for education are determined by the state. For example, in Washington state, there are 33 massage schools approved by the massage board of the Department of Health (E. Oberland, Washington State Department of Health, oral communication, November 15, 2004). In addition to meeting state requirements, massage education programs are accredited by the Commission on Massage Training Accreditation (COMTA). This nonprofit organization, recognized by the US Department of Education, evaluates the quality of entry-level massage therapy training programs.

UTILIZATION

Insurance coverage. Coverage for massage varies widely from one health plan to another:

- Massage is covered by plans such as Aetna, US Healthcare, Kaiser Permanente, and United Healthcare, and is usually covered under workers' compensation and auto insurance personal injury protection (AMTA, 2004).
- Massage is also sometimes available through networks as a discounted or "affinity" benefit.
- In Washington state, under the law that mandates coverage of complementary therapies, therapeutic massage is covered in cases of medical necessity (typically provided in 1-hour sessions).

Availability of practitioners. As of December 2004, it was estimated that there were more than 120,700 American massage therapists in licensed states and more than 100,000 massage therapists in unlicensed states, totaling more than 220,000 practitioners (A. Haller, AMTA, written communication, December 1, 2004). AMTA membership totals more than 47,000 members (AMTA, 2004). ABMP, which also includes various bodywork professions, has more than 52,000 members (ABMP, 2004).

Medical utilization. A national survey of primary care physicians conducted by the State University of New York found that 54% of physicians surveyed said they would recommend therapeutic massage as an adjunct to medical treatment (Grant et al, 1995). In a 2002 national consumer survey, respondents who discussed massage with their physician reported that 96% were favorable or neutral (76% being favorable). Of these consumers, 57% were recommended to massage by a health care practitioner (30% by physicians and 27% by chiropractors) (ORC, 2002). The research literature suggests increased utilization of clinical massage over the past decade (see Table 34–3).

Frequently patients come to massage because they believe it will help them feel better. Over the course of the treatment, they realize that their condition is improving as well. Beyond the benefits of massage in reducing stress and creating a sense of well-being, clinical massage can provide a range of health benefits:

- Direct impact on tissue—We see this clinically in patients who receive medical massage for injuries, such as work-related injuries, accidents, or sports injuries. These benefits are confirmed in the research on circulation, lymphatics, and immune function.
- Immediacy—Massage also offers a certain degree of immediacy in improvement in decreasing stress or physical pain, a welcome secondary benefit.
- Pain relief—When patients report a 50% reduction in pain, that is significant. It may mean the difference between being able to sit or move with comfort—or not.
- Stress reduction—We know from the research that hospitalized patients with major depression experience almost immediate

Table 34–3 Data on the Utilization of Massage Therapy

Source and Universe Surveyed	Parameter	Percent
Interactive Solutions.[1] National survey of consumer preferences with regard to HMO coverage of complementary medicine	Percentage of consumers who would like massage to be covered by their health plan	80.0
Group Health Cooperative, Puget Sound.[2] Survey of physicians, nurses, and physicians' assistants in Washington state	Percentage of health care professionals who perceived massage as effective for purpose for which it was prescribed	74.0
Harvard Center for Alternative Medicine Research.[3] Nationally representative random household survey by telephone (N = 2,055)	Of those who were seen by a massage therapist for back or neck pain, percentage that found massage "very helpful"	65.0
Center for Health Research, Kaiser Permanente Northwest.[4] Survey of patients with temporomandibular joint syndrome (TMJ) (N = 192)	Percentage of respondents with TMJ who used massage and found it "among the most satisfactory and helpful"	62.5
Kaiser Permanente, Division of Research.[5] Kaiser patients surveyed who had severe musculoskeletal pain	• Of 3885 patients, percentage who used massage (1999) • Of 4254 patients, percentage who used massage (1996)	19.4 14.6
Harvard Center for Alternative Medicine Research.[3] Nationally representative random household survey by telephone (N = 2,055)	Percentage of all visits to complementary providers that were made to massage therapists in 1997 (114 million of 629 million)	18.1
National Market Measures.[6] Randomly selected managed care organizations (N = 114 of 449 MCOs in US)	Of MCOs offering complementary therapies, percentage that offered massage	11.0
Kaiser Permanente, Division of Research.[5] Representative sample of a northern California managed care organization	• Percentage of members who used massage (1999) • Percentage of members who used massage (1996)	10.7 7.5
National Center for Complementary and Alternative Medicine, NIH.[7] National Health Interview Survey, a nationally representative sample (N = 31,044)	Percentage of population using massage in past year (2002)	7.5

Source: Nancy Faass, MSW, MPH, San Francisco, CA.

benefit from massage. Stress and depression frequently accompany injury and surgery. Massage can help a patient navigate this stressful time.

Massage is a therapy you can prescribe to your patients that can have an immediate, beneficial effect on their physiology, their experience of pain, and their level of stress.

TABLE REFERENCES

1. Interactive Solutions. Landmark Report I on Public Perceptions of Alternative Care. Sacramento, CA: Landmark Healthcare; 1999.
2. Weeks J. The Integrator for the Business of Alternative Medicine. Atlanta, GA: Integrative Medicine; April 2001.
3. Wolsko PM, Eisenberg DM, Davis RB, Kessler R, Phillips RS. Patterns and perceptions of care for treatment of back and neck pain: results of a national survey. *Spine*. 2003;28(3):292–297, 298.
4. DeBarr LL, Vuckovic N, Schneider J, Ritenbaugh C. Use of complementary and alternative medicine for temporomandibular disorders. *J Orofac Pain*. 2003;17(3):224–236.
5. Gordon NP, Lin TY. Use of complementary and alternative medicine by the adult membership of a large northern California health maintenance organization. *J Ambulatory Care Manager*. 2004; 27(1):12–24.
6. National Market Measures. The Landmark Report II. Sacramento, CA: Landmark Healthcare; 1999.
7. Barnes PM, Powell-Griner E, McFann K, Nahin R. Complementary and alternative medicine use among adults: United States, 2002. *Adv Data*. 2004;343: 1–16.

REFERENCES

Agarwal KN, Gupta A, Pushkarna R, Bhargava SK, Faridi MM, Prabhu MK. Effects of massage and use of oil on growth, blood flow and sleep pattern in infants. *Indian J Med Res*. 2000;112:212–217.

Angus S. Massage therapy for sprinters and runners. *Clin Podiatr Med Surg*. 2001;18:329–336.

American Massage Therapy Association (AMTA). 2004. Available at: www.amta.com. Accessed July 15, 2004.

Associated Bodywork and Massage Professionals (ABMP). Available at www.abmp.com. Accessed July 15, 2004.

Balzer K, Schonebeck I. Edema after vascular surgery interventions and its therapy [Article in German]. *Z Lymphol*. 1993;17(2):41–47.

Birk TJ, McGrady A, MacArthur RD, Khuder S. The effects of massage therapy alone and in combination with other complementary therapies on immune system measures and quality of life in human immunodeficiency virus. *J Altern Complement Med*. 2000;6(5):405–414.

Bodhise PB, Dejoie M, Brandon Z, Simpkins S, Ballas SK. Non-pharmacologic management of sickle cell pain. *Hematology*. 2004;9(3):235–237.

Brefel-Courbon C, Desboeuf K, Thalamas C, et al. Clinical and economic analysis of spa therapy in Parkinson's disease. *Mov Disord*. 2003;18(5): 578–584.

Buonocore M, Manstretta C, Mazzucchi G, Casale R. The clinical evaluation of conservative treatment in patients with the thoracic outlet syndrome [Article in Italian]. *G Ital Med Lav Ergon*. 1998;20(4): 249–254.

Chang MY, Wang SY, Chen CH. Effects of massage on pain and anxiety during labour: a randomized controlled trial in Taiwan. *J Adv Nurs*. 2002;38(1): 68–73.

Chen L, Wu Q. Clinical observation on treatment of 83 cases of posthemiplegic omalgia. *J Tradit Chin Med*. 1998;18(3):215–217.

Chen ML, Lin LC, Wu SC, Lin JG. The effectiveness of acupressure in improving the quality of sleep of institutionalized residents. *J Gerontol A Biol Sci Med Sci*. 1999;54(8):M389–394.

Claire T. *Bodywork*. New York, NY: HarperCollins/ Quill; 1996.

Colledge NR, Barr-Hamilton RM, Lewis SJ, Sellar RJ, Wilson JA. Evaluation of investigations to diagnose the cause of dizziness in elderly people: a community based controlled study. *BMJ.* 1996; 313 (7060):788–792.

Davidson K, Jacoby S, Brown MS. Prenatal perineal massage: preventing lacerations during delivery. *J Obstet Gynecol Neonatal Nurs.* 2000;29(5): 474–479.

De Laat A, Stappaerts K, Papy S. Counseling and physical therapy as treatment for myofascial pain of the masticatory system. *J Orofac Pain.* 2003;17(1): 42–49.

Diego MA, Field T, Hernandez-Reif M, et al. Spinal cord patients benefit from massage therapy. *Int J Neurosci.* 2002;112(2):133–142.

Dieter JN, Field T, Hernandez-Reif M, Emory EK, Redzepi M. Stable preterm infants gain more weight and sleep less after five days of massage therapy. *J Pediatr Psychol.* 2003;28(6):403–411.

Dunn C, Sleep J, Collett D. Sensing an improvement: an experiential study to evaluate the use of aromatherapy, massage, and periods of rest in the intensive care unit. *J Adv Nurs.* 1995;21:34–40.

Ferrari R, Russell AS. Survey of general practitioner, family physician, and chiropractor's beliefs regarding the management of acute whiplash patients. *Spine.* 2004;29(19):2173–2177.

Field T. Massage therapy. In: Jonas W, Levin J, eds. *Essentials of Complementary and Alternative Medicine.* Philadelphia, PA: Lippincott Williams & Wilkins; 1999:383–391.

Field T, Henteleff T, Hernandez-Reif M, et al. Children with asthma have improved pulmonary function after massage therapy. *J Pediatr.* 1998;132:854–858.

Field T, Hernandez-Reif M, La Greca A, et al. Glucose levels decreased after giving massage therapy to children with diabetes mellitus. *Spectrum.* 1997; 10:23–25.

Field T, Hernandez-Reif M, Seligman S, et al. Juvenile rheumatoid arthritis: benefits from massage therapy. *J Pediatr Psychol.* 1997;22(5):607–617.

Field T, Hernandez-Reif M, Taylor S, et al. Labor pain is reduced by massage therapy. *J Psychosom Obstet Gynecol.* 1997;18:286–291.

Field T, Ironson G, Pickens J, et al. Massage therapy reduces anxiety and enhances EEG pattern of alertness and math computations. *Int J Neurosci.* 1996; 86:197–205.

Field T, Peck M, Hernandez-Reif M, Krugman S, Burman I, Ozment-Schenck L. Postburn itching, pain, and psychological symptoms are reduced with massage therapy. *J Burn Care Rehabil.* 2000;21(3): 189–193.

Field T, Peck M, Krugman S, et al. Massage therapy effects on burn patients. *J Burn Care Rehabil.* 1998; 19:241–244.

Field T, Pickens J, Prodromidis M, et al. Targeting adolescent mothers with depressive symptoms for early intervention. *Adolescence.* 2000;35(138):381–414.

Field T, Schanberg S, Cafidi F, et al. Tactile/kinesthetic stimulation effects on preterm neonates. *Pediatrics.* 1986;77:654–658.

Field T, Schanberg S, Kuhn C, et al. Bulimic adolescents benefit from massage therapy. *Adolescence.* 1998;33(131); 555–563.

Field T, Sunshine W, Hernandez-Reif M, et al. Chronic fatigue syndrome: massage therapy effects on depression and somatic symptoms in chronic fatigue syndrome. *J Chronic Fatigue Syndrome.* 1997;3: 43–51.

Friedman MH. The hypomobile temporomandibular joint. *Gen Dent.* 1997;45(3):282–285.

Gehlsen GM, Ganion LR, Helfst R. Fibroblast responses to variation in soft tissue mobilization pressure. *Med Sci Sports Exerc.* 1999;31(4): 531–535.

Gimblett PA, Saville J, Eball P. A conservative management protocol for calcific tendinitis of the shoulder. *J Manipulative Physiol Ther.* 1999;22(9):622–627.

Grant W, Kamps C, Blumberg D, Hendricks S, Dewan M. The physician and unconventional medicine. *Altern Ther Health Med.* 1995;1:31–35.

Greene E. Massage therapy. In: Novey D, ed. *Clinician's Complete Reference to Complementary and Alternative Medicine.* St. Louis, MO: Mosby; 2000:338–348.

Groer M, Mozingo J, Droppleman P, et al. Measures of salivary secretory immunoglobulin A and state anxiety after a nursing back rub. *Appl Nurs Res.* 1994;7(1):2–6.

Guler-Uysal F, Kozanoglu E. Comparison of the early response to two methods of rehabilitation in adhesive capsulitis. *Swiss Med Wkly.* 2004;134(23–24): 353–358.

Hawes MC, Brooks WJ. Reversal of the signs and symptoms of moderately severe idiopathic scoliosis in response to physical methods. *Stud Health Technol Inform.* 2002;91:365–368.

Hernandez-Reif M, Field T, Krasnegor J, Theakston H. Lower back pain is reduced and range of motion increased after massage therapy. *Int J Neurosci.* 2001;106(3–4):131–145.

Hernandez-Reif M, Ironson G, Field T, et al. Breast cancer patients have improved immune and neuroendocrine functions following massage therapy. *J Psychosom Res.* 2004;57(1):45–52.

Hollis N. *Massage for Therapists.* Oxford, England: Blackwell Publishers; 1987.

Ironson G, Field T, Scafidi F, et al. Massage therapy is associated with enhancement of the immune system's cytotoxic capacity. *Int J Neurosci.* 1996;84: 205–218.

Joachim G. The effects of two stress management techniques on feelings of well-being in patients with inflammatory bowel disease. *Nurs Papers.* 1983;15(4): 5–18.

Kaada B, Torsteinbo O. Increase of plasma beta-endorphins in connective tissue massage. *Gen Pharmacol.* 1989;20(4):487–489.

Kantrowitz FG, Farrar DJ, Locke SE. Chronic fatigue syndrome. 2: treatment and future research. *Behav Med.* 1995;21(1):17–24.

Klauser AG, Flaschentrager J, Gehrke A, Muller-Lissner SA. Abdominal wall massage: effect on colonic function in healthy volunteers and in patients with chronic constipation. *Z Gastroenterol.* 1992;30(4):247–251.

Kober A, Scheck T, Greher M, et al. Prehospital analgesia with acupressure in victims of minor trauma: a prospective, randomized, double-blinded trial. *Anesth Analg.* 2002;95(3):723–727.

Kurz W, Kurz R, Litmanovitch YI, Romanoff H, Pfeifer Y, Sulman FG. Effect of manual lymph drainage massage on blood components and urinary neurohormones in chronic lymphedema. *Angiology.* 1981;32(2):119–127.

Labrecque M, Marcoux S, Pinault JJ, et al. Prevention of perinatal trauma by perineal massage during pregnancy: a pilot study. *Birth.* 1994;21:20–25.

Launso L, Brendstrup E, Arnberg S. An exploratory study of reflexological treatment for headache. *Altern Ther Health Med.* 1999;5(3):57–65.

Lowe W. Orthopedic massage: a model for alternative treatment of cumulative trauma disorders. *AAOHN J.* 1999;47(4):175–184.

Luo Z, Luo J. Clinical observations on 278 cases of cervical spondylopathy treated with electroacupuncture and massotherapy. *J Tradit Chin Med.* 1997;17(2):116–118.

Mok E, Pang Woo CP. The effects of slow-stroke back massage on anxiety and shoulder pain in elderly stroke patients. *Complement Ther Nurs Midwifery.* 2004 Nov;10(4):209–216.

Mowen K. Spinal cord injuries and soft tissue rehabilitation. *Massage Bodywork.* Feb/March 2000; 36–44.

Muller-Oerlinghausen B, Berg C, Scherer P, Mackert A, Moestl HP, Wolf J. Effects of slow-stroke massage as complementary treatment of depressed hospitalized patients [Article in German]. *Dtsch Med Wochenschr.* 2004;129(24):1363–1368.

Mur E, Schmidseder J, Egger I, et al. Influence of reflex zone therapy of the feet on intestinal blood flow measured by color Doppler sonography [Article in German]. *Forsch Komplementarmed Klass Naturheilkd.* 2001;8(2):86–89.

Nayak S, Matheis RJ, Agostinelli S, Shifleft SC. The use of complementary and alternative therapies for chronic pain following spinal cord injury: a pilot survey. *J Spinal Cord Med.* 2001;24(1):54–62.

Opinion Research Corporation (ORC). National survey of adult consumers. Chicago, IL: American Massage Therapy Association; 2002. Available at: www.amtamassage.org. Accessed November 15, 2004.

Osborne-Sheets C. *Pre and Perinatal Massage Therapy.* San Diego, CA: Body Therapy Associates; 1998.

Paternostro-Sluga T, Zoch C. Conservative treatment and rehabilitation of shoulder problems [Article in German]. *Radiologe.* 2004;44(6):597–603.

Piotrowski MM, Paterson C, Mitchinson A, Kim HM, Kirsh M, Hinshaw DB. Massage as adjuvant therapy in the management of acute postoperative pain: a preliminary study in men. *J Am Coll Surg.* 2003; 197(6):1037–1046.

Pope MH, Philips RB, Haugh LD, et al. A prospective randomized three-week trial of spinal manipulation, transcutaneous muscle stimulation, massage and corset in the treatment of subacute low back pain. *Spine.* 1994;19:2571–2577.

Puustjarvi K, Airaksinen O, Pontinen PJ. The effects of massage in patients with chronic tension headache. *Acupunct Electrother Res.* 1990;15(2):159–162.

Quinn C, Chandler C, Moraska A. Massage therapy and frequency of chronic tension headaches. *Am J Public Health.* 2002;92(10):1657–1661.

Rattray F, Ludwig L. *Clinical Massage Therapy.* Toronto, Canada: Talus, Inc.; 2000.

Richards KC, Gibson R, Overton-McCoy AL. Effects of massage in acute and critical care. *AACN Clin Issues.* 2000;11(1):77–96.

Rochet JM, Zaoui A. Burn scars: rehabilitation and skin care [Article in French]. *Rev Prat.* 2002;52(20): 2258–2263.

Schachner L, Field T, Hernandez-Reif M, Duarte AM, Krasnegor J. Atopic dermatitis symptoms decreased in children following massage therapy. *Pediatr Dermatol.* 1998;15(5):390–395.

Sheon RP, The Goff Group. Repetitive strain injury. 2. Diagnostic and treatment tips on six common problems. *Postgrad Med.* 1997;102(4):72–78.

Siev-Ner I, Gamus D, Lerner-Geva L, Achiron A. Reflexology treatment relieves symptoms of multiple sclerosis: a randomized controlled study. *Mult Scler.* 2003;9(4):356–361.

Smith WA. Fibromyalgia syndrome. *Nurs Clin North Am.* 1998;33(4):653–669.

Stamp G, Kruzins G, Crowther C. Perineal massage in labour and prevention of perineal trauma: randomised controlled trial. *BMJ.* 2001;322(7297):1277–1280.

Sunshine W, Field T, Schanberg S, et al. Fibromyalgia benefits from massage therapy and transcutaneous electrical stimulation. *J Clin Rheumatol.* 1996;2:18–22.

Tarola GA. Manipulation for the control of back pain and curve progression in patients with skeletally mature idiopathic scoliosis: two cases. *J Manipulative Physiol Ther.* 1994;17(4):253–257.

Ulreich A, Kullich W. Results of a multidisciplinary rehabilitation concept in patients with chronic lumbar syndromes [in German]. *Wien Med Wochenschr.* 1999;149(19–20):564–566.

van den Dolder PA, Roberts DL. A trial into the effectiveness of soft tissue massage in the treatment of shoulder pain. *Aust J Physiother.* 2003;49(3):183–188.

Vendittelli F, Tabaste JL, Janky E. Antepartum perineal massage: review of randomized trials [Article in French]. *J Gynecol Obstet Biol Reprod* (Paris). 2001;30(6):565–571.

Walach H, Guthlin C, Konig M. Efficacy of massage therapy in chronic pain: a pragmatic randomized trial. *J Altern Complement Med.* 2003;9(6):837–846.

Wang HL, Keck JF. Foot and hand massage as an intervention for postoperative pain. *Pain Manag Nurs.* 2004;5(2):59–65.

Warms CA, Turner JA, Marshall HM, Cardenas DD. Treatments for chronic pain associated with spinal cord injuries: many are tried, few are helpful. *Clin J Pain.* 2002;18(3):154–163.

Weinrich SP, Weinrich MC. The effect of massage on pain in cancer patients. *Appl Nurs Res.* 1990;3:140–145.

White-Traut RC, Nelson MN. Maternally administered tactile, auditory, visual, and vestibular stimulation: relationship to later interactions between mothers and premature infants. *Res Nurs Health.* 1988;11:31–39.

Wylie KR, Jackson C, Crawford PM. Does psychological testing help to predict the response to acupuncture or massage/relaxation therapy in patients presenting to a general neurology clinic with headache? *J Tradit Chin Med.* 1997;17(2):130–139.

Yip YB, Tse SH. The effectiveness of relaxation acupoint stimulation and acupressure with aromatic lavender essential oil for non-specific low back pain in Hong Kong: a randomised controlled trial. *Complement Ther Med.* 2004;12(1):28–37.

Zhou XJ, Chen T, Chen JT. 75 infantile palsy children treated with acupuncture, acupressure and functional training [Article in Chinese]. *Zhongguo Zhong Xi Yi Jie He Za Zhi.* 1993;13(4):220–222.

CHAPTER 35

Definitions of Clinical Massage and Bodywork

Karin Olsen, Whitney Lowe, Vickie Ina, Linda Chrisman, and Nancy Faass

INTRODUCTION

This chapter provides a brief overview of some of the most frequently provided massage techniques, among the thousands of modalities available. Within the professional massage community, distinctions are made among massage, bodywork, energy therapies, and movement therapies. This list of definitions, although not exhaustive, includes techniques that may not traditionally be thought of as massage. However, all these disciplines have value as complementary therapies. They reflect the broad range of approaches that utilize the therapeutic benefits of touch and movement. (Research and references on the applications of massage are provided in Chapter 34.)

BASIC MASSAGE TECHNIQUES

Swedish massage. The most familiar form of massage currently in use, Swedish massage is taught in the vast majority of basic 500-hour massage courses. Swedish massage emphasizes long flowing strokes for deep relaxation, nurturance, and sensory awareness. This approach can also involve kneading and friction techniques on the more superficial layers of the muscles, combined with active

Biographies of contributors appear in Chapters 34, 37, 65, 34, and 2, respectively.

and passive movement of the joints. These techniques focus on relieving muscle tension, easing aches and pains, improving range of motion, and supporting better posture. The basic methods of Swedish massage provide the foundation for most other Western massage modalities.

MASSAGE THERAPY IN ADVANCED PRACTICE

Medical massage. This term has taken on a number of meanings. In some cases it simply indicates massage provided by referral from a physician. As a broader term, medical massage describes any type of clinical massage used as an adjunct therapy for a medical condition. Conditions addressed can range from basic muscle aches and soreness to pain management in cancer patients. At the current time, consensus on a specific definition has not yet been established within the massage profession.

Muscle energy technique (MET). A system of manual therapy, MET is utilized in cases of impaired movement and/or musculoskeletal pain—such as low back or neck pain; misalignment of the spine, rib cage, or pelvis; chronic muscle tension; or injuries. One of the primary focuses of MET is assessment and correction of musculoskeletal misalignment. When misalignment results from poor tone (due to lax, overstretched muscles), balance can be restored by strengthening the muscles that support alignment. Misalignment due to chronic tension (and contracted muscles) can be addressed by relaxing and stretching those muscles. Therapy involves the efforts of both practitioner and patient using a series of isometric contractions followed by passive stretching, often reinforced through an individualized exercise program.

Myofascial release. This form of deep tissue massage involves long, stretching strokes to facilitate the release of chronic muscle and fascia tension that may be restricting posture, movement, or circulation. This technique may be performed slowly, applied specifically to one area of the body during a session. The pressure level is generally light and the emphasis of myofascial work is to encourage elongation in the superficial fascia, which in turn, has an effect on reducing muscular tension/hypertonicity.

Neuromuscular therapy. This approach is similar to trigger point therapy and is indicated in conditions of chronic muscle pain and tension. These techniques involve static pressure point therapy and deep tissue massage, to reduce muscular tightness and neutralize the reactivity of trigger points. Neuromuscular therapy is used to address chronic postural problems (such as the classic forward-head posture associated with tension and reactive trigger points). It is also highly effective in the management of many myofascial pain syndromes.

Orthopedic massage. This is not a technique, but a comprehensive system that integrates a variety of methods in the treatment of soft tissue dysfunction, pain, and injury. There is a strong emphasis on proper assessment of the soft tissue disorder in order to choose the most beneficial treatment approach for each client. Practitioners of orthopedic massage frequently work in conjunction with other health professionals.

Sports massage. An approach similar to Swedish and deep-tissue massage, sports massage has adapted these techniques (and others) to address the effects of athletic performance on the body. Sports massage can enhance warm-up and improve range of motion and muscle flexibility. These techniques also increase circulation (to improve absorption of nutrients and oxygen to the tissue) and support recovery from athletic activity. Depending on the therapeutic goal, sports massage may be vigorously applied and may involve cross-fiber friction, compression, pressure points, or techniques to increase circulation. These techniques can be utilized to address muscle cramping, aches, spasms, bruising, tears, pain, or edema.

Strain CounterStrain. This method, originated by Lawrence Jones, DO, can also be described as positional release therapy. Strain CounterStrain utilizes "positions of ease"—stretching postures to relax and elongate muscle fibers and overcome muscle spasms—with the goal of improving range of motion, joint mobility, and balance. This therapy also involves manually addressing tender points in myofascial tissue to neutralize dysfunctional neurological activity.

ACUPRESSURE AND PRESSURE-POINT THERAPIES

Acupressure. This generic term refers to the broad range of Oriental massage techniques that address the flow of Chi or Qi (pronounced "chee") through the body's meridian system. These techniques involve the surface stimulation of acupuncture/acupressure points manually or with tools held in the hand. Related therapies include Jin Shin Do and Jin Shin Jyutsu.

Reflexology. A variation of pressure-point therapy, reflexology is applied to external "reflex points" on the feet, hands, or ears. Energy medicine theory associates these points with acupuncture/acupressure points and meridians, which are massaged to enhance healing. Hand and foot massage also tends to promote relaxation. Reflexology may be incorporated in massage that addresses the entire body, or it may be used as a specific form of therapy that constitutes an entire session.

Shiatsu. This is a Japanese technique whose name literally means "finger-pressure treatment" and may involve finger, thumb, palm, hand, or elbow pressure along the meridians and on acupressure points. Shiatsu is intended to restore energy and balance to the energetic system of the body by promoting the flow of Qi ("ki" in Japanese). There are several styles of this approach, including Zen shiatsu, Oha shiatsu, and Amma therapy, a Korean variation.

Trigger-point or myotherapy. This method utilizes finger or thumb pressure on triggerpoints in the muscle and connective tissue to relieve pain and referred pain patterns, hypersensitivity, muscle spasms, stiffness, or loss of movement. Trigger-point release work can involve deep pressure at specific points to release muscle spasms and break the painspasm-pain cycle. These techniques are applied in a range of conditions including the treatment of sports injuries and chronic back pain.

Tuina (tui na tsang). This form of massage has been used extensively in China for more than 2000 years. A combination of massage, acupressure, and other forms of body manipulation, tuina works by applying pressure to acupoints, meridians, and groups of muscles or nerves to remove blockages and restore the balance of Qi. Tuina is utilized today in hospitals throughout China in conjunction with other forms of traditional Chinese medicine. Tuina techniques are applied in orthopedic and sports massage for the rehabilitation of muscle and joint injuries; in visceral massage as an adjunctive therapy for various digestive disorders; and for the elderly and infants.

DEEP TISSUE TECHNIQUES

Deep tissue massage techniques are intended to release chronic patterns of muscle tension or restriction in connective tissue, using slow strokes and deep finger pressure. These techniques are usually applied following the direction of muscle fibers, tendons, and fascia, with primary focus on the deeper layers of tissue and musculature. Deep tissue work can also involve cross-fiber friction and myofascial release techniques. Rolfing is perhaps the best-known type of deep tissue massage, but deep tissue techniques are an integral aspect of many forms of massage, including:

- Medical, orthopedic, and sports massage
- Myofascial release and neuromuscular therapy
- Rolfing, Hellerwork, soma (somatic neuromuscular integration), and Zentherapy

ENERGY THERAPIES

Energy therapies encompass traditional forms of healing that focus on the life force or vital energy, including the electromagnetic fields of the body. For example, acupressure is a form of energy therapy because, like acupuncture, it is believed to affect the flow of energy along the electromagnetic meridians. Other forms of energy therapy, such as therapeutic touch, do not use physical touch but are intended to affect the energy field around the body.

Polarity therapy. This system of bodywork includes aspects of energy meridian therapies from China and osteopathic techniques. Developed by Randolph Stone, OD, this approach encompasses a range of techniques from light touch to deep tissue massage, as well as pressure-point therapy, stretching postures, and myofascial and structural manipulation. The goal of this work is to promote the unobstructed flow of energy in the body and, like other forms of touch therapy, these techniques appear to reduce stress-related activity in the sympathetic nervous system.

Reiki. This simple laying-on-of-hands technique was formalized as a method of Japanese massage, but is probably one of the oldest forms of comfort known to humanity. The practitioner directs energy ("ki" or "chee") through his hands to the client to balance the body's energy and promote a sense of healing. Clients often experience localized sensations of warmth and relaxation. Some physicians see Reiki as a reasonable palliative adjunct to conventional treatment. Reiki is applied in cases of stress, fatigue, insomnia, headache, anxiety, and pain.

Therapeutic Touch. Derived from the laying on of hands, this method was developed by nurses and does not involve direct contact with the body. The intent of Therapeutic Touch is to balance the patient's energy field with this noncontact approach. This technique is also known as the Krieger-Kunz Method of Therapeutic Touch.

MASSAGE FOR SPECIFIC NEEDS

Chair massage. This approach to back and neck massage is typically performed with the client seated in a specially designed massage chair, fully clothed. Chair massage can be provided in a broad range of environments, including the work site or other public venues, and has been found effective in stress reduction.

Craniosacral therapy. Cranial osteopathy and craniosacral therapy are techniques that focus on the cranium and spine, developed by the osteopaths William Sutherland and John Upledger. These modalities involve gentle, noninvasive touch to enhance functioning of the cerebrospinal system, identifying and releasing critical points of restriction, improving circulation, gently stimulating scalp nerves, and promoting lymph and sinus drainage. The practitioner manually applies subtle pressure to the neck, head, or base of the spine, using a light touch, generally no greater than 5 grams (about the weight of a nickle). Many people report deep relaxation or the unwinding of tension. In infants, craniosacral therapy may focus on correcting distortions in the relationship of the cranial plates due to the effects of birth trauma.

Geriatric massage. Another light form of touch, geriatric massage consists of techniques adapted to the specific physiological needs of older adults, which may include frailty.

Infant massage. These gentle techniques are typically taught to new parents to promote bonding with the infant and are also used in hospitals with premature infants. Infant massage serves to accustom a young child to the positive aspects of touch. Research indicates that touch is essential to proper human development (see Chapter 36).

Manual lymphatic drainage. This is an advanced technique derived from Swedish massage intended to improve lymphatic circulation, thereby decreasing edema. In-depth training in this technique has been developed by Emil Vodder, MD. Manual lymphatic drainage is indicated for a number of disorders, including postmastectomy conditions involving the loss of lymph nodes.

Prenatal and perinatal massage. These advanced techniques are specifically designed to relieve back and hip pain associated with pregnancy. The applications of massage during pregnancy are well-researched and have also been found beneficial in easing the discomforts of labor and postpartum recovery. When referring for pregnancy massage, it is important to identify practitioners with in-depth training and clinical experience in pre- and perinatal massage.

MIND-BODY TECHNIQUES (SOMATIC THERAPIES)

Somatic therapy is a generic term describing techniques that involve touch and movement, and, in some cases, mind-body therapies. Thomas Hanna originated the phrase to distinguish Hanna somatics and other mind-body modalities from massage.

Continuum Movement. Continuum is a method that involves sound, breath, and subtle movement to disrupt habitual patterns and facilitate new movement possibilities. This therapy can be particularly effective in rehabilitation from spinal cord injury and a variety of other neuromuscular conditions.

Rosen Method. This approach, based on the work of Marian Rosen, involves gentle touch and verbal exchange between practitioner and client to draw the client's attention to areas in which tension is frequently held.

The Rosen Method has been found to facilitate the release of chronic muscular tension and, in some cases, suppressed emotions.

Somatic experiencing. Another noninvasive approach to somatic education, this method involves touch, imagery, movement, and dialogue to access and release deeply held emotional or physical tension due to trauma.

Trager psychophysical integration. This technique utilizes rhythmic rocking movements to release deep-seated physical and mental patterns. Its light, gentle, nonintrusive movement relaxes both the body and mind.

MOVEMENT THERAPIES

Alexander Technique. In Alexander work, new patterns of movement and posture are encouraged through coaching, verbal cues, and touch. The goal is to develop and maintain a more effective alignment of the head, neck, and back to improve overall physical and emotional functioning.

Feldenkrais Method. This method of gentle touch developed by Moshe Feldenkrais involves movement reeducation to improve posture and flexibility and to alleviate muscular tension and pain. Clinically, Feldenkrais has been found effective for a wide variety of conditions.

STRUCTURAL INTEGRATION

Aston-Patterning. A mind-body technique that includes deep tissue bodywork, Aston-Patterning also involves analysis of movement patterns to identify areas of ease and discomfort. The goal of this approach is to teach people how to live more optimally in their bodies.

Hellerwork. A form of deep tissue body-work that was developed from Rolfing, Hellerwork also includes movement education and guided verbal dialogue.

Rolfing (structural integration). This system, developed by Ida Rolf, involves deep tissue work and movement education. Rolfing is intended to enhance or restore physical integrity and functionality by reintegrating the body. One of the major goals of this work is to bring the body—head, shoulders, thorax, pelvis, and legs—into a finer alignment with gravity.

Soma (somatic neuromuscular integration). Soma is a deep tissue technique that addresses areas of chronic tension and rigidity to restore ease and freedom of movement to the body. The practitioner may incorporate movement education and relaxation techniques with deep tissue massage.

Zentherapy. This system of massage is intended to release the natural form of the body from the aberrations caused by physical, chemical, psychological, or spiritual trauma. A number of different methods and techniques are used in this highly focused process, which incorporates aspects of the work of Ida Rolf and Moshe Feldenkrais, among others.

GENERAL REFERENCES

American Massage Therapy Association (AMTA). Available at: www.AMTAmassage.com. Accessed July 15, 2004.

American Medical Massage Therapy Association. Available at: www.amma.org. Accessed November 1, 2004.

Claire T. *BodyWork*. New York, NY: Harper-Collins Quill, 1996.

International Zentherapy Institute. Available at: www.zentherapy.org. Accessed November 1, 2004.

Knaster M. *Discovering the Body's Wisdom*. New York, NY: Bantam Books; 1996.

New Seattle Massage: Literature on various massage techniques, Seattle, WA: New Seattle Massage; 2003.

Orthopedic Massage Education and Research Institute. Available at: www.omeri.com. Accessed November 1, 2004.

Peters D, Woodham A. *Encyclopedia of Natural Healing*. New York, NY: Dorling Kindersly Publishing; 2002.

CHAPTER 36

Research on the Effectiveness of Massage

Tiffany M. Field, PhD

INTRODUCTION

The Touch Research Institutes (TRI) at the University of Miami School of Medicine is the first center in the world devoted entirely to the scientific study of touch and its application in the fields of science and medicine. Since 1982, TRI's team of researchers, representing Harvard, Princeton, Duke, McGill, and the University of Maryland, has explored the connection between touch therapy and the effective treatment of disease. Their work has also identified the normalizing effects of massage on a range of physiological mechanisms and functions. For example, massage has been found to measurably normalize biochemistry associated with stress and its potentially damaging effects to the body (see Tables 36–1 and 36–2).

Additional improvements in function have been documented by TRI in a wide range of conditions and populations. A number of these studies are summarized in this chapter.

Tiffany M. Field, PhD, is Director of the Touch Research Institutes (TRI) at the University of Miami School of Medicine. She is recipient of the American Psychological Association Boyd McAndless Distinguished Young Scientist Award and has received a Research Scientist Award from the National Institute of Mental Health for her research career. Dr. Field is the author of *Infancy* (Harvard University Press, 1990), *Touch Therapy* (Churchill Livingstone, 2000), and numerous other books, as well as more than 400 journal articles. She has also served as the editor of a series of volumes on high-risk infants and another series on stress and coping.

Courtesy of Tiffany Field, PhD, Touch Research Institute, University of Miami, Miami, Florida.

THERAPEUTIC MASSAGE: ADULTS

Back pain. This randomized trial assessed the effects on back pain of clinical massage and progressive muscle relaxation (Hernandez-Reif et al., 2001). Twenty-four participants (mean age 39.6 years; 12 women) were randomly assigned to massage therapy or progressive muscle relaxation. The interventions were provided twice a week, in 30-minute sessions, for 5 weeks. Measures included pain, depression, anxiety, and sleeplessness; stress hormones, serotonin, and cortisol; and range of motion. On the first and last day of the 5-week study, participants completed questionnaires, provided urine samples, and were assessed for range of motion.

Results: Participants in the massage group reported less pain, depression, and anxiety, and better sleep. Functional evaluation found improved trunk and pain flexion performance. Laboratory analysis indicated lower levels of stress hormones and higher levels of serotonin and dopamine, also suggesting less pain.

Breast cancer. Stress has been linked to increased tumor development due to lower natural killer (NK) cell activity. In this context, stress reduction for women with breast cancer can be of particular importance, since they are at risk for elevated depression, anxiety, and decreased NK cell levels. This study sought to evaluate the benefits of massage in stress reduction, immune measures, and mood (Hernandez-Reif et al., 2004). Thirty-four

Table 36–1 Mechanisms of Benefit: Clinical Massage

Therapeutic mechanism	Identified in research on the following condition(s)
Functions moderated	
Cortisol levels	Anorexia, bulemia, burn injury, child and adolescent psychiatric disorders, chronic fatigue syndrome, fibromyalgia, HIV, hypertension, job stress, juvenile asthma and rheumatoid arthritis, postpartum depression, and post-traumatic stress
Edema lower	Premenstrual syndrome
Glucose levels more normal	Childhood diabetes
Heart rate normalized	Stress reduction in healthy adults
Norepinephrine lower	Pregnancy and postpartum depression
Substance P lower	Fibromyalgia
Functions stimulated	
CD4 cells elevated, CD4/CD8 ratio improved	HIV
Dopamine levels increased	Back pain and chronic fatigue syndrome
NK cell activity enhanced	HIV and breast cancer
Serotonin levels increased	Back pain, bulemia, migraines, and postpartum depression
White blood cell and neutrophil counts improved	Childhood leukemia

Source: Summarized from clinical trials by the Touch Research Institute, University of Miami. Nancy Faass, MSW, MPH.

women (mean age = 53) diagnosed with Stage 1 or 2 breast cancer, postsurgery, were randomly assigned to massage therapy or a control group. The intervention group received 30-minute massages, 3 times per week for 5 weeks. On the first and last day of the study, participants were assessed for mood, body image, coping style, and functioning. Urine samples were taken to evaluate catecholamines and serotonin levels and a subset of 27 women (N = 15 massage) had blood tests to assess immune measures.

Table 36–2 Improvements in Functioning: Clinical Massage

Functions improved	Identified in research on the following condition(s)
Activities of daily living (ADLs)	Parkinson's
Anger and aggression lowered	Burn injuries, aggression in adolescents, and behavior problems in children
Anxiety and diabetes, depression	Back pain, breast cancer, bulimia, chronic fatigue syndrome, diabetes, fibromyalgia, HIV, job stress, postburn symptoms, postpartum depression, post-traumatic stress, psychiatric disorders (child and adolescent), sexual abuse
Additional findings on reduced anxiety	Anorexia, asthma, AD/HD, atopic dermatitis, hypertension, multiple sclerosis, pregnancy and labor, premenstrual syndrome, rheumatoid arthritis (juvenile)
Blood pressure	Hypertension
Coping ability	Childbirth and burn injuries
Fatigue	Chronic fatigue, fibromyalgia, job stress
Muscle function	Improved flexibility (cerebral palsy), strength (spinal cord injury), tone (Down's syndrome)
Motor function	Cerebral palsy and Down's syndrome
Peak air flow	Childhood asthma and cystic fibrosis
Pain	Back pain, burn injury, carpal tunnel syndrome, chronic fatigue syndrome, fibromyalgia, labor pain, premenstrual syndrome, rheumatoid arthritis (juvenile)
Range of motion	Back pain, spinal cord injury
Sleep and sleep patterns	Autism, back pain, chronic fatigue syndrome, fibromyalgia, infant sleep patterns (preterm infants and infants of depressed mothers), migraines, Parkinson's disease, preschool children, psychiatric disorders (child and adolescent)
Stress	Anorexia, bulimia, burn injury, child and adolescent psychiatric disorders, chronic fatigue syndrome, fibromyalgia, HIV, hypertension, job stress, juvenile asthma and rheumatoid arthritis, postpartum depression, post-traumatic stress

Source: Summarized from clinical trials by the Touch Research Institute, University of Miami. Nancy Faass, MSW, MPH.

Results: Immediate effects reported by participants receiving massage included reduced anxiety, depression, and anger. Urine analysis indicated higher levels of dopamine and serotonin, and blood work showed increased levels of NK cells and lymphocytes.

Burn injury. Twenty-eight adult patients with burns were randomly assigned before debridement to either a massage therapy group or a standard treatment control group (Field, Peck, Krugman et al., 1998).

Results: In the massage group, levels of anxiety and cortisol decreased, and behavior ratings, activity, and anxiety improved after the massage therapy sessions on the first and last days of treatment. Longer-term effects were also significantly better for the massage therapy group, including decreases in depression and anger, and decreased pain on the McGill Pain Questionnaire, the Present Pain Intensity scale, and a Visual Analogue Scale. Although the underlying mechanisms are not known, these data suggest that debridement sessions were less painful after the massage therapy sessions due to a reduction in anxiety, and that the clinical course of treatment was probably enhanced as the result of reduced pain, anger, and depression.

HIV. A group of HIV-positive men were evaluated to determine the effects of massage therapy on the immune system. After 45 minutes of massage therapy, 5 days a week for a month, their anxiety and stress levels were decreased. Of even greater significance were the findings of enhanced immune response. Participants' natural killer cell counts increased, providing increased protection against opportunistic infections such as pneumonia (Ironson et al., 1996).

Migraine headaches. Twenty-six adults with migraine headaches were randomly assigned to a wait-list control group or to a massage therapy group to receive two 30-minute massages per week for five consecutive weeks (Hernandez-Reif, Dieter, Field et al., 1998). The massage therapy subjects reported fewer distress symptoms, less pain, more headache-free days, fewer sleep disturbances, and increased serotonin levels.

Multiple sclerosis. Twenty-four adults with multiple sclerosis were randomly assigned to a standard medical treatment control group or a massage therapy group that received two 45-minute massages a week for 5 weeks (Hernandez-Reif, Field, Field et al., 1998). The massage group reported less depressed mood immediately following the massage sessions and by the end of the study indicated improved self-esteem, better body image, less negative image of disease progression, and enhanced social functional status.

Nicotine cravings. Smoking cessation has been correlated with severe withdrawal symptoms, including intense cigarette cravings, anxiety, and depressed mood (Hernandez-Reif et al., 1999). In this study 20 adult smokers (mean age = 32.6 years) were randomly assigned to a self-massage treatment or a control group. The treatment group was taught to conduct hand or ear self-massage during three periods of cravings each day for 1 month.

Results: Self-reports revealed lower anxiety scores, improved mood, and fewer withdrawal symptoms. In addition, by the last week of the study, the self-massage group smoked fewer cigarettes per day than participants in the control group. The present findings suggest that self-massage may be an effective addition to smoking cessation programs to alleviate smoking-related anxiety and improve mood—and to decrease cravings, withdrawal symptoms, and smoking.

Spinal cord injury. This study assessed the effects of massage therapy on spinal cord injury for depression, functionality, upper body muscle strength, and range of motion (Diego et al., 2003b). Twenty patients with spinal cord injury (C5 through C7) were recruited from a university outpatient clinic and randomly assigned to a massage therapy group or an exercise group. Those in the massage group received 40-minute massage sessions twice a week for 5 weeks. Participants in the control group exercised twice a week for 5 weeks, practicing range of motion exercises focused on the arms, neck, shoulders, and back.

Results: Although measures indicated that both groups benefited from treatment, only the massage group showed lower anxiety and depression scores and significantly increased their muscle strength and wrist range of motion.

THERAPEUTIC MASSAGE: INFANTS AND CHILDREN

The Touch Research Institute has extensive findings on the benefits of massage therapy to premature infants (Field et al., 1986, 1994; Dieter et al., 2003), particularly weight gain, improved sleep, and alertness. At 8-month follow-ups, babies who received massage showed improved cognition and functioning when compared with controls. TRI research has also focused on a broad range of childhood conditions including abuse (sexual and physical), asthma, autism, burns, cancer, developmental delays, dermatitis (psoriasis), diabetes, eating disorders (anorexia and bulimia), juvenile rheumatoid arthritis, post-traumatic stress disorder, and psychiatric problems. Throughout the research, massage therapy typically resulted in lower anxiety, decreases in stress hormones, and improved clinical course. Studies that trained parents, grandparents, and volunteers

to provide the massage also found that the therapy enhanced the well being of caregivers and provided cost-effective benefit for the children.

Preterm infants. In one study preterm infants were randomly assigned to treatment or control groups once they were considered medically stable (Scafidi et al., 1990). The 40 infants averaged a gestational age of 30 weeks with a mean birth weight of 1176 g (2.5 pounds) and mean duration in intensive care, 14 days. The treatment infants (N = 20) received tactile/kinesthetic stimulation for three 15-minute periods per day for a 10-day period. Sleep/awake behavior was monitored and Brazelton assessments were performed at the beginning and end of the treatment period.

Results: The treated infants averaged 21% greater weight gain per day (34 g versus 28 g) and were discharged 5 days earlier. No significant differences were demonstrated in sleep/wake states. The treated infants' performance was superior on the habituation cluster items of the Brazelton scale. The treatment infants were also more active during the stimulation sessions (particularly during the tactile components of the sessions).

A recent study of preterm infants by TRI documented even great gains (Dieter et al., 2003). This research examined the effects of 5 days of massage therapy on the weight gain, sleep, and behavior of stable hospitalized preterm infants. Massage therapy was provided for three 15-minute periods per day to 16 preterm neonates (mean gestational age 30.1 weeks; mean birth weight 1359 g [3 pounds]). Their progress was assessed and compared with that of 16 control infants of similar gestational age (mean birth weight 1421 g [3.14 pounds]). Measures included weight gain, formula intake, kilocalories, stooling, and sleep/awake behavior.

Results: The massage group averaged 53% greater daily weight gain than the control group. This benefit was achieved with just 5 days of massage, in contrast to 10 days in previous studies, indicating that massage can be a cost-effective therapy for medically stable preterm infants.

Aggressive adolescents. A group of aggressive adolescents (N = 17) were randomly assigned to massage or relaxation therapy for 20-minute sessions, twice a week for 5 weeks (Diego et al., 2003a). Measures were taken at the end of the first and last sessions. The adolescents who received massage reported lower anxiety following both sessions. By the end of the study, they also reported feeling less hostile and perceived their parents as less aggressive. Significant differences were not found for the adolescents assigned to the relaxation group.

Childhood asthma. Children with asthma were found to have improved pulmonary function after massage therapy (Field, Henteleff, Hernandez-Reif et al., 1998). Thirty-two children with asthma (sixteen 4- to 8-year-olds and sixteen 9- to 16-year-olds) were randomly assigned to receive either massage therapy or relaxation therapy. The children's parents were taught to provide one therapy or the other for 20 minutes before bedtime each night for 30 days.

Results: The younger children who received massage therapy showed an immediate decrease in anxiety and cortisol levels after massage. Also, their attitude toward asthma and their peak air flow and other pulmonary functions improved over the course of the study. The older children who received massage therapy also reported lower anxiety after the massage. Their attitude toward asthma improved over the study, but only one measure of pulmonary function improved (forced respiratory flow from 25% to 75%). The reason for

the smaller therapeutic benefit in the older children is unknown; however, it appears that daily massage does improve airway caliber and control of asthma.

Attention deficit disorder. Thirty students (ages 7 to 18, mean = 13 years) diagnosed with attention-deficit/hyperactivity disorder were randomly assigned to massage therapy or a wait-list (Khilnani et al., 2003). The massage group received 20-minute sessions twice a week for 4 weeks. Results indicated that participants with AD/HD experienced short-term improvements in mood and long-term benefits in terms of classroom behavior.

Autism. This study involved 20 children (ages 3 to 6) with autism and their families (Escalona et al., 2001). Parents were randomly assigned to read bedtime stories (Dr. Seuss) or provide massage to their children 15 minutes prior to bed every night for a month. In the massage group, parents were trained by a massage therapist to provide massage. Responses were assessed using Conners Teacher and Parent Scales, classroom and playground observations, and sleep diaries, to track hyperactivity, stereotypic and off-task behavior, and sleep problems.

Results: The children in the massage group showed less stereotypic behavior and more on-task and social relatedness behavior during play at school and experienced fewer sleep problems at home.

Childhood insomnia. In this study, preschool children received 20-minute massages twice a week for 5 weeks (Field et al., 1996). They were evaluated after the massage sessions on the first and last days of the study. The behavior of the children who received massage was compared with that of children in the waiting list. The massaged children had better ratings on general state of well-being, vocalization, activity, and cooperation. Their behavior had also improved by the completion of the study, according to ratings by their teachers. At the end of the 5-week period, parents rated their children as having less aversion to touch and more extraverted behaviors.

Pain management in children. Relatively little research has been conducted on pediatric pain management and the crippling effects of pain associated with diseases such as childhood cancers and juvenile rheumatoid arthritis. Traditionally, treatment relies on the use of medications that alter the body's biochemistry, but pediatricians are understandably reluctant to prescribe potentially addictive drugs to children. As a result, children with juvenile arthritis are given anti-inflammatory drugs to reduce pain. Massage is now being evaluated as an alternative therapy because of its capacity to increase serotonin levels with the potential to mediate pain. Researchers are also evaluating the use of massage to offset the need for addictive pain medications (Field et al., 1997).

THERAPEUTIC BENEFITS OF MASSAGE

Studies conducted at TRI have documented a range of therapeutic effects associated with massage therapy, including:

- Long-term benefit—Premature infants who receive early massage therapy continue to do better at 6- to 8-month follow-ups.

- Improved labor and delivery—Women receiving massage during pregnancy reported experiencing fewer obstetric and postnatal complications, including lower prematurity rates.
- Management of childhood illness—In families taught to provide massage for their children (with conditions such as insomnia, autism, insomnia, or leukemia), children benefited and parents also showed decreased stress. (Similarly, volunteers taught to provide massage experienced equal or greater benefit.)
- Reductions in economic and human costs—Preterm newborns receiving massage have been found to improve at a faster rate than those not receiving massage. For example, preterm infants gained 47% more weight, became more socially responsive, and were discharged 6 days earlier at a hospital cost savings of $10,000 per infant or $4.7 billion if the 470,000 preterm infants born each year were massaged (Field et al., 1986).

As the scientific community continues to investigate complementary and adjunctive interventions, ongoing research regarding touch therapies becomes even more vital. This research has demonstrated that touch therapy can play an important role in improving a wide range of medical conditions.

REFERENCES

Diego MA, Field T, Hernandez-Reif M, et al. Aggressive adolescents benefit from massage therapy. *Adolescence.* 2003a;37(147):597–607.

Diego MA, Field T, Hernandez-Reif M, et al. Spinal cord patients benefit from massage therapy. *Int J Neurosci.* 2003b;112(2):133–142.

Dieter JN, Field T, Hernandez-Reif M, Emory EK, Redzepi M. Stable preterm infants gain more weight and sleep less after five days of massage therapy. *J Pediatr Psychol.* 2003;28(6):403–411.

Escalona A, Field T, Singer-Strunk et al. Improvements in the behavior of children with autism. *J Autism and Devel Disorders.* 2001;31: 513–516.

Field T. Massage therapy for infants and children. *J Dev Behav Pediatr.* 1994;16:105–111.

Field T, Henteleff T, Hernandez-Reif M, et al. Children with asthma have improved pulmonary functions after massage. *J Pediatr.* 1998;152: 854–858.

Field T, Hernandez-Reif M, Seligman S et al. Juvenile rheumatoid arthritis: benefits from massage therapy. *J Pediatr Psychol.* 1997;22:607–617.

Field T, Kilmer T, Hernandez-Reif M, Burman I. Preschool children's sleep and wake behavior: effects of massage therapy. *Early Child Dev Care.* 1996;120:39–40.

Field T, Peck M, Krugman S, Tuchel T, Schanberg S, Kuhn C, Burman I. Burn injuries benefit from massage therapy. *J Burn Rehabil.* 1998;19:241–244.

Field T, Schanberg SM, Scafidi F, et al. Tactile/kinesthetic stimulation effects on preterm neonates. *Pediatrics.* 1986;77:654–658.

Hernandez-Reif M, Dieter J, Field T, Swerdlow B, Diego M. Migraine headaches are reduced by massage therapy. *Int J Neurosci.* 1998;96:1–11.

Hernandez-Reif M, Field T, Field T, Theakston H. Multiple sclerosis patients benefit from massage therapy. *J Bodywork Movement Ther.* 1998;2(3):168–174.

Hernandez-Reif M, Field T, Hart S. Smoking cravings are reduced by self-massage. *Prev Med.* 1999;28: 28–32.

Hernandez-Reif M, Field T, Krasnegor J, Theakston H. Lower back pain is reduced and range of motion increased after massage therapy. *Int J Neurosci.* 2001; 106(3–4):131–145.

Hernandez-Reif M, Ironson G, Field T, et al. Breast cancer patients have improved immune and neuroendocrine function following massage therapy. *J Psychosom Res.* 2004;57(1):45–52.

Ironson G, Field T, Scafidi F, et al. Massage therapy is associated with enhancement of the immune system's cytotoxic capacity. *Int J Neurosci.* 1996;84: 205–218.

Khilnani S, Field T, Hernandez-Reif M, Schanberg S. Massage therapy improves mood and behavior of students with attention-deficit/hyperactivity disorder. *Adolescence.* 2003;38(152):623–638.

Scafidi F, Field TM, Schanberg S. Massage stimulates growth in preterm infants: a replication. *Infant Behav Dev.* 1990;13:167–188.

CHAPTER 37

Clinical Massage Resources

Whitney Lowe and Linda Chrisman

RESEARCH ON MASSAGE

Resources for research on clinical massage include the Medline Database and the National Center for Complementary and Alternative Medicine, both affiliates of the NIH, as well as the Touch Research Institute.

Medline Database of the National Library of
    Medicine, NIH
Web site: www.ncbi.nlm.nih.gov

The Medline database is accessed via the PubMed home page. Citations from the peer-reviewed literature can be accessed using the terms *massage* and *therapeutic massage*.

National Center for Complementary and
    Alternative Medicine at the NIH
NCCAM Clearinghouse
PO Box 7923
Gaithersburg, MD 20898
Phone: (888) 644-6226
Web site: www.nccam.nih.gov
Email: info@nccam.nih.gov

Whitney Lowe is director of the Orthopedic Massage Education & Research Institute (OMERI) (www.omeri.com). He is author of the books, *Orthopedic Assessment in Massage Therapy* and *Orthopedic Massage: Theory and Technique*, and a quarterly research newsletter, *Orthopedic & Sports Massage Reviews*. OMERI provides workshops, consultation services, seminars, and educational materials that train massage therapists in the treatment of orthopedic soft tissue pain and injury conditions.

A brief biography of Linda Chrisman appears in Chapter 34.

NCCAM has funded several studies on the benefits of massage, and more research is in progress. NIH-funded studies on therapeutic massage produced findings on both physiologic mechanisms and clinical outcomes. At the time of this writing, the NIH is funding 13 research projects that involve a massage component, including studies that focus on various aspects of back pain, immune function, prostatitis, infant health, and depression in pregnant women.

Touch Research Institute
1400 NW 10th Avenue, Suite 610
Miami, FL 33136
Phone: (305) 243-6781
Web site: www.miami.edu/touch-research

The Touch Research Institute (TRI) at the University of Miami has conducted more than 90 studies and more than 400 papers have been published evaluating the effects of massage therapy, in clinical situations ranging from post-traumatic stress to migraine headache. The Institute works in conjunction with other major universities, including Duke, Harvard, Princeton, and the University of Maryland. (See Chapter 36 for summaries of selected clinical findings.)

NATIONAL ASSOCIATIONS

There are currently two primary national associations and numerous others that focus on specific techniques or populations within the field of massage. The two national associations are ABMP and AMTA. During the past decade, membership has doubled for the major professional bodywork organizations. These associations can assist health care organizations in locating trained, qualified massage therapists.

American Massage Therapy Association
(AMTA)
500 Davis Street, Suite 900
Evanston, IL 60201-4695
Phone: (847) 864-0123
Fax: (847) 864-1178
Web site: www.amtamassage.org
Email: info@amtamassage.org
Referrals: Web site, click on *Find a Massage Therapist*, or call (888) THE-AMTA

AMTA, with more than 47,000 members, sets practice standards for the massage profession. Requirements for membership include:

• Graduation from a massage training program of 500 hours or more
• An appropriate current city, state, or provincial license, or
• Certification by the NCBTMB

Associated Bodywork and Massage Professionals (ABMP)
1271 Sugarbush Drive
Evergreen, CO 80439
Phone: (800) 458-2267
Fax: (800) 667-8260
Web site: www.abmp.com
Email: expectmore@abmp.com
Referrals: Web site, click on *Find a Massage Therapist*, or call (800) 458-2267

ABMP is an association with more than 52,000 members in the fields of massage,

bodywork, and somatic therapy. Member benefits include a directory of resources, publications on marketing and operating a business successfully, comprehensive liability insurance, member certification, and referrals available to the public and to prospective employers at no cost.

CERTIFICATION AND ACCREDITATION PROGRAMS

National Certification Board for Therapeutic
Massage & Bodywork
8201 Greensboro Drive, Suite 300
McLean, VA 22102
Phone: (800) 296-0664 or (703) 610-9015
Fax: (703) 610-9005
Web site: www.ncbtmb.com
Email: info@ncbtmb.com

This is a nationwide certification program for massage therapy and bodywork practitioners which certifies massage practitioners (rather than training programs). While there are numerous training programs that offer certifications in specific techniques, this is the only organization that offers a credential based on a national standard and a legally defensible exam.

Commission on Massage Therapy Accreditation (COMTA)
1007 Church Street, Suite 302
Evanston, IL 60201
Phone: (847) 869-5039
Fax: (847) 869-6739
Web site: www.comta.org

COMTA is a nonprofit accreditation organization recognized by the US Department of Education that evaluates the quality of entry-level massage therapy training programs.

ASSOCIATIONS WITHIN SPECIFIC MASSAGE DISCIPLINES

Craniosacral Therapy

The Upledger Institute
11211 Prosperity Farms Road, Suite D-325
Palm Beach Gardens, FL 33410
Phone: (561) 622-4771
Toll-free registration: (800) 233-5880, ext. 90012
Fax: (561) 622-4771
Web site: www.upledger.com
Email: upledger@upledger.com

Geriatric Massage

Day-Break Geriatric Massage Institute
7434 King George Drive - A
Indianapolis, IN 46240
Phone: (317) 722-9896
Fax: (317) 722-0511
Email: spuszko@juno.com

Infant Massage

International Association of Infant Massage
1891 Goodyear Avenue, Suite 622
Ventura, CA 93003
Phone: (805) 644-8524
Fax: (805) 644-7699
Web site: www.iaim-us.com
Email: IAIM4US@aol.com

Orthopedic Massage

Orthopedic Massage Education & Research Institute (OMERI)
PO Box 1119
Sisters, OR 97759
Phone: (888) 340-1614 or (541) 549-2700
Web site: www.omeri.com

Rolfing

Guild for Structural Integration
PO Box 1559
Boulder, CO 80306
Phone: (800) 447-0150 or (303) 447-0122
Fax: (303) 447-0108
Web site: www.rolfguild.org
Email: gsi@rolfguild.org

Rosen Method

Rosen Method: The Berkeley Center
825 Bancroft Avenue
Berkeley, CA 94710
Phone: (510) 845-6606
Fax: (510) 845-8114
Referrals: (800) 893-2622
National Web site: www.rosenmethod.com/berkschool.htm
Email: rosenmethod@sbcglobal.net
Referrals: www.rosenmethod.org/finding.html

Shiatsu

American Oriental Bodywork Therapy Association
National Headquarters
1010 Haddonfield-Berlin Road, Suite 408
Voorhees, NJ 08043
Phone: (856) 782-1616
Fax: (856) 782-1653
Web site: www.aobta.org
Email: office@aobta.org

Trager Psychophysical Integration

The Trager Institute
21 Locust Avenue
Mill Valley, CA 94941
Phone: (415) 388-2688
Fax: (415) 388-2710

The Trager Approach
24800 Chagrin Boulevard Suite 205
Beachwood, Ohio 44122
Local phone: (250) 337-5556
Fax: (250) 337-5556
Web site: www.trager.com
Email trager@trager.com
Referrals: Web site, click on *Find a Practitioner*

BOOKS

General Overviews

Claire T. *Bodywork*. New York, NY: Harper-Collins/Quill; 1997. (An insightful, well-written introduction to the various fields of clinical and palliative massage.)

Juhan D. *Job's Body: A Handbook for Bodywork*. 3rd ed. Barrytown, NY: Station Hill Press; 2002. (A classic on bodywork.)

Knaster M. *Discovering the Body's Wisdom*. New York, NY: Bantam Books; 1996. (A comprehensive overview of the field of massage.)

Texts

Andrade C, Clifford P. *Outcome-Based Massage*. Philadelphia, PA: Lippincott, Williams & Wilkins; 2001. (An evidence-based approach to clinical massage.)

Chaitow LJ. *Soft Tissue Manipulation: A Practitioner's Guide*. Rochester, VT; Healing Arts Press; 1988. (Another classic, which provides a good introduction to soft tissue treatment for practitioners in the fields of manual therapy.)

Clay J, Pounds D. *Basic Clinical Massage Therapy*. Philadelphia, PA: Lippincott Williams & Wilkins; 2003. (This book provides a basic introduction to the use of massage for muscular disorders and includes excellent illustrations of anatomy that are relevant to clinical work.)

Dychtwald K. *Bodymind*. New York, NY: Jeremy Tarcher/Putnam; 1986. (A clear overview of the field of mind-body massage, intended to encourage emotional release and healing.)

Field T. *Touch Therapy*. Edinburgh, Scotland: Churchill Livingstone; 2000. (An overview of the extensive research by Touch Research Institute on massage, organized by diagnostic area, validating the physiological effects of clinical massage.)

Fritz S. *Mosby's Fundamentals of Therapeutic Massage*. 3rd ed. St. Louis, MO: CV Mosby; 2004.

Johnson DH, ed. *Bone, Breath, and Gesture: Practices of Embodiment*. Berkeley, CA: North Atlantic Books; 1995. (Interviews and writings from the innovators and practitioners of mind-body massage and bodywork.)

Keleman S. *Emotional Anatomy: The Structure of Experience*. Berkeley, CA: Center Press; 1985. (The seminal text on the expression of mind and emotions in the body.)

Loving JE. *Massage Therapy: Theory and Practice*. Englewood Cliffs, NJ; Prentice Hall; 1998. (A basic introductory text to the use of massage for relaxation and stress reduction.)

Lowe W. *Orthopedic Assessment in Massage Therapy*. Sisters, OR: Orthopedic Massage Education and Research Institute; 2005.

Rattray F, Ludwig L. *Clinical Massage Therapy: Understanding, Assessing and Treating over 70 Conditions*. Toronto: Talus Incorporated; 2000. (A thorough, comprehensive text on assessment and treatment.)

Thompson D. *Hands Heal: Communication, Documentation, and Insurance Billing for Manual Therapists*. 2nd ed. Philadelphia, PA: Lippincott Williams & Wilkins; 2002. (A resource that describes massage therapy documentation protocol for communicating with physicians and other health care professionals.)

Werner R, Benjamin B. *A Massage Therapist's Guide to Pathology*. 2nd ed. Philadelphia, PA: Lippincott Williams & Wilkins; 2002. (A comprehensive resource on pathological conditions massage therapists are likely to encounter, so they can make appropriate decisions about treatment or referral.)

Yates J. *A Physician's Guide to Therapeutic Massage*. 3rd ed. Vancouver, BC: Curties-Overzet Publications; 2004.

PERIODICALS

Journal of Bodywork and Movement Therapies
Published by Elsevier
Customer Service Department
6277 Sea Harbor Drive
Orlando, FL 32887-4800
Phone: (877) 839-7126 or (407) 345-4020
Fax: (407) 363-1354
Email: usjcs@elsevier.com

A peer-reviewed publication on massage, bodywork, and various movement therapies, this journal includes contributions from authors worldwide.

Massage and Bodywork Quarterly
Published by American Bodywork and Massage Professionals
Also see the preceding entry for ABMP
Phone: (303) 674-8478
Web site: www.abmp.com

Massage Magazine
1636 W First Avenue Ste. 100
Spokane, WA 99204
Phone: (800) 533-4263 or (509) 324-8117
Web site: www.massagemag.com

This is a bi-monthly publication that covers issues, techniques, and information for practicing massage professionals.

Massage Therapy Journal
Published by the American Massage Therapy Association
See the preceding entry for AMTA
Phone: (847) 864-0123
Web site: www.amtamassage.org

Massage Today
PO Box 4139
Huntington Beach, CA 92605-4139
Phone: (714) 230-3150

Fax: (714) 899-4273
Web site: www.massagetoday.com

This is a monthly publication that targets news and issues of interest to practicing massage therapists; the publication is free and widely distributed throughout the United States.

Orthopedic & Sports Massage Reviews
Published by the Orthopedic Massage Education & Research Institute
See the preceding entry for OMERI
Phone: (888) 340-1614 or (541) 549-2700
Web site: www.omeri.com

This quarterly publication reviews studies published in the medical literature related to the practice of massage in treating pain and injury conditions.

Email discussion lists on massage-related topics are available at www. yahoogroups.com. Go to *Body Work Professional Discussion Forum* and *Orthopedic Massage*. These are lists of threaded discussion that reflect a range of issues affecting practicing professionals within the fields of massage.

Touchpoints
Published by the Touch Research Institute (TRI)
Department of Pediatrics (D-820)
University of Miami School of Medicine
PO Box 016820
Miami, FL 33101
Phone: (305) 243-6781
Fax: (305) 243-6488
Email: tfield@med.miami.edu
Web site: www.miami.edu/touch-research

The Institute's quarterly publication, available for an annual subscription of $10, reviews TRI's current research and that of other research institutions.

PART VII

Acupuncture

Chapter

CHAPTER 38

Overview of Clinical Acupuncture

Efrem Korngold, LAc, OMD, and Nancy Faass, MSW, MPH

ACCESS TO ACUPUNCTURE AND TRADITIONAL CHINESE MEDICINE

In the year 2000 there were more than 14,000 certified or licensed practitioners of acupuncture and Chinese herbal medicine (National Certification Commission on Acupuncture and Oriental Medicine [NCCAOM], 2004) in the United States. The practice of acupuncture is regulated in at least 47 states (Federation of State Medical Boards, 2003). At the time of this writing, there are 45 accredited US schools of Chinese medicine that offer 3- and 4-year programs (Council of Colleges of Acupuncture and Oriental Medicine [CCAOM], 2004). National standards for a doctoral program in Oriental medicine are also in development (Federation of Acupuncture and Oriental Medicine Regulatory Agencies, 2004). In addition, there are also numerous state and national organizations of Chinese medicine professionals, researchers, and educators. (For specific contact information on national organizations, see Chapter 45, Acupuncture Resources.)

Efrem Korngold, LAc, OMD, has been practicing and teaching Chinese traditional medicine since 1973, and has traveled to China on three occasions for advanced study. A founding faculty member of the San Francisco College of Acupuncture and Oriental Medicine, he is currently adjunct faculty at the American College of Traditional Chinese Medicine, and a certification and examination consultant to the National Certification Commission for Acupuncture and Oriental Medicine (NCCAOM). He is coauthor with Harriet Beinfield, LAc, of *Between Heaven and Earth: A Guide to Chinese Medicine*, and maintains a private practice at his San Francisco center, Chinese Medicine Works.

A brief biography for Ms. Faass appears in Chapter 2.

Origins

Acupuncture originated in China millennia ago and soon spread to Japan, the Korean peninsula, and elsewhere in Asia. Descriptions of acupuncture appear in Chinese medical texts dating to approximately 90 BC. Today it is widely used in the health care systems of Asia, where it is officially recognized by national governments, integrated into the health system, and well received by the general public (WHO, 1996).

Acupuncture is based on a comprehensive body of theory and practice. The same procedures and acupuncture points are used throughout China and the world. The location of the points is well established, and acupuncture treatment, although individualized, is highly systematic. An extensive body of literature has developed in Chinese medicine over the past 2000 years. Ancient texts in archives and museums identify acupuncture points that have been in continuous use for centuries and are now part of standard practice. The research and world literature on acupuncture continues to expand.

Research

One of the primary public resources available for information on acupuncture is the Medline database of the NIH National Library of Medicine. At the time of this writing, the PubMed Medline (2004) literature lists 9357 entries on acupuncture dating from 1967 to the present. More than 900 are review articles that originate in medical institutions worldwide. While skepticism is reflected in some of the literature, the majority of the meta-analyses are positive. There are few reports of adverse outcomes.

WORLD HEALTH ORGANIZATION CONSULTATION ON ACUPUNCTURE

In 1996, the World Health Organization (WHO) Consultation on Acupuncture was held in Cervia, Italy, and selection criteria were developed for a review of the world literature on acupuncture. The final report, a review of more than 200 clinical trials, included comments on safety, clinical effectiveness, and conditions benefited (see Table 38–1). The following information is an excerpt from the WHO report:

The past two decades have seen extensive studies on acupuncture, and great efforts have been made to conduct controlled clinical trials that include the use of *sham* acupuncture or *placebo* acupuncture controls. Although still limited in number because of the difficulties of carrying out such trials, convincing reports, based on sound research methodology, have been published. In addition, experimental investigations on the mechanism of acupuncture have been carried out. This research, while aimed chiefly at answering how acupuncture works, may also provide evidence in support of its effectiveness.

Generally speaking, acupuncture treatment is safe if it is performed properly by a well-trained practitioner. Unlike many drugs, it is nontoxic, and adverse reactions are minimal. This is probably one of the chief reasons why acupuncture is so popular in the treatment of chronic pain in many countries. As mentioned previously, acupuncture is comparable with morphine preparations in its effectiveness against chronic pain, but without the adverse effects of morphine, such as dependency. Even [when] the effect of acupuncture therapy is less potent than

that of conventional treatments, acupuncture may still be worth considering because . . . acupuncture treatment does not cause serious side effects.

For example, there are reports of controlled clinical trials showing that acupuncture is effective in the treatment of rheumatoid arthritis, although not as potent as corticosteroids (Man & Barager, 1974; Sun et al., 1992). Because, unlike corticosteroids, acupuncture treatment does not cause serious side effects, it seems reasonable to use acupuncture for treating this condition, despite the difference in effectiveness. [Author's note: While acupuncture has been found to be less potent than corticosteroids for acute, short-term therapy, electroacupuncture has been found as effective or even more effective than conventional therapies in the treatment of osteoarthritis, according to recent research (Stux et al., 2003).]

To date, modern scientific research studies have revealed the following actions of acupuncture:

- Inducing analgesia
- Protecting the body against infections
- Regulating various physiological functions

Numerous examples reveal that the regulatory action of acupuncture is bidirectional. Acupuncture lowers the blood pressure in patients with hypertension and elevates it in patients with hypotension; increases gastric secretion in patients with hypoacidity, and decreases it in patients with hyperacidity; and normalizes intestinal motility under X-ray observation in patients with either spastic colitis or intestinal hypotonia (Stux & Pomeranz, 1987). Therefore, acupuncture itself seldom makes the condition worse (WHO, 1996).

NIH CONSENSUS STATEMENT ON ACUPUNCTURE

In 1997, a consensus panel of the National Institutes of Health met, reviewed the re-

Table 38–1 Diseases and Disorders That Can Be Treated with Acupuncture: WHO

Diseases, symptoms, or conditions for which acupuncture has been proved through controlled trials to be an effective treatment

Adverse reactions to radiotherapy and/or chemotherapy	Knee pain
Allergic rhinitis (including hay fever)	Leukopenia
Biliary colic	Low back pain
Depression (including depressive neurosis and depression following stroke)	Malposition of fetus, correction of
Dysentery, acute bacillary	Morning sickness
Dysmenorrhoea, primary	Nausea and vomiting
Epigastralgia, acute (in peptic ulcer, acute and chronic gastritis, and gastrospasm)	Neck pain
	Pain in dentistry (including dental pain and temporomandibular dysfunction)
Facial pain (including craniomandibular disorders)	Periarthritis of the shoulder
Headache	Postoperative pain
Hypertension, essential	Renal colic
Hypotension, primary	Rheumatoid arthritis
Induction of labor	Sciatica
	Sprain
	Stroke
	Tennis elbow

Diseases, symptoms, or conditions for which the therapeutic effect of acupuncture has been shown but for which further evidence is desirable. Review of clinical trial reports.

Abdominal pain (in acute gastroenteritis or due to gastrointestinal spasm)	Ménière's disease
Acne vulgaris	Neuralgia, postherpetic
Alcohol dependence and detoxification	Neurodermatitis
Bell's palsy	Reflex sympathetic dystrophy
Bronchial asthma	Retention of urine, traumatic
Cancer pain	Schizophrenia
Cardiac neurosis	Sialism, drug-induced
Cholecystitis, chronic, with acute exacerbation	Sjögren's syndrome
Cholelithiasis	Sore throat (including tonsillitis)
Competition stress syndrome	Spine pain, acute
Colitis, chronic	Stiff neck
Craniocerebral injury, closed	Temporomandibular joint dysfunction
Diabetes mellitus, non-insulin-dependent	Tietze's syndrome
Earache	Tobacco dependence
Epidemic haemorrhagic fever	Tourette's syndrome
Epistaxis, simple (without generalized or local disease)	Urolithiasis
	Vascular dementia
	Whooping cough (pertussis)

continues

Table 38–1 continued

Diseases, symptoms, or conditions for which the therapeutic effect of acupuncture has been shown but for which further evidence is desirable. Review of clinical trial reports.

Obesity	Eye pain due to subconjunctival infection
Opium, cocaine, and heroin dependence	Female infertility
Osteoarthritis	Facial spasm
Pain due to endoscopic examination	Female urethral syndrome
Pain in thromboangiitis obliterans	Fibromyalgia and fasciitis
Polycystic ovary syndrome (Stein-Leventhal syndrome)	Gastrokinetic disturbance
	Gouty arthritis
Postextubation in children	Hepatitis B virus carrier status
Postoperative convalescence	Herpes zoster (human [alpha] herpesvirus 3)
Premenstrual syndrome	Hyperlipidemia
Prostatitis, chronic	Hypoovarianism
Pruritus	Insomnia
Radicular and pseudoradicular pain syndrome	Labor pain
Raynaud's syndrome, primary	Lactation, deficiency
Recurrent lower urinary tract infection	Male sexual dysfunction, nonorganic

Source of content: WHO Consultation on Acupuncture. Acupuncture Review and Analysis of Reports on Controlled Clinical Trials. Geneva, Switzerland: World Health Organization, 1996.

---

search on acupuncture, and developed a statement on aspects of its relevant applications. The following quotation is drawn from their report (NIH, 1997).

Participants. A non-Federal, non-advocate, 12-member panel representing the fields of acupuncture, pain, psychology, psychiatry, physical medicine and rehabilitation, drug abuse, family practice, internal medicine, health policy, epidemiology, statistics, physiology, biophysics, and the public. In addition, 25 experts from these same fields presented data to the panel and a conference audience of 1200.

Evidence. The literature was searched through Medline, and an extensive bibliography of references was provided to the panel and the conference audience. Experts prepared abstracts with relevant citations from the literature. Scientific evidence was given precedence over clinical anecdotal experience.

Conclusions. Acupuncture as a therapeutic intervention is widely practiced in the United States. While there have been many studies of its potential usefulness, many of these studies provide equivocal results because of design, sample size, and other factors. The issue is further complicated by inherent difficulties in the use of appropriate controls, such as placebos and sham acupuncture groups. However, promising results have emerged, for example, showing efficacy of acupuncture in adult postoperative and chemotherapy nausea and vomiting and postoperative dental pain. There are other situations . . . in which acupuncture may be useful as an adjunct treatment or an acceptable alternative or be included in a comprehensive management program:

- Addiction
- Asthma
- Carpal tunnel syndrome
- Fibromyalgia
- Headache

- Low back pain
- Menstrual cramps
- Myofascial pain
- Osteoarthritis
- Stroke rehabilitation
- Tennis elbow

THEORY

The contemporary practice of acupuncture has begun to synthesize classical concepts and methods with modern ones. In ancient China the metaphors for the body reflected the development of waterways for commerce that were unifying society during the Han dynasty. Today the overarching concern of societies is the use and acquisition of energy resources. In the context of recent research, acupuncture can now be conceptualized as a bioelectric information-modulating system. As in ancient times, the body continues to be perceived as a miniature projection of its social context. These metaphors are ultimately complementary—the universe of Qi and the fields and forces of quantum physics are only half a step apart (Beinfield & Korngold, 1991).

Acupuncture is a system of healing that activates the body's ability to strengthen and regulate itself. It is based on the theory that life force (Qi or Chi, pronounced "chee") flows continuously in the body through a network of meridians. Life force and Qi are the same. When the heart stops beating and the body becomes cold, the life force, or Qi, is no longer present. Like fresh air, healthy Qi moves freely; like stale air, stagnant Qi is heavy, oppressive, constrictive, and congestive.

The flow of Qi along the meridians may develop blockages or become congested. Since each meridian is associated with a particular internal organ and organ system, any dysfunction in the meridian or in the associated organ system can result in physical disturbances or disease. These dysfunctions can

also produce symptoms or disorders elsewhere in the body.

Acupuncture treatment is intended to remove blockages, restoring the circulation of Qi and coherence to the system. The acupuncturist must determine the significant areas of congestion or depletion to most effectively treat the patient. This involves activating the relevant acupuncture points to move the Qi, thereby increasing circulation in the meridian to restore a homeodynamic condition.

DIAGNOSIS AND TREATMENT

Diagnosis

Traditional Chinese diagnosis is holistic in the sense that it considers a patient's symptoms, history, life circumstances, and environment. Acupuncturists view each patient as a distinct individual.

As part of the patient examination, a unique method of pulse diagnosis is used to obtain information regarding the level of vitality or weakness and the functional status of the various organ systems. The patient's health is also evaluated by inspecting the tongue (tongue diagnosis) and through general observations of posture, demeanor, facial skin color, and other observable reflections of internal function. The practitioner develops skill in acute observation to evaluate the degree of dysfunction and to monitor the patient's subsequent responses to treatment.

Acupuncture Practice

In treatment, the goal is to modulate the flow of Qi, to intensify or diminish it, thereby improving circulation and correcting imbalances. This is achieved by inserting fine, hair-thin sterile needles at specific points along the meridians. (The risk of infection is almost nonexistent when sterile, disposable needles and clean needle technique are used.) Fourteen major pathways traverse the body from the top of the head to the tips of the fingers and toes. While there are between 1000 and 2000 known acupuncture points, the majority of points used in therapy are located on the arms and legs. Acupuncture treatment almost always results in a restored sense of equilibrium and well-being.

The physiological effects of acupuncture include improved detoxification, enhanced resistance to infection, modulation of hormonal secretions, improved metabolism, greater efficiency of cardiovascular function, and activation of endorphin and serotonin release.

Acupuncture points may be stimulated through a variety of techniques. Traditional practitioners who only practice acupuncture-related techniques may also use acupressure, moxibustion, or cupping as adjuncts to needle therapy. Contemporary practitioners may supplement needle therapy with electroacupuncture, laser puncture, or auricular (ear) acupuncture.

Acupressure. Acupressure therapy is based on the same principles as acupuncture and can be used both as a form of self-care and as an expert method of healing performed by a professional. Like other forms of massage, treatment is done without the use of needles. Blockages along meridians and at acupuncture points are dispersed through finger pressure and other manual techniques. In the West, this modality has been integrated into various systems of physical medicine—using the same acupoints—in modalities such as trigger-point therapy provided by physical therapists, physiatrists, osteopaths, and chiropractors.

Moxibustion. Another traditional approach involves the application of heat to an acupoint by burning an herb (moxa—*Artemisia vul-garis*) near the surface of the skin. Moxibustion is used in conjunction with the acupoints to increase circulation and metabolic activity, locally and systemically. This technique is applied when there is poor circulation, coldness, or numbness. In cases of localized weakness, moxibustion is used to strengthen the function of organs or muscles.

Cupping. This is a traditional technique that utilizes a glass or bamboo cup to create suction on the skin over a painful muscle or acupuncture point. The effect is to increase local circulation in order to reduce pain, swelling, and inflammation, in conditions such as muscle strain or trauma.

Electroacupuncture. This contemporary application of acupuncture involves the mild, low-current, low-voltage electric stimulation of acupuncture points with or without needles, to amplify the effect. Electroacupuncture is primarily used to treat neuromuscular and musculoskeletal pain, neuropathies, and paralysis. Research has shown that constant stimulation for 20 to 30 minutes is often necessary to induce the analgesic effects of acupuncture. By generating a continuous stimulus, electroacupuncture frees the practitioner from the need to manually manipulate the needles for long periods of time in order to sustain the required level of stimulation.

Laser puncture. Another modern innovation, laser puncture, is the use of low-intensity "cool" lasers to stimulate acupuncture points on the body and the ear. This technique is especially useful in pediatrics and with needle-sensitive patients.

Auricular acupuncture. This technique employs specific points exclusively on the external ear to alleviate pain, dysfunction, or illness. Auricular therapy was introduced to the West in France (Nogier, 1972) and has been extensively researched and developed in both France and mainland China (PRC). There is now a substantial amount of evidence that documents the effectiveness and safety of this approach for a great variety of conditions, and it is used extensively worldwide in the treatment of disorders of addiction and substance abuse.

ADJUNCTIVE THERAPIES AND APPLICATIONS

Although we have focused our discussion primarily on acupuncture in this chapter, Chinese traditional medicine is a comprehensive system of healing that includes acupuncture, herbal medicine, dietetics, exercises such as Qigong and tai chi, massage, and manipulation.

Dietetics. An improper diet is considered to be one of the primary causes of illness and disease along with psychological, constitutional, and environmental factors. Therefore, the preparation and consumption of foods that are in accord with a person's constitution, diagnosis, and treatment goals are essential to a successful outcome. Determinations about the correct diet are made based on the same principles used for selecting acupuncture points and medicinal herbs: according to the Five Phase and Yin/Yang theories of traditional Chinese medicine briefly summarized in Table 38–2. For additional insight into these approaches, see *Between Heaven and Earth* (Korngold and Beinfeld), *Foundations of Chinese Medicine* (G. Maciocoa), and *The Web That Has No Weaver* (T. Kaptchuk).

Herbal therapy. Medicinal herbs are taken in a variety of forms. The most common methods of administration are the decocting of loose herbs in water by the patient at home and the ingestion of commercially prepared medicines in the form of liquid or powdered extracts, syrups, pills, or tablets. Chinese me-

dicinal herbs are low in toxicity, and the guidelines for their use have been established over many centuries.

Tui na. Tui na literally means "pushing and pulling." This is the practice of traditional Chinese physical therapy based on acupuncture theory as well as a deep understanding of functional and structural anatomy. It is to a large extent comparable to what might be termed a synthesis of Western practices such as massage, chiropractic, osteopathy, and trigger-point therapies.

Qigong and tai chi. These are integrated forms of exercise that require mental concentration, regulation of breathing, and precise sequences of physical movement. Both forms of practice are intended to activate and regulate the circulation of Qi, thereby invigorating the entire body, promoting recovery from illness, and enhancing resistance to stress and disease.

Acupuncture detoxification. Acupuncture detoxification is a modern application of acupuncture techniques, first developed in Hong Kong by a Dr. Wong, who used electroacupuncture. This technique was further developed by Michael Smith, MD, and others who preceded him at Lincoln Hospital in New York City. Acupuncture detoxification utilizes auricular acupuncture to ease the stress of drug withdrawal by reducing cravings, anxiety, and sleep disorders (Smith, 1988). Currently, there are more than 2000 acupuncture detoxification programs worldwide and more than 1000 certified practitioners in the United States (J. Renaud, National Acupuncture Detoxification Association, written communication, October 1, 2004). Auricular therapy has proven an effective treatment even for people who have had problems with drugs or alcohol for years. A number of studies report success rates

Table 38–2 Basic Diagnostic Categories in Traditional Chinese Medicine

Syndrome	Process	Symptoms
Internal	Conditions that affect basic vital functions and internal organs; brain or spinal cord, bones, blood vessels, middle and inner ear, lining of body cavities, internal reproductive organs	No specific symptoms
External	Conditions that affect surface tissue or skin, peripheral blood vessels or nerves, muscles, tendons, ligaments, joints, eyes, ears, nose, mouth, teeth, breasts, anus, or external reproductive organs	No specific symptoms
Deficiency	Impaired or diminished capacity of an organ or physiological process; decreased resistance to stress or infection; deficiency in basic nutrients or biological secretions	Systemic or localized sensation of fatigue, weakness, or low-grade pain
Excess	Acceleration or obstruction of organ function or physiological process; increased reactivity to stress or infection	Systemic or localized sensations of tension, agitation, or intense pain; edema, elevated blood pressure, swelling of lymph nodes or muscles, blood clots, or intestinal obstructions
Cold	Compromised metabolic activity	Measurable decrease in body temperature; pallid complexion, skin, or mucous membranes; systemic or localized sensations of cold or chill; impaired circulation, usually due to some internal organ deficiency (e.g., adrenal, thyroid, or cardiac) or exposure such as hypothermia
Heat	Increased metabolic activity	Measurable increase in body temperature; reddening or flushing of complexion, skin, or mucous membranes, systemic or localized sensations of heat or burning; inflammation

continues

Table 38–2 continued

Syndrome	Process	Symptoms
Yin	Cold, deficient, and internal syndromes and disease processes that reflect these syndromes	
Yang	Heat, excess, and external syndromes and disease processes that reflect these syndromes	

Source: Courtesy of Efrem Korngold, OMD, San Francisco, CA.

---

ranging from 50% to better than 80% and rates of relapse are unusually low, even in 2-year follow-up studies. Typically auricular acupuncture is provided as one component of a comprehensive program that includes group support, case management, and frequent drug testing. These programs tend to have significantly lower rates of relapse or recidivism when compared to conventional protocols. (See Acupuncture Resources, Chapter 45, for contact information.)

LICENSING AND CERTIFICATION

For the practice of acupuncture in the United States, training and licensing requirements are defined by state and vary significantly from state to state. However, the vast majority of states base their statutes on the guidelines of the NCCAOM (2004). For specific information on individual state li-

censing and academic requirements, contact the appropriate state agency. (Contact information for a range of certification and accrediting agencies is provided in Chapter 45, Acupuncture Resources.)

CONCLUSION

Within the Chinese medicine worldview, the acupuncturist is a practical ecologist—a systems analyst who never loses sight of the whole while attending to any of the parts. Since this model assumes the synchronicity of response throughout the organism, it is reasonable that stimulation of a local site will have global impact and that stimulation of an array of sites can have specific outcomes. In the approach of Chinese medicine, global changes in the whole organism to improve overall health are applied to resolve specific symptoms.

REFERENCES

Beinfield H, Korngold E. *Between Heaven and Earth: A Guide to Chinese Medicine.* New York, NY: Ballantine Books; 1991.

Council of Colleges of Acupuncture and Oriental Medicine (CCAOM). Available at: www.ccaom.org. Accessed August 1, 2004.

Federation of Acupuncture and Oriental Medicine Regulatory Agencies. Available at: www.faomra.com. Accessed August 1, 2004.

Federation of State Medical Boards of the United States (FSMB). Health professions regulated and legislative schedules. In 1999–2000 Exchange. Euless, TX: FSMB; 2003.

Man SC, Barager FO. Preliminary clinical study of acupuncture in rheumatoid arthritis. *J Rheumatol.* 1974;1(1):126–129.

National Certification Commission on Acupuncture and Oriental Medicine (NCCAOM). Available at: www.nccaom.org. Accessed August 1, 2004.

National Institutes of Health. *Acupuncture: NIH Consensus Statement Online.* 1997 Nov 3–5;15(5): 1–34.

Nogier PFM. Treatise of auriculotherapy. Moulin-les-Metz, Maisonneuve, France; 1972.

PubMed/Medline Database, National Library of Medicine, NIH. Available at: www.ncbi.nlm.nih.gov/PubMed. Accessed September 1, 2004.

Smith MO. Acupuncture treatment for crack cocaine; clinical survey of 1,500 patients. *Am J Acupuncture.* 1988;16(3):241–247.

Stux G, Berman B, Pomeranz B. *The Basics of Acupuncture,* 5th ed. New York, NY: Springer; 2003.

Stux G, Pomeranz B. *Acupuncture: Textbook and Atlas.* Berlin, Germany: Springer-Verlag, 1987.

Sun LQ, et al. Observation of the effect of acupuncture and moxibustion on rheumatoid arthritis in 434 cases [in Chinese]. *Chinese Acupuncture and Moxibustion,* 1992;12(1):9–11.

WHO Consultation on Acupuncture. *Acupuncture: Review and Analysis of Reports on Controlled Clinical Trials.* Geneva, Switzerland: World Health Organization; 1996. Available at: http://www.who.int/medicines/library/trm/acupuncture/acupuncture_trials.doc. Accessed August 21, 2004.

CHAPTER 39

Research on Acupuncture Safety

Stephen Birch, PhD, MBAc, LAc; Jan Keppel Hesselink, MD, PhD, FFPM;
Fokke A.M. Jonkman, MD, PhD; Thecla A.M. Hekker, MD; and Aat Bos, PhD

SYSTEMATIC REVIEWS

In recent years acupuncture has received a great deal of attention in peer-reviewed journals and through several national reviews such as the British Medical Association report (2000) and the National Institutes of Health Consensus Conference on Acupuncture (1998). Hundreds of clinical trials of acupuncture have been conducted in the West since the early 1970s. More than 45 systematic reviews or meta-analyses of acupuncture have also been conducted to date.

In addition to these attempts to summarize the scientific knowledge on the efficacy of acupuncture in systematic reviews, various government bodies, professional bodies, and government-sponsored research groups have undertaken official reviews and summaries of the literature (Alpert, 1996; British Medical Association, 2000; Ernst,

1999; Linde et al., 2001; Monckton et al., 1998; NIH Consensus Conference, Acupuncture, 1998; Tait et al., 2002; Vickers, 2001; Vickers et al., 2002). Some of these have been more descriptive summaries of the literature and some more formal reviews. (See Table 39–1.)

SAFETY

There have been a number of adverse events reported in association with acupuncture treatment. The most serious events such as cardiac tamponade (Halvorsen et al., 1995), punctured organs such as pneumothorax (Ramnarain & Braams, 2002), and transmission of disease such as hepatitis (Rampes & James, 1995), are rare but do occur and generally are associated with poorly trained unlicensed acupuncturists (Vickers et al., 2002). Reviewers who have examined these problems have concluded that knowledge of anatomy and proper handling of needles are sufficient to guarantee that these problems will not recur or will be minimized in normal practice (Alpert, 1996; British Medical Association, 2000; Lao et al., 2003; Lytle, 1993; Norheim, 1996; Vickers, 2001).

No serious adverse events were found in four recent surveys in Japan, Sweden, and the United Kingdom of 140,229 treatments (MacPherson et al., 2001; Oldsberg et al., 2001; White et al., 2001; Yamasita et al., 1999). Ernst and White (2001) reviewed

Stephen Birch, PhD, is coauthor of a number of books on acupuncture, including *Understanding Acupuncture* with Robert Felt (New York: Harcourt Health Sciences, 1999), *Chasing the Dragon's Tail, Extraordinary Vessels,* and *Essentials of Japanese Acupuncture.* He has been a practicing clinician for more than a decade. Active in acupuncture research, he is cofounder and past president of the Society for Acupuncture Research, has been research director of the New England School of Acupuncture, and has performed acupuncture research at Yale University.

Source: This chapter is excerpted from: Birch S, Hesselink JK, Jonkman FA, Hekker TA, Bos A. Clinical research on acupuncture: part I. What have reviews of the efficacy and safety of acupuncture told us so far? *Journal of Alternative and Complementary Medicine.* 2004;10(3):468–480. Courtesy of Mary Ann Liebert Inc., Publishers.

Table 39–1 Conclusions About Safety and Adverse Effects of Acupuncture

Lytle, US—FDA, 1993	"Considering the number of patients treated (estimated 9–12 million treatments per year [in the US]) and the number of needles used per treatment (estimated average of 6–8) . . . 'there are, however, remarkably few serious complications' (American Medical Association, 1981)."
Alpert, US—FDA, 1996	"The clinical studies and safety information included in support of these acupuncture petitions report few risks to health associated with the use of acupuncture needles and those that are reported have been clearly identified, documented and characterized. FDA's own search of the literature supports this finding."
Lytle, US—NIH Consensus Conf., 1997	"The present level of information on the low-level risks of acupuncture . . . should provide reasonable assurance of safety during use of acupuncture needles."
NIH Consensus Conference, 1997 (1998)	"One of the advantages of acupuncture is that the incidence of adverse effects is substantially lower than that of many drugs or other accepted procedures for the same conditions."
Rampes and Peuker, 1999	"Previous surveys with differing methodologies indicate that there is a significant but low risk of serious side effects of acupuncture from 1:10,000 to 1:100,000 (White et al., 1997)." Given the number of practitioners around the world "these figures suggest a very low prevalence of adverse reactions."
British Medical Association, 2000	"In terms of safety, few major adverse reactions to acupuncture treatment are reported in comparison to adverse reactions to orthodox interventions." "Many of the injuries can be avoided by ensuring acupuncturists are fully trained in anatomy and physiology."
Prospective surveys, 1999–2001	No serious adverse events were found in a Japanese study of 65,000 treatments (Yamashita et al., 1999), a Swedish study of 9000 treatments (Oldsberg et al., 2001), a U.K. study of 34,407 treatments (MacPherson et al., 2001), and another U.K. study of 31,822 treatments (White et al., 2001). "Although the incidence of minor adverse events associated with acupuncture may be considerable, serious adverse events are rare" (Ernst & White, 2001).
Incidence of adverse reactions—British Medical Association, 2000	"Norheim and Fonnebo (1995) estimated that for each year of full-time acupuncture practice in Norway, 0.21 complications would arise (complications were classified as mechanical organ injuries, infections and other adverse effects, not including point-bleeding or small haematomas). Bensoussan and Myers' Australian study (1996) estimated that the average number of adverse events per year of full-time

continues

Table 39–1 continued

	traditional Chinese medicine practice was one every eight months. Umiani's (1988) study of acupuncture treatments and found 8.9% (approximately 12,459 treatments) resulted in adverse events (faintness, fainting, haematoma, pneumothorax, and retained needles). Considering that the Medicines Control Agency receives approximately 17,000–18,000 U.K. reports of suspected adverse reactions to all medicines each year, of which 35% are serious and 3% are fatal, the incidence of adverse reactions to acupuncture appears relatively low."
Vickers, UK—NHS, 2001, and Vickers et al., 2002	"Acupuncture appears a relatively safe treatment in the hands of suitably qualified practitioners, with serious adverse events being extremely rare" (2001). "Serious adverse effects including pneumothorax, spinal lesions, and hepatitis B transmission have been reported in the literature, but these are rare and generally associated with poorly trained unlicensed acupuncturists" (2002)
Tait et al. Canadian/Alberta Health Authorities Report, 2002	"The studies' conclusions are consistent in that they found that the rate or incidence of serious adverse events due to acupuncture treatment is low but that they do occur. MacPherson and colleagues stated that the adverse event rate, when compared with primary care drugs, suggests that acupuncture is a relatively safe treatment, and many researchers concur that it is a relatively safe technique."
Lao et al., 2003	"Declines in adverse reports may suggest that recent practices, such as clean needle techniques and more rigorous acupuncturist training requirements, have reduced the risks associated with the procedure. Therefore, acupuncture performed by trained practitioners using clean needle techniques is a generally safe procedure."

these and five other surveys and found two cases of pneumothorax in nearly a quarter of a million treatments. From their review they concluded that serious adverse events are rare.

Table 39–1 summarizes conclusions from several of the major reviews of the acupuncture literature. It is clear that the general consensus is that acupuncture is relatively safe, especially when provided by properly trained individuals. (In addition to the references cited in Table 39–1, see also Bensoussan & Myers, 1996 and Vincent, 2001.) The adverse effect rate of acupuncture is lower in comparison to standard conventional treatment (British Medi-

cal Association, 2000; NIH Consensus Conference, Acupuncture, 1998).

CONCLUSION

There is general agreement that acupuncture is a relatively safe therapy. While serious adverse events can occur, they are extremely rare and can be avoided with proper training. Minor, transitory adverse events occur more often, but are well tolerated by patients. Overall, the incidence of serious adverse effects from acupuncture is lower than that of many medications or therapeutic procedures used for the same conditions for which acupuncture is used.

REFERENCES

Alpert S. Letter: Reclassification order, Docket No. 94P–0443. Acupuncture needles for the practice of acupuncture. Reproduced in: Birch S, Hammerschlag R. *Acupuncture Efficacy: A Compendium of Controlled Clinical Trials.* New York: National Academy of Acupuncture and Oriental Medicine; 1996:76–78.

Bensoussan A, Myers SP. *Towards a Safer Choice: The Practice of Traditional Chinese Medicine in Australia.* MacArthur: Faculty of Health, University of Western Sydney; 1996.

British Medical Association Board of Science and Education. *Acupuncture: Efficacy, Safety, and Practice.* London, UK: Harwood Academic Publishers; 2000.

Ernst E. Clinical effectiveness of acupuncture: an overview of systematic reviews. In Ernst E, White A, eds. *Acupuncture: A Scientific Appraisal.* Oxford, UK: Butterworth-Heinemann; 1999:107–127.

Ernst E, White AR. Prospective studies of the safety of acupuncture: a systematic review. *Am J Med.* 2001; 110:481–485.

Halvorsen TB, Anda SS, Naess AB, Levang OW. Fatal cardiac tamponade after acupuncture through congenital sternal foramen. *Lancet.* 1995;345:1175.

Lao LX, Hamilton GR, Fu JP, Berman BM. Is acupuncture safe? A systematic review of case reports. *Altern Ther Health Med.* 2003;9:72–83.

Linde K, Vickers A, Hondras M, et al. Systematic reviews of complementary therapies—an annotated bibliography. Part 1: Acupuncture. *BMC Complement Altern Med.* 2001;1:4.

Lytle CD. *An Overview of Acupuncture.* Bethesda, MD: US Department of Health and Human Services, Public Health Service, Food and Drug Administration, Center for Devices and Radiological Health; 1993.

Lytle CD. Safety and regulations of acupuncture needles and other devices. Bethesda, MD: Presentation to the NIH Consensus Development Conference on Acupuncture on behalf of the US Food and Drug Administration; November 3, 1997.

MacPherson H, Thomas K, Walters S, Filter M. The York acupuncture safety study: a prospective survey of 34,000 treatments by traditional acupuncturists. *BMJ.* 2001;323:486–487.

Monckton J, Belicza B, Betz W, Engelbart H, van Wassenhoven M, eds. European Commission COST B4: Unconventional Medicine. Final Report of the Management Committee 1993–1998. Brussels, Belgium: Directorate-General Science, Research and Development. 1998:49–51.

National Institutes of Health. NIH Consensus Conference: Acupuncture. *JAMA.* 1998;280: 1518–1524.

Norheim AJ. Adverse effects of acupuncture: a study of the literature for the years 1981–1994. *J Altern Complement Med.* 1996;2:291–297.

Norheim AJ, Fonnebo V. Adverse effects of acupuncture [letter to the editor]. *Lancet.* 1995;345:1576.

Oldsberg A, Schill U, Haker E. Acupuncture treatment: side effects and complications reported by Swedish physiotherapists. *Complement Ther Med.* 2001;9: 17–20.

Ramnarain D, Braams R. Bilateral pneumothorax by acupuncture in a young woman. *Ned Tijdschr Geneeskd.* 2002;146:172–174.

Rampes H, James R. Complications of acupuncture. *Acupunct Med.* 1995;13:26–33.

Rampes H, Peuker E. Adverse effects of acupuncture. In Ernst E, White A, eds. *Acupuncture: A Scientific Appraisal.* Oxford, England: Butterworth Heinemann; 1999:128–152.

Tait PL, Brooks L, Harstall C. Acupuncture: Evidence from Systematic Reviews and Meta-analyses. Alberta, Canada: Alberta Heritage Foundation for Medical Research; 2002.

Umlauf R. Analysis of the main results of the activity of the acupuncture department of faculty hospital. *Acupuncture in Medicine.* 1988;5:16–18.

Vickers A. Acupuncture. *Eff Health Care.* 2001;7: 1–12.

Vickers A, Wilson P, Kleijnen J. Effectiveness bulletin: acupuncture. *Qual Saf Health Care.* 2002;11: 92–97.

Vincent C. Editorial: the safety of acupuncture. *BMJ.* 2001;323:467–468.

White A, Hayhoe S, Hart A, Ernst E. Adverse events following acupuncture: prospective survey of 32,000 consultations with doctors and physical therapists. *BMJ.* 2001;323:485–486.

Yamashita H, Tsukayama H, Tanno Y, Nishijo K. Adverse events in acupuncture and moxibustion treatment: a six-year survey at a national clinic in Japan. *J Altern Complement Med.* 1999;5:229–236.

CHAPTER 40

Controlled Clinical Trials of Acupuncture

Richard Hammerschlag, PhD; Ryan Milley; and Stephen Birch, PhD, MBAc, LAc

A review of the clinical research on acupuncture affirms its value in the treatment of a variety of illnesses. While far from perfect or exhaustive, these studies clearly indicate that acupuncture, properly done and applied, can aid in the alleviation of pain and discomfort. In addition, the overwhelmingly convincing conclusion that can be drawn from the research is that acupuncture must be done in a manner which is informed by its own body of theory, and appropriate to the overall therapeutic approach.

The literature clearly highlights the need for more research into the clinical applications of correctly performed acupuncture and

---

Richard Hammerschlag, PhD, is research director at the Oregon College of Oriental Medicine in Portland. He served from 1997–2003 as copresident of the Society for Acupuncture Research, an organization whose mission is to increase the quality, scope, and awareness of acupuncture research. He also coedited with Gabriel Stux *Clinical Acupuncture: Scientific Basis* (Berlin: Springer-Verlag, 2001) and is an associate editor of the *Journal of Alternative and Complementary Medicine.*

Ryan Milley is completing the master's degree program at the Oregon College of Oriental Medicine.

A brief biography of Stephen Birch appears in Chapter 39.

The Oregon College of Oriental Medicine is a nationally accredited college offering a master's degree in Acupuncture and Oriental Medicine, and is one of the first US acupuncture colleges approved to also offer a postgraduate clinical doctorate degree. Students receive academic and clinical training in all modalities of Oriental medicine and upon graduation are qualified to take national licensing examinations. The research program at the college includes studies on acupuncture and Chinese herbal therapies, and participation in federally funded collaborative research with Oregon Health Sciences University, Kaiser Permanente Center for Health Research, the National College of Naturopathic Medicine, Western States Chiropractic College, and the Oregon School of Massage.

underscores the possibilities that acupuncture presents if it were more readily available. While acupuncture is little used in inpatient settings in this country, the evidence indicates that it could offer much to hospital patients in alleviating pain and postoperative discomfort, and in improving the speed and quality of recovery (Kotani et al., 2001; Wong et al., 2001).

ACUTE AND CHRONIC PAIN

Pain management is the most widely investigated use of acupuncture (Birch et al., 1996; Ezzo et al., 2000). The explosion of interest in acupuncture in the West, triggered by James Reston's article in the *New York Times* and Richard Nixon's trip to China in the early 1970s, focused almost entirely on the use of the needles to produce analgesia. Not only were numerous clinical trials conducted, but many studies investigated the mechanisms by which acupuncture alleviates pain. The initial progress in explaining the analgesic action in Western scientific terms provided a measure of credibility for acupuncture within the biomedical community. But it also had the inappropriate effect of focusing the clinical testing on acupuncture largely within the framework of the drug model.

Slow in coming were the realizations that, in many of the clinical trials for pain, what were designed as "placebo acupuncture" treatments were causing significant non-placebo effects (Vickers et al., 2004; Wonderling et al., 2004). Needling of supposed nonpoints ("irrelevant acupuncture") as a sham control was often producing effects intermediate between placebo responses and the effects of true needling. The design of clinical trials of acupuncture has only recently begun to receive the necessary attention to ensure that it is tested by methods that on the one hand are rigorous enough to satisfy scientific standards, while on the other, do not distort the diagnostic and treatment principles that are unique to this therapeutic tradition.

The best designed and most clinically promising studies in the use of acupuncture for relief of acute and chronic pain reflect a wide range of pain conditions for which acupuncture has been effectively applied. These conditions include headache; facial, dental, neck, and low back pain; and pain disorders that include tennis elbow, osteoarthritis, renal colic, dysmenorrhea, fibromyalgia, athletic injury, endoscopy-associated pain, labor pain, and postsurgical pain. In a number of the clinical trials, acupuncture proved as good as or better than current standard care (Junnila, 1982; Ahonen et al., 1983; Johansson et al., 1991; Allais et al., 2002; Leibing et al., 2002; Ramnero et al., 2002; Vickers et al., 2004) and usually without the side effects commonly associated with the standard therapies (Wang et al., 1992; Hesse et al., 1994; Allais et al., 2002).

The cumulative evidence, supported by recent large-scale clinical trials for headache (Vickers et al., 2004; Wonderling et al., 2004) and osteoarthritis (Berman et al., 2004), suggests that acupuncture represents a therapeutically beneficial, cost-effective treatment option for a broad spectrum of acute and chronic pain conditions. Patients unable to tolerate standard therapies for pain management or non-responsive to them, as well as those who desire other treatment options could be offered the opportunity to receive an adequate course of acupuncture treatment for their conditions.

NAUSEA AND VOMITING

These conditions are regularly experienced following general anesthesia and cancer chemotherapy as well as during pregnancy. While partial success in moderating unpleasant side effects is usually achieved with antiemetic drugs, medication frequently provides inadequate relief, especially if anesthesia is prolonged or if chemotherapy is in the high-dose range. This has encouraged the testing of acupuncture as an alternative, and as a supplement, to standard antiemetic care (Aglietti et al., 1990; Parfitt, 1996; Vickers, 1996; Carlsson et al., 2000; Shen et al., 2000; Kotani et al., 2001; Somri et al., 2001; Smith et al., 2002).

A unique aspect of research on this condition is that most of the clinical trials of acupuncture have tested only a single point. The collective evidence from the research indicates that stimulation of the acupuncture point called Neiguan or PC6, located on the inner side of the wrist, provides effective therapy for nausea related to the postoperative state, chemotherapy, and pregnancy. In several of the studies, PC6 acupuncture provided significantly better relief from nausea and vomiting than stimulation at a "dummy" point (Dundee, Ghaly, Bill et al., 1989; Dundee, Ghaly, Fitzpatrick et al., 1989; Smith et al., 2002), while in others, PC6 needling was at least as beneficial as antiemetic drugs (Ghaly et al., 1987; Dundee, Ghaly, Bill et al., 1989; Ho et al., 1990; Somri et al., 2001) or was an effective adjunct to medication (Dundee, Ghaly, Fitzpatrick et al., 1989; Aglietti et al., 1990; Dundee & Yang, 1990; Carlsson et al., 2000; Shen et al., 2000).

Acupressure at point PC6, provided manually or by wearing the commercially available Sea Bands, was also found to suppress nausea and vomiting beyond the level of placebo (Barsoum et al., 1990; Harmon et al., 1999; Stern et al., 2001; Werntoft & Dykes, 2001), to prolong the effectiveness of acupuncture (Dundee & Yang, 1990) and was as effective as standard care (Stein et al., 1997). Additional studies found that acupressure at PC6 was effective as a nondrug alternative for alleviating nausea and vomiting of pregnancy-related morning sickness, postoperative pain, and visually induced motion sickness. Advantages of acupressure are that it requires only a brief instruction period and can be applied as needed by the patient without additional office or clinic visits.

STROKE

The conclusion of the 1997 NIH Consensus Panel that acupuncture "may be useful" for recovery from poststroke paralysis was based on the promising outcomes of at least four controlled trials, two treating in the acute phase, less than 2 weeks poststroke (Hu et al., 1993; Johansson, 1993) and two in the subacute phase, 2 weeks to 3 months poststroke (Naeser et al., 1992; Sallstrom et al., 1996). However, since 1997, the preponderance of evidence has weighed in against the efficacy of acupuncture for stroke rehabilitation. For example, four well-designed trials, providing acute-phase acupuncture treatment, resulted in little if any improved motor function (Gosman-Hedstrom et al., 1998; Wong et al., 1999; Johansson et al., 2001; Sze, Wong, Yi et al., 2002). There are no obvious study design variables, e.g., type or number of treatments, or choice of control groups, that appear to correlate with treatment outcomes. The conclusion of a recent meta-analysis of 14 trials of acupuncture for stroke rehabilitation is that acupuncture has no added effect to that of conventional physical therapy and occupational therapy treatment (Sze, Wong, Or et al., 2002). Additional information has been generated on the value of neurological function tests and CT scans for predicting which patients were most likely to benefit from acupuncture. Of particular interest is that acupuncture appears to increase the effectiveness of physical therapy when treatment is provided as soon as patients are medically stabilized (within 1 to 10 days of stroke). Benefits are observed even when treatment is not begun until 1 to 3 months poststroke, but they are not as great as those following early intervention. It is also of interest that acupuncture has been found effective in treating the sequelae of stroke in animal models, including a hypertensive strain of rats (Cho et al., 2004; Inoue et al., 2002).

RESPIRATORY DISEASE

Clinical trials of acupuncture for the treatment of respiratory diseases have been extensively reviewed (Jobst, 1995). A major reason for assessing the benefits of acupuncture for chronic conditions such as asthma and disabling breathlessness is that long-term use of corticosteroids and other commonly prescribed inhalants can result in a variety of adverse side effects (Lane & Lane, 1991). In the studies reviewed, acupuncture was found to be effective for reversing the acute effects of bronchoconstriction induced by either pharmacological means or exercise. It was also found to alleviate the chronic effects of asthma.

In two of the studies, acupuncture was performed at a standard set of points, while in the third study, patients were needled at individualized sets of points chosen on the basis of traditional Chinese medicine diagnosis.

Control needling was always matched to acupuncture in terms of number of needles, region of the body needled, and frequency and duration of treatments. In all three blinded studies, acupuncture significantly outperformed control needling under conditions designed to keep the patients as well as the treatment assessors unaware of whether true or control points had been needled.

Five small-scale controlled trials performed since the Lane and Lane (1991) review have produced conflicting claims of acupuncture efficacy for asthmatics. Respiratory function was not significantly improved relative to sham acupuncture in patients with moderate persistent asthma (Biernacki & Peake, 1998; Medici et al., 2002; Shapira et al., 2002). In contrast, patients with "mild to moderately severe bronchial allergic asthma" benefited to a significantly greater extent from acupuncture at asthma-specific points than at acupoints not specific for asthma (Joos et al., 2000). Improvement was observed in general well-being as well as in several biomarkers of immune system function. As well, a recent report indicated that quality-of-life parameters, measured with standardized questionnaires, significantly improved with the addition of acupuncture or acupressure (Maa et al., 2003).

SUBSTANCE ABUSE

At present in the United States, acupuncture is used in several hundred government-supported and private clinics as adjunctive therapy for the treatment of persons dependent on opiates, cocaine, tobacco, alcohol, and other substances (Brewington et al., 1994). Acupuncture treatment programs are also being increasingly instituted in the legal and prison systems (Brumbaugh, 1993). Despite the growth of acupuncture as a viable treatment option for substance abuse (Culliton &

Kiresuk, 1996), and the formation of the National Acupuncture Detoxification Association that promotes acupuncture for treating addictions, relatively few clinical trials have examined this aspect of acupuncture use (D'Alberto, 2004). Several "early" trials have focused on chronic cigarette smoking, alcoholism, and cocaine dependence. In a study of nicotine addiction, acupuncture and nicotine gum achieved a similar modicum of success in enabling chronic smokers to abstain from cigarettes (Clavel et al., 1985). Positive outcomes of a trial of acupuncture for chronic alcohol consumption, the focus of a 1989 study published in *Lancet*, galvanized interest in the use of acupuncture to treat chemical dependency (Bullock et al., 1989). Acupuncture therapy compared favorably to a previous trial of medication for treating methadone-maintained cocaine addicts (Margolin et al., 1993). Acupuncture also outperformed control needling for decreasing cocaine use, as determined by urinalysis (Lipton et al., 1994). Of particular recent note are two trials demonstrating effectiveness of acupuncture for smoking cessation (He et al., 2001; Bier et al., 2002), a positive outcome trial of acupuncture for treatment of methadone-maintained cocaine addicts (Avants et al., 2000), and a negative outcome, large scale multicenter trial, again for treating methadone-maintained cocaine abusers (Margolin, Kleber, Avants et al., 2002). In puzzling out the possible design differences between the latter two trials, which may have bearing on their respective outcomes, it seems important to recognize that clinical research should be based as much as possible on clinical practice. In this regard, virtually all substance abuse programs involving acupuncture use it as adjunctive treatment to 12-step or other psychotherapeutic counseling sessions and not as a stand-alone treatment (Margolin,

Avants, & Holford, 2002; Kaptchuk, 2002). The added cost notwithstanding, the multi-center study results would have been far more useful to the public health community if acupuncture and sham acupuncture groups had been compared to a third group receiving acupuncture plus counseling sessions, based on real-world treatment protocols.

WOMEN'S REPRODUCTIVE HEALTH

Evaluation of acupuncture for obstetric and gynecologic-related conditions is a rapidly growing area of clinical research. The past 5 years have seen a range of trials testing its efficacy for reducing nausea and vomiting in early pregnancy, relieving low back and pelvic pain during pregnancy, and decreasing the duration and pain of labor. Acupuncture has also been tested as adjunctive care in trials of fertility-promoting techniques. Overall, the results have been promising. As described above, acupuncture—performed either at a single traditionally used acupoint or at multiple acupoints informed by individualized Chinese medicine pattern differentiations—consistently produced intragroup reductions in early pregnancy-related nausea (Carlsson et al., 2000; Knight et al., 2001; Smith et al., 2002), but only in one of these trials was it found to significantly outperform sham acupuncture (Carlsson et al., 2000). When tested for relieving pregnancy-related low back and pelvic pain, acupuncture was significantly more effective than physiotherapy (Wedenberg et al., 2000). Acupuncture reduced the time of active labor in three trials (Tempfer et al., 1998; Zeisler et al., 1998; Skilnand et al., 2002); in a fourth trial the overall time from "estimated date of confinement" to delivery was shortened but not the duration of labor (Rabl et al., 2001).

Acupuncture was also more effective than sham needling in reducing labor-related pain (Skilnand et al., 2002). In in vitro fertilization trials, women receiving electroacupuncture had significantly higher rates of implantation and pregnancy than those receiving the opioid analgesic, alfentanil (Stener-Victorin et al., 1999); a higher rate of clinical pregnancy was also documented in women receiving acupuncture relative to those in a no-acupuncture group (Paulus et al., 2002).

PROBLEMS IN THE DESIGN AND REPORTING OF ACUPUNCTURE RESEARCH

In reviewing clinical trials of acupuncture, several frequently occurring problems have been identified that can create difficulties when assessing results of the studies (Hammerschlag, 1998). Several examples of these methodological issues follow:

1. Lack of information on the training of the acupuncturist(s): Since, in some medical circles, acupuncture is regarded, inappropriately, as a "technique" that can be learned in several short sessions, insufficient training may be an inadvertent factor contributing to a negative outcome.

2. Inadequate description of the points needled or the frequency and duration of acupuncture treatment: Without sufficient information on the nature of the treatment, it is difficult to assess whether a negative outcome indicates that the acupuncture treatment was truly ineffective or was, instead, inadequately provided.

3. The implicit assumption that needling at control points equates to a placebo treatment: Invasive needling at points inap-

propriate to the treatment is likely to produce nonspecific effects as well as placebo effects. Such nonspecific effects include local responses to the microtrauma of needling (Kendall, 1989) as well as neurally mediated responses to noxious stimuli (Le Bars et al 1991). As a result, control needling often produces effects that are intermediate between those of real acupuncture and no treatment (Vincent & Lewith, 1995).

4. Underenrollment of patients: Dropouts can reduce group size to an extent where statistical significance of treatment is lost, particularly in studies involving treatment of outpatients.

5. Variability in acupuncture point selection strategy: While some studies administered acupuncture at a fixed set of treatment points (following a Western medicine-style research design), in other studies acupuncture points were chosen on an individualized basis (in keeping with traditional Chinese medicine diagnostic principles). Ulcers, for example, in an acupuncturist's

view can arise from at least a half dozen different underlying conditions, each requiring a distinctly different treatment plan. Unless the fixed-protocol patients have been preselected for the same Chinese medicine diagnosis, such a study design may contribute to a poor treatment outcome. This variable of fixed versus individualized treatment plans is a particular problem when attempting to compare results from different clinical trials.

These five, and other recurring methodological problems in acupuncture research, have been addressed in a set of guidelines called Standards for Reporting Interventions in Controlled Trials of Acupuncture (STRICTA) (MacPherson et al., 2002). The STRICTA guidelines, adopted by an increasing number of journals when reviewing controlled trials of acupuncture submitted for publication, are also of value during the design phase of trials planned to assess the efficacy of the traditional medical practice of acupuncture.

REFERENCE LIST

Aglietti L, Roila F, Tonato M, Basurto, et al. A pilot study of metoclopramide, dexamethasone, diphenhydramine and acupuncture in women treated with cisplatin. *Cancer Chemother Pharmacol.* 1990;26: 239–240.

Ahonen E, Hakumaki M, Mahlamaki S, et al. Acupuncture and physiotherapy in the treatment of myogenic headache patients: pain relief and EMG activity. *Adv Pain Res Ther.* 1983;5:571–576.

Allais G, De Lorenzo C, Quirico PE. Acupuncture in the prophylactic treatment of migraine without aura: a comparison with flunarizine. *Headache.* 2002; 42:855–861.

Avants SK, Margolin A, Holford TR, Kosten TR. A randomized controlled trial of auricular acupuncture for cocaine dependence. *Arch Intern Med.* 2000;160:2305–2312.

Barsoum G, Perry EP, Fraser IA. Postoperative nausea is relieved by acupressure. *J R Soc Med.* 1990;83: 86–89.

Berman BM, Lao L, Langenberg P, Lee WL, Gilpin AMK, Hochberg MC. Effectiveness of acupuncture as adjunctive therapy in osteoarthritis of the knee. *Ann Intern Med.* 2004;141:901–910.

Bier ID, Wilson J, Studt P, Shakleton M. Auricular acupuncture, education, and smoking cessation: a randomized, sham-controlled trial. *Am J Public Health.* 2002;92:1642–1647.

Biernacki W, Peake MD. Acupuncture in treatment of stable asthma. *Respir Med.* 1998;92:1143–1145.

Birch S. Clinical research on acupuncture: part 2. Controlled clinical trials, an overview of their methods. *J Altern Complement Med.* 2004;10: 481–498.

Birch S, Hammerschlag R, Berman BM. Acupuncture in the treatment of pain. *J Altern Complement Med.* 1996;2:101–124.

Brewington V, Smith M, Lipton D. Acupuncture as a detoxification treatment: an analysis of controlled research. *J Subst Abuse Treat.* 1994;11:289–307.

Brumbaugh AG. Acupuncture: new perspectives in chemical dependency treatment. *J Subst Abuse Treat.* 1993;10:35–43.

Bullock ML, Culliton PD, Olander RT. Controlled trial of acupuncture for severe recidivist alcoholism. *Lancet.* 1989;1:1435–1439.

Carlsson CP, Axemo P, Bodin A, et al. Manual acupuncture reduces hyperemesis gravidarum: a placebo-controlled, randomized, single-blind, cross-over study. *J Pain Symptom Manage.* 2000;20: 273–279.

Cho NH, Lee JD, Cheong BS et al. Acupuncture suppresses intrastriatal hemorrage-induced apoptotic neuronal cell death in rats. *Neurosci Lett.* 2004; 362:141–145.

Clavel F, Benhamou S, Company-Huertas A, Flamant R. Helping people to stop smoking: randomised comparison of groups being treated with acupuncture and nicotine gum with control group. *Br Med J (Clin Res Ed).* 1985;291:1538–1539.

Culliton PD, Kiresuk TJ. Overview of substance abuse acupuncture treatment research. *J Altern Complement Med.* 1996;2:149–159.

D'Alberto A. Auricular acupuncture in the treatment of cocaine/crack abuse: a review of the efficacy, the use of the National Acupuncture Detoxification Association protocol, and the selection of sham points. *J Altern Complement Med.* 2004;10:985–1000.

Dundee JW, Ghaly RG, Bill KM, Chestnutt WN, Fitzpatrick KT, Lynas AG. Effect of stimulation of the P6 antiemetic point on postoperative nausea and vomiting. *Br J Anaesth.* 1989;63:612–618.

Dundee JW, Ghaly RG, Fitzpatrick KT, Abram WP, Lynch GA. Acupuncture prophylaxis of cancer chemotherapy-induced sickness. *J R Soc Med.* 1989;82:268–271.

Dundee JW, Yang J. Prolongation of the antiemetic action of P6 acupuncture by acupressure in patients having cancer chemotherapy. *J R Soc Med.* 1990;83: 360–362.

Ezzo J, Berman B, Hadhazy VA, Jadad AR, Lao L, Singh BB. Is acupuncture effective for the treatment of chronic pain? A systematic review. *Pain.* 2000; 86:217–225.

Ghaly RG, Fitzpatrick KT, Dundee JW. Antiemetic studies with traditional Chinese acupuncture. A comparison of manual needling with electrical stimulation and commonly used antiemetics. *Anaesthesia.* 1987;42:1108–1110.

Gosman-Hedstrom G, Claesson L, Klingenstierna U, et al. Effects of acupuncture treatment on daily life activities and quality of life: a controlled, prospective, and randomized study of acute stroke patients. *Stroke.* 1998;29:2100–2108.

Hammerschlag R. Methodological and ethical issues in clinical trials of acupuncture. *J Altern Complement Med.* 1998;4:159–171.

Harmon D, Gardiner J, Harrison R, Kelly A. Acupressure and the prevention of nausea and vomiting after laparoscopy. *Br J Anaesth.* 1999;82: 387–390.

He D, Medbo JI, Hostmark AT. Effect of acupuncture on smoking cessation or reduction: an 8-month and 5-year follow-up study. *Prev Med.* 2001;33:364–372.

Hesse J, Mogelvang B, Simonsen H. Acupuncture versus metoprolol in migraine prophylaxis: a randomized trial of trigger point inactivation. *J Intern Med.* 1994;235:451–456.

Ho RT, Jawan B, Fung ST, Cheung HK, Lee JH. Electro-acupuncture and postoperative emesis. *Anaesthesia.* 1990;45:327–329.

Hu HH, Chung C, Liu TJ, et al. A randomized controlled trial on the treatment for acute partial ischemic stroke with acupuncture. *Neuroepidemiology.* 1993;12:106–113.

Inoue I, Chen L, Zhou L et al. Reproduction of scalp acupuncture therapy on strokes in the model rats, spontaneous hypertensive rats-stroke prone (SHR-SP). *Neurosci Lett.* 2002;333:191–194.

Jobst KA. A critical analysis of acupuncture in pulmonary disease: efficacy and safety of the acupuncture needle. *J Altern Complement Med.* 1995;1: 57–85.

Johansson A, Wenneberg B, Wagersten C, Haraldson T. Acupuncture in treatment of facial muscular pain. *Acta Odontol Scand.* 1991;49:153–158.

Johansson BB. Has sensory stimulation a role in stroke rehabilitation? *Scand J Rehabil Med.* 1993;29(Suppl): 87–96.

Johansson BB, Haker E, von Arbin M, et al. Acupuncture and transcutaneous nerve stimulation in stroke rehabilitation: a randomized, controlled trial. *Stroke.* 2001;32:707–713.

Joos S, Schott C, Zou H, Daniel V, Martin E. Immunomodulatory effects of acupuncture in the treatment of allergic asthma: a randomized controlled study. *J Altern Complement Med.* 2000;6: 519–525.

Junnila SYT. Acupuncture therapy for chronic pain: a randomized comparison between acupuncture and pseudo-acupuncture with minimal peripheral stimulus. *Amer J Acupunct.* 1982;10:259–262.

Kaptchuk TJ. Acupuncture for the treatment of cocaine addiction. *JAMA.* 2002;287:1801–1802.

Kendall DE. Part I, a scientific model for acupuncture. *Am J Acupunct.* 1989;17:251–268.

Knight B, Mudge C, Openshaw S, White A, Hart A. Effect of acupuncture on nausea of pregnancy: a randomized, controlled trial. *Obstet Gynecol.* 2001;97: 184–188.

Kotani N, Hashimoto H, Sato Y, et al. Preoperative intradermal acupuncture reduces postoperative pain, nausea and vomiting, analgesic requirement, and sympathoadrenal responses. *Anesthesiology.* 2001; 95:349–356.

Lane DJ, & Lane TV. Alternative and complementary medicine for asthma. *Thorax.* 1991;46:787–797.

Le Bars D, Villaneuva L, Willer JC, Bouhassira D. Difuse noxious inhibitory control (DNIC) in man and animals. *Acupunct Med.* 1991;9:47–57.

Leibing E, Leonhardt U, Koster G, et al. Acupuncture treatment of chronic low-back pain—a randomized, blinded, placebo-controlled trial with 9-month follow-up. *Pain.* 2002;96:189–196.

Lipton DS, Brewington V, Smith M. Acupuncture for crack-cocaine detoxification: experimental evaluation of efficacy. *J Subst Abuse Treat.* 1994;11: 205–215.

Maa SH, Sun MF, Hsu KH, et al. Effect of acupuncture or acupressure on quality of life of patients with chronic obstructive asthma: a pilot study. *J Altern Complement Med.* 2003;9:659–670.

MacPherson H, White A, Cummings M, Jobst K, Rose K, Niemtzow R. Standards for reporting interventions in controlled trials of acupuncture: the STRICTA recommendations. Standards for reporting interventions in controlled trials of acupuncture. *Acupunct Med.* 2002;20:22–25.

Margolin A, Avants SK, Chang PL, et al. Acupuncture for the treatment of cocaine dependence in methadone-maintained patients. *Am J Addic.* 1993;2: 194–201.

Margolin A, Avants SK, Holford TR. Interpreting conflicting findings from clinical trials of auricular acupuncture for cocaine addiction: does treatment context influence outcome? *J Altern Complement Med.* 2002;8:111–121.

Margolin A, Kleber HD, Avants SK, et al. Acupuncture for the treatment of cocaine addiction: a randomized controlled trial. *JAMA.* 2002;287:55–63.

Medici TC, Grebski E, Wu J, Hinz G, Wuthrich B. Acupuncture and bronchial asthma: a long-term randomized study of the effects of real versus sham acupuncture compared to controls in patients with bronchial asthma. *J Altern Complement Med.* 2002;8:737–750.

Naeser MA, Alexander MP, Stiassny-Eder D, et al. Real versus sham acupuncture in the treatment of paralysis in acute stroke patients: a CT scan lesion site study. *J Neuro Rehab.* 1992;6:163–173.

Parfitt A. Acupuncture as an antiemetic treatment. *J Altern Complement Med.* 1996;2:167–174.

Paulus WE, Zhang M, Strehler E, El Danasouri I, Sterzik K. Influence of acupuncture on the pregnancy rate in patients who undergo assisted reproduction therapy. *Fertil Steril.* 2002;77:721–724.

Rabl M, Ahner R, Bitschnau M, Zeisler H, Husslein P. Acupuncture for cervical ripening and induction of labor at term—a randomized controlled trial. *Wien Klin Wochenschr.* 2001;113:942–946.

Ramnero A, Hanson U, Kihlgren M. Acupuncture treatment during labour—a randomised controlled trial. *BJOG.* 2002;109:637–644.

Sallstrom S, Kjendahl A, Osten PE, Stanghelle JK, Borchgrevink CF. Acupuncture in the treatment of stroke patients in the subacute stage: a randomized, controlled study. *Compl Ther Med.* 1996;4:193–197.

Shapira MY, Berkman N, Ben David G, Avital A, Bardach E, Breuer R. Short-term acupuncture therapy is of no benefit in patients with moderate persistent asthma. *Chest.* 2002;121:1396–1400.

Shen J, Wenger N, Glaspy J, Hays RD, Albert PS, Choi C, Shekelle PG. Electroacupuncture for control of myeloablative chemotherapy-induced emesis: a randomized controlled trial. *JAMA.* 2000;284: 2755–2761.

Skilnand E, Fossen D, Heiberg E. Acupuncture in the management of pain in labor. *Acta Obstet Gynecol Scand.* 2002;81:943–948.

Smith C, Crowther C, Beilby J. Acupuncture to treat nausea and vomiting in early pregnancy: a randomized controlled trial. *Birth.* 2002;29:1–9.

Somri M, Vaida SJ, Sabo E, Yassain G, Gankin I, Gaitini LA. Acupuncture versus ondansetron in the prevention of postoperative vomiting. A study of children undergoing dental surgery. *Anaesthesia.* 2001;56:927–932.

Stein DJ, Birnbach DJ, Danzer BI, Kuroda MM, Grunebaum A, Thys DM. Acupressure versus intravenous metoclopramide to prevent nausea and vomiting during spinal anesthesia for cesarean section. *Anesth Analg.* 1997;84:342–345.

Stener-Victorin E, Waldenstrom U, Nilsson L, Wikland M, Janson PO. A prospective randomized study of electro-acupuncture versus alfentanil as anaesthesia during oocyte aspiration in in-vitro fertilization. *Hum Reprod.* 1999;14:2480–2484.

Stern RM, Jokerst MD, Muth ER, Hollis C. Acupressure relieves the symptoms of motion sickness and reduces abnormal gastric activity. *Altern Ther Health Med.* 2001;7:91–94.

Sze FK, Wong E, Or KK, Lau J, Woo J. Does acupuncture improve motor recovery after stroke? A meta-analysis of randomized controlled trials. *Stroke.* 2002;33:2604–2619.

Sze FK, Wong E, Yi X, Woo J. Does acupuncture have additional value to standard poststroke motor rehabilitation? *Stroke.* 2002;33:186–194.

Tempfer C, Zeisler H, Heinzl H, Hefler L, Husslein P, Kainz C. Influence of acupuncture on maternal serum levels of interleukin-8, prostaglandin F2alpha, and beta-endorphin: a matched pair study. *Obstet Gynecol.* 1998;92:245–248.

Vickers AJ. Can acupuncture have specific effects on health? A systematic review of acupuncture antiemesis trials. *J R Soc Med.* 1996;89:303–311.

Vickers AJ. Placebo controls in randomized trials of acupuncture. *Eval Health Prof.* 2002;25:421–435.

Vickers AJ, Rees RW, Zollman CE, et al. Acupuncture for chronic headache in primary care: large, pragmatic, randomised trial. *BMJ.* 2004; 328(7442):744.

Vincent C, Lewith GT. Placebo controls for acupuncture studies. *J Roy Soc Med.* 1995;88:192–202.

Wang HH, Chang YH, Liu DM. A study in the effectiveness of acupuncture analgesia for colonoscopic examination compared with conventional premedication. *Am J Acupunct.* 1992;20:217–221.

Wedenberg K, Moen B, Norling A. A prospective randomized study comparing acupuncture with physiotherapy for low-back and pelvic pain in pregnancy. *Acta Obstet Gynecol Scand.* 2000;79: 331–335.

Werntoft E, Dykes AK. Effect of acupressure on nausea and vomiting during pregnancy: a randomized, placebo-controlled, pilot study. *J Reprod Med.* 2001;46:835–839.

Wonderling D, Vickers AJ, Grieve R, McCarney R. Cost effectiveness analysis of a randomised trial of acupuncture for chronic headache in primary care. *BMJ.* 2004;328(7442):747.

Wong AM, Su TY, Tang FT, Cheng PT, Liaw MY. Clinical trial of electrical acupuncture on hemiplegic stroke patients. *Am J Phys Med Rehabil.* 1999;78: 117–122.

Wong R, Sagar CM, Sagar SM. Integration of Chinese medicine into supportive cancer care: a modern role for an ancient tradition. *Cancer Treat Rev.* 2001; 27:235–246.

Zeisler H, Tempfer C, Mayerhofer K, Barrada M, Husslein P. Influence of acupuncture on duration of labor. *Gynecol Obstet Invest.* 1998;46:22–25.

CHAPTER 41

Six-Center Study of Acupuncture Outcomes

Claire M. Cassidy, PhD, LAc

RESEARCH DESIGN

This study was the first in-depth survey of acupuncture users. It was conducted among patients of six large clinics in five states, using a mixed qualitative-quantitative written questionnaire format. The final sample size consisted of 575 respondents to the quantitative segment of the research questionnaire. In addition, 460 participants responded to requests for written narrative. The study gathered data on the following issues:

- Who attends acupuncture clinics?
- Why do they seek Chinese medicine?
- What is their self-reported response to Chinese medicine care?
- What other forms of health care do they use?
- How satisfied are they with Chinese medicine?

- What motivates them to continue its use and (usually) pay for it out of their own pockets?

Methodology:

- Using a menu of 30 items, 575 respondents marked any condition for which they had ever received Chinese medicine.
- Respondents could choose to report up to four changes in symptoms or conditions: 95 people did not answer the question: 478 named one symptom; 303 named two symptoms; 167 named three symptoms; and 58 named four symptoms. Choices included symptoms that disappeared, improved, did not change, or got worse, indicated by the headings "Condition resolved," "Improved," "Same," and "Worse." The results of the quantitative research questionnaire are reflected in the table.

Claire M. Cassidy, PhD, LAc, is a medical anthropologist and acupuncturist with a professional interest in the development of research methodology. She served for 6 years as research director at a premier US acupuncture school, taught at universities for more than 15 years, and heads her own consulting firm and acupuncture clinic. She has an extensive publications list and is author of *Contemporary Chinese Medicine and Acupuncture*, Philadelphia, PA: W. B. Saunders, 2002.

Courtesy of Claire M. Cassidy, PhD, LAc, Bethesda, Maryland.

Table 41–1 Survey of Complaints and Resolution in Response to Acupuncture Treatment: Study of 575 patients in total, from 6 centers, located in 5 states

Condition	Sample size/ percentage of sample		Response condition resolved	Improved	Same	Worse
	N	%	%	%	%	%
Stress, anxiety, depression, fatigue, chronic fatigue	381	66.3	10.7	82.7	6.2	0.4
Well care	362	63.0	7.1	91.1	—	1.8
Musculoskeletal system	321	58.8	15.1	74.6	9.9	0.4
Respiratory system	231	40.2	17.6	68.2	7.1	—
Head and neck conditions	182	31.7	17.5	76.3	5.0	1.3
Digestive system	129	22.4	7.5	85.1	7.5	—
Urinary and male reproductive system	117	20.3	11.6	58.8	29.4	—
Female reproductive system	100	17.4	13.3	78.3	6.7	1.7
Infectious illness	77	13.4	43.2	54.1	2.7	—
Autoimmune dysfunctions	72	12.5	9.5	66.7	23.8	—
Weight problems	62	10.8	—	61.1	33.3	5.6
Other	254	44.2	12.8	82.6	3.7	0.9

Conditions benefited:

• Stress or fatigue category includes: all reports of mood support; those seeking Chinese medicine to relieve stress, anxiety, or depression; and those reporting fatigue or chronic fatigue syndrome.
• Well care category includes all reports of using Chinese medicine care for maintaining well-being and health, as well as illness prevention.
• Musculoskeletal system category includes all reports of pain and other disability in bones, muscles, joints, and ligaments.
• Head and neck category includes all reports of headache, all types of chronic neck or head pain, learning disabilities, epilepsy, and insomnia; it excludes cancers.
• Respiratory system category includes all reports of allergies, asthma, tinnitis, emphysema, and multiple chemical sensitivities; it excludes respiratory infections and cancers.
• Digestive system category includes all reports of painful and nonpainful, noninfectious, digestive system conditions.
• Urinary and male reproductive system category includes all reports relative to the urinary system as well as the male reproductive system.

continues

Table 41–1 continued

- Female reproductive system category includes all reports of menstrual pain or discomfort, menopausal symptoms, infertility, endometriosis, uterine fibroids, and other reproductive system complaints.
- Infectious illness category includes all reports of infections, including colds, sinusitis, pneumonia, cystitis, hepatitis (N = 7), and HIV (N = 10).
- Autoimmune dysfunctions category includes all reports of immune dysfunctions including diabetes (N = 8), thyroiditis (N = 5), and multiple sclerosis (N = 3); it excludes reproductive system complaints.
- Weight problems category includes all reports of anorexia, bulimia, low weight, and high weight.
- "Other" category includes all conditions with fewer than 10% of sample reporting that complaint. These disorders related to circulation (N = 53); eyes and ears (N = 48); skin (N = 45); substance abuse (N = 43); mouth or jaw (N = 30); sleep disturbance (N = 21, a respondent-created category); cancer and radiation chemotherapy (N = 14); and complaints phrased in Chinese medical terms (N = 10).

Source: Courtesy of Claire Cassidy, PhD, LAc, Bethesda, Maryland.

CHAPTER 42

Acupuncture Analgesia: Basic Research

Bruce Pomeranz, MD, PhD and Brian Berman, MD

OVERVIEW

In recent years in the West, acupuncture analgesia (AA) has been restricted mainly to the treatment of chronic pain and has not been used for surgical procedures except for demonstration purposes. However, even for the treatment of chronic pain, many Western physicians were skeptical at first, despite a vast body of anecdotal evidence from both China and Europe.

How could an acupuncture needle inserted in the hand possibly relieve a toothache? Because such phenomena did not conform to physiological concepts, scientists were puzzled and skeptical. Many explained it by the well-known placebo effect, which works through suggestion, distraction, or even hypnosis (Wall, 1972, 1974). In 1945, Beecher (1955) had shown that morphine relieved pain in 70% of patients, while sugar injections (placebo) reduced pain in 35% of patients who believed they were receiving morphine. Thus, many medical scientists in the early 1970s assumed that acupuncture analgesia worked by the placebo (psychological) effect. However, there were several problems with this idea.

How does one explain the use of acupuncture analgesia in veterinary medicine over the past 1000 years in China and for approximately 100 years in Europe, and its growing use on animals in America? Animals are not suggestible, and only a very few species are capable of the still reaction (so-called animal hypnosis). Similarly, small children respond to acupuncture analgesia. Moreover, several studies in which patients were given psychological tests for suggestibility did not show a good correlation between acupuncture analgesia and suggestibility (Liao, 1978). Hypnosis has also been ruled out as an explanation, as there have been two studies (Barber & Mayer, 1977; Goldstein & Hilgard, 1975) showing that hypnosis and acupuncture analgesia respond differently to naloxone, AA being blocked and hypnosis being unaffected by this endorphin antagonist.

Up to 1973, the evidence for AA was mainly anecdotal, with a huge collection of

Bruce Pomeranz, MD, PhD, is a researcher in the neurophysiology of acupuncture and a member of the neuroscience faculty at the University of Toronto, where he has taught for more than two decades. Dr. Pomeranz has published more than 66 papers on acupuncture research and 8 acupuncture textbooks. He has served as president of the American Society of Acupuncture and served on the advisory boards of the World Federation of Acupuncture Societies, Harvard Medical School, NIH Center for Alternative Medicine, and the University of Maryland.

Brian Berman, MD, is founder and director of the University of Maryland Center for Integrative Medicine (CFIM); he is board certified in family medicine, which he teaches at the University; and has extensive training in acupuncture and in pain management. Dr. Berman is chair of the steering committee of the Consortium of Academic Medical Centers, principal investigator of an NIH center grant for complementary medicine research, and investigator on other large NIH-funded randomized controlled trials in CAM. He also coordinates the Complementary Medicine Field of the international Cochrane Collaboration.

Courtesy of Springer-Verlag, Berlin and Heidelberg, Germany, and New York, New York.

case histories from one quarter of the world's population. Unfortunately, there were few scientifically controlled experiments to convince the skeptics. In the past 20 years, however, the situation has changed considerably. Scientists have been asking two important questions. First, does acupuncture analgesia really work (that is by a physiological rather than a placebo/psychological effect)? Second, if it does work, what is the mechanism?

DOES ACUPUNCTURE WORK?

The first question (does it work?) had to be approached by way of controlled experiments to remove variables such as placebo effects and spontaneous remissions. These have been carried out in clinical practice on patients with chronic pain, in the laboratory on humans studying acute laboratory-induced pain, and on animals. From these numerous studies it can be concluded that AA works much better than placebo.

Hence AA must have some physiological basis. But what are the possible mechanisms? Only the answer to the second question (how does AA work?) could possibly dispel the deep skepticism toward acupuncture. More than three decades of research has provided evidence for acupuncture effects that include neurological mechanisms, stimulation of endorphins, stimulation of monoamines such as serotonin, and influences on the pituitary-hypothalamic axis.

EVIDENCE FOR ENDORPHINS DUE TO ACUPUNCTURE ANALGESIA

Research Studies

Perhaps the most exciting experiments, which opened up the field of acupuncture analgesia to scientific research, were those in which endorphin antagonists (e.g., naloxone, naltrexone) were used. That naloxone could antagonize AA was reported initially by two groups (Mayer et al., 1977; Pomeranz & Chiu, 1976).

Mayer et al. (1977), studying acute laboratory-induced tooth pain in human volunteers, produced AA by manual twirling of needles at the LI4 acupoint (first dorsal interosseus muscle of the hand). In a double-blind design they gave one group of subjects intravenous naloxone, while another group received IV saline. The saline group achieved AA with a time-course typical of clinical reports (30 minutes to onset of analgesia and effects lasting for over 1 hour). The naloxone-treated group showed no AA.

Mayer et al. (1977) also studied a control group of subjects receiving placebo injections. The placebo subjects were told to expect a strong analgesic effect, but none was observed (as predicted from Beecher's work [1955] on acute pain, where only 3% of subjects reported placebo analgesia).

The other early naloxone study was by Pomeranz and Chiu (1976) in awake mice; they used the mouse squeak latency paradigm and gave electroacupuncture at the LI4 acupoint. Numerous control groups were used in this latter experiment in an attempt to pick out some of the possible artifacts. Each group received one of the following treatments: electroacupuncture alone, electroacupuncture plus saline, electroacupuncture plus IV naloxone, sham electroacupuncture in a non-acupuncture point, naloxone alone, saline alone, or no treatment at all (just handling, restraint, and repeated pain testing). The results were unequivocal: naloxone completely blocked acupuncture analgesia; sham electroacupuncture produced no effect; and naloxone alone produced very little hyperalgesia (not enough to explain reduction of acupuncture analgesia by subtraction).

Moreover, the results in mice and in humans indicated, first, that AA was not a psychological effect, and secondly, that AA was truly blocked by naloxone. In a later study, Cheng and Pomeranz (1979) produced a dose-response curve for naloxone and found that increasing doses produced increasing blockade. In a third study in anesthetized cats, Pomeranz and Cheng (1979), recording from layer-5 cells (pain transmission cells) in the spinal cord, completely prevented the electroacupuncture effects with IV naloxone.

Since these early papers, there have been numerous studies in which systematically administered endorphin antagonists have been used to test the endorphin-AA hypothesis. The majority of researchers reported naloxone antagonism (Boureau et al., 1979; Chapman & Benedetti, 1977; Charlton, 1982; Chen et al., 1996; Cheng & Pomeranz, 1979, 1980a, 1980b; Chung et al., 1983; Fu et al., 1980; Ha et al., 1981; He et al., 1991; Lagerweij et al., 1984; Lee & Blitz, 1992; Lee et al., 1978; Peets & Pomeranz, 1985, 1978; Pomeranz & Chiu, 1976; Pomeranz & Paley, 1979; Pomeranz & Warma, 1988; Sato & Takeshige, 1986; Shimizu et al., 1981, 1986; Sjolund & Erikson, 1979; Sodipo et al., 1981; Takagi et al., 1996; Takahashi et al., 1986; Thoren et al., 1989; Tsunoda et al., 1980; Willer et al., 1982; Woolf et al., 1977; Zhou et al., 1981; Zou et al., 1980).

However, a few did not find any effects of naloxone (Abrams et al., 1981; Chapman et al., 1980, 1983; Pertovaara et al., 1982; Tay et al., 1982; Walker & Katz, 1981; Woolf et al., 1978).

- Three of these seven failures were obtained with high-frequency, low-intensity stimulation using a TENS (transcutaneous electrostimulation) unit, a method that does not involve acupuncture needles and is probably not endorphinergic (Abrams et al., 1981; Walker & Katz, 1981; Woolf et al., 1978). In one of the failures (Chapman et al., 1983)

in which this low-intensity stimulation was used, in spite of this, 4 of 7 subjects in that study showed naloxone antagonism.
- While the reasons for the other three negative papers (Chapman et al., 1980; Pertovaara et al., 1982; Tay et al., 1982) are not entirely clear, a possible explanation has recently emerged. Antagonists work best when given before the treatment (Pomeranz & Bibic, 1988; Watkins & Mayer, 1982) and fail to reverse analgesia that has already been initiated. Thus, naloxone can prevent but often cannot reverse AA. (In the three failed experiments researchers tried to reverse AA, giving the endorphin antagonist after, not before, the acupuncture treatments.) Taken together, the overwhelming weight of evidence shows that naloxone antagonizes AA and that the few negative results may be due to poor timing of the naloxone administration.

THE ACUPUNCTURE-ENDORPHIN HYPOTHESIS

Support for the Hypothesis

Seventeen different lines of experimentation have emerged which have independently provided support for the AA-endorphin hypothesis:

1. Many different opiate antagonists block AA (Chen & Han, 1992; Chen et al., 1996; Cheng & Pomeranz, 1979).

2. Naloxone has a stereospecific effect (Cheng & Pomeranz, 1979).

3. Microinjection of naloxone (or antibodies to endorphins) blocks AA only if given into analgesic sites in the central nervous system (Bing et al., 1991; Chou et al., 1984; Han & Xie, 1984; Han et al., 1982, 1985; Peets & Pomeranz, 1985; Pomeranz

& Bibic, 1988; Pomeranz & Warma, 1988; Xie et al., 1983; Zao et al., 1987; Zhou et al., 1981).

4. Mice genetically deficient in opiate receptors show poor AA (Peets & Pomeranz, 1978; Roy et al., 1980).

5. Rats deficient in endorphin show poor AA (Murai et al., 1986; Takahashi et al., 1986).

6. Endorphin levels rise in blood and CSF during AA and fall in specific brain regions during AA (Avants et al., 2000; Chou et al., 1984; Facchinetti et al., 1981; Hardebo et al., 1989; He et al., 1985; Ho & Hen, 1989; Kiser et al., 1983; Malizia et al., 1979; Masala et al., 1983; Nappi et al., 1982; Pert et al., 1981; Sjolund et al., 1977; Vacca-Galloway et al., 1985; Zou et al., 1980).

7. AA is enhanced by protecting endorphins from enzyme degradation (Cheng & Pomeranz, 1980a; Chou et al., 1984; Ehrenpreis, 1985; Fujishita et al., 1986; Hachisu et al., 1986; Hishida et al., 1986; Kishioka et al., 1994; Murai et al., 1986; Takahashi et al., 1986; Zou et al., 1980).

8. AA can be transmitted to a second animal by CSF transfer or by cross-circulation, and this effect is blocked by naloxone (Lee et al., 1978; Lung et al., 1978; Research Group Peking Med Coll, 1974).

9. Reduction of pituitary endorphins suppresses AA (Cheng, Pomeranz, & Yu, 1979; Masala et al., 1983; Pomeranz et al., 1977; Takeshige, Kobori et al., 1992; Takeshige, Nakamura et al., 1992; Takeshige et al., 1993; Takeshige, Tsuchiya et al., 1991).

10. There was a rise in messenger RNA for proenkephalin in brain and pituitary: this

lasted 24–48 hours after 30 minutes of electroacupuncture indicating a prolonged increased rate of synthesis of enkephalin. This could explain the enduring effects of electroacupuncture and the potentiation of repeated daily treatments (Guo, Tian et al., 1996; Zheng et al., 1988).

11. There is cross-tolerance between AA and morphine analgesia, implicating endorphins in AA (Chen & Han, 1992; Han et al., 1981).

12. AA is more effective against emotional aspects of pain; this is typical of endorphins (Yang et al., 1989).

13. Lesions of the accurate nucleus of hypothalamus (the site of beta endorphins) abolishes AA (Takeshige, Tsuchiya et al., 1991; Takeshige, Zhao et al., 1991; Wang et al., 1990a).

14. Lesions of the periaquaductal gray (containing endorphins) abolishes AA (Wang et al., 1990b).

15. The level of e-fos gene protein (which measures increased neural activity) is elevated in endorphin-related areas of the brain during AA (Guo, Cui et al., 1996; Lee & Beitz, 1993).

16. Recent evidence suggests that in addition to monoamines mediating 100 Hz electroacupuncture effects, dynorphin (one of the three endorphins) may also be involved. At 100 Hz there is an elevation of dynorphin levels in the dorsal horn of rat spinal cord (Xue et al., 1995). In lumbar punctures in humans receiving 100 Hz electroacupuncture, there is an elevation of dynorphin A (Han et al., 1991). Moreover, rats given electroacupuncture at 100 Hz show AA, which is blocked by the dynorphin Kappa antagonist (nor-binaltorphimine), while the electroacupuncture at 2 Hz is blocked by

mu and delta antagonists suggesting involvement of enkephalins and beta endorphin at these lower frequencies (Chen et al., 1996).

17. Electroacupuncture in rats elevated precursors of the three endorphins: preproenkephalin, preprodynorphin, and preproendorphina mRNA. Moreover, antisense nucleotides for c-fos or c-jun successfully blocked the electroacupuncture-induced preprodynorphin mRNA (Guo, Tian et al., 1996).

In summary, 17 different lines of research strongly support the AA-endorphin hypothesis.

Objections to the Hypothesis

With so much convergent evidence for this hypothesis, why are there still a few skeptics?

1. Some skeptics cite the few failures of naloxone to reverse AA (Chapman et al., 1983). It has already been suggested previously that naloxone reversal experiments are prone to difficulty because naloxone prevents, but does not reverse, AA. Moreover, the number of successful naloxone antagonisms of AA far exceeds the number of failures (28 successes versus 7 failures).

2. Skeptics state that naloxone antagonism is necessary but not sufficient evidence (Hayes et al., 1977). That is why we have presented 17 different lines of evidence.

3. Some skeptics attack animal studies of AA as being unrelated to AA in humans (Chapman et al., 1983). First, there have been numerous experiments in humans, which have had the same AA-endorphin outcome as in lower animals. Second, the similarity of results across many species proves the generality of the phenomenon.

Third, there is no proper objective measure of pain in man. Fourth, if skeptics are correct, then the entire animal "pain" literature should be discarded, a literature which gave us our initial insights into endorphins, brain stimulation analgesia, TENS, and other results that have been highly applicable to human pain.

4. Some skeptics are concerned that AA in animals may merely be stress-induced analgesia (which also releases endorphins) and hence has nothing to do with acupuncture in humans (Chapman et al., 1983). At a conference on stress-induced analgesia at the New York Academy of Sciences we gave a lecture entitled "Relation of stress-induced analgesia to acupuncture analgesia." Some of the points made in that paper (Pomeranz, 1985) were:

• Sham electroacupuncture on nearby nonacupuncture points in animals induces no AA, thus controlling for stress (Chan & Fung, 1975; Cheng et al., 1980; Fung et al., 1975; Fung & Chan, 1976; Liao et al., 1979; Pomeranz & Chiu, 1976; Takeshige, 1985; Toda & Ichioka, 1978).

• AA elicited in anesthetized rats and cats, or decerebrate cats, does not involve psychological stress (Chan & Fung, 1975; Fung et al., 1975; Fung & Chan, 1976; Peets & Pomeranz, 1987; Pomeranz, 1988; Pomeranz, 1979; Pomeranz, 1986; Pomeranz & Warma, 1988; Pomeranz et al., 1977; Toda & Ichioka, 1978).

• AA at one frequency is endorphin mediated, while at another it is seratonin mediated, yet both give similar levels of stress (Cheng et al., 1980; Sjolund & Erikson, 1979).

• Many mechanisms of stress analgesia are very different from those of AA.

- Results in mice and rats were obtained with mild stimulation activating A beta nerve fibers, a nonpainful procedure which is no more stressful than sham point stimulation (Peets & Pomeranz, 1985; Pomeranz & Paley, 1979; Toda & Ichioka, 1978).

In conclusion, overwhelming evidence supports the acupuncture analgesia-endorphin hypothesis.

ACUPUNCTURE POINTS (DO THEY REALLY EXIST?)

The question of the existence of acupuncture points has been explored in several ways:

- By comparing the effects of needling at true points versus sham points
- By studying the unique anatomical structures at acupoints
- By studying the electrical properties of skin at acupoints
- By studying the nerves being activated by acupuncture at acupoints

Does needling at true points work better than needling at sham points? Several experimenters have shown, for acute laboratory-induced pain in human subjects, that needling of true points produces marked analgesia while needling of sham points produces very weak effects (Brockhaus & Elger, 1990; Chapman, Chen, & Bonica, 1977; Stacher et al., 1975). These results were clear-cut because effects elicited by sham point stimulation are nonexistent in acute laboratory pain (placebo pills also have poor efficacy in acute pain, causing analgesia in only 3% of cases).

In contrast to these clear-cut results, the work on chronic pain patients has been less convincing. As mentioned earlier, placebo analgesia in chronic pain has a strong effect, working in 30–35% of patients. Moreover, needling in sham points seems to work in about 33–50% of patients, while true points are effective in about 55–85% of cases (Vincent & Richardson, 1986). Therefore, to show statistical significance in the differences between sham-point needling and true-point needling requires huge numbers of patients (at least 122 per study), and experiments that would allow definitive conclusions have not yet been done (Vincent & Richardson, 1986).

It is puzzling that sham acupuncture works in 33–50% of patients with chronic pain, while not working at all in acute laboratory-induced pain. Because of these problems, the specificity of acupoints has only been shown in acute pain studies in humans but has yet to be properly studied in patients with chronic pain, where the number of patients studied has never exceeded the required statistical minimum of 122 (Vincent & Lewith, 1995).

In animal studies in mouse (Pomeranz & Chiu, 1976), cat (Chan & Fung, 1975; Fung & Chan, 1976), horse (Cheng et al., 1980), rat (Takeshige, 1985; Toda & Ichioka, 1978), and rabbit (Fung et al., 1975; Liao et al., 1979), many researchers have shown that true acupuncture works better than sham needling in acute pain studies. These results are consistent with the research on acute pain in humans. It is important in such studies to use mild stimulation in awake animals to avoid inducing stress; strong stimulation of sham sites could cause stress-induced analgesia (Pomeranz, 1985). Stress analgesia is a well-documented phenomenon (Madden et al., 1977) and is often mediated by endorphins. If the stimulation used is very strong, animals are highly stressed by both true- and sham-point needling.

Hence, numerous studies on acute pain in animals and humans clearly demonstrate that

AA from needling true points is far superior to AA from needling sham points. However, more studies are needed on chronic pain to see whether true points are more effective than sham points.

In sum, although much needs to be accomplished, the emergence of plausible mechanisms for the therapeutic effects of acupuncture is encouraging. The introduction of acupuncture into the choices of treatment modalities that are readily available to the public is in its early stages. Issues of training, licensure, and reimbursement remain to be clarified. There is sufficient evidence, however, of acupuncture's value to expand its use into conventional medicine and to encourage further studies of its physiology and clinical value.

REFERENCES

Abrams SE, Reynolds AC, Cusick JF. Failure of naloxone to reverse analgesia from TENS in patients with chronic pain. *Anesth Analg*. 1981;60:81–84.

Avants SK, et al. A randomized controlled trial of auricular acupuncture for cocaine dependence. *Arch Intern Med*. 2000;160:2305–2312.

Barber J, Mayer DJ. Evaluation of the efficacy and neural mechanism of a hypnotic analgesia procedure in experimental and clinical dental pain. *Pain*. 1977; 4:41–48.

Beecher HK. Placebo analgesia in human volunteers. *JAMA*. 1955;159:1602–1606.

Bing Z, Le Bars D, et al. Acupuncture-like stimulation induces a heterosegmental release of Met-enkephalin-like material in the rat spinal cord. *Pain*. 1991;47: 71–77.

Boureau P, Willer JC, Yamaguchi Y. Abolition par la naloxone de l'effect inhibiteur d'une stimulation électrique péripherique sur la composante tardive du reflex clignement. *EEG Clin Neurophysiol*. 1979; 47:322–328.

Brockhaus A, Elger CE. Hypalgesic efficacy of acupuncture on experimental pain in men. Comparison of laser acupuncture and needle acupuncture. *Pain*. 1990;43:181–185.

Chan SHH, Fung SJ. Suppression of polysynaptic reflex by electroacupuncture and a possible underlying presynaptic mechanism in the spinal cord of the cat. *Exp Neurol*. 1975;48:336–342.

Chapman CR, Benedetti C. Analgesia following TENS and its partial reversal by a narcotic antagonist. *Life Sci*. 1977;21:1645–1648.

Chapman CR, Benedetti C, et al. Naloxone fails to reverse pain thresholds elevated by acupuncture: acupuncture analgesia reconsidered. *Pain*. 1983;16: 13–31.

Chapman CR, Chen AC, Bonica JJ. Effects of intrasegmental electrical acupuncture on dental pain: evaluation by threshold estimation and sensory decision theory. *Pain*. 1977;3:213–227.

Chapman CR, Colpitts YM, et al. Evoked potential assessment of neupuncture analgesia: attempted reversal with naloxone. *Pain*. 1980;9:183–197.

Charlton G. Naloxone reverses electroacupuncture analgesia in experimental dental pain. *South Afri J Sci*. 1982;78:80–81.

Chen XH, Geller EB, et al. Electrical stimulation at traditional acupuncture sites in periphery produces brain opioid-receptor-mediated antiociceptin in rats. *J Pharm Exper Ther*. 1996;277:654–660.

Chen XH, Han JS. All three types of opioid receptors in the spinal cord are important for 2/15 Hg electroacupuncture analgesia. *Eur J Pharmacol*. 1992; 211:203–210.

Cheng R, Pomeranz B. Electroacupuncture analgesia is mediated by stereospecific opiate receptors and is reversed by antagonists of type 1 receptors. *Life Sci*. 1979;26:631–639.

Cheng R, Pomeranz B. A combined treatment with D-amino acids and electroacupuncture produces a greater anesthesia than either treatment alone: naloxone reverses these effects. *Pain*. 1980a;8: 231–236.

Cheng R, Pomeranz B. Electroacupuncture analgesia could be mediated by at least two pain-relieving mechanisms: endorphin and nonendorphin systems. *Life Sci*. 1980b;25:1957–1962.

Cheng RS, Pomeranz B, Yu G. Dexamethasone partially reduces and 2% saline treatment abolishes electroacupuncture analgesia: these findings implicate pituitary endorphins. *Life Sci*. 1979;24: 1481–1486.

Cheng R, Pomeranz B, et al. Electroacupuncture elevates blood cortisol levels in naive horses: sham treatment has no effect. *Int J Neurosci*. 1980; 10:95–97.

Chou J, Tang J, Yang HY, Costa E. Action of peptidase inhibitors on methionine5-enkephalin-arginine-phenylalanine7 (YGGFMRF) and methionine5-enkephalin (YGGFM) metabolism and on electroacupuncture antiociception. *J Pharmacol Exp Ther.* 1984;230:349–352.

Chung JM, Willis WD, et al. Prolonged naloxone-reversible inhibition of the flexion reflex in the cat. *Pain.* 1983;15:35–53.

Ehrenpreis S. Analgesic properties of enkephalinase inhibitors: animal and human studies. *Prog Clin Biol Res.* 1985;192:363–370.

Facchinetti F, Nappi G, et al. Primary headaches: reduced circulating beta-lipotropin and beta-endorphin levels with impaired reactivity to acupuncture. *Cephalalgia.* 1981;1:195–201.

Fu TC, Halenda SP, Dewey WL. The effect of hypophysectomy on acupuncture analgesia in the mouse. *Brain Res.* 1980;202:33–39.

Fujishita M, Hisantsu M, Takeshige C. Difference between non-acupuncture point stimulation and AA after D-phenylalanine treatment [in Japanese]. In: Takeshige C, ed. *Studies on the Mechanism of Acupuncture Analgesia Based Animal Experiments.* Tokyo, Japan: Showa University Press; 1986:638.

Fung DTH, Chan SHH, et al. Electroacupuncture suppression of jaw depression reflex elicited by dentalgia in rabbits. *Exp Neurol.* 1975;47:367–369.

Fung SF, Chan SHH. Primary afferent depolarization evoked by electroacupuncture in the lumbar cord of the cat. *Exp Neurol.* 1976;52:168–176.

Goldstein A, Hilgard EF. Failure of the opiate antagonist naloxone to modify hypnotic analgesia. *Proc Natl Acad Sci USA.* 1975;72:2041–2043.

Guo HF, Cui X, et al. C-Fos proteins are not involved in the activation of preproenkephalin gene expression in rat brain by peripheral electric stimulation (electroacupuncture). *Neurosci Lett.* 1996;207:163–166.

Guo HF, Tian J, et al. Brain substrates activated by electroacupuncture (EA) of different frequencies (II): role of Fos/Jun proteins in EA-induced transcription of preproenkephalin and preprodynorphin genes. *Brain Res Mol Brain Res.* 1996;43:167–173.

Ha H, Tan EC, Fukunaga H, Aochi D. Naloxone reversal of acupuncture analgesia in the monkey. *Exp Neurol.* 1981;73:298–303.

Hachisu M, Takeshige C, et al. Abolishment of individual variation in effectiveness of acupuncture analgesia [in Japanese]. In: Takeshige C, ed. *Studies on the Mechanism of Acupuncture Analgesia Based Animal Experiments.* Tokyo, Japan: Showa University Press; 1986:549.

Han JS, Ding XZ, Fen SG. Is cholecystokinin octapeptide (CCK-8) a candidate for endogenous antiopioid substrates? *Neuropeptides.* 1985;5:399–402.

Han JS, Li SJ, Tang J. Tolerance to acupuncture and its cross-tolerance to morphine. *Neuropharmacology.* 1981;20:593–596.

Han JS, Terenius L, et al. Effect of low- and high-frequency TENS on niet-enkephalin-arg-phe and dynorphin A immunoreactivity in human lumbar CSF. *Pain.* 1991;47:295–298.

Han JS, Xie GX. Dynorphin: important mediator for electroacupuncture analgesia in the spinal cord of the rabbit. *Pain.* 1984;18:367–377.

Han JS, Xie GX, Terenius L, et al. Enkephalin and beta endorphin as mediators of electroacupuncture analgesia in rabbits: an antiserum microinjection study. In: Costa E, ed. *Regulatory Peptides: From Molecular Biology to Function.* New York, NY: Raven; 1982:369–377.

Hardebo JE, Ekmin R, Eriksson M. Low CSF Met-enkephalin levels in cluster headache are elevated by acupuncture. *Headache.* 1989;29:494–497.

Hayes R, Price DD, Dubner R. Naloxone antagonism as evidence for narcotic mechanisms. *Science.* 1977;196:600.

He L, Le R, Zhuang S, et al. Possible involvement of opioid peptides of caudate nucleus in acupuncture analgesia. *Pain.* 1985;23:83–93.

He LF, Doug WQ, Wang MZ. Effects of iontophoretic etorphine, naloxone and electroacupuncture on nociceptive responses from thalamic neurones in rabbits. *Pain.* 1991;44:89–95.

Herget HF, L'Allemand H, et al. Combined acupuncture analgesia and controlled respiration. A new modified method of anesthesia in open heart surgery. *Anaesthesist.* 1976;25:223–230.

Hishida F, Takeshige C, et al. Effects of D-phenylalanine on individual variation of analgesia and on analgesia inhibitory system in their separated experimental procedures [in Japanese]. In: Takeshige C, ed. *Studies on the Mechanism of Acupuncture Analgesia Based Animal Experiments.* Tokyo, Japan: Showa University Press; 1986:51.

Ho UK, Hen HL. Opioid-like activity in the cerebrospinal fluid of pain patients treated by electroacupuncture. *Neuropharmacology.* 1989;28:961–966.

Kho HG, Eijk RI, et al. Acupuncture and transcutaneous stimulation analgesia in comparison with moderate-dose fentanyl anesthesia in major surgery.

Clinical efficacy and influence on recovery and morbidity. *Anesthesia.* 1991;46:129–135.

Kiser RS, Khatam MJ, et al. Acupuncture relief of chronic pain syndrome correlates with increased plasma met-enkephalin concentrations. *Lancet.* 1983;2:1394–1396.

Kishioka S, Miyamoto Y, et al. Effects of a mixture of peptidase inhibitors of met-enkephalin, beta-endorphin, dynorphin (1–13) and electroacupuncture induced antinociception in rats. *Jpn J Pharm.* 1994;66:337–345.

Lagerweij E, Van Ree J, et al. The twitch in horses: a variant of acupuncture. *Science.* 1984;225:1172–1173.

Lee JH, Beitz AJ. The distribution of brain-stem and spinal nuclei associated with different frequencies of electroacupuncture analgesia. *Pain.* 1993;52: 11–28.

Lee JH, Beitz AJ. Electroacupuncture modifies the expression of c-fos in the spinal cord induced by noxious stimulation. *Brain Res.* 1992;577:80–91.

Lee Peng CH, Yang MMP, et al. Endorphin release: a possible mechanism of AA. *Comp Med East West.* 1978;6:57–60.

Liao SJ. Recent advances in the understanding of acupuncture. *Yale J Biol Med.* 1978;51:55–65.

Liao YY, Seto K, Seito H, et al. Effect of acupuncture on adrenocortical hormone production: variation in the ability for adrenocortical hormone production in relation to the duration of acupuncture stimulation. *Am J Chin Med.* 1979;7:362–371.

Lung CH, Sun AC, Tsao CJ, et al. An observation of the humoral factor in acupuncture analgesia in rats. *Am J Chin Med.* 1978;2:203–205.

Madden J, Akil H, Barchas JD, et al. Stress-induced parallel changes in central opioid levels and pain responsiveness in rat. *Nature.* 1977;265:358–360.

Malizia E, Andreucci G, Paolucci D, et al. Electroacupuncture and peripheral beta-endorphin and ACTH levels. *Lancet.* 1979;2:535–536.

Masala A, Satta G, Alagna S, et al. Suppression of electroacupuncture (EA)-induced beta-endorphin and ACTH release by hydrocortisone in man. Absence of effects on EA-induced anaesthesia. *Acta Endocrinol (Copenh).* 1983;103:469–472.

Mayer DJ, Price DD, Raffii A. Antagonism of acupuncture analgesia in man by the narcotic antagonist naloxone. *Brain Res.* 1977;121:368–372.

Murai M, Takeshige C, et al. Correlation between individual variations in effectiveness of acupuncture analgesia and that in contents of brain endogenous morphine-like factors [in Japanese]. In: Takeshige C,

ed. *Studies on the Mechanism of Acupuncture Analgesia Based Animal Experiments.* Tokyo, Japan: Showa University Press; 1986:542.

Nappi G, Faccinetti F, et al. Different releasing effects of traditional manual acupuncture and electroacupuncture on propiocortin-related peptides. *Acupunct Electrother Res Int J.* 1982;7:93–103.

Peets J, Pomeranz B. Acupuncture-like transcutaneous electrical nerve stimulation analgesia is influenced by spinal cord endorphins but not serotonin: an intratheral pharmacological study. In: Fields H, et al., eds. *Advances in Pain Research and Therapy.* New York, NY: Raven; 1985:519–525.

Peets J, Pomeranz B. CXB mice deficient in opiate receptors show poor electroacupuncture analgesia. *Nature.* 1978;273:675–676.

Peets J, Pomeranz B. Studies in suppression of nocifensive reflexes measured with tail flick electromyograms and using intrathecal drugs in barbiturate anaesthetized rats. *Brain.* 1987;416:301–307.

Pert A, Dionne R, Ng L, Pert C, et al. Alterations in rat central nervous system endorphins following transauricular electroacupuncture. *Brain Res.* 1981;224: 83–93.

Pertovaara A, Kemppainen P, et al. Dental analgesia produced by non-painful, low-frequency stimulation is not influenced by stress or reversed by naloxone. *Pain.* 1982;13:379–384.

Pomeranz B. Relation of stress-induced analgesia to acupuncture analgesia. In: Kelly DD, ed. *Stress-Induced Analgesia.* New York, NY: New York Academy of Science; 1985:1444–1447.

Pomeranz B, Bibic L. Naltroxone, an opiate antagonist, prevents but does not reverse the analgesia produced by electroacupuncture. *Brain Res.* 1988; 452:227–231.

Pomeranz B, Cheng R. Suppression of noxious responses in single neurons of cat spinal cord by electroacupuncture and its reversal by the opiate antagonist naloxone. *Exp Neurol.* 1979;64:327–341.

Pomeranz B, Cheng R, Law P. Acupuncture reduces electrophysiological and behavioural responses to noxious stimuli: pituitary is implicated. *Exp Neurol.* 1977;54:172–178.

Pomeranz B, Chiu D. Naloxone blocks acupuncture analgesia and causes hyperalgesia: endorphin is implicated. *Life Sci.* 1976;19:1757–1762.

Pomeranz B, Nyguyen P. Intrathecal diazepam suppresses nociceptive reflexes and potentiates electroacupuncture effects in pentobarbital rats. *Neurosci Lett.* 1986;77:316–320.

Pomeranz B, Paley D. Electroacupuncture hyalgesia is mediated by afferent nerve impulses: an electrophysiological study in mice. *Exp Neurol.* 1979;66: 398–402.

Pomeranz B, Stux G. *Scientific Bases of Acupuncture.* Berlin, Germany: Springer; 1989.

Pomeranz B, Warma N. Potentiation of analgesia by two repeated electroacupuncture treatments: the first opioid analgesia potentiates a second non-opioid analgesia response. *Brain Res.* 1988;452:232–236.

Research Group Peking Med Coll. The role of some neurotransmitters of brain in finger acupuncture analgesia. *Sci Sin.* 1974;17:112–130.

Roy BP, Cheng R, Pomeranz B, et al. Pain threshold and brain endorphin levels in genetically obese ob/ob and opiate receptor deficient CXBK mice. In: E. Leong Way, ed. *Exogenous and Endogenous Opiate Agonists and Antagonists.* New York: Pergamon Press; 1980:297.

Sato T, Takeshige C. Morphine analgesia caused by activation of spinal acupuncture afferent pathway in the anterolateral tract [in Japanese]. In: Takeshige C, ed. *Studies on the Mechanism of Acupuncture Analgesia Based Animal Experiments.* Tokyo, Japan: Showa University Press; 1986:673.

Shimizu S, Takeshige C, et al. Relationship between endogenous morphine-like factor and serotonergic system in analgesia of acupuncture anesthesia [in Japanese]. In: Takeshige C, ed. *Studies on the Mechanism of Acupuncture Analgesia Based Animal Experiments.* Tokyo, Japan: Showa University Press; 1986:700.

Shimizu T, Koja T, et al. Effects of methysergide and naloxone on analgesia produced by peripheral electrical stimulation in mice. *Brain Res.* 1981;208: 463–467.

Sjolund B, Terenius L, Eriksson M. Increased cerebrospinal fluid levels of endorphins after electroacupuncture. *Acta Physiol Scand.* 1977;100: 382–384.

Sjolund BH, Erikson BE. The influence of naloxone on analgesia produced by peripheral conditioning stimulation. *Brain Res.* 1979;173:295–301.

Sodipo JG, Gilly H, Pauser G. Endorphins: mechanism of acupuncture analgesia. *Am J Chin Med.* 1981;9:249–258.

Stacher G, Wancura I, et al. Effect of acupuncture on pain threshold and pain tolerance determined by electrical stimulation of the skin: a controlled study. *Am J Chin Med.* 1975;3:143–146.

Stux G, Hammerschlag R. *Clinical Acupuncture Scientific Basis.* Berlin, Germany: Springer; 2001.

Takagi J, Sawada T, et al. A possible involvement of monoaminergic and opioidergic systems in the analgesia induced by electroacupuncture in rabbits. *Jpn J Pharm.* 1996;70:73–80.

Takahashi G, Mera H, Kobori M. Inhibitory action on analgesic inhibitory system and augmenting action on naloxone reversal analgesia of D-phenylalanine [in Japanese]. In: Takeshige C, ed. *Studies on the Mechanism of Acupuncture Analgesia Based Animal Experiments.* Tokyo, Japan: Showa University Press; 1986:608.

Takeshige C. Differentiation between acupuncture and non-acupuncture points by association with an analgesia inhibitory system. *Acupunct Electrother Res.* 1985;10:195–203.

Takeshige C, Kobori M, et al. Analgesia inhibitory system involvement in nonacupuncture point stimulation produced analgesia. *Brain Res Bull.* 1992;28: 379–391.

Takeshige C, Nakamura A, et al. Positive feedback action of pituitary beta-endorphin on acupuncture analgesia afferent pathway. *Brain Res Bull.* 1992;29: 37–44.

Takeshige C, Oka K, et al. The acupuncture point and its connecting central pathway for producing acupuncture analgesia. *Brain Res Bull.* 1993;30: 53–67.

Takeshige C, Tsuchiya M, et al. Dopminergic transmission in the arcuate nucleus to produce acupuncture analgesia in correlation with the pituitary gland. *Brain Res Bull.* 1991;26:113–122.

Takeshige C, Zhao WH, Guo SY. Convergence from the preoptic area and arcuate nucleus to the median eminence in acupuncture and nonacupuncture stimulation analgesia. *Brain Res Bull.* 1991;26: 771–778.

Tay AA, Tseng CK, Pace NL, et al. Failure of narcotic antagonist to alter electroacupuncture modification of halothane anaesthesia in the dog. *Can Anaesth Soc J.* 1982;29:231–235.

Thoren P, Floras JS, et al. Endorphins and exercise: physiological mechanisms and clinical implications. *Med Sci Sports Exerc.* 1989;22:417–428.

Toda K, Ichioka M. Electroacupuncture: relations between forelimb afferent impulses and suppression of jaw opening reflex in the rat. *Exp Neurol.* 1978; 61:465–470.

Tsunoda Y, Ikezonu E, et al. Antagonism of acupuncture analgesia by naloxone in unconscious men. *Null Tokyo Med Dent.* 1980;27:89–94.

Vacca-Galloway LL, et al. Alterations of immunoreactive substance P and enkephalins in rat spinal cord after electroacupuncture. *Peptides*. 1985;6(Suppl 1):177–188.

Vincent C, Lewith G. Placebo controls for acupuncture studies. *J R Sec Med*. 1995;88:199–202.

Vincent CA, Richardson PH. The evaluation of therapeutic acupuncture: concepts and methods. *Pain*. 1986;24:1–13.

Walker JB, Katz RL. Non-opioid pathways suppress pain in humans. *Pain*. 1981;11:347–354.

Wall PD. Acupuncture revisited. *New Sci*. 1974:31–34.

Wall PD. An eye on the needle. *New Sci*. 1972: 129–131.

Wang Q, Mao L, Han J. The arcuate nucleus of hypothalamus mediates low- but not high-frequency electroacupuncture in rats. *Brain Res*. 1990a;513:60–66.

Wang Q, Mao L, Han J. The role of periaqueductal grey in mediation of analgesia produced by different frequencies of electroacupuncture stimulation in rats. *Int J Neurosci*. 1990b;53:167–172.

Watkins LR, Mayer DJ. Organization of endogenous opiate and non-opiate pain control systems. *Science* 1982;216:1185–1192.

Willer JC, Boureau F, et al. Comparative effects of EA and TENS on the human blink reflex. *Pain*. 1982; 14:267–278.

Woolf CJ, Barrett G, et al. Naloxone reversible peripheral electroanalgesia in intact and spinal rats. *Eur J Pharmacol*. 1977;451:311–314.

Woolf CJ, Mitchell D, et al. Failure of naloxone to reverse peripheral TENS analgesia in patients suffering from trauma. *S Afr Med J*. 1978;53: 179–180.

Xie GX, Han JS, Hollt V. Electroacupuncture analgesia blocked by microinjection of anti-beta-endorphin antiserum into periaqueductal grey of the rabbit. *Int J Neurosci*. 1983;18:287–291.

Xue JI, Yu YX, et al. Changes in the content of immunoreactive dynorphin in dorsal and ventral spinal cord of the rat in three different conditions. *Int J Neurosci*. 1995;82:95–104.

Yang ZL, Cai TW, Wu JL. Acupuncture and emotion: the influence of acupuncture anesthesia on the sensory and emotional components of pain. *J Gen Psychol*. 1989;116:247–258.

Zao FY, Han JS, et al. Acupuncture analgesia in impacted last molar extraction. Effect of clomipramine and pargyline. In: Han JS, ed. *The Neurochemical Basis of Pain Relief by Acupuncture: A Collection of Papers 1973–1989*. Beijing, China: Beijing Medical Science; 1987:96–97.

Zheng M, Yang SG, Zou B. Electroacupuncture markedly increases proenkephalin mRNA in rat striatun and pituitary. *Sci Sin*. 1988;B31:81–86.

Zhou ZF, Du MY, Han JS, et al. Effect of intracerebral microinjection of naloxone on acupuncture- and morphine-analgesia in the rabbit. *Sci Sin*. 1981; 24:1166–1178.

Zou K, Yi QC, Wu SX, Lu YX, et al. Enkephalin involvement in acupuncture analgesia. *Sci Sin*. 1980;23:1197–1207.

CHAPTER 43

Referring Patients to Acupuncture

Efrem Korngold, OMD, LAc

INDICATIONS FOR REFERRAL AND CONTRAINDICATIONS

Reviews of conditions benefited by acupuncture have been performed by consensus panels of both the National Institutes of Health and the World Health Organization. For a summary of these conditions, see the overview, Chapter 38.

Major contraindications for acupuncture include the following:

THE PATIENT'S EXPERIENCE

Treatment. Most people experience acupuncture as pleasant, even pleasurable and many fall asleep during treatment. When the treatment session is completed, patients often report feeling very relaxed and/or energized.

Experience of the needles. Acupuncture needles are extremely fine (the thickness of a strand of hair), so minimal pain accompanies insertion. The needle itself goes unnoticed or feels like a small pinch accompanied by warmth, tingling, numbness, ache, or heaviness at the site. These sensations are not only common but desirable, indicating that the Qi is present. This is the vital power that animates all life functions. Sensations may occur around the acupuncture point and along the channel of which it is a part or possibly in areas of the body far from the point of insertion.

A brief biography of Efrem Korngold appears in Chapter 38.

Response to treatment is highly individual. A sense of well-being and relaxation is usual, as is an elevation of mood. Research shows that feelings of relaxation are experienced by as many as 86% of patients (Ernst & White, 2001). Following acupuncture treatment, many patients wish to continue resting, while others report feeling energized. In some cases, this sense of invigoration is delayed until the days following treatment. Most people are relieved to find that treatments are not especially uncomfortable and, in fact, look forward to the experience (Beinfield & Korngold, 1991).

Extent of treatment. The duration and frequency of treatment may vary, since each person's health is a unique riddle to be solved. Some require only a few sessions, while others need the accumulated benefit of weeks or months of treatment. This depends on factors such as the severity of the complaint, how long the person has experienced symptoms, and the extent to which lifestyle exacerbates the condition. A session lasts approximately an hour and is scheduled as often as every day or as little as once or twice a month. As symptoms improve, fewer visits are required, individual progress being the yardstick (Beinfield & Korngold, 1991).

By the end of the acupuncture session, some of the patient's presenting symptoms may be diminished or even gone within the course of the hour or by the time they return home. Improvement may continue in the days following an acupuncture treatment, but the rate

Table 43–1 Acupuncture Contraindications and Cautions

Contraindications in use of acupuncture:
- When inebriated
- When there is evidence or suspicion of overdose of psychotropic drugs, opiate analgesics, or barbiturates
- In any type of brain trauma, stroke, or concussion during the first 48 hours. Acupuncture is quite beneficial following a stroke, once the condition has stabilized.
- Acute poisoning
- Any condition in which the individual is suddenly unconscious

Contraindications in the use of electroacupuncture:
- Pregnancy
- Individuals who have a cardiac pacemaker or some other electronic device attached to or within their bodies
- Individuals who are highly sensitive may prefer traditional acupuncture.

Caution in the use of traditional acupuncture:
- Highly sensitive, unstable individuals, or those who are nervous about or frightened of acupuncture needles
- Individuals who are extremely upset emotionally or have suffered a sudden emotional or physical trauma
- During pregnancy, especially in the first and third trimesters
- Immune compromised patients for whom there is increased risk of infection

Caution in the use of electroacupuncture:
- Individuals with cardiac arrhythmias
- Individuals suffering from epilepsy or other seizure disorders
- Individuals with sensory deficits (as in diabetic neuropathy, multiple sclerosis, or paralysis)

Courtesy of Efrem Korngold, OMD, LAc, San Francisco, CA.

---

at which that occurs for an individual is not predictable. In some cases, symptoms may appear aggravated for a day or two, after which the patient improves and feels better than before the treatment. Others may not feel any change, but gradually, over the course of a series of treatments, discover that their symptoms or complaints have diminished or disappeared altogether. Sometimes, a person's original complaints are replaced by newer or even earlier ones, but these tend to be milder in nature. It is also common for patients to improve so gradually, they only realize the magnitude of their improvement in hindsight, after they review how they felt when they first came for treatment.

Assessment. Traditional modes of assessment include the qualities of the pulse, the appearance of the tongue, the overall color and vibrancy of the person's complexion, the quality of the voice, and how he carries himself. Does he look tired and collapsed or is his bearing upright and lively? Assessment involves broad observation and examination of the general and specific aspects of the patient's physical, mental, and emotional character and behavior. Contemporary acupuncturists also incorporate information derived from modern diagnostic methods such as lab tests, imaging studies, and postoperative reports, as well as EKG and EEG studies. For example, under California law, licensed acupuncturists are permitted to request lab tests in the same manner as MDs, DOs, DCs, DPMs, and DDSs, although this may differ from state to state. It is also quite common for licensed acupuncturists to request copies of the results of diagnostic tests and studies from other providers. Well-educated and well-trained acupuncturists tend to use all of the traditional and contemporary assessment tools at their disposal.

Most practitioners favor direct observation of the patient, which is the basis of Chinese traditional medicine. Others use electronic instruments for measuring physiological changes such as the Voll machine (EAV), developed in Germany in the 1970s. These instruments measure electrical resistance and/or conductivity at specific acupuncture points. We know from many years of physiological research that acupuncture points are characterized by distinct areas of low electrical resistance compared to other areas of the skin's surface. Voll's model adapts the meridian theory to a Western model of diagnosis using such instrumentation. While it assesses information using the acupuncture points, it does not apply the physiological paradigm or treatment that has developed within the historical tradition of Chinese medicine. Applied Kinesiology (AK) is another practice based on the meridian theory of Chinese medicine, but adapted to a Western chiropractic model of neuromuscular systems and interactions.

One approach to electroacupuncture diagnosis and treatment is to compare one side of the body to the other in terms of skin resistance at a given point. The principle is to equalize the bioelectric current in the body between the right and the left side. This is one among many modern and effective acupuncture methodologies.

Possible Short-Term Side Effects

- Acupuncture syncope—This is one of the side effects that occurs, although rarely, in a small percentage of sensitive patients who faint or swoon during or following needle insertion. Feelings of faintness and syncope are uncommon, with a reported incidence of 0% to 0.3% (Ernst & White, 2001). This type of physiological reaction typically triggers a sudden drop in blood pressure. When people are overtired, in a weakened condition, too hungry, or too nervous, they are more susceptible to this reaction. Consequently, it is generally best for patients to lie down when receiving treatment. There are, however, effective techniques for reviving a patient if a syncope reaction occurs.
- Bruising—Small hematomas and bruising can result from the puncture of a small vein or capillary by the acupuncture needle; this occurs in approximately 10% of cases.
- Momentary discomfort—Some degree of discomfort may occur when the needles are first inserted and includes sensations such as tingling, numbness, aching, swelling, itching, or burning. In the majority of cases these effects usually diminish or resolve quickly. When this occurs, it is helpful for the patient to communicate with the practitioner so the needles can be adjusted.
- Temporary irritation of peripheral nerves— Rarely, an acupuncture needle may puncture a small nerve, and this occurs in approximately 1% of cases. This can be accompanied by neuralgia in the form of mild local soreness and tingling; if a nerve in the wrist or ankle is affected, movement

will aggravate the discomfort. These injuries are rarely serious and typically resolve within two weeks.

- Collapsed lung—This is a serious injury and occurs in approximately one in a million acupuncture treatments. When it does occur, it is almost always due to a lack of training, experience, and prudence on the part of the practitioner.

OUTCOMES

Clinical outcomes. Acupuncture has an exceptional track record in the treatment of many disorders including acute and chronic illnesses, whether simple or complex. For additional information on clinical research, see the overview in Chapter 38, as well as Chapter 40 on research.

Long-term treatment. Long-term treatment usually refers to a course of acupuncture therapy that lasts more than 3 months. This is typical in the treatment of many longstanding conditions, from chronic lumbago to chronic colitis or arthritis, which may require a year or more of treatment to achieve optimum recovery. In some cases, symptom management and the retardation of a disease process or stabilization of health is a realistic expectation, for example, in conditions such as HIV/AIDS, cancer, multiple sclerosis, emphysema, ileitis, chronic fatigue or chronic postsurgical pain. This type of condition requires ongoing treatment for months or years with occasional "treatment holidays" along the way.

Self-care. One of the major traditions of Chinese medicine was the emphasis on prevention. A traditional doctor became closely affiliated with a particular community of people who were all potentially his patients. He learned enough about the health and the conditions of that community so that he or she

would intervene early to prevent individuals or groups from getting sick. Ideally he would be so successful, he would ultimately have little work to do, because he would have cultivated a healthy community that was essentially capable of caring for itself.

A preventive approach involves educating patients about what they can do for themselves to complement and enhance the effects of their treatment. Consider the situation of ulcer patients. While being treated with acupuncture, their condition is likely to improve. However, if they continue to eat the wrong foods or to indulge in behaviors that exacerbate their condition (for example, drinking coffee or alcohol, and/or eating spicy foods) the results of the acupuncture treatment will not be fully effective or lasting. To promote patient self-care, the practitioner must determine how to gain the cooperation of patients in changing the habits that contribute to their illness.

There are many things patients can do for themselves that can be beneficial. Some patients learn to perform simple acupressure techniques or moxibustion. Acupressure self-massage can help to relieve headaches, joint and muscle pain, constipation or indigestion, and even asthmatic wheezing. Indirect moxibustion with a "moxa stick," used once or twice daily, can be very helpful to patients suffering from muscle strains and sprains, the pain of osteoarthiritis, or from weakness and fatigue. Clearly the patient's efforts with diet and exercise can make an enormous difference. In addition, there are numerous home therapies that are safe and effective. For example, dry brushing of the skin is a technique that can be used to improve circulation. It is a simple technique that involves brushing the skin briskly with a natural bristle brush once, twice, or even three times a day. The skin is brushed until it feels invigorated and warm, and the color is pink. This is a good method for combating fatigue and improving the health of the skin itself. In essence, it is a way to stimulate all the acupuncture channels. Some people readily adopt this habit and enjoy it a great deal.

Insurance coverage. Approximately 20–30% of patients receive insurance reimbursement. Acupuncture is often paid for by workers' compensation plans and auto accident coverage. More and more HMOs and other third-party payers are reimbursing patients and/or practitioners for acupuncture treatment, although the categories of diagnoses and the number of treatments allowed are often limited. Blue Cross/Blue Shield, Prudential, Aetna, and some municipal employee health plans cover acupuncture to some extent. There are probably others as well, depending on the state and the policies.

Acupuncture referrals. Periodically a formal referral may be required for insurance coverage, in which case the licensed primary provider (MD, DO, ND, DC, DDS, or DPM) writes a requisition. Communication with regard to patient progress is made by mail, email, or telephone, and periodic updates are provided.

The majority of professional acupuncture organizations maintain a list of practitioners to whom patients can be referred. The NCCAOM Web site provides access to an updated list of practitioners who are nationally certified in acupuncture, Chinese herbal medicine, or Oriental body therapy. There are also several other Web sites that specialize in information and referrals for interested patients and health care providers. (For specific contact information, see Chapter 45 on Acupuncture Resources.)

REFERENCES

Beinfield H, Korngold E. *Between Heaven and Earth.* New York, NY: Ballantine Books; 1991.

Ernst E, White AR. Prospective studies of the safety of acupuncture: a systematic review. *Am J Med.* 2001; 110:481–485.

CHAPTER 44

Acupuncture Training for Physicians

American Board of Medical Acupuncture

OVERVIEW

Definitions of Medical Acupuncture

Medical acupuncture is a medical discipline having a central core of knowledge embracing the integration of acupuncture from various traditions into contemporary biomedical practice.

A physician acupuncturist is one who has acquired specialized knowledge and experience related to the integration of acupuncture within a biomedicine practice.

Education and Training in Medical Acupuncture

The World Health Organization and the World Federation of Acupuncture and Moxibustion Societies (WFAS) have promulgated acupuncture training and education standards for all acupuncture practitioners, including Western-trained physicians. Those standards were first adopted in Beijing,

China, in 1987 and reaffirmed at the WFAS conference in Milan, Italy, in 1996.

These standards are considered to reflect the minimum level of training necessary for acupuncturists and for Western-trained physicians to enter the practice of medical acupuncture. The WFAS standards (Section 4.2.1) state, "For licensed graduates of modern Western medical colleges, who already have had education and training in anatomy, physiology, neurology, and all the other basic and clinical sciences involved in medical diagnosis and treatment, training in acupuncture can be accomplished following a different training pathway for them to master acupuncture as a special medical modality. . . . The whole course should be devoted to acquiring the knowledge and skill in acupuncture as well as the related basic theory for at least 200 hours of formal training. By the end of the course the participants should be able to integrate acupuncture into their medical practices. The proficiency of training and practice should be evaluated through an official examination by health authorities to ensure safety, competence, and efficacy."

Note: The WFAS standards set training criteria for acupuncturists (non-medical), for other health care practitioners, and for Western trained physicians . . . most US states have training standards for licensed acupuncturists (2–3 years of full time study) that are closely based on the WFAS standards. The portion related to physicians is only one aspect of those standards.

The mission of the American Board of Medical Acupuncture is to promote safe, ethical, efficacious medical acupuncture to the public by maintaining high standards for the examination and certification of physician acupuncturists as medical specialists. Physicians and osteopaths who are candidates for certification in medical acupuncture must meet minimum requirements in education, training, and experience, and must successfully pass a board examination in order to acquire certification. At the time of this writing, the Amercian Academy of Medical Acupuncture lists more than 1800 members and the Board has certified more than 400 diplomates in acupuncture.

Courtesy of the American Board of Medical Acupuncture, Los Angeles, California.

The American Board of Medical Acupuncture (ABMA) has established standards of training and education that exceed those established by WFAS as the entry-level standards. The ABMA will not accept into the process of certification anyone who has not met the board's standards for training, education, and experience.

REQUIREMENTS FOR CERTIFICATION IN MEDICAL ACUPUNCTURE

Candidates for certification in medical acupuncture must meet minimum general requirements, education and training requirements, and experience requirements and must successfully pass the board examination in order to achieve certification.

General Requirements

1. Graduation from an accredited allopathic or osteopathic medical school in the United States or Canada, or possession of final certification by the Educational Commission for Foreign Medical Graduates (ECFMG) if graduated from a medical school in some other country.
2. Possession of a current, valid, unrestricted license to practice medicine or osteopathy in a state or jurisdiction of the United States or province of Canada.

Acupuncture Education and Training Requirements

1. Subsequent to graduation from medical school, the applicant must have satisfactorily completed a minimum of 300 hours of systematic acupuncture training acceptable to the ABMA. Such training shall include a formal course of study of not less than 200 hours in a program that meets the WFAS standards for such courses as determined by the ABMA.
2. At least 100 hours of the minimum 300 hours of training shall have been clinical training acceptable to the ABMA.
3. All training hours must be acupuncture-specific training.
4. Applicants should obtain a current list of ABMA-approved training programs by contacting the ABMA office or from the Board Web site.
    (See www.medicalacupuncture.org or the Resources at the end of the chapter.)
5. Applicants who have obtained training through means other than through an ABMA approved training course must have the Board review their training to determine acceptability in lieu of an approved course of study. Detailed information regarding the content and curriculum of the course, the faculty, and the teaching methodologies employed in addition to appropriate certificates documenting successful completion of said training must accompany the application. The Board, in its sole judgment, shall determine the acceptability of any such training, on a case-by-case basis.
6. For applicants who obtained training from programs not previously approved by the ABMA, the Board may determine that an oral interview of the applicant is necessary, in order for the Board to determine the adequacy of training.

Examination Requirements

1. Applicants who have submitted an application for certification documenting that the applicant has met the education requirement established by the ABMA will receive notice of eligibility to sit for the written board examination.

2. The written examination will be conducted in the spring each year and at such additional times during the year as may be determined by the Board.
3. Applicants who have passed the proficiency examination offered by the American Academy of Medical Acupuncture prior to May 15, 2000, have met the examination process requirement of the ABMA.

ACUPUNCTURE CERTIFICATION REQUIREMENTS

1. Applicants for certification must submit an affidavit attesting that the applicant has had a minimum of 2 years of medical acupuncture clinical experience subsequent to the completion of the basic 200-hour medical acupuncture training and an acupuncture case history of not less than 500 medical acupuncture treatments.
2. The Board reserves the right to require documentation sufficient to verify the applicant has provided the minimum medical acupuncture treatments.
3. Acupuncture practice should involve more than one of the following acupuncture paradigms, including but not limited to energetic acupuncture, neuroanatomic acupuncture, Five Elements, traditional Chinese medicine, auricular, scalp, or hand acupuncture.
4. Applicants for certification must provide confidential letters of reference from three physicians pertaining to the applicant's character, professionalism, and standards of clinical practice.

Certification

Upon approval of the application and the candidate's successful completion of the examination and completion of the clinical experience requirements, the ABMA will grant a certificate to the effect that the candidate has met the requirements of the Board. The recipient of a certificate will be known as a diplomate of the American Board of Medical Acupuncture (DABMA) and may use such title or initials in his or her professional name.

All certificates issued are time-limited, expiring on June 30th of the 10th year following the date issued. Recertification is available. A certificate granted by the ABMA does not of itself confer or purport to confer any degree or legal qualifications, privileges, or license to practice medical acupuncture. The ABMA does not limit or interfere with the professional activity of any duly licensed physician who is not certified by the board. Privileges granted physicians in the practice of medical acupuncture in any hospital or clinic are the prerogatives of that hospital or clinic, not of the Board. The names of diplomates of the American Board of Medical Acupuncture appear in the official roster of diplomates of the ABMA available from the Board office and on the Academy's Web site. (See the Resources section that follows.)

RESOURCES

Additional Information

For additional information about the American Board of Medical Acupuncture, board certification requirements and procedures, or a board certification application, please contact the ABMA Executive Office at the following location:

American Board of Medical Acupuncture
4929 Wilshire Boulevard, Suite 428
Los Angeles, California 90010
Phone: (323) 937-5514
Fax: (323) 937-0959
Email: jdowden@prodigy.net
Web site: www.medicalacupuncture.org

PHYSICIAN ACUPUNCTURE TRAINING PROGRAMS

Acupuncture Foundation of Canada Institute
Course: Medical Acupuncture: Level I & II
2131 Lawrence Ave. E., # 204
Scarborough, Ontario M1R 5G4 Canada
Phone: (416) 752-3988
Fax: (416) 752-4398
Web site: www.afcinstitute.com

Brigham Women's Hospital
Course: Clinical Acupuncture for Physicians
Division of Education and Training
Department of Radiology
PO Box 470617
Brookline Village, MA 02447-0617
Phone: (617) 525-7330
Fax: (617) 525-3320

McMaster University School of Medicine
Course: Contemporary Medical Acupuncture
  for Health Professionals
Department of Anesthesia, Office of Contin-
  uing Medical Education
1200 Main St. West
Hamilton, ON L8N 3Z5 Canada
Phone: (905) 521-2100, ext. 75175
Fax: (905) 523-1224
Email: acupuncturecourses@mcmaster.ca
Web site: www.acupuncturecourses.com

New York Medical College
Course: Acupuncture Training Program
Department of Community and Preventive
  Medicine

Munger Pavilion
Valhalla, NY 10595
Phone: (914) 594-4253
Fax: (914) 594-4576
Web site: www.nymc.edu/cpm

SUNY Downstate Medical Center
Course: Medical Acupuncture for Physicians
Office of Continuing Medical Education
450 Clarkson Ave., Box 1244
Brooklyn, NY 11203
Phone: (718) 270-2422
Fax (718) 270-4563
Email: ocme@downsate.edu
Web site: www.downstate.edu/ocme

University of California, Los Angeles
Course: Medical Acupuncture for Physicians
c/o Helms Medical Institute
2520 Milvia Street
Berkeley, CA 94704
Phone: (510) 649-8488
Fax: (510) 649-8692
Email: Phil@HMIeducation.com
Web site: www.HMIeducation.com

University of Miami
Course: The Art and Science of Acupuncture:
  Basic and Advanced
The General Acupuncture Research and
  Training Clinic
PO Box 016960 (D-79)
Miami, FL 33101
Phone: (305) 243-4751
Fax: (305) 243-3648
Web site: med.miami.edu/psychiatry/acu
  puncture.html

Wilson Memorial Regional Medical Center
Course: Acupuncture for Physicians
40 Arch Street
Johnson City, NY 13790
Phone: (607) 763-5334
Fax: (607) 763-5415

CHAPTER 45

Acupuncture Resources

Efrem Korngold and Michael Devitt

ACCREDITATION AND CERTIFICATION

Accreditation

Accreditation Commission for Acupuncture and Oriental Medicine (ACAOM)
Maryland Trade Center #3
7501 Greenway Center Drive, Suite 820
Greenbelt, MD 20770
Phone: (301) 313-0855
Fax: (301) 313-0912
Email: info@acaom.org
Web site: www.acaom.org

Many states require that the practitioner have training from an accredited institution. Schools of acupuncture are accredited by the ACAOM, a peer-review group recognized by the US Department of Education Council for Higher Education Accreditation and the Commission on Recognition of Postsecondary Accreditation. Formed in 1982 for the purpose of advancing the profession, the ACAOM has developed academic and clinical guidelines and core curriculum requirements for master's-level programs in acupuncture and Oriental medicine, as well as for doctorate-level programs. Information on the accreditation or candidacy status of any particular program can be obtained directly from the ACAOM.

Council of Colleges of Acupuncture and Oriental Medicine (CCAOM)
3909 National Drive, Suite 125
Burtonsville, MD 20866
Phone: (301) 476-7790
Fax: (301) 476-7792
Email: executivedirector@ccaom.org
Web site: www.ccaom.org

The CCAOM provides a list of accredited training programs and a course on clean-needle technique. Accreditation information is particularly important. For example, some states will not license practitioners who have been trained at institutions located outside the United States.

National Oriental Medicine Accreditation Agency (NOMAA)
3445 Pacific Coast Highway, Suite 300
Torrance, CA 90505
Phone: (213) 820-2045
Email: needle.drs@verizon.net
Web site: www.nomaa.org

Certification

National Certification Commission for Acupuncture and Oriental Medicine (NCCAOM)
11 Canal Center Plaza, Suite 300
Alexandria, VA 22314
Phone: (703) 548-9004

A brief biography of Efrem Korngold appears in Chapter 38.

Michael Devitt has worked for more than a decade in the field of publishing as a writer and editor. He is currently managing editor of *Acupuncture Today*, a monthly publication for the acupuncture and Oriental medicine profession, and their affiliated Web site *AcupunctureToday.com*.

Fax: (703) 548-9079
Email: info@nccaom.org
Web site: www.nccaom.org

The NCCAOM currently administers both written and practical certification examinations in acupuncture (more than 11,000 diplomates certified to date) and in Chinese herbology (3300 certified). Certification is also available in Oriental medicine (which combines acupuncture and Chinese herbology) and in Asian bodywork therapy. The Commission, founded in 1982, is a member of the National Organization for Competency Assurance and accredited by the National Commission for Certifying Agencies. At this writing, 42 states have practice standards in acupuncture and of those, more than 75% require NCCAOM certification. However, it is important to check the licensing requirements of each state regarding examinations and training requirements. A few states, such as California, provide their own examination or require additional testing on clinical competence.

American Academy of Medical Acupuncture
4929 Wilshire Boulevard, Suite 428
Los Angeles, CA 90010
Phone: (323) 937-5514
Fax: (323) 937-0959
Email: jdowden@prodigy.net
Web site: www.medicalacupuncture.org

The mission of the American Academy of Medical Acupuncture is to promote the integration of paradigms and methods from traditional and modern forms of acupuncture with Western medical training and thereby advance a more comprehensive approach to health care. Physicians and osteopaths who are candidates for certification in medical acupuncture must meet minimum requirements in education, training, and experience,

and must successfully pass a board examination in order to acquire certification. Specific information on prerequisites and training is available on the Academy's Web site. State law requirements for physician acupuncturists can be confirmed through the relevant state licensing agency, frequently the health department. At the time of this writing, the Academy lists more than 1800 members and has certified more than 300 diplomates in acupuncture.

PROFESSIONAL ORGANIZATIONS

Acupuncture and Oriental Medicine Alliance
6405 43rd Avenue Ct. NW, Suite B
Gig Harbor, WA 98335
Phone: (253) 851-6896
Fax: (253) 851-6883
Email: info@aomalliance.org
Web site: www.aomalliance.org

The AOM Alliance publishes a quarterly newsletter, sponsors an annual conference the first weekend of each May, and maintains a referral service of more than 10,000 state-licensed or national board-certified practitioners.

American Association of Oriental Medicine
    (AAOM)
PO Box 162340
Sacramento, CA 95816
Phone: (866) 455-7999 or (916) 451-6950
Email: info@aaom.org
Web site: www.aaom.org

The AAOM provides practitioner referrals over the phone and online, as well as information on malpractice insurance, HIPAA-office kits, patient brochures, a journal, and CEU opportunities.

Federation of Acupuncture and Oriental Medicine Regulatory Agencies (FAOMRA)
c/o Maryland Board of Acupuncture
4201 Patterson Avenue
Baltimore, MD 21215
Phone: (800) 530-2481 or (410) 764-4766
Email: contact@faomra.com
Web site: www.faomra.com

International Veterinary Acupuncture Society
PO Box 271395
Fort Collins, CO 80527-1395
Phone: (970) 266-0666
Fax: (970) 266-0777
Email: office@ivas.org
Web site: www.ivas.org

The International Veterinary Acupuncture Society (IVAS) is a nonprofit organization that provides training in veterinary acupuncture, supports research in this field, and sponsors an annual international conference.

National Acupuncture Detoxification Association (NADA)
PO Box 1927
Vancouver, WA 98668-1927
Phone: (360) 254-0186
Fax: (360) 260-8620
Email: nadaoffice@acudetox.com
Web site: www.acudetox.com

NADA is an international organization with more than 1200 active US members that conducts a training program for health professionals in acupuncture as an adjunctive treatment for addictions. Acupuncture detoxification is currently used worldwide in more than 2000 comprehensive addiction treatment programs. NADA sponsors an annual conference, publications, and a Web site.

RESEARCH

Medical Acupuncture Research Foundation (MARF)
Web site: www.medicalacupuncture.org/aama_marf/marf.html

The Medical Acupuncture Research Foundation (MARF) was founded in 1988 as a charitable, nonprofit organization that serves as the research arm of the American Academy of Medical Acupuncture to promote and support acupuncture research.

Medline/PubMed Biomedical Journal Literature
Web site: www.ncbi.nlm.nih.gov/PubMed

Medline/PubMed, a service of the NIH National Library of Medicine, includes more than 15 million searchable citations, abstracts, and links from biomedical journals, dating from 1967 to the present.

National Center for Complementary and Alternative Medicine (NCCAM)
Web site: http://nccam.nih.gov

The National Center for Complementary and Alternative Medicine (NCCAM) at the NIH, established by Congress in 1998, is dedicated to exploring complementary and alternative healing practices in the context of rigorous science and disseminating evidence-based information to the public and professionals.

Society for Acupuncture Research
Email: info@acupunctureresearch.org
Web site: www.acupunctureresearch.org

The Society is a nonprofit organization whose mission is to promote scientifically sound inquiries into the clinical efficacy, physiological mechanisms, patterns of use, and theoretical foundations of acupuncture, herbal therapy, and other modalities of Oriental medicine.

BOOKS AND BOOKSELLERS

Regulatory Information

Books on acupuncture law and regulatory issues are available through the National Acupuncture Foundation (NAF) at (800) 814-5956 and their Web site:
www.nation alacupuncturefoundation.org

Cohen MH. *Legal Issues in Integrative Medicine*. Gig Harbor, WA: National Acupuncture Foundation; 2005.

Mitchell B. *Acupuncture and Oriental Medicine Laws*. Gig Harbor, WA: National Acupuncture Foundation; 2005.

National Acupuncture Foundation. *Clean Needle Technique Manual*, 5th ed. Gig Harbor, WA: National Acupuncture Foundation; 2004. (Also available in Chinese and Korean.)

Overviews of Acupuncture

Beinfield H, Korngold E. *Between Heaven and Earth*. New York, NY: Ballantine Books; 1992.

Birch S, Felt B. *Understanding Acupuncture*. London, UK: Elsevier; 1999.

Cassidy C. *Contemporary Chinese Medicine and Acupuncture*. Philadelphia, PA: W. B. Saunders; 2002.

Kaptchuk T. *The Web That Has No Weaver: Understanding Chinese Medicine*. New York, NY: Congdon and Weed; 1992.

Kendall D. *Dao of Chinese Medicine: Understanding an Ancient Healing Art*. Oxford, UK: Oxford University Press; 2002.

Stux G, Berman B, Pomeranz B. *The Basics of Acupuncture*, 5th ed. New York, NY: Springer; 2003. (Written in the vocabu-

lary of Western medicine for physicians, acupuncturists, and medical students.)

Stux G, Hammerschlag R. eds. *Clinical Acupuncture: Scientific Basis*. Berlin, Germany: Springer-Verlag; 2000.

General References

Birch S, Hammerschlag R. *Acupuncture Efficacy: A Compendium of Controlled Clinical Studies*. The National Academy of Acupuncture and Oriental Medicine; 1996. (Can be ordered through Redwing Books at (800) 873-3946.)

British Medical Association Board of Science and Education. *Acupuncture: Efficacy, Safety and Practice*. London, UK: Harwood Academic Publishers; 2000.

Brumbaugh AG. *Transformation and Recovery: A Guide for the Design and Development of Acupuncture-Based Chemical Dependency Treatment Programs*. New York, NY: Stillpoint Press; 1994.

Chaitow L. *The Acupuncture Treatment of Pain: Safe and Effective Methods for Using Acupuncture in Pain Relief*. Rochester, VT: Healing Art Press; 1990.

Deadman P, Baker K, Al-Khafaji M. *A Manual of Acupuncture*. Seattle, WA: Eastland Press; 1998. (An extensive reference on acupuncture points.)

Hecker H, Steveling A, Peuker E, et al. *Color Atlas of Acupuncture*. Stuttgart, Germany: Thieme; 2001. (Another compendium of acupuncture points with anatomical illustrations.)

Huan ZY, Rose K. *Who Can Ride the Dragon? An Exploration of the Cultural Roots of Traditional Chinese Medicine*. St. Paul, MN: EMC-Paradigm Publishing; 1999.

Loo M. *Pediatric Acupuncture*. Edinburgh, Scotland: Churchill Livingstone; 2002. (A physician's view of medical acupuncture in the treatment of children.)

MacPherson H, Kaptchuk T. *Acupuncture in Practice: Case History Insights from the West*. London, UK: Elsevier; 1996.

Micozzi MS. *Fundamentals of Complementary and Alternative Medicine*. 2nd ed. Edinburgh, Scotland: Churchill Livingstone; 2001.

Mitchell ER. *Fighting Drug Abuse with Acupuncture: The Treatment That Works*. Berkeley, CA: Pacific View Press; 1995.

Oleson T. *Auriculotherapy Manual: Chinese and Western Systems of Ear Acupuncture*, 3rd ed. Edinburgh, Scotland: Churchill Livingstone; 2002.

Stux G, Hammerschlag R, eds. *Clinical Acupuncture: Scientific Basis*. Berlin, Germany: Springer; 2001.

Stux G, Pomeranz B. *Acupuncture Textbook and Atlas*. Berlin, Germany: Springer-Verlag; 1987.

Unschuld P. *Huang Di Nei Jing Su Wen: Nature, Knowledge, Imagery in an Ancient Chinese Medical Text*. Berkeley, CA: University of California Press; 2003.

Unschuld P. *Medicine in China: A History of Ideas*. Berkeley, CA: University of California Press; 1988.

Veith I. *The Yellow Emperor's Classic of Internal Medicine*. Berkeley, CA: University of California Press; 2002.

Wiseman N, Feng Y. *A Practical Dictionary of Chinese Medicine*, 2nd ed. Boston, MA: Paradigm Publications; 1998.

Booksellers

Blue Poppy Press
5441 Western Avenue, Suite 2
Boulder, CO 80301
Phone: (303) 447-8372 or (800) 487-9296
Fax: (303) 245-8362
Email: bob@bluepoppy.com or honora@bluepoppy.com
Web site: www.bluepoppy.com

Eastland Press
1240 Activity Drive, Suite D
Vista, CA 92081
Phone: (800) 453-3278 or (760) 598-9695
Fax: (800) 241-3329 or (760) 598-6083
Email: info@eastlandpress.com
Web site: www.eastlandpress.com

Elsevier (Churchill Livingstone)
Customer Service Department
11830 Westline Industrial Drive
St. Louis, MO 63146 USA
Phone: (800) 545-2522 or (314) 453-7010
Fax: (800) 568-5136
Email: usbkinfo@elsevier.com
Web site: www.elsevier.com

Redwing Books
202 Bendix Drive
Taos, NM 87571
Phone: (800) 873-3946 or (505) 758-7758
Fax: (505) 758-7768
Email: info@redwingbooks.com
Web site: www.redwingbooks.com

JOURNALS

Acupuncture in Medicine
Published by the British Medical Acupuncture Society
Web site: www.medical-acupuncture.co.uk/aimintro.htm

Alternative Therapies in Health and Medicine
Published bimonthly by InnoVision
Phone: (866) 828-2962 or (760) 633-3910
Fax: (760) 633-3918
Email: alternative.therapies@innerdoorway.com
Web site: www.alternative-therapies.com

Acupuncture Today
A monthly publication mailed to acupuncture and Oriental medicine practitioners in the United States

Phone: (714) 230-3150
Fax: (714) 899-4273
Web site: www.acupuncturetoday.com.

American Journal of Acupuncture
Published from 1973 to 1999; back issues (hardcover and softbound) still available.
Phone: (408) 475-1700
Fax: (408) 475-1439
Web site: www.acupuncturejournal.com

American Journal of Chinese Medicine: An International Journal of Comparative Medicine, East and West
Published four times a year
Web site: www.worldscinet.com/ajcm/ajcm.shtml

Guidepoints: Acupuncture in Recovery
A publication of the National Acupuncture Detoxification Association
Phone: (888) 765-6232
Fax: (360) 260-8620
Web site: www.acudetox.com

Journal of Alternative and Complementary Medicine
Official journal of the Society of Acupuncture Research
Mary Ann Liebert Publishers
Phone: (800) 654-3237 or (914) 834-3100
Fax: (914) 834-3688
Web site: www.liebertpub.com

Journal of Traditional Chinese Medicine
Published quarterly in the US through the American Center of Chinese Medicine
Email: accm@jtcm.com
Web site: www.jtcm.com

Medical Acupuncture
Published three times a year by the American Academy of Medical Acupuncture
Phone: (323) 937-5514
Fax: (323) 937-0959
Web site: www.medicalacupuncture.org

WEB SITE INFORMATION AND REFERRAL SOURCES

AcuFinder
Contact information on acupuncture practitioners
Referrals: www.acufinder.com

Acupuncture.com
Extensive information resource on acupuncture
Web site: www.acupuncture.com

AcupunctureToday.com
Referrals and resources: www.acupuncture-today.com

National Certification Commission for Acupuncture and Oriental Medicine (NCCAOM)
(See earlier entry.)
Phone: (703) 548-9004
Email: info@nccaom.org
Referrals: www.nccaom.org

PART VIII

Chiropractic

Chapter

CHAPTER 46

Overcoming Barriers to the Integration of Chiropractic

J. Michael Menke. MA, DC

Low-back pain is the third most common acute condition seen by primary care providers (Bigos et al., 1994, Deyo, 1998). This condition and its sequelae tend to generate high utilization of outpatient medical services. These conditions are typically chronic, involving recurring symptoms for which there is little intervention except medication and exercise.

The treatment of back pain is an area of health care in which chiropractic can make a major contribution. Chiropractors currently provide 94% of all spinal manipulation services in the United States (Shekelle, 1994). Numerous controlled clinical trials and meta-analyses have found spinal manipulation to be one of the most effective treatments for low-back pain. Research over two decades has also consistently identified high patient satisfaction with chiropractic treatment.

Michael Menke is on the faculty of University of Arizona Program in Integrative Medicine, Palmer College of Chiropractic-West, National University of Health Sciences, and Palmer Center for Chiropractic Research. He is a member of the Stanford University Spinal Research Group, a content advisor for the Osher Center for Integrative Medicine at the University of California, San Francisco, and a research methodologist for women's health issues at the Harvard University Osher Center—New England School of Acupuncture. In 2003, his two-part series on chiropractic appeared in Johns-Hopkins' *Integrative Select*. He is pursuing a PhD in health services research at the University of Arizona.

Courtesy of Michael Menke, MA, DC, Tucson, Arizona.

As an indication of the extent of the clinical research, in a recent meta-analysis, 69 randomized controlled clinical trials on low-back and neck pain met the study selection criteria, of which 43 met the more stringent admissibility criteria for evidence (Bronfort et al., 2004). More than 50 systematic reviews have been published since 1979, and have found chiropractic efficacious for uncomplicated, mechanical back pain (Shekelle, 1994; Assendelft et al. 2003).

Spinal manipulation is consistently at least as effective as other conservative back treatments. Economically, chiropractic also has great potential to lower health care costs and ancillary expenses, when applied to common musculoskeletal problems (Branson, 1999, Legorreta et al., 2004, Metz et al., 2004). In addition, chiropractic offers major potential in the treatment of serious spine disorders in the context of highly successful multidisciplinary programs such as the Texas Back Institute in Plano, Texas (Triano, 2001, Ness & Nisly, 2004).

However, despite this promising potential, there are certain health care environments in which chiropractic is not yet considered as a treatment option. It is valuable to identify factors that tend to impede the full expression of chiropractic in a health system, as well as the chiropractic practitioners who are most likely to interface successfully in a mainstream environment. This chapter addresses these issues.

BARRIERS TO CHIROPRACTIC

Perceptions of the Research

Currently, there is a perception that there is little or no research on chiropractic. In reality, there are at least a thousand studies on chiropractic manipulation and manual therapy. Of these, more than 100 are randomized controlled clinical trials of high enough research quality to provide useful clinical and health policy information (see Chapter 49). In terms of the quality issue, in the clinical trials on back pain, chiropractic research has received quality scores comparable to evaluations of conventional therapies. Additional informative and critical chiropractic discussion, appraisals, and research are cited in the Medline databases of the National Institutes of Health (NIH) in more than 3,000 journal articles with the keyword chiropractic.

It is also noteworthy that this research is predominantly published in peer-reviewed medical journals, such as the *Journal of the American Medical Association*, the *New England Journal of Medicine*, the *British Medical Journal*, and *Spine*. For example, in a recent systematic review of the literature, more than 91% of the 43 studies that met the admissibility criteria were published in medical journals (Bronfort et al., 2004). Some studies have interdisciplinary principal investigators, including physicians and medical researchers. The legitimate nature of this research inquiry and its reporting of negative outcomes is an important aspect of its credibility.

Data on Safety

Chiropractic safety has been well established through research, and the safety record of chiropractic is exceptional. What is known in quantitative terms about the safety of chiropractic? Researchers have reported serious complications to occur at a rate of approximately 1 in 1 million manipulations (Hurwitz et al., 1996; Klougart et al., 1996). Extensive meta-analysis by the RAND Corporation also places the incidence of fatalities due to chiropractic treatment conservatively at less than approximately 1 in 3 million treatments (Shekelle, 1994). Reported safety rates are reflected in Table 46–1.

Table 46–1 Complication Rates Associated with Chiropractic Treatment

Stroke (caused by vertebrobasilar accident)[1]	1 in 3,000,000
Major impairment[2]	1 in 3,000,000
Death[3]	< 3 in 10,000,000
Low back (lumbar) nerve damage[4]	1 in approximately 100,000,000

Courtesy of J. Michael Menke, MS, DC, Tucson, Arizona.

1. Rothwell DM, Bondy SJ, Williams JI. Chiropractic manipulation and stroke: a population-based case-control study. *Stroke*. 2001;32:1054.
2. Assendelft WJ, Bouter LM, Knipschild PG. Complications of spinal manipulation: a comprehensive review of the literature. *J Fam Pract*. 1996;42:475–480.
3. Hurwitz EL, Aker PD, Adams AH, Meeker WC, Shekelle P. Manipulation and mobilization of the cervical spine: a systematic review of the literature. *Spine*. 1996;21:1746–1760.
4. Shekelle PG, Adams AH, Chassin MR, et al. Spinal manipulation for low-back pain. *Ann Int Med*. 1992;117:590.

Comparison with other forms of treatment for the same condition provides an additional frame of reference. For example, with respect to side effects and complications, chiropractic has been found to be far safer than the use of nonsteroidal, anti-inflammatory medications and cortisone therapies.

Chiropractic Education

Many of the concerns regarding chiropractic practice can be addressed through a better understanding of chiropractic education. At this point in time, chiropractic education is extensive and rigorous. Medical education and chiropractic education both require 4 years of study, with chiropractic education requiring 4822 class hours, comparable to medical education's 4667 hours.

For the most part, textbooks, course requirements, and objectives are equivalent for the same courses in chiropractic and medical education. However, chiropractic does not currently offer a postgraduate residency, whereas medical education has a residency requirement. Graduation from an accredited college of chiropractic is required of any and all chiropractors who are licensed in any of the 50 United States; Washington, DC; and territories. Chiropractic educational institutions must undergo a rigorous review process biannually, which is conducted by the Council on Chiropractic Education of the US Department of Health and Human Services.

Schools of chiropractic provide coursework in differential diagnosis that train practitioners to identify conditions that are more appropriately treated by medical doctors and should be referred out. Coursework in differential diagnosis is comparable to that of medical schools. These classes involve the same curriculum design, have the same number of credit hours, and use the same textbooks as those of medical schools.

ALTERNATIVE OR INTEGRATIVE CHIROPRACTIC?

Scope of Practice

Issues regarding scope of practice may surface when chiropractic is considered for inclusion in a mainstream medical environment. There may be a concern that chiropractors treat beyond their scope of practice. There is also the fear that they may not detect more serious underlying pathology and delay critical referral to appropriate medical care. The profession has matured to recognize the value of medical care in cases that are beyond the benefits of chiropractic treatment. The integrative chiropractic approach—chiropractic as a part of the health care system—is being taught more frequently in the chiropractic college curriculum as part of differential diagnosis, pathology classes, and chiropractic treatment classes.

Some physicians have concerns that chiropractors might co-opt patients, in the capacity of primary care providers. Physicians do not want to work in a competitive environment but may be willing to work in a collaborative and integrative mode, mutually referring and co-managing patient conditions as appropriate.

Two Styles of Practice

On the Web site of the National Center for Complementary and Alternative Medicine (2004), the distinction is made between complementary treatment and alternative therapies. The distinction may sound subtle, given that the two terms are often used interchangeably to describe therapies not typically taught in medical education. However, in England and Europe, there has been an emphasis on the inclusion of non-medical therapies in conventional treatment, which are therefore described as complementary.

In the United States, non-medical treatments are usually considered alternative.

Both distinctions are relevant to chiropractic, which encompasses two general styles of practice within the discipline. Complementary or integrative chiropractic practitioners can be distinguished by their willingness to work in conjunction with physicians and other practitioners. This requires a different emphasis on patient care and a different scope and style of practice (Menke, 2003).

Central to all chiropractic is treatment utilizing spinal manipulation. The clinical effectiveness of spinal manipulative therapy has been verified through more than a hundred studies. This treatment is focused on musculoskeletal functionality of the spine—addressing biomechanical dysfunction—and associated neurological dysfunction.

However, spinal health is a challenge for both conventional medicine and chiropractic. Given the current state of imaging and evaluation, there is no reliable testing available to verify the causal status of many back conditions that practitioners see in the day-to-day clinical environment—in either medical or chiropractic treatment.

We do know from X-rays, MRIs, and cadaver studies that biomechanical dysfunction does occur, but is not always visible on X-rays or MRIs (Carragee et al., 1997, 2000; Carragee & Kim, 2001). Associated neurological sequelae—inflammation, damage, or dysfunction of spinal nerves—are only detectable through surgical biopsy, so we have little direct evidence of this type of condition beyond that provided by animal models. At this time, our best evidence regarding the nature of many back disorders is the evaluation of functional clinical indicators. In assessing the result of spinal interventions, the primary focus is on clinical outcomes:

- Has function been restored or improved in terms of range of motion and mobility?

- Is there a decrease in subjective pain?
- Are there any indications of adverse reactions to the intervention?
- Is there an improvement in quality of life and ability to perform activities of daily living?
- Which type of treatment will provide maximal benefit at the least cost?
- What is the level of patient satisfaction with care?

In the absence of specific indicators for biomechanical or neurological phenomena, the integrative chiropractor observes response to care, and whether musculoskeletal health and function are progressing towards specific clinical endpoints or outcomes. In contrast, the alternative clinician treats the same biomechanical dysfunction, but focuses on the broader implications for overall health. Treatment is more likely to lack specific clinical endpoints. It should be noted that the alternative chiropractic approach continues to help thousands of patients each year. However, for insurers and consumers who want a finite treatment schedule, and empirical evaluations of progress, this approach does not provide the kind of data that allows the tracking of treatment effectiveness. The key questions to ask chiropractors to determine if their practice style is alternative or integrative include:

1. Do you X-ray every new patient?
2. When do you release a patient from care?
3. How do you decide that a treatment plan has been completed?

An alternative approach is suggested by a response such as, "The patient is never released from care because patients need maintenance treatment in order to preserve good health." Another indicator of alternative practice is over-reliance on X-rays to diagnose a patient condition. This is an approach that measures subtle malpositions of adjacent vertebrae over the course of treatment. The following aspects of practice style are characteristic of integrative chiropractic.

In contrast, integrative chiropractic protocol is typically more empirically defined. It involves monitoring patients' symptoms periodically throughout the course of treatment and at the endpoint. This is symptom-based care: the patient is discharged when the symptoms are resolved or maximum benefit has been achieved. If the condition has not resolved, appropriate referral is made to a specialist. Integrative practitioners use outcome measures to assess patient status, including the level of pain, functionality, ability to perform activities of daily living, and quality of life as evidence of response to treatment. The following aspects of practice style are characteristic of integrative chiropractic (Table 46–2).

The profile of the integrative chiropractor is one who uses X-rays judiciously, works in the context of a finite treatment schedule, and provides empirical evaluations of prognosis, progress, and outcomes with the goal of promoting maximal benefit. If a condition has not resolved or progressed satisfactorily at a particular milestone in treatment, immediate referral is made to a specialist. There is a commitment to cost containment and effectiveness. The practitioner also educates patients thoroughly in prevention and self-care. This is a genuine value-added service in an integrated environment, particularly for those patients with chronic conditions such as pain.

CHIROPRACTIC AND PHYSICAL THERAPY

Although chiropractic is currently experiencing high utilization in managed care networks, the integration of chiropractic into hospitals, spine centers, and university

Table 46–2 Integrative Chiropractic

- Provides care based on empirical evidence, assessments, and response to treatment
- Encourages patient independence and self-care
- Refers the patient to an appropriate specialist when patient progress is slow or stalls

Competencies
- Uses differential diagnosis to rule out underlying pathology or clinical red flags
- Is knowledgeable about other medical and health care disciplines
- Consults with other health care providers regarding treatment, as appropriate
- Uses standard protocol for making professional referrals

Scope of Practice
- Limits intervention primarily to musculoskeletal pain and dysfunction
- Bases assessment on physical examination and standard diagnosis using current ICD-9 or ICD-10 diagnostic codes, or ABC Codes (Alternative Link, 2005)
- Uses X-rays and other types of diagnostic imaging judiciously, for high-risk cases
- Communicates in standard medical nomenclature

Practice Guidelines
- All conditions should show some degree of improvement within a month
- Reassessment after 6 to 8 visits should indicate at least 50% to 75% improvement. Given signs of progress, the chiropractor may continue treatment for another 6 to 8 visits (using the same care plan or a different approach, as appropriate) and again reevaluate.
- With stable maximum treatment benefit or a failure to progress, the integrative chiropractor discharges or refers patient out, as indicated.

Courtesy of J. Michael Menke, MA, DC, Tucson, Arizona.

medical centers is occurring at a slower rate. One of the major barriers to the integration of chiropractic in these environments has been the perception that chiropractors and physical therapists provide similar services.

Key differences. In conversations with medical and managed care directors about the inclusion of chiropractic, the response to these issues has often been, "We have no need for chiropractors—we already have a physical therapy department." The question then is, "Does chiropractic provide a type of intervention not performed by physical therapists? Is there a fundamental difference between these disciplines that would suggest a rationale for the inclusion of chiropractic?"

The focus of chiropractic. Chiropractic focuses primarily on conditions of the spine and chiropractors perform approximately 94% of all spinal manipulation procedures in the United States. The effectiveness of this approach has been borne out in a large body of research in the peer-reviewed journals. In a review of more than 10,000 studies on treatment for back pain with a meta-analysis by the Agency for Health Care Policy and Research, spinal manipulation was found to be one of three therapies most efficacious in the treatment of low-back pain (Bigos et al., 1994). The other two were anti-inflammatory medications and bed rest not to exceed 4 days duration. From the first day of chiropractic education, the majority of didactic and clinical instruction focuses on the spine and its structure, function, diagnosis, imaging, anatomy, and treatment. No other profession currently retains this depth of focus and training on spinal health.

The focus of physical therapy. In contrast, physical therapists perform less than 5% of the spinal manipulation in the United States (Bigos et al., 1994). Physical therapy education focuses broadly on a range of conditions and therapeutic methodologies. Clinically it has a record of particular effectiveness in rehabilitation of shoulders, hips, and knee joints; in post-surgical conditions; and a wide range of conditions caused by physical trauma, including stroke and burns. Physical therapists use a variety of therapeutic techniques that include exercise, body mechanics, ergonomics, manual therapy, patient education, and self-care.

Complementary disciplines. In sum, physical therapy has a record of extensive benefit for a wide range of conditions, whereas chiropractic treatment addresses the health and function of the spine. (See Table 46–3 for a comparative review of scope of practice for these two disciplines.) Physical therapy and chiropractic interventions are potentially very compatible in integrative treatment for musculoskeletal conditions. Both professions share the goal of empowering patients through coaching and self-care and have a commitment to patient education, exercise, and rehabilitation.

CONCLUSION

The safety and popularity of chiropractic and its effectiveness for certain conditions make it a viable candidate for greater inclusion in health care. Back pain is among the most frequent complaints patients brought to the primary care doctor. Chiropractic is the ultimate complementary discipline—with the potential to interface cohesively with all other disciplines. In multidisciplinary spine centers and sports medicine programs, medical and managed care directors find it beneficial to include an integrative chiropractor on the clinical team. With professions working shoulder-to-shoulder, new protocols and care algorithms will be developed.

New benchmarks of excellence will evolve to provide the context for the systematic and

Table 46–3 Practice Style

Physical Therapists	Integrative Chiropractors
Use wide range of techniques including exercise, body mechanics, ergonomics, manual therapy, patient education, and self-responsibility, but do not specialize in spinal manipulation	Perform spinal manipulation (94% of all US procedures). Almost all patients receive spinal manipulation, when indicated. Refer out patients not appropriate for manipulation
Evaluate the condition and define treatment plan May also determine the condition (over half the states allow patients to attend physical therapy without a physician referral)	Determine the condition and define treatment plan Are trained in differential diagnosis
Have wide range in education and competencies: —Nonspinal musculoskeletal conditions —Postsurgical rehabilitation —Sports injuries Are trained in treatment of spinal conditions	Focus primarily on treatment of spinal conditions since that is the focus of therapeutic intervention May treat joint problems in shoulders, knees, or hips, but chiefly those related to spinal dysfunction
Employ adjunctive therapies including spinal manipulation, but only for certain indications Select from broad range of adjunctive therapies, as appropriate	Employ adjunctive therapies including nutrition and exercise Use physiotherapy modalities to support spinal manipulation, such as light, heat, water, ice or cold packs, electrical stimulation, ultrasound, massage, and office- or home-based traction
See wider variety of patients, such as burn or stroke victims, and other patients with serious conditions that result from major trauma to the body	See patients with spinal problems; they tend to have less serious conditions and some ambulatory capacity
Use various approaches to manipulation, in the context of mobilization Use manipulation as required by the situation	Use spinal manipulation as mainstay of chiropractic practice; procedure involves high-velocity, low-amplitude short thrust
Apply regional approach to soft tissue, focusing on muscles and ligaments with skeletal structure as supportive Focus primarily on musculoskeletal system and related soft tissue	Focus on skeletal juxtaposition—joints and lack of mobility and how that affects the soft tissue Include role of nerve supply to the region in diagnosis and treatment
In rehabilitation, emphasize active patient participation	Require patient to be passive during the treatment; active participation is required only for posttreatment rehabilitation

Courtesy of J. Michael Menke, MA, DC, Tucson, AZ.

relevant measurement of outcomes in response to single therapies and combination treatments. Then perhaps the safest and best

that each profession has to offer can truly be integrated for improved patient care and lower costs.

REFERENCES

Alternative Link. *ABC Coding Manual for Integrative Health Care*. 7th ed. Albuquerque, NM: Alternative Link; 2005. Available at www.alternativelink.com

Assendelft WJ, Bouter LM, Knipschild PG. Complications of spinal manipulation: a comprehensive review of the literature. *J Fam Pract*. 1996;42:475–480.

Assendelft WJ, Morton SC, Yu EI, Suttorp MJ, Shekelle PG. Spinal manipulative therapy for low back pain. A meta-analysis of effectiveness relative to other therapies. *Ann Intern Med*. 2003;138: 871–881.

Bigos S, Bowyer O, Braen G, et al. *Acute Low Back Problems in Adults. Clinical Practice Guideline No. 14*. AHCPR publication 95-0642. Rockville, MD: Agency for Health Care Policy and Research; 1994.

Branson RA. Cost comparison of chiropractic and medical treatment of common musculoskeletal disorders: a review of the literature after 1980. *Top Clin Chiro*. 1999;6(2):157–168.

Bronfort G, Haas M, Evans RL, Bouter LM. Efficacy of spinal manipulation and mobilization for low back pain and neck pain: a systematic review and best evidence synthesis. *Spine J*. 2004;4:335–356.

Carragee EJ, Kim DH. A prospective analysis of magnetic resonance imaging findings in patients with sciatica and lumbar disc herniation: correlation of outcomes with disc fragment and canal morphology. *Spine*. 1997;22(14):1650–1660.

Carragee EJ, Paragioudakis SJ, Khurana S, 2000 Volvo Award winner in clinical studies: lumbar high-intensity zone and discography in subjects without low back problems. *Spine*. 2000;25(23):2987–2992.

Carragee EJ, Tanner CM, Khurana S, et al. The rates of false-positive lumbar discography in select patients without low back symptoms. *Spine*. 2001;26(8): 994–996.

Deyo RA. Low-back pain. *Sci Am*. 1998;279(2): 48–53.

Eisenberg D, Davis R, Ettner S, et al. Trends in alternative medicine use in the United States, 1990–997:

results of a follow-up national study. *JAMA*. 1998:280:1569–1575.

Hurwitz EL, Aker PD, Adams AH, Meeker WC, Shekelle P. Manipulation and mobilization of the cervical spine: a systematic review of the literature. *Spine*. 1996;21:1746–1760.

Klougart N, LeBoeuf-Y de C, Rasmussen LR. Safety in chiropractic practice. Part I. The occurrence of cerebrovascular accidents following cervical spine adjustment in Denmark during 1978–1988. *J Manipulative Physiol Ther*. 1996:19:371–377.

Legorreta AP, Metz RD, Nelson CF, Ray S, Chernicoff HO, Dinubile NA. Comparative analysis of individuals with and without chiropractic coverage: patient characteristics, utilization, and costs. *Arch Intern Med*. 2004;164(18):1985–1992.

Menke JM. Principles in integrative chiropractic. *J Manipulative Physiol Ther*. 2003;26(4):254–272.

Metz RD, Nelson CF, LaBrot T, Pelletier KR. Chiropractic care: is it substitution care or add-on care in corporate medical plans? *J Occup Environ Med*. 2004;46(8):847–855.

National Center for Complementary and Alternative Medicine. Available at: www.nccam.nih.gov. Accessed July 1, 2004.

National Market Measures. *The Landmark Report II*. Sacramento, CA: Landmark Healthcare; 1999.

Ness J, Nisly N. Cracking the problem of back pain: is chiropractic the answer? *Arch Intern Med*. 2004; 164(18):1953–1954.

Shekelle PG. *The Use and Costs of Chiropractic Care in the Health Insurance Experiment*. Santa Monica, CA: RAND Corporation; 1994.

Triano JJ, Rashbaum RF, Hansen DT, Raley B. The integrative multidisciplinary spine center: the Texas Back Institute. In: Faass N, ed. *Integrating Complementary Medicine into Health Systems*, Sudbury, MA: Jones and Bartlett/Aspen; 2001.

CHAPTER 47

Overview of the Chiropractic Profession

David Chapman-Smith, LLB

DEFINITION AND LEGAL SCOPE OF PRACTICE

Chiropractic (from Greek, meaning treatment by hand) is a health profession concerned with the diagnosis, treatment, and prevention of disorders of the musculoskeletal system and the effects of these disorders on the nervous system and general health. Chiropractic practice emphasizes clinical interventions that support the natural ability of the body to heal itself (homeostasis) and includes:

- Manipulation and mobilization of spinal and other joints, also known as joint adjustment
- Soft tissue techniques
- Exercise and rehabilitative programs
- Other supportive methods, such as the use of back supports and orthotics, interferential therapies, and ultrasound
- Patient education on spinal health, posture, nutrition, and other lifestyle modifications

---

David Chapman-Smith, LLB, received his honors degree in law from Auckland University, New Zealand, and was a litigation partner there in the firm of Holmden Horrocks & Co. until his move to Toronto, where he now has his legal practice. He currently serves as secretary-general for the World Federation of Chiropractic and general counsel for the Ontario Chiropractic Association. A recognized author and spokesman for the profession, he is coeditor of national chiropractic clinical guidelines in the United States and Canada, has been editor of the newsletter *The Chiropractic Report* for the past 18 years, and is the author of *The Chiropractic Profession*.

Source: Adapted and updated content provided courtesy of NCMIC Group, Clive, IA. From: Chapman-Smith D. *The Chiropractic Profession*. Des Moines, IA: NCMIC Group Inc.; 2000.

The legally defined scope of practice of chiropractic is not the same in every country, state, or province, but always has these common features:

1. Primary contact or care—meaning patients can consult a chiropractor directly without any requirement of medical referral
2. The right and duty to perform a diagnosis, including the right to perform and/or order diagnostic skeletal X-rays and other imaging studies
3. The use of spinal manipulation and a range of other manual and physical therapeutics
4. No use of prescription drugs or surgery

The legal scope of practice may appear in one or more of three levels of legislation:

1. Statute
2. Regulations or rules under that statute enacted by government
3. In-practice standards issued by the chiropractic board or regulatory authority established under the statute

An annual directory of all US state scope-of-practice laws and other licensure requirements can be obtained from:

Federation of Chiropractic Licensing Boards (FCLB)
901 54th Avenue, Suite 101
Greeley, CO 80634
Phone: (970) 356-3500
Email: fclb@fclb.org
Web site: www.fclb.org

EPIDEMIOLOGY AND TREATMENT

Various studies on the use of chiropractic services, including a recent large survey in the United States and Canada (Hurwitz et al., 1998), report that approximately 95% of chiropractic patients seek care for neuromusculoskeletal pain or disorders. Approximately 65% of patients have low back pain and/or leg pain. Approximately 10% have headache. (See Table 47–1 for a summary of conditions treated in chiropractic practice.) Nonmusculoskeletal conditions constitute approximately 5% of the chiropractic case load and include circulatory, digestive, gynecological, and respiratory problems that may improve or resolve completely when a related spinal problem is corrected. A recent national survey in Sweden (Leboeuf-Yde et al., 1999) indicates that 23% of patients receiving chiropractic treatment for musculoskeletal pain report significant nonmusculoskeletal benefits after chiropractic treatment, primarily with respect to digestive and respiratory problems.

Table 47–1 Patient Complaints Seen in Chiropractic Practice

Complaint	Percentage
Back pain70%	
Low back pain	65%
Midback pain	5%
Other neuro-	
musculoskeletal pain	25%
Head/neck pain	15%
Extremity pain	10%
Nonneuromusculoskeletal	
disorders: allergies, asthma, etc.	5%

Source: Adapted with permission from D. Chapman-Smith, *The Chiropractic Profession*, © 2000, NCMIC Group Inc., Des Moines, IA.

Goals of Chiropractic Practice

Following from the above, the goals of chiropractic practice are to:

1. Meet the patient's immediate needs, often the relief of pain.
2. Address the cause of the symptoms by restoring normal ranges of movement and function to the joints, muscles, and other structures of the musculoskeletal or locomotor system.
3. Thereby allow the nervous system to function without interference, better regulating the various body systems and general health.

Within their scope of practice, chiropractors employ a range of techniques of spinal adjustment as described in Exhibit 47–1.

Safety and Effectiveness

There is now good research evidence of the safety and effectiveness of chiropractic treatment for the conditions most commonly seen in practice—acute and chronic back pain (Manga et al., 1993; Meade et al., 1990; van Tulder et al., 1997; Bronfort et al., 2004), neck pain (Coulter et al., 1996; Hurwitz et al., 1996), and headache (Nilsson et al., 1997; Boline et al., 1995).

The only risk of significant harm is vertebral artery injury and stroke as the result of cervical manipulation, but that is a very remote risk at 1 to 2 incidents per 1 million treatments (Haldeman et al., 1999), a much lesser risk than the morbidity and mortality arising from medications and surgeries given to equivalent patients in medical practice (Coulter et al., 1996; Terrett, 2001). The scientific literature on the safety and effectiveness of spinal manipulation and mobilization has been reviewed in studies by the RAND

Exhibit 47–1 Classification System for Chiropractic Manipulative/Adjustive Techniques

Manual Articular Manipulative and Adjustive Procedures
- Specific contact thrust procedures
  1. High-velocity thrust
  2. High-velocity thrust with recoil
  3. Low-velocity thrust
- Nonspecific contact thrust procedures
- Manual force, mechanically assisted procedures
  1. Drop-table and terminal point adjustive thrust
  2. Flexion-distraction table adjustment
  3. Pelvic block adjusting
- Mechanical force, manually assisted procedures
  1. Fixed stylus, compression wave adjustment
  2. Moving stylus instrument adjustment

Manual Nonarticular Manipulative and Adjustive Procedures
- Manual reflex and muscle relaxation procedures
  1. Muscle energy techniques
  2. Neurologic reflex techniques
  3. Myofascial ischemic compression procedures
  4. Miscellaneous soft tissue techniques
- Miscellaneous procedures
  1. Neural retraining techniques
  2. Conceptual approaches

Source: Reprinted from S. Haldeman et al., eds., *Quality Assurance and Practice Parameters, Guidelines for Chiropractic Quality Assurance,* © 1993, 2004, Jones and Bartlett Publishers.

Corporation, which has reported that these procedures are appropriate for many forms of back pain (Shekelle & Adams, 1991), neck pain, and headache (Coulter et al., 1996). See Chapter 48 for reviews of safety and Chapter 49 for research on effectiveness.

EDUCATION AND LICENSURE

Qualifications for the Right to Practice

Many countries and jurisdictions, including all US states and Canadian provinces, have legislation regulating the practice of chiropractic. To practice, a chiropractor must have a license or registration with the licensing board with the following preconditions:

1. Graduation with a doctor of chiropractic degree from a duly accredited chiropractic college
2. Completion of national board examinations
3. Completion of state/provincial licensing board examinations
4. Satisfaction of various conditions common to licensed health professions, such as being of sound character, holding malpractice insurance, and completing mandatory continuing education and/or practice review requirements

Education

In North America, there is a minimum of 7 years full-time, university-level education, which includes 3 years of college credits in qualifying subjects and then a 4-year program at chiropractic college. This training is followed by national and state/provincial licensing board examinations. Postgraduate specialties include chiropractic sciences, neurology, nutrition, orthopedics, radiology, rehabilitation, and sports chiropractic.

Although many chiropractic colleges are private institutions, they are not free to establish their own entrance requirements, curricula, faculty, staff, governance, facilities, research, or patient care. In these and other areas, uniform minimum requirements are established through an official accreditation system. In the United States, the accrediting agency for the chiropractic profession is the Council on Chiropractic Education (CCE). It is based in Scottsdale, Arizona, and has been recognized by the US Department of Education since 1974. In Canada, the accrediting agency is the Canadian Council on Chiropractic Education (CCE Canada), which is formally affiliated with the CCE and has reciprocal standards. There are 17 chiropractic colleges in the United States, and all have accredited status with the CCE. Additionally, 13 of them are accredited by nonchiropractic regional accrediting agencies such as the North Central Association of Schools and Colleges.

Licensure Examinations

A doctor of chiropractic seeking a license to practice must pass the following board exams:

- Part I—Basic science in seven areas (general anatomy, spinal anatomy, physiology, chemistry, pathology, microbiology, and public health)
- Part II—Clinical science in six areas (general diagnosis, neuromusculoskeletal diagnosis, radiography, principles of chiropractic, chiropractic practice, and associated clinical sciences)
- Part III—Clinical competency in 9 areas (case history, physical examination, neuromusculoskeletal examination, X-ray examination, clinical laboratory and special studies examination, diagnosis/clinical impression, chiropractic techniques, supportive techniques, and case management)

Prior to 1965, at a time when chiropractic examining boards had fewer resources, chiropractors in most US states took the same basic science board examinations as medical doctors. Accordingly, they were required to meet the same standard. Since that time, chiropractic examinations have become separate, while remaining at an equivalent standard with medicine.

The regulatory process for chiropractic practice has created two national organizations in the United States. The Federation of Chiropractic Licensing Boards (FCLB), established in 1933, seeks to unify standards and requirements of individual state boards and publishes their state licensure requirements annually. It is affiliated with and has appointed members on the National Board of Chiropractic Examiners (NBCE). The NBCE, established in 1963, administers the state and national board licensing examinations. It has developed examination systems that are now used nationally and internationally, including the 3-part exam referred to above. At this writing, 46 states require or accept NBCE exams for licensure, and others have requirements modeled on the NBCE exams. Information available at:

National Board of Chiropractic Examiners
901 54th Avenue Greeley, CO 80634
Phone: (970) 356-9100
Email: nbce@nbce.org
Web site: www.NBCE.org/nbce

APPROPRIATE COURSE OF TREATMENT

Reporting on the appropriateness of spinal manipulation for low back pain, a 1991 RAND Corporation expert panel, was composed of 3 chiropractors, 2 medical orthopedists, an internist, a family practitioner, a neurologist, and an osteopath, unanimously concluded, "An adequate trial of spinal manipulation is a course of 2 weeks for each of two different types of spinal manipulation (4 weeks total); after which, in the absence of documented improvement, spinal manipulation is no longer indicated" (Shekelle & Adams, 1991).

Typically, a patient is given manipulation 3 times weekly at first, then less frequently. This amounts to approximately 12 treatments over 4 weeks. This approach to frequency and duration of care has been endorsed in subsequent formal evidence-based chiropractic practice guidelines in the United States (Haldeman et al., 1993) and Canada (Henderson et al., 1994).

Some patients will only require 1 or a few treatments. If there is documented improvement after 4 weeks, but not complete relief of symptoms or restored function, the course of manipulations may continue. Typically, it will end within 8 weeks for uncomplicated conditions, within 16 weeks for other conditions unless there has been major trauma and/or complications. Some patients, because of lasting effects of trauma and/or the demands of their work and lifestyle, will require long-term supportive care. Others elect to have preventive or maintenance care.

REIMBURSEMENT AND INSURANCE COVERAGE

Since the level of government and private third-party payment for chiropractic services constantly changes according to time and jurisdiction, the following is a summary overview only.

Government Funding

Worldwide over the past 20 years, four government commissions have been asked to study and report on whether there should be government funding for chiropractic services.

These commissions were convened in Australia (1986) (Thompson, 1986), New Zealand (1978) (Hasselberg, 1979), Sweden (1987) (Commission on Alternative Medicine, 1987), and Ontario, Canada (1993) (Manga et al., 1993)—all said yes. These recommendations have led to varying degrees of coverage in Australia (veterans only), Canada (partial funding for all patients in most provinces), and Sweden (partial funding for all patients in approximately one third of the health regions). There is also government funding in:

- Denmark (nationally, for all patients)
- Israel (nationally through health maintenance organizations for all patients)
- Italy (only on medical referral in designated interdisciplinary clinics)
- Norway (nationally for all patients)
- Switzerland (Switzerland was the first country to establish government funding for chiropractic services)
- United Kingdom (for patients receiving chiropractic services through National Health Service contracts)
- United States (for seniors under Medicare, military veterans, and in some cases for the disadvantaged under Medicaid)

Workers' Compensation and Automobile Insurance

These plans typically include coverage of chiropractic services on a similar basis to medical services in US states, Canadian provinces, Australian states, and several European countries.

Employee Benefit Plans

Private insurance coverage under employee benefit plans has become available wherever the profession has become established (Jensen et al., 1997). In the United

States, HMO coverage for chiropractic appears to be increasing, as reflected in the findings of the Landmark Report II (National Market Measures, 1999), which indicated that approximately 67% of managed care organizations surveyed offered chiropractic benefits. In conventional insurance plans, preferred provider organizations (PPOs), and point-of-service plans, more than 80% of employees have full or partial coverage for chiropractic services. Jensen et al. (1997) reported that chiropractic coverage was provided by a range of insurers:

- Conventional insurance plans—84%
- Preferred provider organizations—83%
- Point-of-service plans—81%
- Managed care plans—44%

As mentioned, coverage in managed care plans expanded from 44% to 67% by 1999.

Professional Expertise

Skilled spinal manipulation requires extended training and full-time practice. "The art of manipulation depends on the ability of the practitioner to combine the forces he uses such that the maximum leverage occurs precisely at the level of the restricted joint. Such skill takes a great deal of practice to perfect. Clearly those engaged in continuous practice are likely to be more skilled than those who provide manipulation only on rare occasions. The concert pianist practices his art daily to maintain a high standard. This applies equally to the art of spinal manipulation" (Stoddard, 1979).

REFERENCES

Boline PD, Kassak K, Bronfort G, Nelson C, Anderson A. Spinal manipulation versus amitriptyline for the treatment of chronic tension-type headaches: a randomized clinical trial. *J Manipulative Physiol Ther*. 1995;18:148–154.

Bronfort G, Haas M, Evans RL, Bouter LM. Efficacy of spinal manipulation and mobilization for low back pain and neck pain: a systematic review and best evidence synthesis. *Spine J*. 2004;4:335–356.

Commission on Alternative Medicine, Social Departementete. Legitimization for Vissa Kiropraktorer. Stockholm, SOU (English Summary). 1987;12–16.

Coulter ID, Hurwitz EL, Adams AH, et al. *The Appropriateness of Manipulation and Mobilization of the Cervical Spine*. Document No. MR-781-CR. Santa Monica, CA: RAND Corporation; 1996.

Haldeman S, Chapman-Smith D, Petersen D, eds. *Guidelines for Chiropractic Quality Assurance and Practice Parameters. Proceedings of the Mercy Center Consensus Conference*. Gaithersburg, MD: Aspen Publishers; 1993:179–184.

Haldeman S, Kohlbeck FJ, McGregor M. Risk factors and precipitating neck movements causing vertebrobasilar artery dissection after cervical trauma and spinal manipulation. *Spine*. 1999;24(8):785–794.

Hasselberg PD. *Chiropractic in New Zealand, Report of a Commission of Inquiry*. Wellington, New Zealand: Government Printer; 1979.

Henderson D, Chapman-Smith D, Mior S, Vernon H, eds. *Clinical Guidelines for Chiropractic Practice in Canada*. Suppl. to JCCa. 1994;38(1).

Hurwitz EL, Aker PD, Adams AH, Meeker, WC, Shekelle P. Manipulation and mobilization of the cervical spine: a systematic review of the literature. *Spine*. 1996;21:1746–1760.

Hurwitz EL, Coulter I, Adams A, Genovese B, Shekelle P. Utilization of chiropractic services in the United States and Canada: 1985–1991. *Am J Pub Health*. 1998;88(5):771–776.

Jensen G, Morrisey M, Gaffney S, Liston DK. The new dominance of managed care: insurance trends in the 1990s. *Health Affairs*. 1997;16:125–136.

Leboeuf-Yde C, Axen I, Ahlefeldt G, Lidefelt P, Rosenbaum A, Thurnherr T. The types and frequencies of improved nonmusculoskeletal symptoms reported after chiropractic spinal manipulative therapy. *J Manipulative Physiol Ther*. 1999;22(9):559–564.

Manga P, Angus D, Papadopoulos C, Swan W. *The Effectiveness and Cost-Effectiveness of Chiropractic Management of Low-Back Pain*. Ottawa, Ontario:

Pran Manga and Associates, University of Ottawa; 1993:65–70.

Meade TW, Dyer S, Browne W, Townsend J, Frank AO. Low back pain of mechanical origin: randomized comparison of chiropractic and hospital outpatient treatment. *Br Med J.* 1990;300:1431–1437.

National Market Measures. *The Landmark Report II.* Sacramento, CA: Landmark Healthcare; 1999.

Nilsson N, Christensen HW, Hartvigsen J. The effect of spinal manipulation in the treatment of cervicogenic headache. *J Manipulative Physiol Ther.* 1997;20(5): 326–330.

Shekelle P, Adams A. *The Appropriateness of Spinal Manipulation for Low-Back Pain: Indications and Ratings by a Multidisciplinary Expert Panel.* Monograph No. R-4025/2-CCR/FCER. Santa Monica, CA: RAND Corporation; 1991.

Stoddard A. *The Back: Relief from Pain.* Canada: Prentice Hall; 1979:17.

Terrett AGJ. *Current Concepts in Vertebrobasilar Complications Following Spinal Manipulation,* 2nd ed. West Des Moines, IA: NCMIC; 2001: 118–119.

Thompson C. *Second Report, Medicare Benefits Review Committee.* Canberra, Australia: Commonwealth Government Printer; June 1986: Chapter 10 (Chiropractic).

van Tulder MW, Koes BW, Bouter LM. Conservative treatment of acute and chronic nonspecific low back pain: a systematic review of randomized controlled trials of the most common interventions. *Spine.* 1997;22(18):2128–2156.

CHAPTER 48

Safety of Chiropractic Spinal Manipulation

William J. Lauretti, DC

Doctors of chiropractic are highly trained professionals who have an excellent track record of providing the public with safe and effective treatments. Their dedication to conservative treatment approaches has resulted in some of the lowest malpractice insurance rates of any licensed health care profession.

In spite of their favorable record of safety, cases of injuries from chiropractic treatments occasionally make the news. The most serious potential complication from chiropractic treatment is secondary to manipulation of the neck. In very rare cases, cervical manipulation may damage one of the vertebral arteries—the two small arteries that pass through the upper cervical vertebrae into the base of the brain—resulting in a stroke to the brainstem.

These events appear to have received a disproportionate amount of attention in the medical literature and in the popular media, considering how infrequently they occur. Based on current research, the best estimates of the odds of suffering a serious complication from a chiropractic neck treatment are about 1 incident out of every 2 million treatments (see Table 48–1).

William J. Lauretti, DC is a practicing chiropractor from Gaithersburg, Maryland, who has written and lectured extensively on the risks and benefits of chiropractic treatments. He is a Fellow of the International College of Chiropractors, a recipient of the American Chiropractic Association President's Award, and was named "Chiropractor of the Year 2000" by the Maryland Chiropractic Association.

APPROPRIATENESS OF CERVICAL MANIPULATION

Many scientific studies and expert reviews show that neck manipulation (chiropractic cervical adjustment) is safe, effective, and appropriate for patients with common forms of neck pain and headache. Examples include:

Duke University Evidence Report (McCrory et al., 2001)

The Duke University Evidence-Based Practice Center performed a systematic review of the scientific evidence for treatments of headache. It found cervical manipulation appropriate for both tension-type headache and cervicogenic headache—a subcategory of tension headache that is associated with specific neck symptoms. In addition, it noted that "cervical spinal manipulation has a very low risk of serious complications" which may be "one of its appeals over drug treatment."

RAND Corporation Report (Coulter et al., 1996)

This report, based on the work of a multidisciplinary expert panel including primary care physicians, chiropractors, neurologists, a neurosurgeon, and an orthopedic surgeon, concluded that, "Manipulation is probably slightly more effective than mobilization or physical therapy for some patients with

Table 48–1 Studies That Have Estimated the Probability of Stroke Following Cervical Manipulation

Source and Investigator	Findings
Swiss Society of Manual Medicine (survey of 203 members), Dvorak & Orelli, 1985	1 serious complication per 400,000 cervical manipulations; no reported deaths
Extensive literature review to formulate practice guidelines, Haldeman et al., 1993	1–2 incidences of stroke per 1,000,000 neck manipulations
Survey of Danish Chiropractors' Association members cross-referenced against cerebrovascular occurrences from case records, Klougart et al., 1996	1 cerebrovascular accident (CVA) per 1,320,000 cervical spine treatment sessions; 1 CVA per 414,000 sessions using rotation techniques in the upper cervical spine
Review of the world literature on chiropractic by the RAND Corporation, Shekelle et al., 1992	1 CVA per 3,000,000 chiropractic treatments
Review of Canadian malpractice figures, Carey, 1993	1 CVA per 3,000,000 neck manipulations
Case control study (review of hospital records for vertebral artery stroke and insurance billing records for chiropractic visits), Rothwell et al., 2001	1 CVA per 3–4,000,000 chiropractic visits for neck symptoms
Canadian malpractice figures (updated review), Haldeman et al., 2001	1 CVA per 5,850,000 chiropractic visits

Courtesy of William J. Lauretti, DC, Bethesda, MD.

subacute or chronic neck pain, and all three treatments are probably superior to usual medical care." It also concluded that, "Manipulation and/or mobilization may be beneficial for muscle tension headache."

Quebec Task Force Report on Whiplash Injuries (Spitzer et al., 1995)

A multispecialty panel of leading researchers and clinicians from North America and Europe reviewed the scientific literature and provided treatment guidelines for whiplash-type injuries to the neck. Joint manipulation and mobilization were recommended to improve range of motion and reduce pain, and as part of a management strategy based on early return to function and activities as opposed to rest or use of a cervical collar.

Chiropractic neck manipulation has also been shown to have specific physiological benefits. Studies have shown that cervical manipulation produces a consistent and significant increase in the active range of motion, and that this benefit remains for many weeks after the treatment is complete (Whittingham & Nilsson, 2001).

OTHER FINDINGS ON MANIPULATION

The safety record regarding other aspects of spinal manipulation is equally strong.

Although minor reactions to manipulative treatment are relatively common, they tend to be self-limiting and relatively benign in nature (see Table 48–2). For example, one study of Norwegian chiropractors (Senstad et al., 1997) found that 55% of patients reported at least one unpleasant reaction during the course of a maximum of six visits, most commonly local discomfort, headache, or tiredness. However, among the 4712 treatments followed in this study, no serious complications were reported.

Cauda equina syndrome is usually described as the most serious accident that can result from lumbar spine manipulation. In a detailed literature review of spinal manipulation for low back pain, Shekelle et al. (1992) estimated the occurrence of cauda equina syndrome from lumbar manipulation to be less than 1 case per 100 million manipulations.

Terrett and Kleynhans (1992) analyzed other disc-related complications from low back manipulation, and found only 65 cases reported in the worldwide literature in the 80 years from 1911–1991. They also noted that this complication is more common with manipulation under anesthesia (usually performed by orthopedic surgeons), accounting for more than 44% of the reported cases.

Contraindications to spinal manipulation have been very well described in the chiropractic literature and are covered in the curriculum of every chiropractic college. Major contraindications include the presence of a tumor, fracture, bone infection, or severe osteoporosis in the area being treated. A suspected mild disc herniation or disc bulge is not necessarily a contraindication to manipulation, unless it is accompanied by signs of true radiculopathy (nerve root damage), such as severe and progressive muscle weakness or loss of sensation.

Even in cases in which there is a contraindication to high-velocity chiropractic manipulation, other types of chiropractic treatment may be appropriate. Almost all chiropractors are also trained in conservative methods such as soft tissue massage, physiological therapeutics, or low-force manual techniques that do not involve manipulation.

Table 48–2 Studies That Have Estimated the Probability of Major Injury Following Spinal Manipulation

Source and Investigator	Findings
Extensive review of the English language literature, Hurwitz et al., 1996	1–3 per 3,000,000 treatments: risk of major impairment due to spinal manipulation
Systematic review of the literature to 1995 on serious complications, reversible and irreversible, including case reports in all other languages, Assendelft et al., 1996	1 per 3,000,000 treatments: risk of major complication
Extensive review of the English language literature, Hurwitz et al., 1996	< 1 in 3,000,000 treatments: risk of fatality due to spinal manipulation
Review of the world literature on chiropractic by the RAND Corporation and reviews by others, Shekelle et al., 1992; Haldeman et al., 1992	1 per 100,000,000 treatments: risk of irreversible cauda equina syndrome (neurological damage) following lumbar manipulation

Courtesy of William J. Lauretti, DC, Bethesda, Maryland.

Keep in mind also that a carefully applied manipulation uses a minimal amount of force; a skillful manipulation is usually quite gentle and painless.

In conclusion, chiropractic treatments are associated with an extremely low incidence of major complications, and chiropractic treatments for mechanical neck and back pain compare favorably in safety and efficacy to other available treatments for similar conditions (Lauretti, 2003).

REFERENCES

Assendelft WJ, Bouter LM, Knipschild PG. Complications of spinal manipulation: a comprehensive review of the literature. *J Fam Pract.* 1996;42: 475–480.

Carey PF. A report on the occurrence of cerebral vascular accidents in chiropractic practice. *J Canadian Chiropractic Assoc.* 1993;37(2):104.

Coulter ID, Hurwitz EL, et al. *The Appropriateness of Manipulation and Mobilization of the Cervical Spine.* Document No. MR-781-CR: Santa Monica, CA: RAND Corporation. 1996.

Dvorak J, Orelli F. How dangerous is manipulation to the cervical spine? *Manual Medicine.* 1985;2:1.

Haldeman S, Carey P, Townsend M, Papadopoulos C. Arterial dissections following cervical manipulation: the chiropractic experience. *CMAJ.* 2001;165: 905.

Haldeman S, Chapman-Smith D, Petersen DM. *Guidelines for Chiropractic Quality Assurance and Practice Parameters.* Gaithersburg, MD: Aspen Publishers; 1993.

Haldeman S, Rubinstein SM. Cauda equina syndrome in patients undergoing manipulation of the lumbar spine. *Spine.* 1992;17:1469–1473.

Hurwitz EL, Aker PD, Adams AH, Meeker WC, Shekelle P. Manipulation and mobilization of the cervical spine. A systematic review of the literature. *Spine.* 1996;21:1746–1760.

Klougart N, Leboeuf-Yde C, Rasmussen LR. Safety in chiropractic practice part I: the occurrence of cerebrovascular accidents after manipulation to the neck in Denmark from 1978–1988. *J Manipulative Physiol Ther.* 1996;19:371.

Lauretti WJ. The comparative safety of chiropractic. In: Redwood D, Cleveland C, eds. *Fundamentals of Chiropractic.* St. Louis, MO: Mosby; 2003.

McCrory DC, Penzien DB, et al. *Evidence Report: Behavioral and Physical Treatments for Tension-Type and Cervicogenic Headache.* Des Moines, IA: Foundation for Chiropractic Education and Research; 2001.

Rothwell DM, Bondy SJ, Williams JI. Chiropractic manipulation and stroke: a population-based case-control study. *Stroke.* 2001;32:1054.

Senstad O, Leboeuf-Yde C, Borchgrevink C. Frequency and characteristics of side effects of spinal manipulative therapy. *Spine.* 1997;22:435.

Shekelle PG, Adams AH, Chassin MR, et al. Spinal manipulation for low-back pain. *Ann Int Med.* 1992;117(7):590.

Spitzer WO, Skovron ML, et al. Scientific monograph of the Quebec Task Force on whiplash-associated disorders: redefining whiplash and its management. *Spine.* 1995;20:8S.

Terrett AGJ, Kleynhans AM. Complications from manipulation of the low back. *Chiropractic J Aust.* 1992;22:129.

Whittingham W, Nilsson N. Active range of motion in the cervical spine increases after spinal manipulation. *J Manipulative Physiol Ther.* 2001;24(9):552–555.

CHAPTER 49

Efficacy of Spinal Manipulation

Gert Bronfort, PhD, DC; Mitchell Haas, DC, MA;
Roni L. Evans, DC, MS; Lex M. Bouter, PhD

The current literature includes many published randomized clinical trials on spinal manipulative therapy and mobilization, as well as a substantial number of reviews, and several national clinical guidelines. However, there is not yet clear consensus regarding the evidence for or against efficacy of spinal manipulation for low back pain and neck pain.

STUDY DESIGN

A review by Bronfort et al. (2004) reassessed the literature on the efficacy of spinal manipulative therapy and mobilization for the management of low back pain and neck pain. The review applied more stringent criteria than earlier reviews, both with regard to study admissibility into evi-

Gert Bronfort, DC, PhD, professor and director of Clinical Biomechanics and Extramural Research at Northwestern Health Sciences University, received his PhD from Vrije University of Amsterdam. He is principle or co-investigator on several NIH clinical trials: a major randomized controlled trial on chiropractic care for acute neck pain; two studies on back pain and neck pain with the University of Minnesota and Hennepin County Medical Center; and a project with the Minnesota Consortium Program to train future clinical researchers. Dr. Bronfort is currently director of the Chiropractic Clinical Practice Guidelines Project in Denmark, a reviewer for NCCAM, and an active member of the Cochrane Collaboration's Cervical Overview Group, and has served as consultant for the World Health Organization.

Source: The following content is adapted from Bronfort G., et al. Efficacy of spinal manipulation and mobilization for low back pain and neck pain: a systematic review and best evidence synthesis. *Spine J.* 2004;4:335–356. Courtesy of Elsevier Sciences.

dence and for isolation of the effect of spinal manipulative therapy and/or mobilization.

Inclusion criteria included clinical trials with 10 or more subjects per group receiving spinal manipulative therapy or mobilization and those using patient-oriented primary outcome measures (e.g., patient-rated pain, disability, global improvement, and recovery time). Articles in English, Danish, Swedish, Norwegian, and Dutch reporting on randomized trials were identified by a comprehensive search of computerized and bibliographic literature databases up to the end of 2002. Two reviewers independently abstracted data and assessed study quality according to eight explicit criteria.

A best-evidence synthesis incorporating explicit, detailed information regarding outcome measures and interventions was used to evaluate treatment efficacy. The strength of evidence was assessed by a classification system that incorporated study validity and statistical significance of study results. Sixty-nine randomized controlled trials met the study selection criteria and were reviewed and assigned validity scores varying from 6 to 81 on a scale of 0 to 100. Forty-three randomized controlled trials met the admissibility criteria for evidence.

RESULTS: BACK PAIN

We identified 46 low back pain trials of spinal manipulation/mobilization. Of these, 31 studies with a total of 5202 participants met the inclusion criteria. Spinal manipulation was investigated in 25 trials, mobilization in 3 trials, and a combination in 3 trials. Chiropractors in 14 trials, medical doctors in 7 trials, physical therapists in 6 trials, and osteopaths in 4 trials provided spinal manipulation/mobilization. Comparison therapies included acupuncture, back school, bed rest, corset, diathermy, education advice, electrical modalities, exercise, heat, injections, massage and trigger-point therapy, medication, no treatment, placebo, physical therapy, sham spinal manipulation, and ultrasound. The number of treatments varied from 1 to 24, and outcomes were measured from immediate posttreatment to 3 years after commencement of therapy. Among the studies in evidence, 6 trials (sample size, N = 662) evaluated acute low back pain, 11 trials (N = 1472) assessed chronic low back pain, and 14 trials (N = 3068) investigated a mix of acute and chronic low back pain patients.

Acute Low Back Pain

There is now moderate evidence that spinal manipulative therapy provides more short-term pain relief than mobilization and detuned diathermy. There is limited evidence of faster recovery than a commonly used physical therapy treatment strategy (see Table 49–1).

Chronic Low Back Pain

There is moderate evidence that spinal manipulative therapy has an effect similar to an efficacious prescription nonsteroidal anti-inflammatory drug (see Table 49–2).

- Spinal manipulative therapy/mobilization is effective in the short term when compared with placebo and general practitioner care, and in the long term compared to physical therapy.

- There is limited to moderate evidence that spinal manipulative therapy is better than physical therapy and home back exercise in both the short and long term.
- There is limited evidence that spinal manipulative therapy is superior to sham therapy in the short term and superior to chemonucleolysis for disc herniation in the short term.
- However, there is also limited evidence that mobilization is inferior to back exercise after disc herniation surgery.

Mix of Acute and Chronic Low Back Pain

Spinal manipulative therapy/mobilization provides either similar or better pain outcomes in the short and long term when compared with placebo and with other treatments, such as McKenzie therapy, medical care, management by physical therapists, soft tissue treatment, and back school (see Table 49–3).

RESULTS: NECK PAIN

We identified 23 neck pain trials of spinal manipulation/mobilization. Of these, 12 studies with a total of 1172 participants met the inclusion criteria. Spinal manipulation was investigated in 7 trials, mobilization in 4 trials, and a combination in 1 trial. Therapy was provided by a doctor of chiropractic in 5 trials, a medical doctor in 2 trials, a physical therapist in 4 trials, and a manual therapist in 1 trial. Comparison therapies included acupuncture, cervical collar, education, electrical exercise, heat, modalities, medication, no treatment, physical therapy, placebo, and rest. The number of treatments varied from 1 to 24, and outcomes were evaluated from immediately after the first treatment to 1 year after commencement of therapy.

With regard to *acute* neck pain, there are few studies, and the evidence is currently inconclusive. For *chronic* neck pain, there is moderate evidence that spinal manipulative therapy/mobilization is superior to general practitioner management for short-term pain reduction. There is moderate evidence that spinal manipulative therapy offers at most pain relief similar to high-technology rehabilitative exercise in the short and long term. For conditions that involve both acute and chronic neck pain, the overall evidence is not clear. There is moderate evidence that mobilization is superior to physical therapy and family physician care, and similar to spinal manipulative therapy in both the short and long term. There is limited evidence that spinal manipulative therapy, in both the short and long term, is inferior to physical therapy (see Table 49–4).

CONCLUSION

Our data synthesis suggests that recommendations can be made with some confidence regarding the use of spinal manipulative therapy and/or mobilization as a viable option for the treatment of both low back pain and neck pain. There have been few high-quality trials distinguishing between acute and chronic patients, and most are limited to shorter-term follow-up. Future trials should examine well-defined subgroups of patients, further address the value of spinal manipulative therapy and mobilization for acute patients, establish the optimal number of treatment visits, and consider the cost-effectiveness of care.

Table 49–1 Acute Low Back Pain

First author, date, sample size (N)	Finding
Farrell, 1982 N = 48	Patients receiving spinal manipulative therapy recovered faster than patients receiving a combination of diathermy, exercise, and ergonomic instruction.
Glover, 1974 N = 84	One session of spinal manipulative therapy was found to be superior to detuned diathermy 1 week after treatment.
Godfrey, 1984 N = 90	Spinal manipulation combined with low-level electrical stimulation was nonsignificantly better in terms of pain reduction than low-level electrical stimulation alone after 2 weeks.
Hadler, 1987 N = 54	One session of spinal manipulative therapy was superior to one session of mobilization.
MacDonald, 1990 N = 95	Spinal manipulative therapy was nonsignificantly better than low back education in a subgroup of patients 1 week after the start of treatment.
Mathews, 1987 N = 291	Patients with low back pain accompanied by sciatica improved faster with spinal manipulative therapy than with heat after 2 weeks of treatment.

Table 49–2 Chronic Low Back Pain

First author, date, sample size (N)	Finding
Bronfort, 1996 N = 174	The combination of spinal manipulation and exercise was similar in effect to the combination of nonsteroidal anti-inflammatory drugs (NSAIDs) and exercise.
Burton, 2000 N = 40	Spinal manipulation had a higher short-term reduction in pain and disability for disc herniation than chemonucleolysis.
Coxhead, 1981 N = n.a.	Spinal manipulation was superior to traction, exercise, corset, and no treatment in the short term.
Gibson, 1985 N = 109	Detuned diathermy was found to be better than spinal manipulation/ mobilization and active diathermy. Baseline dissimilarity between groups rendered the results of this trial questionable.
Hemmilä, 1997, 2002 N = 114	Spinal manipulation resulted in greater short- and long-term disability reduction than home back exercise or physical therapy. Spinal manipulation was superior to physical therapy for pain in the long term.
Herzog, 1991 N = 37	No significant short-term differences found between spinal manipulation, back education, and exercise in pain and disability reduction.
Koes, 1992 N = 144	Spinal manipulation/mobilization was shown to have an advantage over general medical practice and placebo for severity of main complaint and perceived global improvement in the long term.
Pope, 1994 N = 164	Spinal manipulation was superior to TENS (transcutaneous electrical nerve stimulation) in pain improvement.
Timm, 1994 N = 250	Mobilization resulted in slightly more short-term disability reduction than physical therapy and no-treatment control. Exercise resulted in more disability reduction than mobilization.
Triano, 1995 N = 209	Spinal manipulation had more short-term pain and disability reduction than sham spinal manipulation.
Waagen, 1986 N = 29	Reported an advantage of spinal manipulation over placebo in pain reduction after 2 weeks of treatment.

Table 49–3 Mix of Acute and Chronic Low Back Pain

First author, date, sample size (N)	*Finding*
Andersson, 1999 N = 155	Small but nonsignificant short-term benefit of spinal manipulation over standard medical care for pain and no difference for disability.
Bronfort, 1989 N = 21	Spinal manipulation was nonsignificantly better than medical general practice in improvement and sick leave, both in the short and long term.
Cherkin, 1998 N = 321	Short-term advantage reported for spinal manipulation over a booklet and no difference between spinal manipulation and McKenzie therapy for pain in the short term.
Doran, 1975 N = 452	Spinal manipulation resulted in greater improvement than physiotherapy, corset, or analgesics after treatment. No important differences were seen subsequently.
Evans, 1978 N = 32	Nonsignificantly more pain and disability reduction favoring SMT after 3 to 4 weeks of treatment compared with acupuncture and medication.
Giles, 1999 N = 69	Substantially higher proportion of patients receiving spinal manipulation than patients receiving analgesics rated treatment effective. The advantage in pain reduction for spinal manipulation was nonsignificant.
Hoehler, 1981 N = 95	Nonsignificant but greater pain reduction for spinal manipulation than placebo massage. A significantly higher proportion in the spinal manipulation group reported effective treatment.
Hsieh, 2002 N = 200	Nonsignificant advantage for spinal manipulation over myofascial therapy and for back school over spinal manipulation in terms of pain and disability reduction.
Hurwitz, 2002 N = 339	Spinal manipulation was almost identical to medical care for pain and disability in the short and long term. Adding the use of physical modalities to spinal manipulation did not improve any outcomes.
Meade, 1990, 1995 N = 741	Small, significant advantage reported for spinal manipulation over hospital outpatient management for disability in the short and long term.

continues

Table 49–3 Mix of Acute and Chronic Low Back Pain (continued)

First author, date, sample size (N)	Finding
Postacchini, 1988 N = 168	Greater global improvement was found for spinal manipulation than for placebo ointment.
Skargren, 1997 N = 253	Equal effectiveness was found for spinal manipulation and physical therapy in terms of pain and disability reduction in the short and long term.
Wreje, 1992 N = 46	One session of spinal manipulation produced a lower number of sick-leave days than friction massage.
Zylbergold, 1981 N = 28	Spinal manipulation and heat were nonsignificantly better than flexion exercise and heat for pain and disability.

Table 49–4 Neck Pain

First author, date, sample size (N)	Finding
Acute Neck Pain	
Howe, 1983 N = 52	A higher proportion of patients receiving spinal manipulation experienced short-term pain improvement after the first treatment than a no-treatment control.
Nordemar, 1981 N = 30	A regimen with mobilization was nonsignificantly better than the regimen without mobilization in the short term for pain. Mobilization was no better than TENS.
Chronic Neck Pain	
Bronfort, 2001 N = 191	High-technology rehabilitative exercise produced more long-term pain reduction than spinal manipulation.
David, 1998 N = 30	Nonsignificantly higher reduction in pain for mobilization than acupuncture in the short and long term; disability was similar.
Jordan, 1998 N = 119	Small, nonsignificant differences found between spinal manipulation, intensive exercise, and physical therapy in the short and long term.
Koes, 1992 N = 65	Spinal manipulation/mobilization found to be superior to massage and to medical care for physical functioning in the short term.

continues

Table 49–4 Chronic Neck Pain (continued)

First author, date, sample size (N)	Finding
Chronic Neck Pain	
Sloop, 1982 N = 39	A nonsignificant advantage was found for spinal manipulation over placebo in the short term for pain reduction and improvement.
Acute and Chronic Neck Pain	
Brodin, 1982 N = 63–71	Greater short-term pain reduction found for a combination therapy including mobilization than for a combination therapy including massage or for analgesics alone.
Giles, 1999 N = 50	Spinal manipulation produced nonsignificantly more pain and disability improvement in the short term than acupuncture or analgesic medication.
Hoving, 2001 N = 119	Patients receiving mobilization had faster improvement and less pain than patients receiving physical therapy or general practice care in the short and long term.
Hurwitz, 2002 N = 336	Essentially no differences found between the effect of spinal manipulation and mobilization in terms of pain and disability reduction in the short and long term.
Skargren, 1997 N = 70	Physical therapy resulted in greater pain reduction than spinal manipulation in the short and long term.

REFERENCES

Andersson GB, Lucente T, Davis AM, Kappler RE, Lipton JA, Leurgans S. A comparison of osteopathic spinal manipulation with standard care for patients with low back pain. *N Engl J Med.* 1999;341: 1426–1431.

Brodin H. Cervical pain and mobilization. *Manuelle Med.* 1982;20:90–94.

Bronfort G. Chiropractic versus general medical treatment of low back pain: a small scale controlled clinical trial. *Am J Chiro Med.* 1989;2:145–150.

Bronfort G, Evans R, Nelson B, Aker P, Goldsmith C, Vernon H. A randomized clinical trial of exercise and spinal manipulation for patients with chronic neck pain. *Spine.* 2001;26:788–799.

Bronfort G, Goldsmith CH, Nelson CF, Boline PD, Anderson AV. Trunk exercise combined with spinal manipulative or NSAID therapy for chronic low back pain: a randomized, observer-blinded clinical trial. *J Manipulative Physiol Ther.* 1996;19:570–582.

Burton AK, Tillotson KM, Cleary J. Single-blind randomised controlled trial of chemonucleolysis and manipulation in the treatment of symptomatic lumbar disc herniation. *Eur Spine J.* 2000;9:202–207.

Cherkin DC, Deyo RA, Battie M, Street J, Barlow W. A comparison of physical therapy, chiropractic manipulation, and provision of an educational booklet for the treatment of patients with low back pain. *N Engl J Med.* 1998;339:1021–1029.

Coxhead CE, Inskip H, Meade TW, North WR, Troup JD. Multicentre trial of physiotherapy in the management of sciatic symptoms. *Lancet.* 1981;1:1065–1068.

David J, Modi S, Aluko AA, Robertshaw C, Farebrother J. Chronic neck pain: a comparison of acupuncture treatment and physiotherapy. *Br J Rheumatol.* 1998;37:1118–1122.

Doran DM, Newell DJ. Manipulation in treatment of low back pain: a multicentre study. *BMJ.* 1975; 2:161–164.

Evans DP, Burke MS, Lloyd KN, Roberts EE, Roberts GM. Lumbar spinal manipulation on trial. Part I: clinical assessment. *Rheumatol Rehabil.* 1978;17: 46–53.

Farrell JP, Twomey LT. Acute low back pain. Comparison of two conservative treatment approaches. *Med J Aust.* 1982;1:160–164.

Gibson T, Grahame R, Harkness J, Woo P, Blagrave P, Hills R. Controlled comparison of short-wave diathermy treatment with osteopathic treatment in non-specific low back pain. *Lancet.* 1985;1: 1258–1261.

Giles LGF, Muller R. Chronic spinal pain syndromes: a clinical pilot trial comparing acupuncture, a nonsteroidal anti-inflammatory drug, and spinal manipulation. *J Manipulative Physiol Ther.* 1999; 22:376–381.

Glover JR, Morris JG, Khosla T. Back pain: a randomized clinical trial of rotational manipulation of the trunk. *Br J Industr Med.* 1974;31:59–64.

Godfrey CM, Morgan PP, Schatzker J. A randomized trial of manipulation for low-back pain in a medical setting. *Spine.* 1984;9:301–304.

Hadler NM, Curtis P, Gillings DB, Stinnett S. A benefit of spinal manipulation as adjunctive therapy for acute low-back pain: a stratified controlled trial. *Spine.* 1987;12:703–706.

Hemmilä HM, Keinänen-Kiukaanniemi SM, Levoska S, Puska P. Does folk medicine work? A randomized clinical trial on patients with prolonged back pain. *Arch Phys Med Rehabil.* 1997;78:571–577.

Hemmilä HM, Keinänen-Kiukaanniemi SM, Levoska S, Puska P. Long-term effectiveness of bone-setting, light exercise therapy, and physiotherapy for prolonged back pain: a randomized controlled trial. *J Manipulative Physiol Ther.* 2002;25:99–104.

Herzog W, Conway PJ, Willcox BJ. Effects of different treatment modalities on gait symmetry and clinical measures for sacroiliac joint patients. *J Manipulative Physiol Ther.* 1991;14:104–109.

Hoving JL. *Neck Pain in Primary Care: The Effects of Commonly Applied Interventions:* The Netherlands Institute for Research in Extramural Medicine (EMGO Institute) of the Vrije Universiteit; 2001.

Howe DH, Newcombe RG, Wade MT. Manipulation of the cervical spine—a pilot study. *J R Coll Gen Pract.* 1983;33:574–579.

Hsieh CY, Adams AH, Tobis J, et al. Effectiveness of four conservative treatments for subacute low back pain: a randomized clinical trial. *Spine.* 2002;27: 1142–1148.

Hsieh CY, Phillips RB, Adams AH, Pope MH. Functional outcomes of low back pain: comparison of four treatment groups in a randomized controlled trial. *J Manipulative Physiol Ther.* 1992;15:4–9.

Hurwitz EL, Morgenstern H, Harber P, Kominski GF, Yu F, Adams AH. A randomized trial of chiropractic manipulation and mobilization for patients with neck pain: clinical outcomes from the UCLA neck-pain study. *Am J Public Health.* 2002;92:1634–1641.

Jordan A, Bendix T, Nielsen H, Hansen F, Host D, Winkel A. Intensive training, physiotherapy, or manipulation for patients with chronic neck pain. A prospective single-blinded randomized clinical trial. *Spine.* 1998;23:311–319.

Koes BW, Bouter LM, van Mameren H, et al. The effectiveness of manual therapy, physiotherapy, and treatment by the general practitioner for nonspecific back and neck complaints. A randomized clinical trial. *Spine.* 1992;17:28–35.

Koes BW, Bouter LM, van Mameren H, et al. Randomised clinical trial of manipulative therapy and physiotherapy for persistent back and neck complaints: results of one year follow-up. *BMJ.* 1992;304:601–605.

MacDonald RS, Bell CMJ. An open controlled assessment of osteopathic manipulation in nonspecific low-back pain. *Spine.* 1990;15:364–370.

Mathews JA, Mills SB, Jenkins VM, et al. Back pain and sciatica: controlled trials of manipulation, traction, sclerosant and epidural injections. *Br J Rheumatol.* 1987;26:416–423.

Meade TW, Dyer S, Browne W, Townsend J, Frank AO. Low back pain of mechanical origin: randomised comparison of chiropractic and hospital outpatient treatment. *BMJ.* 1990;300:1431–1437.

Meade TW, Dyer S, Browne W, Frank AO. Randomised comparison of chiropractic and hospital outpatient management for low back pain: results from extended follow up. *BMJ.* 1995;311:349–351.

Nordemar R, Thorner C. Treatment of acute cervical pain—a comparative group study. *Pain.* 1981;10: 93–101.

Pope MH, Phillips RB, Haugh LD, Hsieh CY, MacDonald L, Haldeman S. A prospective random-ized three-week trial of spinal manipulation, transcutaneous muscle stimulation, massage and corset in the treatment of subacute low back pain. *Spine.* 1994;19:2571–2577.

Postacchini F, Facchini M, Palieri P. Efficacy of various forms of conservative treatment in low back pain. A comparative study. *Neuro Orthop.* 1988;6: 28–35.

Skargren EI, Oberg BE, Carlsson PG, Gade M. Cost and effectiveness analysis of chiropractic and physiotherapy treatment for low back and neck pain. Six-month follow-up. *Spine.* 1997;22:2167–2177.

Sloop PR, Smith DS, Goldenberg E, Dore C. Manipulation for chronic neck pain. A double-blind controlled study. *Spine.* 1982;7:532–535.

Timm KE. A randomized-control study of active and passive treatments for chronic low back pain following L5 laminectomy. *J Orthop Sports Phys Ther.* 1994;20:276–286.

Triano JJ, McGregor M, Hondras MA, Brennan PC. Manipulative therapy versus education programs in chronic low back pain. *Spine.* 1995;20:948–955.

Waagen GN, Haldeman S, Cook G, Lopez D, DeBoer KF. Short term trial of chiropractic adjustments for the relief of chronic low back pain. *Manual Med.* 1986;2:63–67.

Wreje U, Nordgren B, Aberg H. Treatment of pelvic joint dysfunction in primary care—a controlled study. *Scand J Prim Health Care.* 1992;10: 310–315.

Zylbergold RS, Piper MC. Lumbar disc disease: comparative analysis of physical therapy treatments. *Arch Phys Med Rehabil.* 1981;62:176–179.

CHAPTER 50

Biomechanical Mechanisms of Chiropractic

John Triano, DC, PhD

INTRODUCTION

Statistics indicate that chiropractic deals primarily with musculoskeletal problems, predominantly of the spine, some of the extremities, and with headache disorders. Forms of treatment include manipulation, manual therapy, physical therapy, nutrition, lifestyle change, and other types of preventive health care.

Two fundamental questions are frequently asked with regard to chiropractic. How can chiropractors treat multiple kinds of pathologies—and how can they use the same treatment (manipulation) and still achieve good results? There are two aspects to these inquiries. First is the issue of multiple pathologies, and the second is the question of whether the same treatment is always applied. The actual nature of pathology and its treatment is often far more subtle and complex than these questions might imply.

EXPANDING THE MODEL OF SPINAL PATHOLOGY

The classic pathoanatomical model is to identify specific pathology that will dictate a specific treatment, likely to produce a specific outcome. In the discussion of the spine the classical model does not work as well as it does for conditions such as heart or lung disease. This model fails to account for clinical observation, the complexity of spinal anatomy, and the limitations of current diagnostic technology.

Complex neurophysiological spinal phenomena. Diagnosis and treatment of spinal disorders represents a significant challenge to both conventional medicine and chiropractic. The spine is exceptionally formed and complex. When injury or dysfunction occur, classic models of treatment are often not sufficient. We need to turn to models of disease that are more descriptive and account for clinical experience.

John J. Triano, DC, PhD, FCCS, is codirector of Conservative Medicine and director of the Chiropractic Division for the Texas Back Institute, and he also serves as research professor for the University of Texas, Biomedical Engineering Program in Arlington. He is a member of the North American Spine Society and serves as an editorial advisor to *Spine*, *The Spine Journal,* and the *Journal of Manipulative and Physiological Therapeutics*. Dr. Triano's publications in the peer-reviewed medical literature number more than 65, with an additional 15 book chapters.

Courtesy of John Triano, PhD, DC, Texas Back Institute, Plano, Texas.

The spinal column is a multisegmented link system composed of 24 vertebrae, 23 discs, the base of the skull, and the sacrum within the pelvis. Each functional spinal unit (FSU) is composed of two vertebrae with an interposing disc (except for the unique c1/c2 joint) that permits a pair of nerves to exit and serve the body within the local region. In general, each bone forms a part of at least six joints. Its role is to give solid structural support for daily activities and to permit a wide range of movements, while protecting the spinal cord and nerve roots. In all, the spine involves 96 joints.

Limitations of diagnostic evidence. Imaging is often not useful in the early stages of treatment since up to 50% of otherwise healthy adults have significant anatomical abnormalities of the spine that are clinically unrelated to their symptoms. Frequently, spine and back dysfunctions and their symptoms resolve quickly. Of those that persist, the majority resolve within a month of conservative treatment. However, a percentage of these conditions do not respond well to treatment or recur if concerted efforts to restore fitness are not pursued.

Unfortunately, many of the subtle dysfunctions and injuries that occur to the spine are not perceptible with X-ray or sometimes even with MRI. Examples include nerve inflammation; damaged, torn, or bruised muscles; buckling phenomena; impingement within the functional spinal unit; and damage to specific areas within the disc.

No Single Model of Disease

The complex and subtle nature of spinal injuries that undermines the classic model of disease are borne out in our clinical observations of treatment and response. In the case of the spine, a specific pathology may be identified. Yet, this pathology may not have any negative affect on the individual—or across the population statistically. Moreover in those with symptoms and presence of the pathology, treatment designed to address that anatomy (e.g., surgical ablation or prosthetic replacement) may or may not achieve good outcome. On the other hand, pathology may be detected, but the patient may have no symptoms and no need for treatment. This is true for a substantial portion of our population. In short, there is no single model of spinal injury or dysfunction.

Multifactorial etiology. For example, if a herniated disk is the source of pain, why can it be successfully treated with either manipulation, pain therapy, or an epidural injection and still achieve a good outcome? Moreover when the patient is symptom free and functional, why does follow-up imaging demonstrate that the herniation still exists? This suggests that we are dealing with a multifactorial etiology of symptoms. Much of spinal pathology in its early stage may or may not be symptomatic. It may become symptomatic only after it has been overstressed to a degree that exceeds a threshold effect. If that is the case, then a successful strategy may be to prevent it from reaching threshold level or to reduce excessive stress back to a level below the threshold.

Effects of biomechanical stress. The modern evidence suggests that excessive biomechanical stress is a key factor that can result in many symptoms, both for normal and abnormal anatomical structures. We call the result of that overstressing event a subluxation, and its panorama of potential symptoms a subluxation complex. An evidence-based definition of subluxation describes it as a buckling of the functional spinal unit within the bounds of its normal range of motion, resulting in the concentration of stress in one or more of the local tissues (disc, ligament, joint, nerve, or muscle). Subluxation can arise from:

• Single overload events
• Prolonged static stress followed by small movements
• Rapid loads to the spine
• Vibration environments

Manipulation and other forms of treatment used in chiropractic are designed to release the overstress in the tissues, and then the symptoms improve. Therefore, regardless of concurrent pathoanatomy, we see clinically that altering the local biomechanical stresses through treatment frequently results in decreased swelling and general improvement of symptoms. Evidence suggests that this successful outcome occurs not due to the treatment of the pathology directly, but by addressing the associated mechanical problem that increased the stress in the tissues beyond threshold.

Late stage pathology. We also know from this model that there is a stage in the development of pathology at which patients can no longer benefit from treatment. Research from the latter 20th century on extremity joints (Dhert et al., 1988; Salter, 1989) and recent animal work (Cramer et al., 2004) show that altered joint stress can result in classical pathoanatomical changes resulting in adhesions and degenerative joint disease. If the biomechanical dysfunction and resulting inflammatory/degenerative processes have been present for too long or become too severe, changes in the local tissue may become too difficult to attenuate or reverse.

BIOMECHANICAL PHENOMENA OF THE SPINE

Buckling Phenomena Defined

Buckling is a mechanical term that is applied in materials science and engineering to describe a type of structural failure. Any type of material or structure can buckle. For example, on impact a car door buckles, a tin roof buckles, and the supports of a building can buckle. This term is also relevant in discussing the biomechanics of the human spine, its structures, configuration, and function. Technically, the spine is a kinetic chain that poses multiarticular, multiple muscle stability problems.

The notion of buckling is not complex—it involves a sudden shift in the shape or configuration of a structure under load that exceeds acceptable functional limits. Technically it has three fundamental characteristics.

- First, it occurs after reaching a critical load that is unique, based on the configuration and stiffness of the structure.
- Second, it results in an unacceptable deformation, meaning that the shift in shape causes the structure to become nonfunctional or dysfunctional.
- As implied by characteristic number two, the structure may remain intact but *deformed* with increased strain at the site of buckling. *Deformation* in this sense is not in the orthopedic sense of scoliosis or misshapen bone; rather in a mechanical sense, a shift of configuration has occurred within the bounds of normal range of motion that results in increased local tissue strain. Essentially, structural failure can be a result of separation (fracture or tearing) or by unacceptable deformation as in buckling.

Buckling Phenomena in Musculoskeletal Pathology

When a tissue buckles, increased localized mechanical stress occurs, involving adjacent tissues. That tissue may be the disc, the joint, capsules within the joint, the ligament around it, or the adjacent muscles—whichever structure exceeded its injury threshold. This is an actual phenomenon that occurs, for example, in the wrist where it has been called a *z-joint collapse*. In the functional spinal unit, in its more subtle form, it is termed subluxation and when more extensive damage occurs, is described as frank instability.

Structural changes and buckling deformation within the spine increase stress in the tissues, typically resulting in inflammation, pain, and swelling. Additional local symptoms frequently follow and may include increased muscle tension to guard and limit the joint activity, resulting in loss of motion. More remote symptoms may include radiating pain into the head or extremities and even nerve irritation with radicular symptoms, depending on the comorbid pathology and central reflex changes. Central reflex changes may arise due to altered stimuli from joint proprioceptor input (Pickar, 2002; Pickar et al., 2004). Pain symptoms typically occur in the tissues where the greatest strain occurred during the buckling phenomena. Therefore, it is not surprising that if the stress exceeded the injury threshold for the facet joint, the symptoms resemble facet disease. If it occurred in the disc, it resembles discogenic pain. If irritation spills over to the nerve by means of a concurrent bone spur or disc bulge/protrusion, the patient evinces pain in the dermatome or sclerotome where that nerve traverses.

The inflammatory cascade may be triggered by two pathways:

- The frank tearing of tissue with release of local agents that stimulate pain and promote the vascular dilation and chemotactic stimuli necessary for formation of swelling within the tissues
- Reflex changes that promote neurogenic inflammation

Causes of Buckling Phenomena

These phenomena can occur in a number of specific circumstances:

Stress within the range of motion. In the progression of movement, the spinal joint must maintain a balance between the loads acting on the body and its ability to sustain that load. If the muscles that provide the stiffness to control the spine posture and motion during activity are ill timed in their re-

sponse, or if the load simply overwhelms them, buckling will occur. Evidence also shows that preexisting tissue damage or disease may promote buckling and lower the load-bearing capacity of the functional spinal unit. A number of basic stressors can trigger a buckling event.

Effects of prolonged static posture. Evidence suggests that buckling can occur when one remains in a single posture for an extended period of time and then makes even a small movement that changes the balance at the spine. This is described as a prolonged static posture followed by an incremental load. The classic example is the person who gets underneath the car to make a repair, remains there for a while, and comes out stiff and uncomfortable. This is an awkward posture at extremes of position. The resulting symptoms are usually reversible through stretching and conscious change of posture. However, if upon standing, the body does not come out of that posture, that is a buckling event.

Rapid loading. When very rapid loading occurs, a buckling event or buckling phenomena can result. For example, rapid loading of 500 pounds per second or more can trigger a buckling event. Just 500 pounds per second is not much: consider that simply jumping off the floor and landing on one's heels applies pressure to the spine of about half the body weight. In the case of a 200-pound man, that is approximately 100 pounds of load on his spine above the L5 vertebrae. That represents 1000 pounds of pressure per second. The effects of this rapidly applied force, under certain circumstances, can trigger biomechanical buckling.

Vibration. A third condition, vibration, can potentiate buckling as shown by biomechanical studies. This is consistent with observations in practice. For example, a moving car vibrates at ten times per second, which happens to be approximately the natural frequency of the spine. We know clinically that people who experience that vibration a great deal, such as truck and taxi drivers, have more back problems than those who do not.

Excessive localized stress. When the system is fatigued or struck by a rapid unexpected load for which it is unprepared, buckling can occur because there has been a mismatch between the task and the coordination of the individual vertebra in performing that task—resulting in increased localized stress. Symptoms of pain reflect the location and degree of damage.

REGIONAL AND LOCAL MUSCULATURE IN THE BACK

The spinal column is divided into four regions: the neck (cervical), the upper back (thoracic), the lower back (lumbar), and the pelvis. Each region has widely different functions and the transition point between them must accommodate the different stresses of each area to which it joins. The cervical region gives rise to the brachial plexus of nerves serving the upper extremity, the thoracic region delivers nerves to control the trunk and influences internal organ function, and the lumbar region eminates from the lumbar plexus to the pelvis and lower extremity. Each functional spinal unit is influenced directly by small intrinsic muscles of the spine and indirectly by longer regional muscles that cross over it but do not necessarily attach to it.

The spine is a multiarticular, multiple muscle structure that attempts to maintain stability. Balance control is provided by two separate muscular control systems (McGill, 2002)—a regional control that drives posture and trunk movement and a local control system that coordinates the individual functional spinal units in that region to form a consistent configuration. This consistency minimizes local stress during the desired task. For any activity to occur, there must be coordination between these two control systems.

Regional control—The large muscles of the trunk, such as the abdominal and large back muscles, control the overall choice of posture at any given moment. Tasks can be performed using many different postures. Under normal situations, we choose postures that are the most comfortable, those causing lower tissue stress.

Posture is an example of regional control and a very useful tool for self-care. One can sit in a good posture, which reduces the stress on the back, or an awkward one, which increases these stresses. We know that the back is capable of assuming a great many postures, appropriate or stressful, but it is not as adapted to maintain the awkward postures for an extended period of time or under stress or weight bearing. In certain circumstances a buckling event can occur—for example, when we are fatigued and a sudden, unexpected load is placed on the system.

Local control—The small muscles that traverse one or two functional spinal units provide local coordination of the joint structures. This configures the vertebrae consistently with posture or movement, while attempting to keep local tissue stress reduced (Bergmark, 1987). Think of the spine as a series of links. For example, when the pelvis is stationary and the upper trunk bends forward, that requires adaptation by the five vertebrae that provide the linkage between the pelvis and the rib cage. Each one of those links must coordinate its movement in order to facilitate effective, low-stress activities such as bending.

DIAGNOSIS

Correlating Pathology and Symptoms

There are a great many people who appear to have various forms of abnormal structure on MRIs such as bulging discs, protrusion, tears, stenosis, or other phenomena. As mentioned, the data suggest that as many as 50% of us have some type of spinal abnormality. We typically manage without problems on a day-to-day basis. However, under certain circumstances we may suddenly develop pain or impaired function. Why? Frequently, the answer is that a buckling event occurred to that structure. We also know that if a structure is already injured, it will buckle more readily.

Spinal and musculoskeletal phenomena are incredibly complex. All the disciplines that provide musculoskeletal interventions recognize this: orthopedic surgery and orthopedics, rheumatology, sports medicine, and chiropractic. In clinical practice, we all see patients who present with subtle and challenging pathologies that are difficult to diagnose and to treat.

Given the current level of imprecision in available imaging technology, diagnosis in chiropractic continues to be based in part on clinical symptoms and response. Diagnosis is utilized to determine the limits of what the practitioner can safely and effectively do. Diagnostic analysis is used to provide guidance on the appropriate use of treatment methods, their modification to accommodate local pathology, the effects of aging, and other issues with regard to patient status (Triano et al., 2004). The purpose of diagnosis in chiropractic is to determine what the boundaries are for a trial therapy and to provide a guide for that therapy.

TREATMENT

The second question regarding chiropractic involves the definition of treatment. Spinal manipulation is generally conceived of as a single form of therapy, whereas in reality, it involves a number of subtle variations in velocity, force, and the application of the treatment procedures.

To regard manipulation and manual methods as a single form of treatment would be comparable to the suggestion that anti-inflammatories, all having the same in-tent, work through one common mechanism. Yet in reality, there is an extensive variety of over-the-counter and prescription anti-inflammatories, as well as botanicals and nutrients (nutraceuticals) with anti-inflammatory properties. While these tools have a common intent, it is clear that pharmaceutical differences encompass wide variability. This offers opportunities to meet the challenges of biological individuality and sensitivities among patients that make them more or less responsive to one preparation over another. Medical doctors are familiar with this variability because it is within the realm of their daily clinical experience.

Comparably, manipulation encompasses a range of therapeutic procedures designed to achieve various clinical effects and meet the needs of the individual situation. In any given treatment, the choice of technique will be based on the therapeutic goal and the nature of biomechanical phenomena. Some forms of manipulation appear to be similar superficially but have different effects. Other procedures within manipulation appear quite different, but have similar effects due to the specific application. In sum, manipulation is not a single technique but a rich and varied set of procedures available to alter biomechanical stress within the tissue, reduce symptoms, and promote normal function.

As described earlier, the discipline of chiropractic has historically used the term "subluxation" to describe the biomechanical phenomena amenable to manipulation and manual methods. It is important to understand the unique characteristics of a subluxation. What evidence exists that defines and describes it?

As in any other field, this is an evolving science. Historically, the theory with regard to subluxation has not been complete and did not account for some of what we were observing clinically. Over the past two decades, applying existing and emerging scientific evidence, the theory has been revised and is now capable of explaining clinical observations more accurately, accounting for current clinical practice (Triano, 2000, 2001). This enables us to more fully define and describe some of the underlying mechanisms of chiropractic. It also increases understanding of how and why patients with different symptoms and underlying pathology can benefit from manual manipulative procedures.

When treatment is successful that is excellent. If a series of treatments are not successful within a reasonable time frame, then it is time to try a different therapy. Ultimately, this approach is not different from medicine. Medical treatment for back pain frequently involves a course of medication—either an anti-inflammatory, a muscle relaxant, or an analgesic—with the purpose of relieving pain and reducing inflammation and muscle spasms. If that is not successful, the patient is referred to physical therapy to strengthen the muscles in that region of the spine. Chiropractic provides patients with a biomechanical procedure for a mechanical disorder: the goal is to reduce local stress in order to decrease the pain and inflammation, and initiate healing. Frequently exercise and physical therapy are also recommended. In summary, conventional medicine applies a chemical approach; we apply a mechanical approach. We are simply utilizing different tools to accomplish the same thing.

Case study. When a patient develops a mildly symptomatic herniated disk, if the tissue pathology is not too severe, chiropractic treatment can often shift and remove the mechanical stress through spinal manipulation. Once the mechanical stress is removed, the tissue begins to heal, swelling is reduced, and the pain decreases.

As in any type of therapy, a certain dosage and duration of treatment is necessary to create a threshold effect. In manipulation, a certain level of biomechanical force is necessary to alter the buckling event—the biomechanical displacement or dysfunction. Initially, the therapy must occur frequently enough to keep the swelling under control. However, once patients have been treated, they are not usually immobilized, since patients generally feel better and immobility has no proven benefit. As they go about their daily lives, obviously their physical activities involve movement and that movement can be irritating. As a result, the swelling and the buckling tends to recur. This means that the intervention must occur periodically to counter the recurrences of biomechanical stress.

The role of exercise and lifestyle. While passive treatment using manipulation and manual methods may be useful to reduce symptoms and promote function, only analysis of risk factors in the patient's lifestyle to minimize future events and the use of exercise to help strengthen and stiffen the control systems for spinal function can bring about long-term recovery.

Using medication and manipulation together. We know from clinical outcomes at integrative treatment centers such as the Texas Back Institute that sometimes it is important to utilize both medication and manipulation to achieve the desired outcome. It is not uncommon for a buckling event to irritate the tissues or nerve of the disk. That irritation may develop to the extent that the patient may not be able to tolerate the manipulation procedure. In these cases, the next step is the use of an anti-inflammatory—a nonsteroidal anti-inflammatory, oral steroid, or even an injection—to calm that inflammation. Once the inflammation is reduced, the chiropractor applies spinal manipulation to alter the mechanical stress that initiated the inflammation. If the response does not occur in a timely manner, the case can become a failed therapy that may require surgery.

Medication or manipulation. In some cases, an anti-inflammatory is not sufficient. As long as the patient is on the anti-inflammatory they feel better, but the medication alone does not remove the mechanical irritant. Consequently, once the anti-inflammatory effect wears off, the mechanical irritant is still present and reirritates the tissues. At that point, the case is frequently considered a failed therapy.

When does the case become a failed therapy? In some cases, patients have exceeded their capacity to heal and require surgery. Others may have incurred too much damage to completely stabilize the situation and will have to restrict their activities and change their work or their lifestyle to accommodate the damage that has been done. Anyone working with spine patients encounters such situations. However, long before the inflammatory process and the spinal pathology reach that point, many patients can benefit from biomechanical treatment.

For some, anti-inflammatory medication is sufficient to address the biomechanical issue. A patient with an inflammatory condition, given anti-inflammatories, may begin to move more comfortably and more easily. The restored movement may be sufficient to shift the biomechanical stress, which removes the cause of inflammation and the patient improves.

The effects of previous surgery can become another form of coexisting pathology. Patients who have had prior surgery may still undergo buckling events at other levels or at the same level, depending on the type of surgery that was involved. Patients who have had surgery need to be evaluated carefully with regard to limitations that would impose on the appropriate use of manipulation procedures.

SAFETY

Chiropractors have been very good at educating the world that what they do is relatively safe and not too difficult. The problem is that they have been too convincing—there is now an impression that spinal manipulation, particularly high-velocity procedures, is a very simple thing to do and that anyone should be able to do it. Current evidence suggests that health care practitioners and physicians who take weekend training programs in spinal manipulation do not gain enough expertise to be effective (Curtis, et al., 2000) in administering these procedures and changing clinical outcomes. Any effective intervention, used on the wrong person or used without sufficient in-depth training, can result in adverse effects.

Medical school and chiropractic education involve approximately the same number of classroom hours. However, in chiropractic the vast majority of that training focuses on the care and treatment of the spine. While chiropractors are responsible for 94% of spinal procedures using high-velocity techniques, they are only responsible for approximately 65% of the serious adverse reactions in reviewed case series (Triano et al., 2004). These procedures should be performed only after adequate training in differential diagnosis and extensive supervised training and practice in the use of the procedures (McGregor, 2004).

CONCLUSION

The human body is amazingly resilient: sometimes it needs a chemical push, sometimes a mechanical push, and sometimes both. In a few cases neither is adequate and other interventions are necessary to solve the problem. Clearly, from a dispassionate perspective, there is the need for both conventional medicine and chiropractic in the treatment of spinal dysfunction and damage.

REFERENCES

Bergmark A. *Mechanical Stability of the Human Lumbar Spine*. Lund University, Department of Solid Mechanics. Thesis/Dissertation; 1987:1–85.

Cramer GD, Fournier JT, Henderson CN, Wolcott CC. Degenerative changes following spinal fixation in a small animal model. *JMPT*. 2004;27:141–154.

Curtis P, Carey TS, Evans P, Rowane MP, Mills-Garrett J, Jackman A. Training primary care physicians to give limited manual therapy for low back pain: patient outcomes. *Spine*. 2000;25(22):2954–2960.

Dhert WJ, O'Driscoll SW, Salter RB. Effects of immobilization and continuous passive motion on postoperative muscle atrophy in mature rabbits. *Can J Surg*. 1988;31:185–188.

McGill SM. *Low Back Disorders*. Champaign, IL: Human Kinetics; 2002.

McGregor, M. Musculoskeletal complications of chiropractic practice. In: Haldeman S, ed. *Principles and Practice of Chiropractic*. New York, NY: McGraw-Hill; 2004:1127–1148.

Pickar JG. Neurophysiological effects of spinal manipulation. *Spine J*. 2002;2:357–371.

Pickar JG, Sung PS, Kang Y. The effect of a spinal manipulation's impulse speed on low-threshold mechanoreceptors in lumbar paraspinal muscles. *J Chiro Educat*. 2004;18:25–26.

Salter RB. The biologic concept of continuous passive motion of synovial joints: the first 18 years of basic research and its clinical application. *Clin Orthop*. 1989;242:12–25.

Triano J. Biomechanics of spinal manipulation. *Spine*. 2001;1:121–130.

Triano J. The mechanics of spinal manipulation. In: Herzog W, ed. *Clinical Biomechanics of Spinal Manipulation*. New York, NY: Churchill Livingstone; 2000:92–190.

Triano JJ, Bougie J, Rogers C. Procedural skills in spinal manipulation: do prerequisites matter? *Spine J*. 2004;4(5):557–563.

CHAPTER 51

Research on Spinal Physiology

Joel G. Pickar, DC, PhD

Much of the initial basic science research in the field of chiropractic focused on biomechanical changes in the spine because these changes were thought to contribute to spinal dysfunction in general and to low back and neck pain specifically. In some cases, biomechanical changes are visible on X-ray as abnormal anatomical or functional relationships between vertebrae. However, signs from imaging studies, including X-ray, do not necessarily correlate with clinical symptoms, particularly in relation to low back pain (Witt et al., 1984; Carragee & Hannibal, 2004). There are people whose lumbar spine on X-ray looks relatively normal, yet who have low back pain. There are others whose X-rays demonstrate pathological changes, yet these individuals experience no pain. This raises the possibility that more subtle, non-pathological biomechanical, neurophysiological, or biochemical factors contribute to the etiology of spinal dysfunction. In this context, research over the past 15 years has begun to elucidate the role of the physiological changes that can occur in the spine.

Joel G. Pickar, DC, PhD is a professor at the Palmer Center for Chiropractic Research in Davenport, IA. His research laboratory is studying neurophysiological issues related to the vertebral column and to chiropractic manipulation. Dr. Pickar serves on the Advisory Editorial Board for *The Spine Journal* and is a member of the NIH Advisory Council for Complementary and Alternative Medicine.

Courtesy of Joel Pickar, DC, PhD, Palmer Chiropractic Center, Davenport, Iowa.

BIOMECHANICAL PROCESSES

Almost all definitions of chiropractic treatment agree that chiropractic addresses biomechanical dysfunction and neurological changes in the spine. A number of biomechanical processes can lead to spinal dysfunction:

Adhesions. These tissue changes can develop in collagen, the protein in connective tissue that provides its structure, strength, and flexibility/rigidity. Adhesions most often take the form of cross-linking between adjacent collagen fibers. This can occur within the collagenous sheets that comprise the fascia (a network of fibrous connective tissue attached to the deepest layer of skin and investing all deeper tissue, including muscle and bone). Adhesions are present in scar tissue and are also known to occur when a joint is immobilized for an extended period of time, resulting in restricted range of motion.

- Synovial adhesions (those within the joint space) are due to many causes. Even slight injury and some decreased joint movement (due to "favoring" the injury) can result in the development of adhesions. Adhesions within the facet joints of the spine that cause some restriction to intersegmental movement are a possible cause of segmental dysfunction (Haldeman, 1978; Farfan, 1980; Giles, 1989; Lewit, 1991).
- Myofascial adhesions can occur within muscle and soft connective tissue. They restrict or alter normal movement as well as

the relative position of one musculoskeletal segment to another.

Occlusions. In the knee joint it is known that pieces of the meniscus can break off, wedge between the femur and tibia, and cause pain, inflammation, and abnormal motion. Meniscoids are also present in facet joints of the lumbar spine (Giles, 1989). These synovial meniscoids may become trapped between the joint surfaces and potentially interfere with intervertebral motion. In addition, occlusions can occur when redundant folds of the neurally innervated facet capsule become trapped between surfaces of the joint (Haldeman, 1978; Farfan, 1980; Giles, 1989; Lewit, 1991).

Muscle tension. Palpatory findings from clinical experience suggest that muscle tension is frequently present in individuals with low back pain. Because muscle forces contribute substantially to spinal stability and movement, muscle tautness may alter the dynamics of vertebral movement and position and predispose one to spinal injury. Paradoxically, however, clinical studies of muscle activity in individuals with low back pain do not consistently show increased muscle activity when assessed by EMG (electromyography) (Nouwen & Bush, 1984; Ahern et al., 1988; Arena et al., 1991).

However, some research indicates that increased neural activity from sensory receptors responding to injury may evoke active muscle contractions. The mechanism by which this occurs is described as the "pain-spasm-pain cycle" (Roland, 1986). Several studies provide support for this hypothetical cycle in neck muscles of the cervical spine (Pedersen et al., 1997; Wenngren et al., 1998), but not in the lumbar spine (Kang et al., 2001) and inconsistently in studies of leg muscle (Anastasijevic et al., 1987; Jovanovic et al., 1990; Mense & Skeppar, 1991).

Dysfunction in spinal facet joints. Vertebral facet joints may become restricted, disturbed, or functionally asymmetric due to adhesions, occlusions, or dysfunction of paraspinal muscles. Buckling phenomena may occur leaving the segment in a new and abnormal equilibrium or position, which adversely affects intervertebral motion (Wilder et al., 1988; Cholewicki & McGill, 1996).

Dysfunction within the disc. Intervertebral discs, shaped somewhat like ovoid hockey pucks, are positioned between contiguous vertebrae and are composed of three components: an outer portion (anulus fibrosus), an inner portion (nucleus pulposus), and vertebral endplates.

• The outer portion—the anulus fibrosus—is somewhat ovoid-shaped with a structure comparable to that of a radial tire, composed of concentric layers of collagen. This structure provides strength as well as flexibility similar to that of a braided finger puzzle. The anulus fibrosus encloses the nucleus pulposus and attaches to the vertebral endplates, which are composed of cartilage.
• The inner portion—nucleus pulposus—is a pressurized, hydrated gel enclosed and contained by the anulus. It functions like a ball bearing between vertebrae, resisting compression and preventing kinking of the anulus fibrosus, and cushioning movement.
• The vertebral endplates connect the outer layers to the vertebrae above and below. The structure of the disc provides each vertebral body with substantial freedom of motion including bending, twisting, and sliding.

We know from MRI imaging and cadaver studies that tears or rents occur between collagen layers of the anulus fibrosus. The nucleus pulposus can ooze or migrate through and into these fissures (disc disruption). When the disruption is substantial (disc herniation/prolapse) the nucleus pulposus causes the outermost layers to bulge (protrusion) or escapes from the outermost layers altogether (extrusion). These mechanical changes in the disc can alter the biomechanics of spinal motion, release inflammatory mediators, and have neurological effects.

BIOCHEMICAL MECHANISMS

Causal factors leading to spinal dysfunction and potentially to back pain also include a number of biochemical mechanisms. These, in turn, have been associated with both deranged biomechanical processes and neural dysfunction.

Enzymatic action of inflammatory mediators. Studies indicate that herniated intervertebral discs produce and elaborate various proinflammatory chemicals, including phospholipase A_2 (McCarron et al., 1987; Nygaard et al., 1997). At high levels, phospholipase A_2 will silence and even kill nerve cells. At moderate levels, phospholipase A_2 increases the excitability and mechanical sensitivity of nerve cell bodies in the dorsal root ganglia (Chen et al., 1997; Ozaktay et al., 1998), which lie in close physical proximity to the intervertebral disc.

Inflammatory mediators. Extruded nucleus pulposus can become detached from the remainder of the intervertebral disc in a process called sequestration. This displaced tissue may evoke neurological consequences. In an experimental model, simulating a sequestered, herniated intervertebral disc, the application of nucleus pulposus directly to a lumbar nerve root caused hyperalgesia in the limbs, swelling, and decreased blood flow to nerve cell bodies in the dorsal root ganglia (Kawakami et al., 2000; Yabuki et al., 2000).

NEUROLOGICAL MECHANISMS

More than a decade of basic research has contributed to our understanding of the physiological role played by neural innervation of the spinal column.

Neurological responses to mechanical pressures.
- The dorsal roots and dorsal root ganglia which lie close to the spinal column are responsive to mechanical pressure (Howe et al., 1977; Rydevik, 1992).
- The dorsal roots are more responsive compared with their more peripheral processes located at a distance from the spinal column.
- Mechanical pressure can impede the transmission of neural information.

The sensitivity of dorsal roots and the dorsal root ganglia may reflect their structural characteristics. The density of ion channels for Na^+ (sodium) is higher in the dorsal root ganglia than in their axons (Devor & Obermayer, 1984). Connective tissue in dorsal roots is weaker and sparser, thus providing less mechanical protection and support (Berthold et al., 1984; Beel et al., 1986; Thomas et al., 1993) compared with the peripheral processes of these sensory neurons. Since the dorsal roots travel close to the intervertebral disc, these nerves can be irritated by compressive forces arising from a herniated disc (Takahashi et al., 1999).

Abnormal proprioceptive input. Obvious functions of the spinal column are to protect the spinal cord, support the limbs, and impart mobility to the trunk. To enable these functions, the spinal column must be stable, yet flexible. Stability is provided by passive tissues (spinal ligaments, intervertebral discs, and paraspinal muscles) and active spinal tissues (again, paraspinal muscles). Substantial evidence shows that active muscle contraction is especially important for spinal stability (Panjabi et al., 1989; Cholewicki & McGill, 1996). Neural input from paraspinal muscles and facet joints are thought to provide sensory information to help regulate muscle stiffness and provide spinal stability (Panjabi, 1992; Ianuzzi et al., 2004).

Recent work suggests that stimulation of sensory nerves from the intervertebral disc can induce reflex muscle activity in the lumbar multifidus muscle (Indahl et al., 1997). Other studies demonstrate that the sensitivity of paraspinal neurons (muscle spindles) to vertebral movement can increase or decrease depending upon a vertebra's position relative to its neighboring vertebrae (Pickar & Kang, 2001; Ge et al., 2004). Thus proprioceptive input from muscle spindles in the longissimus and multifidus muscles may provide unreliable information depending upon spinal posture.

Increased sensitivity/central facilitation.

Neurons of the spinal cord can become sensitized to incoming sensory messages in a phenomenon of increased sensitivity known as central facilitation (Cook et al., 1987). Increased sensitivity can manifest in several ways:

- Spinal cord neurons can become spontaneously active.
- These neurons can become hyperexcitable, developing an increased responsiveness to sensory input from the periphery.
- Spinal cord neurons may respond to stimuli to which they were previously unresponsive.
- Receptive fields of spinal cord neurons can broaden, responding to sensory input from parts of the body to which they were previously unresponsive.

Sensitivity to subthreshold stimuli.

Another aspect of increased sensitization relates to the concept of subthreshold stimuli. Spinal cord neurons continually receive sensory input from different kinds of sensory receptors, receptors sensitive to mechanical, chemical, and temperature changes. However, neurons within the spinal cord do not always respond to these sensory inputs. An input is considered subthreshold when it increases a spinal cord neuron's excitability without actually exciting the neuron. Altered spinal biomechanics may contribute to greater sensitization by increasing the number of subthreshold inputs to the spinal cord.

Activation of the stress response/ sympathetic system.

When tissues of the spine are inflamed or when mechanical changes occur in the spine during inflammation, neural reflexes appear to trigger the sympathetic nervous system. Research in experimental animal models, for example, indicates that sympathetic nerve activity to the adrenal glands (Budgell et al., 1995) and to the spleen and kidneys (Kang et al., 2003) can increase when tissues of the lumbar spine are inflamed. When mechanical changes in the spine are accompanied by the chemical changes of inflammation, the sympathetic responses can be prolonged (Kang et al., 2003).

A general impression from the literature suggests that noxious inputs from paraspinal tissues have an excitatory effect on the sympathetic system, but it is not clear if mechanical and inflammatory-type inputs produce different effects (Sato & Swenson, 1984; Deboer et al., 1988; Brennan et al., 1994; Budgell et al., 1995, 1997, 2000; Kang et al., 2003). Additional research is needed to understand the relationship between neural input from axial tissues and changes in the autonomic nervous system. It is of special interest that sympathetic outflow to different organ beds such as the kidney, spleen, heart, and vascular system can be differentially controlled. The sympathetic nervous system does not necessarily respond in an all-or-none fashion (Kenney et al., 1991).

Immune suppression. In general, pain and inflammation can have immune suppressive effects. This phenomenon may be basic to all mammalian physiology (Selye, 1978). As the organism responds to stress, the immune system can become less responsive. Once the stress response has abated, rest and repair can resume as the immune system is reactivated. If specific stressors are prolonged or severe, immune suppression may be long lasting.

Animal studies have shown that increased sympathetic nerve activity to the spleen is immune suppressive, decreasing the number of natural killer cells released by the spleen (Katafuchi et al., 1993). Interestingly, depressed levels of natural killer cells have also been measured in individuals with low back pain (Brennan et al., 1994). This raises the question as to whether inflammatory changes in paraspinal tissues that reflexively affect sympathetic outflow to the spleen (Kang et al., 2003) could depress the immune system.

EFFECTS OF SPINAL MANIPULATION

The research described in the following section, drawn from the international literature, provides a brief overview of a body of work that investigates the neurophysiological impact of spinal manipulation. The author's own research is in the area of basic neurophysiology related to the spinal column and is on understanding how primary sensory neurons respond to the mechanical forces delivered during spinal manipulation.

Effects on paraspinal neurons. Research in an animal model indicates that one of the mechanisms by which spinal manipulation may affect the nervous system is through direct mechanical stimulation of sensory receptors in paraspinal tissues. Table 51–1 enumerates the four classes of sensory nerve endings found in paraspinal tissues. A recent study (Pickar & Wheeler, 2001) examined the effect of spinal manipulation on two types of sensory receptors in muscle: muscle spindles and Golgi tendon organs. The manipulation was delivered in a manner that closely imitated the preload and impulse load delivered clinically to the lumbar spine. The activity of both types of receptors increased by more than two-fold in response to manipulation, when compared with the resting state. The magnitude of this increase often depended upon the direction in which the spinal manipulation was applied.

Effect of the speed of manipulation on neural discharge. In general, manual therapies can be characterized by their force-time profile. The change in mechanical input during manipulation is very fast compared with other approaches such as mobilization and massage therapy. Manipulation involves a thrusting motion, which typically occurs in less than 1/4 of a second and is difficult to voluntarily resist. Mobilization involves a nonthrusting motion that can be applied singly or repetitively, and which occurs over the course of seconds. It is of interest, therefore, to know if the speed with which a manipulation is delivered makes a difference in the neurological outcome.

To gain insight into this issue, we (Pickar et al., 2004; Sung et al., 2004) experimentally applied spinal manipulation at six different durations. The force and time profiles were identical except for the manipulation's duration. The response of low threshold mechanoreceptors and proprioceptors (see table) located in lumbar paraspinal muscles was measured. Changes in neural discharge

Table 51–1 Classification of Receptive Nerve Endings and Their Parent Nerve Fibers

Type of Receptive Ending	Location	Enervation	Conduction Velocity (meters/second)	Conduction Velocity (miles/hour)
Proprioceptors (muscle spindles and Golgi tendon organs)	Muscle	Group Ia, Ib (Aα); Group II (Aβ)	80–120 35–65	179–269 78–146
Low-threshold mechanoreceptors	Muscles, joints, ligaments, skin	Group II (Aβ) Group III (Aδ) Possibly Group IV (C)	35–65 2.6–30 2.5	78–146 6–67 <6
High-threshold mechanoreceptors	Muscles, joints, ligaments, skin	Group II Group III (Aδ) Group IV (C)	35–65 2.6–30 2.5	78–146 6–67 <6
Chemoreceptors and thermoreceptors	Muscles, joints, ligaments, skin	Group III (Aδ) Group IV (C)	2.6–30 2.5	6–67 <6

occurred as the manipulation's duration approached the duration typically used clinically (≤200 ms, approximately 1/4 second). The manner of the change suggested a threshold effect wherein the manipulation, when delivered with sufficient speed, elicited a novel response from paraspinal muscle mechanoreceptors. Thus, spinal manipulation may provide a novel neurological input to the central nervous system compared with that of slower types of manual therapies. Further work is necessary to determine the neurophysiological consequences and potential therapeutic benefit of this input.

Decreased area of pain sensitivity. Spinal manipulative therapy has been found to decrease sensitivity to pain. In one study of pain responses (Glover et al., 1974), the effects of spinal manipulation were evaluated based on changes in sensitivity to pinpricks applied to skin over the lumbar area. The control group received de-tuned shortwave therapy; no change was experienced in this group. The treatment group received spinal manipulation: in this group of patients, the size of the area from which pain could be evoked by pinpricks was reduced for 15 minutes following spinal manipulation.

Decreased sensitivity to pain. In another study, pain sensitivity was measured using a handheld electrical stimulator that delivered controlled current. The activated device evoked the sensation of pain when touching the skin (Terrett & Vernon, 1984). The higher the current required to evoke pain, the less sensitive the subject was to pain. The magnitude of current necessary to evoke the sensation of pain was monitored in 25 individuals who received spinal manipulation and in a control group of 25 individuals who did not and were simply resting quietly. Measurements were taken in both groups at the start of the experiment and periodically over the next 10 minutes. Following manipulation, the amount of current that could be tolerated by those in the treatment group increased within 30 seconds and continued to increase over the 10 minutes of monitoring. In the nonmanipulated group no change in pain tolerance was observed.

Changes in pressure/pain thresholds. In a case study, pressure/pain thresholds were assessed before and after spinal manipulation using a handheld pressure algometer (Vernon, 1988). The threshold measurement indicated the amount of pressure at which the perception of pressure changed to the perception of pain. The algometer was applied to six tender points in the neck region. The participant identified his own specific tender points. Spinal manipulation increased pressure-pain thresholds and decreased his sensitivity to pain by approximately 45% on average.

In an effort to extend the findings from this case study to the lumbar spine area, a study was undertaken that focused on chronic mechanical low back pain (Cote et al., 1994). A pressure algometer was applied to three sensitive points, but in this study, identical points were studied in all participants. These were standardized myofascial trigger points associated with low back pain. Unlike the earlier case study, these trigger points were not necessarily clinical relevant: they were not identified as tender by participants, nor were they the most sensitive points for each individual. Unlike the earlier case

study, no changes in pressure-pain thresholds were observed.

In these studies, the mechanisms underlying the observed changes in pain tolerance or threshold level is unknown. Research on the effects of spinal manipulation indicates that it:

- May alter sensory input to the central nervous system.
- May affect central processing of pain-producing signals.
- May activate the neuroendocrine system, stimulating the release of endogenous opiates (Vernon et al., 1986; Christian et al., 1988; Rosner, 2001).

CONCLUSION

The research in this chapter highlights biomechanical and neurophysiological aspects of vertebral function and begins to build a rational foundation for the clinical intervention of spinal manipulation. The vertebral column protects the nervous system and, from a biomechanical perspective, supports and literally enables nearly all activities of daily living. Therefore our understanding of these mechanisms is vital. The recent neurophysiological studies presented in this chapter demonstrate physiological mechanisms of spinal column function and dysfunction, as well as the neurophysiological impact of spinal manipulation. Substantial work is necessary to better understand the mechanisms that underlie the integrated function of the spinal column and the impact of therapeutic interventions directed to the spine.

REFERENCES

Ahern DK, Follick MJ, Council JR, Laser-Wolston N, Litchman H. Comparison of lumbar paravertebral EMG patterns in chronic low back pain patients and non-patient controls. *Pain.* 1988;34(2): 153–160.

Anastasijevic R, Jocic M, Vuco J. Discharge rate and reflex responses of fusimotor neurons during muscle ischemia. *Exp Neurol.* 1987;97:340–344.

Arena JG, Sherman RA, Bruno GM, Young TR. Electromyographic recordings of low back pain subjects and non-pain controls in six different positions: effect of pain levels. *Pain.* 1991;45:23–28.

Beel JA, Stodieck LS, Luttges MW. Structural properties of spinal nerve roots: biomechanics. *Exp Neurol.* 1986;91:30–40.

Berthold CH, Carlstedt T, Corneliuson O. Anatomy of the nerve root at the central-peripheral transitional region. In: Dyck PJ, ed. *Peripheral Neuropathy.* 1st ed. Philadelphia, PA: WB Saunders Company; 1984:156–170.

Brennan PC, Graham MA, Triano JJ, Hondras MA, Anderson RJ. Lymphocyte profiles in patients with chronic low back pain enrolled in a clinical trial. *J Manipulative Physiol Ther.* 1994;17:219–227.

Budgell B, Hotta H, Sato A. Spinovisceral reflexes evoked by noxious and innocuous stimulation of the lumbar spine. *J Neuromusculoskel Sys.* 1995;3:122–130.

Budgell B, Sato A, Suzuki A, Uchida S. Responses of adrenal function to stimulation of lumbar and thoracic interspinous tissues in the rat. *Neurosci Res.* 1997;28:33–40.

Budgell B, Suzuki A. Inhibition of gastric motility by noxious chemical stimulation of interspinous tissues in the rat. *J Autonom Nerv Sys.* 2000;80:162–168.

Carragee EJ, Hannibal M. Diagnostic evaluation of low back pain. *Orthop Clin North Am.* 2004;35(1):7–16.

Chen C, Cavanaugh JM, Ozaktay AC, Kallakuri S, King AI. Effects of phospholipase A$_2$ on lumbar nerve root structure and function. *Spine.* 1997;22:1057–1064.

Cholewicki J, McGill SM. Mechanical stability of the *in vivo* lumbar spine: implications for injury and chronic low back pain. *Clin Biomech.* 1996;11:1–15.

Christian GF, Stanton GJ, Sissons D, et al. Immunoreactive ACTH, b-endorphin, and cortisol levels in plasma following spinal manipulative therapy. *Spine.* 1988;13:1411–1417.

Cook AJ, Woolf CJ, Wall PD, McMahon SB. Dynamic receptive field plasticity in rat spinal cord dorsal horn following C-primary afferent input. *Nature.* 1987;325:151–153.

Cote P, Silvano AM, Vernon H, Mior SA. The short-term effect of a spinal manipulation on pain/pressure threshold in patients with chronic mechanical low back pain. *J Manipulative Physiol Ther.* 1994;17:364–368.

Deboer KF, Schutz M, McKnight ME. Acute effects of spinal manipulation on gastrointestinal myoelectric activity in conscious rabbits. *Manual Med.* 1988;3:85–94.

Devor M, Obermayer M. Membrane differentiation in rat dorsal root ganglia and possible consequences for back pain. *Neurosci Letters.* 1984;51:341–346.

Farfan HF. The scientific basis of manipulation procedures. In: Buchanan WW, Kahn MF, Laine V, et al., eds. *Clinics in Rheumatic Diseases.* Philadelphia, PA: WB Saunders Company; 1980:159–177.

Ge W, Cobb T, Pickar, JG. Changes in lumbar paraspinal muscle spindle response due to the history of vertebral position. *Society for Neuroscience.* 2004; Presentation Number 672.13.

Giles LGF. *Anatomical Basis of Low Back Pain.* Philadelphia, PA: Williams and Wilkins; 1989.

Glover JR, Morris JG, Khosla T. Back pain: a randomized clinical trial of rotational manipulation of the trunk. *Br J Indust Med.* 1974;31:59–64.

Haldeman S. The clinical basis for discussion of mechanisms of manipulative therapy. In: Korr IM, ed. *The Neurobiologic Mechanisms in Manipulative Therapy.* New York, NY: Plenum; 1978:53–75.

Howe JF, Loeser JD, Calvin WH. Mechanosensitivity of dorsal root ganglia and chronically injured axons: a physiological basis for the radicular pain of nerve root compression. *Pain.* 1977;3:27–41.

Ianuzzi A, Little JS, Chiu JB, Baitner A, Kawchuk G, Khalsa PS. Human lumbar facet joint capsule strains: I. During physiological motions. *Spine J.* 2004;4(2):141–152.

Indahl A, Kaigle AM, Reikeras O, Holm SH. Interaction between the porcine lumbar intervertebral disc, zygapophysial joints, and paraspinal muscles. *Spine.* 1997;22(24):2834–2840.

Jovanovic K, Anastasijevic R, Vuco J. Reflex effects on gamma fusimotor neurones of chemically induced discharges in small-diameter muscle afferents in decerebrate cats. *Brain Res.* 1990;521:89–94.

Kang, YM, Kenney MJ, Spratt KF, Pickar JG. Somatosympathetic reflexes from the low back in the anesthetized cat. *J Neurophysiol.* 2003;90:2548–2559.

Kang, YM, Wheeler JD, Pickar JG. Stimulation of chemosensitive afferents from multifidus muscle does not sensitize multifidus muscle spindles to vertebral loads in the lumbar spine of the cat. *Spine.* 2001;26(14):1528–1536.

Katafuchi T, Take S, Hori T. Roles of sympathetic nervous system in the suppression of cytotoxicity of splenic natural killer cells in the rat. *J Physiol.* 1993;465:343–357.

Kawakami M, Tamaki T, Hayashi N, et al. Mechanical compression of the lumber nerve root alters pain-related behaviors induced by the nucleus pulposus in the rat. *J Orthop Res.* 2000;18:257–264.

Kenney MJ, Barman SM, Gebber GL, Zhong S. Differential relationships among discharges of post-ganglionic sympathetic nerves. *Am J Physiol.* 1991; 29:R1159–R1167.

Lewit K. *Manipulative Therapy in Rehabilitation of the Locomotor System.* Oxford, UK: Butterworth-Heinemann; 1991.

McCarron RF, Wimpee MW, Hudkins PG, Laros GS. The inflammatory effect of nucleus pulposus. A possible element in the pathogenesis of low-back pain. *Spine.* 1987;12:760–764.

Mense S, Skeppar P. Discharge behaviour of feline gamma-motoneurones following induction of an artificial myositis. *Pain.* 1991;46:201–210.

Nouwen A, Bush C. The relationship between paraspinal EMG and chronic low back pain. *Pain.* 1984; 20:109–123.

Nygaard OP, Mellgren SI, Osterud B. The inflammatory properties of contained and noncontained lumbar disc herniation. *Spine.* 1997;22:2484–2488.

Ozaktay AC, Kallakuri S, Cavanaugh JM. Phospholipase A_2 sensitivity of the dorsal root and dorsal root ganglion. *Spine.* 1998;23:1297–1306.

Panjabi, MM. The stabilizing system of the spine. Part 1. Function, dysfunction, adaptation, and enhancement. *J Spinal Disord.* 1992;5(4):383–389.

Panjabi MM, Kuniyoshi A, Duranceau J, Oxland T. Spinal stability and intersegmental muscle forces: a biomechanical model. *Spine.* 1989;14:194–199.

Pedersen J, Sjolander P, Wenngren BI, Johansson H. Increased intramuscular concentration of bradykinin increases the static fusimotor drive to muscle spindles in neck muscles of the cat. *Pain.* 1997;70: 83–91.

Pickar JG, Kang YM. Short-lasting stretch of lumbar paraspinal muscle decreases muscle spindle sensitivity to subsequent muscle stretch. *J Neuromusculoskel Sys.* 2001;9(3):88–96.

Pickar JG, Kang YM, Cobb T. Discharge of paraspinal muscle spindles to impulse loading of a spinal manipulation. *Society for Neuroscience.* 2004; Presentation Number 672.18.

Pickar JG, Wheeler JD. Response of muscle proprioceptors to spinal manipulative-like loads in the anesthetized cat. *J Manipulative Physiol Ther.* 2001; 24:2–11.

Roland MO. A critical review of the evidence for a pain-spasm-pain cycle in spinal disorders. *Clin Biomech.* 1986;1:102–109.

Rosner A. Endocrine disorders. In: Masarsky CS, Todres-Masarsky C, eds. *Somatovisceral Aspects of Chiropractic: An Evidence-Based Approach.* Edinburgh, UK: Churchill-Livingstone; 2001:187–202.

Rydevik BL. The effects of compression on the physiology of nerve roots. *J Manipulative Physiol Ther.* 1992;15:62–66.

Sato A, Swenson RS. Sympathetic nervous system response to mechanical stress of the spinal column in rats. *J Manipulative Physiol Ther.* 1984;7:141–147.

Selye H. *The Stress of Life.* New York, NY: McGraw-Hill; 1978.

Sung PS, Kang YM, Pickar JG. Effect of spinal manipulation duration on low threshold mechanoreceptors in lumbar paraspinal muscles: a preliminary report. *Spine.* 2004; (in press).

Takahashi K, Shima I, Porter RW. Nerve root pressure in lumbar disc herniation. *Spine.* 1999;24:2003–2006.

Terrett ACJ, Vernon HT. Manipulation and pain tolerance: a controlled study of the effect of spinal manipulation on paraspinal cutaneous pain tolerance levels. *Am J Phys Med.* 1984;63:217–225.

Thomas PK, Berthold CH, Ochoa J. Microscopic anatomy of the peripheral nervous system. In: Dyck PJ, ed. *Peripheral Neuropathy.* 1st ed. Philadelphia, PA: WB Saunders Company; 1993:28–91.

Vernon HT. Pressure pain threshold evaluation of the effect of spinal manipulation on chronic neck pain: a single case study. *JCCA.* 1988;32:191–194.

Vernon HT, Dhami MSI, Howley TP, Annett R. Spinal manipulation and beta-endorphin: a controlled study of the effect of a spinal manipulation on plasma beta-endorphin levels in normal males. *J Manipulative Physiol Ther.* 1986;9:115–123.

Wenngren BI, Pedersen J, Sjolander P, Bergenheim M. Bradykinin and muscle stretch alter contralateral cat neck muscle spindle output. *Neurosci Res.* 1998;32: 119–129.

Wilder DG, Pope MH, Frymoyer JW. The biomechanics of lumbar disc herniation and the effect of overload and instability. *J Spinal Disord.* 1988;1(1): 16–32.

Witt I, Vestergaard A, Rosenklint A. A comparative analysis of X-ray findings of the lumbar spine in patients with and without lumbar pain. *Spine.* 1984;9(3):298–300.

Yabuki S, Igarashi T, Kikuchi S. Application of nucleus pulposus to the nerve root simultaneously reduces blood flow in dorsal root ganglion and corresponding hind paw in the rat. *Spine.* 2000;25: 1471–1476.

CHAPTER 52

Referring Patients to Chiropractic Care

Charles A. Simpson, DC

REFERRING FOR CHIROPRACTIC CARE

Indications for referral. Chiropractors treat the spectrum of mechanical problems of the musculoskeletal system. Many conditions involving the spine or the extremities are appropriate for referral. In general, if the structure is intact, but the function is impaired, chiropractic treatment is an appropriate alternative. Conditions frequently treated by chiropractic physicians include sprains and strains of the spine and extremities, back pain, neck pain, muscle tension and migraine headaches, extremity symptoms, referred and radicular problems, and peripheral neuropathies such as carpal tunnel syndrome. There is also some evidence that chiropractic care is useful for conditions such as hypertension, asthma, infantile colic, and other nonmusculoskeletal conditions.

Contraindications. Chiropractic care is generally quite safe compared to other routine clinical procedures. However, there are situations in which patients are not appropriate for referral. Contraindications can be considered in two categories: relative and ab-

solute contraindications. There are a few very important absolute contraindications, and it is essential that referring practitioners are familiar with them. These include conditions that feature destruction of bone such as primary and metastatic lesions of bone. There are also serious neurological conditions that are not appropriate for referral including lesions of the spinal cord and cauda equina syndrome. The following information provides the guidelines from Medicare on relative and absolute contraindications to chiropractic manipulation.

CHIROPRACTIC CONTRAINDICATIONS

Medicare Document 2251.3

Dynamic thrust is the therapeutic force or maneuver delivered by the physician during manipulation in the anatomic region of involvement. A relative contraindication is a condition that adds significant risk of injury to the patient from dynamic thrust, but does not rule out the use of dynamic thrust. The doctor should discuss this risk with the patient and record this in the chart. The following are *relative contraindications* to dynamic thrust:

- Articular hypermobility and circumstances where the stability of joint is uncertain
- Severe demineralization of bone
- Benign bone tumors (spine)
- Bleeding disorders and anticoagulant therapy
- Radiculopathy with progressive neurological signs

Charles A. Simpson, DC, has been a practicing chiropractor for over 25 years. He is a founder of Complementary Healthcare Plans (CHP) of Beaverton, Oregon, and currently serves as their vice president and medical director. CHP provides integrative acupuncture, chiropractic, naturopathic medicine, and massage therapy services for health plans, health maintenance organizations, and preferred-provider organizations in Oregon and Washington state.

Dynamic thrust is *absolutely contraindicated* near the site of demonstrated subluxation and proposed manipulation in the following:

- Acute arthropathies characterized by acute inflammation and ligamentous laxity and anatomic subluxation or dislocation; including acute rheumatoid arthritis and ankylosing spondylitis
- Acute fractures and dislocations or healed fractures and dislocations with signs of instability
- An unstable os odontoideum
- Malignancies that involve the vertebral column
- Infection of bones or joints of the vertebral column
- Signs and symptoms of myelopathy or cauda equina syndrome
- For cervical spinal manipulations, vertebrobasilar insufficiency syndrome
- A significant major artery aneurysm near the proposed manipulation

Source: Medicare Administration, 2003; 10-01-04.

Osteoporosis provides an example of a relative contraindication. Manipulation of an osteoporotic patient can cause a fracture. However, it is only a relative contraindication, since there are many low-force chiropractic techniques that do not put an osteoporotic patient at risk. In fact, many people with osteoporosis can obtain real benefit from certain chiropractic techniques. For a more thorough discussion of relative and absolute contraindications, see Haldeman S, *Principles and Practices of Chiropractic.*

Complications of cervical manipulation. Manipulation of the upper cervical spine bears a very small, but very serious potential for harm. Due to the anatomical structure of the upper cervical region, there is a greater risk associated with upper cervical chiropractic manipulative therapy (CMT) than that involved with manual manipulation gener-

ally. The anatomy of the cervico-cranial junction places the vascular supply to the brain at potential risk of compromise from inappropriate upper cervical manipulation. That said, the material risk is a very small one, especially in the context of risk from all routine health care interventions. Unfortunately at this point, there are no identifiable risk factors or screening tests that can reliably be used to assess contraindications to upper cervical manipulation. Risk can be minimized by use of manipulative procedures that avoid rotation of the upper cervical complex.

Short-term side effects. Short-term side effects of chiropractic treatments are common and a referring provider should be aware of the usual reactions to chiropractic adjusting both to prepare patients and to differentiate more serious side effects. Three studies have evaluated the types of short-term discomfort that patients report to chiropractors. Although approximately half of patients reported some discomfort (44% to 55%), all three studies found that symptoms resolved in the majority of cases within 24 to 48 hours. Senstad et al. (1997) found that discomfort was mild to moderate in 85% of cases. Specifics of these studies follow.

Senstad et al. (1997) studied "unpleasant" side effects experienced after adjusting by 1058 new patients. After a cumulative 4712 adjustment sessions, 55% of patients reported to their chiropractors some type of reaction. "Unpleasant reactions" included "local discomfort, which accounted for more than half of the symptoms, followed by headache, tiredness, and radiating discomfort which accounted for another one third." Patients reported these reactions to be mild (35%), moderate (50%), definitely unpleasant (11%), and unbearable (1%). Most (74%) of these unpleasant side effects disappeared within 24 hours. There were no reports of serious complications by any participant.

Lebouf-Yde and colleagues (1997) studied 625 patients prospectively. Throughout a total of 1858 visits, 44% of patients reported at least one unpleasant reaction. The most common reaction was local discomfort at the treatment site of these cases; 75% of unpleasant symptoms resolved in 48 hours. However, patients with long-lasting problems (> 3 months) generally experienced more adverse, though short-lived effects from adjusting. No serious complications were noted by any patient in this study.

Barrett and Breen (2000) studied a small sample (N = 68) of chiropractic patients; fifty-three percent of patients reported some sort of adverse effect up to 2 days posttreatment. Extra pain, radiating pain, and stiffness were the most commonly reported side effects. These on average were reported by patients to be only mild to moderate. Throughout the study the authors noted, "No serious adverse side effects were reported."

In conclusion, it is probably useful to inform patients that chiropractic adjusting is likely to cause some discomfort, especially after the first few treatments, but that the soreness is almost always mild and short term.

Writing a prescription for chiropractic services. There are several ways to approach a chiropractic referral:

- One is to refer with directions to "evaluate and treat." This approach is most appropriate in the context of a referral to a provider already familiar to the referral source.
- Prescribing chiropractic. If the referring physician is comfortable prescribing chiropractic in the same way they prescribe a medication, the referral could specify the treatment including dosage, frequency and duration, goals, patient limitations, and specific manipulative or physical therapy techniques to be used.

- Utilizing existing referral protocols. Many health plans, medical groups, and other organizations have developed referral protocols that specify parameters for chiropractic treatment. The best of these guidelines are evidence-based, focused on specific clinical conditions, and define the length and scope of treatment, and expected outcomes, as well as requirements for reevaluation (for example, after 5 visits and again after 10 visits).

WHAT TO LOOK FOR IN A PRACTITIONER

Training and licensure. Chiropractic training is provided in 4- to 5-year programs with a residency supervised by the chiropractic college. Accreditation of chiropractic colleges in the United States and abroad is accomplished by the Council on Chiropractic Education, which is certified by the US Office of Education. Chiropractic programs are also accredited by regional higher-education accrediting agencies. In addition, national board examinations assure academic and clinical competency. Chiropractic licensing occurs in all 50 states and more than 35 foreign countries.

Skill set. The skills that chiropractors acquire are primarily diagnosis and treatment in manual medicine. In addition, a variety of physical medicine modalities are provided in conjunction with musculoskeletal practice, such as traction, heat, ultrasound, and electrical stimulation. The treatment process also involves engaging the patient in self-care, activity modification, exercise, proper biomechanics, and ergonomics.

Mindset. One of the qualities that makes an effective chiropractor is a willingness to understand how chiropractic fits in with the rest of a patient's health care. An integrative approach entails patient-focused, outcomes-based services that include objective indicators of patient progress. An effective chiropractor is consistent in involving each patient in clinical decision making and engaging patients in the treatment process and in their own care.

Communication with the referring practitioner. The integrative chiropractor is aware of the value offered by each member of the health care team and the need for effective communication among team members. A referring practitioner should expect back a written summary of the patient's case, the treatment plan, expected outcomes, current status, and future treatment recommendations. (For more information on basic referral protocol, see Chapter 68.) This is now standard operating procedure among chiropractors who interface with conventional medicine providers.

THE PATIENT'S EXPERIENCE

Patient satisfaction. The literature indicates that patients are extremely satisfied with chiropractic care. In terms of what the patient is likely to experience (Simpson, 2001), treatments include a clinical interview similar to that conducted in a medical office, a physical and neurological examination, a chiropractic evaluation for dysfunction, and, when appropriate, special studies such as diagnostic imaging. The treatment itself requires cooperation by the patient, primarily by relaxing during the process of spinal manipulation.

Treatment plan. An integrative chiropractor individualizes each treatment plan to the patient, the condition, and patient preferences. Depending on the patient and the nature of the condition, the treatment plan will be different. The fact that two patients both have back pain does not necessarily mean that they will both have the same treatment plan. For example, a healthy young weightlifter who just pulled a back muscle and needs a few adjustments will have a very different treatment plan from that of someone who has had a lifetime of low back pain with frequent flare-ups. In the first instance, relief may occur within minutes, while patients with chronic conditions may require treatment over a course of a month or two to achieve results.

Outcomes. A chiropractor accustomed to focusing on specific clinical endpoints will establish explicit goals or outcomes targets in terms of both symptomatic relief and improved physical function. The actual outcomes are assessed over an established number and duration of treatments (typically five or six treatments over 2 weeks for most acute conditions). At that point, the patient's progress is reevaluated to determine 1) whether another series of treatments is potentially beneficial, 2) if maximum benefit has been reached, or 3) if the patient should be referred out for a different course of care.

There is growing evidence on clinical outcomes in chiropractic with regard to specific conditions. The research is very favorable on the utilization of chiropractic for management of back pain—both chronic and acute. (See Chapter 49 for a summary of research outcomes.) With regard to neck pain, we also have research evidence of the effectiveness for acute conditions. Additional positive outcomes studies have been published on muscle tension headaches. Positive outcomes with those three conditions are increasingly confirmed as new studies are published. When comparing the relative risks of common interventions, we now know that patients have less risk from chiropractic treatment than, for example, from taking over-the-counter nonsteroidal anti-inflammatory medication.

Long-term treatment. To date, the research has focused on acute conditions and only to a limited degree on chronic conditions. Treatment interventions studied so far have all been primarily short term. There have been few long-term treatment studies. For example, we do not know whether going to a chiropractor once a month enhances overall health and quality of life for certain populations. There is some evidence that Medicare patients who see chiropractors have lower health expenses in total and therefore possibly better health status. That does not answer the question, "Does chiropractic adjustment at intervals make any difference in the average person's health or in their health care expenses?"

Self-care. Chiropractors recognize the importance of self-care in the physical, nutritional, and psychological realms. Ultimately, all those aspects of function need to be maintained by the patient for long-term good health. While chiropractors are primarily focused on the musculoskeletal system, chiropractic care also logically encompasses exercise, nutrition, and lifestyle management.

INSURANCE COVERAGE AND UTILIZATION

Chiropractic treatment is included in more health plans and managed care networks than any other complementary discipline (see Table 52–1). A recent survey of 1800 visits to complementary practitioners in four states found that most visits to chiropractors were covered by insurance, in contrast to less than one third for most other types of complementary practitioners (Cherkin et al., 2002).

CONCLUSION

Generally speaking, medical doctors in the mainstream who are willing to intelligently make referrals to disciplines such as chiropractic can enhance their own clinical practice by providing patients access to effective early interventions. There is good evidence in the research literature that chiropractic is one of the safest, most cost-effective forms of treatment for back pain and many other conditions.

It has become apparent that biomedicine, chiropractic, and other complementary disciplines really are genuinely complementary. Each discipline has different strengths. Each concentrates on a particular area of treatment that can be beneficial for certain diagnoses. Effective patient comanagement, focused on the best outcome for the patient, provides the basis for the positive professional relationships that are emerging between chiropractors and medical doctors. Integrative practice expands the tools we all have available at every stage in the continuum.

Table 52–1 Data on the Utilization of Chiropractic

Source and Universe Surveyed	Parameter	Percent
National Market Measures.[1] Randomly selected managed care organizations (N = 114 of 449 MCOs in US)	Of MCOs offering complementary therapies, percentage that offer chiropractic	65.0
Madigan Army Medical Center.[2] Patients in a family practice (N = 177)	Of patients using complementary medicine, percentage using chiropractic	64.0
Kaiser Permanente, Division of Research.[3] Percentage of clinicians who used or recommended chiropractic	• OB/Gyn clinicians (N = 157) • Primary care clinicians (N = 624)	37.6 33.6
Harvard Center for Alternative Medicine Research.[4] Nationally representative random household survey by telephone (N = 2055)	Percentage of all visits to complementary providers which were made to chiropractors in 1997 (192 million of 629 million)	30.5 approx.
Kaiser Permanente, Division of Research.[5] Kaiser patients surveyed who had severe musculoskeletal pain	• Of 3885 patients, the percentage who used chiropractic (1999) • Of 4254 patients, the percentage who used chiropractic (1996)	21.5 18.4
Stanford Center for Research.[6] Demographically representative random survey (N = 1035)	Of those using all forms of complementary medicine in previous year, percentage who used chiropractic	15.7
Harvard University, Center for Alternative Medicine Research.[7] Nationally representative random household survey by telephone (N = 2055)	Prevalence and frequency of use of chiropractic among adult respondents	11.0
National Center for Complementary and Alternative Medicine, NIH.[8] Data from 2002 National Health Interview Survey, a nationally representative sample (N = 31,044)	Percentage of population using chiropractic in past year	7.5
Yale University, Departments of Psychiatry and Public Health.[9] Participants in 1996 Medical Expenditure Panel Survey (N = 16,068)	From broader population in survey, statistics on visits to chiropractors in past year	3.3

Source: Charles A. Simpson, DC, Complementary Healthcare Plans, Beaverton, Oregon, 2004.

TABLE REFERENCES

1. National Market Measures. *The Landmark Report II*. Sacramento, CA: Landmark Healthcare; 1999.
2. Drivdahl CE, Miser WF. The use of alternative health care by a family practice population. *J Am Board Fam Pract*. 1998;11(3):193–199.
3. Gordon N, Sobel D, Tarazona E. Use of and interest in alternative therapies among adult primary care clinicians and adult members in a large health maintenance organization. *WJM*. 1998;169(3): 153–161.
4. Wolsko PM, Eisenberg DM, Davis RB, Kessler R, Phillips RS. Patterns and perceptions of care for treatment of back and neck pain: results of a national survey. *Spine*. 2003;28(3):292–297, 298.
5. Gordon NP, Lin TY. Use of complementary and alternativce medicine by the adult membership of a large northern California health maintenance organ-ization. *J Ambulatory Care Manager*. 2004;27(1): 12–24.
6. Astin J. Why patients use alternative medicine: results of a national study. *JAMA*. 1998;279(19): 1548–1553.
7. Eisenberg D, Davis R, Ettner S, Appel S, Wilkey S, Van Rompay M, Kessler R. Trends in alternative medicine use in the United States, 1990–1997: results of a follow-up national survey. *JAMA*. 1998;280(18):1569–1575.
8. Barnes PM, Powell-Griner E, McFann K, Nahin R. Complementary and alternative medicine use among adults: United States, 2002. *Adv Data*. 2004;343:1–16.
9. Druss B, Rosenheck R. Association between use of unconventional therapies and conventional medical services. *JAMA*. 1999;282(7):651–656.

REFERENCES

Barrett A, Breen A. Adverse effects of spinal manipulation. *J R Soc Med*. 2000;93:258–259.

Cherkin DC, et al. Characteristics of visits to licensed acupuncturists, chiropractors, massage therapists, and naturopathic physicians. *J Am Board Fam Pract*. 2002;15(6):463–472.

Haldeman S. *Principles and Practices of Chiropractic*. 3rd ed. New York, NY: McGraw-Hill/Appleton & Lange; 2004.

Leboueuf-Yde C, et al. Side effects of chiropractic treatment: a prospective study. *J Manipulative Physiol Ther*. 1997;20:511–515.

Medicare Administration. Revised Requirements for Chiropractic Billing of Active/Corrective Treatment and Maintenance Therapy; CR3449. Washington, DC: US Department of Health and Human Services; 2004.

Senstad O, et al. Frequency and characteristics of side effects of spinal manipulative therapy. *Spine*. 1997;22(4):435–440.

Simpson CA. Utilization data: chiropractic utilization and cost-effectiveness. In: Faass N, ed. *Integrating Complementary Medicine into Health Systems*. Sudbury, MA: Jones and Barlett/Aspen; 2001.

CHAPTER 53

Six Perspectives on Herniated Disc Treatment

Kelli Pearson, DC

STUDY METHOD

Design. This study was conducted as a form of conference, an informal think tank of mainstream and complementary practitioners. A group of clinicians were identified in Spokane, Washington, and the surrounding locality and a series of meetings were held to develop protocols for treatment. The goal was to gain a greater depth of understanding of the treatment approach of various disciplines. Discussion focused on the day-to-day realities of clinical decision making and treatment.

Participants. Practitioners participated from a range of disciplines: acupuncture, chiropractic, family practice medicine, massage therapy, nutrition, occupational medicine, orthopedic surgery, physical therapy, psychology, rheumatology, and therapeutic exercise (strength training).

Inquiry. A series of fundamental questions were considered with regard to diagnosis and treatment:

- What is the process used to diagnose common conditions?
- What are the criteria for appropriate diagnosis?
- What are the interventions (what do we do, why, and in what time frame)?
- What are the clinical expectations and definitions of success?
- To whom are patients referred and why?

The focus. Ultimately the research focused on practitioners from six disciplines, whose perspectives were the most clear cut: physical therapy, orthopedic surgery, and rheumatology, as well as chiropractic, acupuncture, and massage therapy. We asked each practitioner to describe typical responses, define clinical success, suggest a time line for rehabilitation, and indicate the level of confidence in their ability to correct the condition. Table 53–1 summarizes their reports. The brief reference list included amplifies clinical outcomes reported by study participants.

Kelli Pearson DC, DABCO, is a chiropractor in clinical practice in Spokane, Washington.

Table 53–1.1 Treatment of Herniated Disc Conditions from the Perspective of Six Practitioners

Treatment Approach	Time Line	Expected Outcomes	Patient Outcomes
Physical therapy			
Physical modalities, mobilization, and exercise	Expects major pain relief in 4 to 6 weeks to continue care; will refer out as appropriate	Expects positive outcomes in 70% of these cases	Research evidence of positive outcomes in treatment of herniated disc conditions[1,2,3]
Orthopedic surgery			
Variety of approaches, including medication; then a variety of surgical interventions to match the pathology	Initially 30–90 days of conservative therapy; then considers surgery	Expects 80% recovery in 6 to 10 weeks if the patient was properly screened initially	Evidence of success at 10-year follow-ups[4] Appropriate rehab measures following surgery increase clinical success
Rheumatology			
Primarily medication and case management (also refers to other disciplines)	Long-term treatment for patients with difficult and chronic illness (some for life)	Disease management for severe, chronic disorders, often with multiple physiological challenges	Outcomes are variable, based on the degree of complication in clinical presentations[5]

Table 53–1.2 Treatment of Herniated Disc Conditions from the Perspective of Six Practitioners

Treatment Approach	Time Line	Expected Outcomes	Patient Outcomes
Chiropractic			
Spinal manipulative therapy, soft tissue work, and exercise	Expects major pain relief in 4 to 6 weeks, in order to continue care; will refer out as appropriate	Expects positive outcomes in 70% of these cases	Research evidence of positive outcomes in treatment of herniated disc conditions[6,7,8]
Acupuncture			
Acupuncture, moxibustion heat treatments, sometimes massage, and herbs	Dependent on progress on objective measures and pain remediation	Better success with patients who have acute rather than chronic pain	Research evidence of positive outcomes in treatment of pain associated with herniated disc conditions[9,10,11]
Clinical massage			
A range of massage techniques	Dependent on progress on objective measures and pain remediation	Intervention focuses on pain relief, may be palliative rather than curative	Research evidence of positive outcomes in the general treatment of pain[12]

REFERENCES

1. Kladny B, Fischer FC, Haase I. Evaluation of specific stabilizing exercise in the treatment of low back pain and lumbar disk disease in outpatient rehabilitation [in German]. *Z Orthop Ihre Grenzgeb.* 2003;141(4):401–405.

2. Lie H, Frey S. Mobilizing or stabilizing exercise in degenerative disk disease in the lumbar region? [in Norwegian]. *Tidsskr Nor Laegeforen.* 1999; 119(14):2051–2053.

3. Nwuga VC. Ultrasound in treatment of back pain resulting from prolapsed intervertebral disc. *Arch Phys Med Rehabil.* 1983;64(2):88–89.

4. Weber H. Lumbar disc herniation. A controlled, prospective study with ten years of observation. *Spine.* 1983;8(2):131–140.

5. Berthelot JM, Rodet D, Guillot P, Laborie Y, Maugars Y, Prost A. Is it possible to predict the efficacy at discharge of inhospital rheumatology department management of disk-related sciatica? A study in 150 patients. *Rev Rhum Engl Ed.* 1999; 66(4):207–213.

6. Oliphant D. Safety of spinal manipulation in the treatment of lumbar disk herniations: a systematic review and risk assessment. *J Manipulative Physiol Ther.* 2004;27(3):197–210.

7. Floman Y, Liram N, Gilai AN. Spinal manipulation results in immediate H-reflex changes in patients with unilateral disc herniation. *Eur Spine J.* 1997;6(6):398–401.

8. Pustaver MR. Mechanical low back pain: etiology and conservative management. *J Manipulative Physiol Ther.* 1994;17(6):376–384.

9. Yi-Kai L, Xueyan A, Fu-Gen W. Silver needle therapy for intractable low-back pain at tender point after removal of nucleus pulposus. *J Manipulative Physiol Ther.* 2000;23(5):320–323.

10. Wang RR, Tronnier V. Effect of acupuncture on pain management in patients before and after lumbar disc protrusion surgery: a randomized control study. *Am J Chin Med.* 2000;28(1):25–33.

11. Longworth W, McCarthy PW. A review of research on acupuncture for the treatment of lumbar disk protrusions and associated neurological symptomatology. *J Altern Complement Med.* 1997;3(1):55–76.

12. Ulreich A, Kullich W. Results of a multidisciplinary rehabilitation concept in patients with chronic lumbar syndromes [in German]. *Wien Med Wochenschr.* 1999;149(19–20):564–566.

CHAPTER **54**

Chiropractic Resources

David Chapman-Smith, LLB

PROFESSIONAL ASSOCIATIONS

The two largest national associations in the world are the American Chiropractic Association (ACA) and the Canadian Chiropractic Association (CCA). In the United States, there is a second national association, the International Chiropractors' Association (ICA). The ACA and ICA conduct an increasing number of joint professional and public education and political action initiatives. Since health care laws and rights and funding arrangements are mainly matters of state/provincial law rather than national law in the United States and Canada, chiropractors' first professional memberships are often with their state or provincial associations.

The organization representing state associations in the United States is the Congress of Chiropractic State Associations (COCSA). The organization representing national associations throughout the world is the World Federation of Chiropractic (WFC), a member of the Council of International Organizations of Medical Sciences (CIOMS) and in official relations with the World Health Organization (WHO).

A brief biography of David Chapman-Smith, LLB, appears in Chapter 47.

Source: Adapted and updated content provided courtesy of NCMIC Group, Clive, IA. From: Chapman-Smith D., *The Chiropractic Profession.* Des Moines, IA: NCMIC Group Inc.; 2000.

American Chiropractic Association (ACA)
1701 Clarendon Boulevard
Arlington, VA 22209
Phone: (800) 986-4636, (703) 276-8800
Fax: (703) 243-2593
Web site: www.amerchiro.org

Canadian Chiropractic Association (CCA)
1396 Eglinton Avenue
West Toronto, Ontario M6C 2E4, Canada
Phone: (416) 781-5656
Fax: (416) 781-7344
Email: ccachiro@inforamp.net
Web site: www.ccachiro.org

Congress of Chiropractic State Associations
(COCSA)
PO Box 2054
Lexington, SC 29071-2054
Phone: (803) 356-6809
Fax: (803) 356-6826
Web site: www.cocsa.org

International Chiropractors' Association
(ICA)
1110 Glebe Road, Suite 1000
Arlington, VA 22201
Phone: (703) 528-5000
Fax: (703) 528-5023
Web site: www.chiropractic.org

World Federation of Chiropractic
1246 Yonge Street, Suite 203
Toronto, Ontario M4T 1W5, Canada
Phone: (416) 484-9978
Fax: (416) 484-9665
Email: info@wfc.org
Web site: www.wfc.org

PROFESSIONAL LIABILITY INSURANCE

Chiropractors may obtain their professional liability/malpractice insurance from many private companies. The National Chiropractic Mutual Insurance Company (NCMIC Insurance) was established by the profession and is by far the largest carrier for chiropractors in the United States.

NCMIC Insurance
14001 University Avenue
Clive, IA 50325-8258
Phone: (800) 321-7015 or (515) 313-4500
Fax: (515) 313-4475
Web site: www.ncmic.com

RESEARCH ORGANIZATIONS

Leading research organizations are the Foundation for Chiropractic Education and Research (FCER), which funds research and awards for postgraduate education from private funding, and the Consortial Center for Chiropractic Research (CCCR), which has significant funding support from the US government through the National Center for Complementary and Alternative Medicine, National Institutes of Health, and the Bureau of Health Professions, Health Resources and Services Administration.

The Foundation for Chiropractic Education and Research (FCER)
P.O. Box 400 or 380 Wright Road
Norwalk, IA 50211
Phone: (800) 622-6309 or (515) 981-9888
Fax: (515) 981-9427
Email: FCER@fcer.org
Web site: www.fcer.org

FCER Research Offices
1330 Beacon Street #315

Brookline, MA 02446
Phone: (888) 690-1378 or (617) 734-3397
Fax: (617) 734-0989
Email: RosnerFCER@aol.com

The Foundation for Chiropractic Education and Research (FCER) is the oldest chiropractic research-funding institution in the world. Since 1980, FCER has funded grants, fellowships, and residencies totaling nearly $10 million. The foundation publishes research-based information for physicians, the health care industry, and the public at large.

Consortial Center for Chiropractic Research
c/o Palmer Center for Chiropractic Research
741 Brady Street
Davenport, IA 52803-5287
Phone: (563) 884-5150
Fax: (563) 884-5227
Email: research@palmer.edu
Web site: www.palmer.edu

The Consortial Center for Chiropractic Research is a coalition of seven chiropractic colleges, five state-supported universities, and Harvard Medical Center. The Center supports a multidisciplinary group of researchers and clinicians in the performance of basic preclinical, clinical, epidemiological, and/or health services research on chiropractic.

SOURCES OF FURTHER INFORMATION

Clinical Texts

Bergmann T, Peterson D, Lawrence D, eds. *Chiropractic Technique*. St. Louis, MO: Mosby Yearbook Inc.; 1998.

Bougie J, Morgenthal A, eds. *The Aging Body: Conservative Management of Common*

Neuromusculoskeletal Conditions; New York, NY: McGraw-Hill Medical; 2001.

Cramer GD, Darby SA, eds. *Basic and Clinical Anatomy of the Spine: Spinal Cord and ANS.* St. Louis, MO: Mosby Yearbook; 1995.

Curl DD, ed. *Chiropractic Approach to Head Pain.* Baltimore, MD: Williams & Wilkins; 1994.

Foreman SM, Croft CA, eds. *Whiplash Injuries: The Cervical Acceleration/ Deceleration Syndrome.* Baltimore, MD: Williams & Wilkins; 1988.

Haldeman S, ed. *Principles and Practice of Chiropractic.* 3rd ed. New York, NY: McGraw-Hill/Appleton and Lange; 2004.

Hammer WI, ed. *Functional Soft-Tissue Examination and Treatment of Manual Methods.* 2nd ed. Gaithersburg, MD: Aspen Publishers; 1999.

Herzog W, ed. *Clinical Biomechanics of Spinal Manipulation.* Edinburgh, Scotland: Churchill Livingstone; 2000.

Hyde TE, Gengenbach M, eds. *Conservative Management of Sports Injuries.* Baltimore, MD: Williams & Wilkins; 1997.

Liebenson C, ed. *Rehabilitation of the Spine: A Practitioner's Manual.* Baltimore, MD: Williams & Wilkins; 1996.

Marchiori DM, ed. *Clinical Imaging: With Skeletal Chest and Abdomen Patterned Differentials.* St. Louis, MO: Mosby; 1999.

Murphy DR, ed. *Conservative Management of Cervical Spine Syndromes.*New York, NY: McGraw-Hill/Appleton & Lange; 1999.

Peterson DH, Bergmann TF. *Chiropractic Technique: Principles and Procedures.* 2nd ed. St. Louis, MO: C.V. Mosby; 2002.

Redwood D, Cleveland C. *Fundamentals of Chiropractic.* St. Louis, MO: C.V. Mosby; 2003.

Souza TA, ed. *Differential Diagnosis for the Chiropractor: Protocols and Algorithms.*

2nd ed. Gaithersburg, MD: Aspen Publishers; 2001.

Stude DE, ed. *Spinal Rehabilitation.* Stamford, CT: Appleton and Lange; 1999.

Vernon H, ed. *Upper Cervical Syndrome: Chiropractic Diagnosis and Treatment.* Baltimore, MD: Williams & Wilkins; 1998.

Wyatt L. *Handbook of Clinical Chiropractic Care.* 2nd ed. Sudbury, MA: Jones and Bartlett Publishers, Inc.; 2004.

Yochum TR, Rowe LJ, eds. *Essentials of Skeletal Radiology.* Baltimore, MD: Williams & Wilkins; 1996.

Newsletter

The Chiropractic Report
Phone: (416) 484-9601, Toronto
Web: www.chiropracticreport.com

Peer-Reviewed Journals

Journal of Manipulative and Physiological Therapeutics
Published by Mosby/Elsevier for the National College of Chiropractic
Phone: (314) 453-4351
Web site: www.us.elsevierhealth.com

Indexed on Index Medicus and included in the Medline database, this journal reports on chiropractic and other manual therapy interventions.

The Spine Journal
Published by Elsevier for the North American Spine Society
Subscriptions from Elsevier: (877) 774-6337
Subscriptions from the Society: (708) 588-8080
Email: info@spine.org
Web site: www.spine.org

The Spine Journal is an international, multidisciplinary publication with original, peer-reviewed articles on research and treatment related to the spine and spine care. The journal is published six times a year and is indexed in Index Medicus/Medline.

Spine
Published by Lippincott Williams & Wilkins
Phone: (800) 408-5353
Web site: www.spinejournal.com

Spine is an international, peer-reviewed, biweekly periodical (24 issues per year) that considers original articles in the field of spine care for publication for a range of disciplines including chiropractic, manual therapy, surgery and orthopedics.

PART IX

Herbal Therapy

Chapter

CHAPTER 55

Access to Botanical Therapy

Carlo Calabrese, ND, MPH

Many conventional physicians are seeking a greater understanding of botanical treatments. There are at least five different levels on which a physician can focus:

1. Access to information on safety and drug interactions
2. Maximizing clinical interventions
3. Responding to patient interest
4. Comanaging patients with chronic illness
5. Inclusion of botanical practitioners into settings integrated with physicians

At each level, educational programs are available that address the particular goals and area of interest. For medical students, for example, NCCAM has put forth an initiative to increase the amount of information available on complementary medicine (NCCAM, 2004). For physicians currently in practice, resources are available that address interest at any level.

FIVE APPROACHES TO BOTANICAL THERAPY

Level 1. Access to information on safety and drug interactions. Many physicians want to educate themselves about botanicals in order to assure patient safety and avoid botanical in-

Carlo Calabrese, ND, MPH, is a research professor at National College of Naturopathic Medicine in Portland, Oregon, where his professional focus is the development of research methods for the investigation of complementary and alternative therapies. He has served as codirector of the Research Institute at Bastyr University, and also as product development manager for Nutricia, Inc., at that time the largest dietary supplement manufacturer in the world. A member of the Advisory Council for the NIH National Center for Complementary and Alternative Medicine and NCCAM's Data Safety Monitoring Board, he is a graduate of National College and holds a master's degree in public health from the University of Washington.

teractions with medication. A survey of Denver physicians found that 77% of those interested in complementary medicine CME were motivated because they "want to dissuade a patient if the alternative method is unsafe and/or ineffective" (Winslow & Shapiro, 2002). Physicians want and need to know about botanicals because patients are using them.

Level 2. Maximizing clinical interventions. At another level, many physicians want to educate themselves about the use of herbs, to become more knowledgeable about the research literature, and to gain skill in the clinical application of herbal therapy.

Most physicians are pleasantly surprised to learn that botanicals are medically valuable. We know, for example, that approximately 40% of all medications are derived from the active constituents of herbs. Informed and focused use of botanicals expands the continuum of treatment options. Botanical therapy provides a less intensive form of intervention that can be appropriate for specific, mild acute conditions; early intervention; and the management of particular chronic disorders.

Physicians who review the research and find this approach of interest may want to seek CME training in the use of herbs. This can provide an initial introduction to botanical therapy, in order to become knowledgeable in this type of prescribing and its clinical applications.

Level 3. Responding to patient interest. A third reason for educating oneself in greater depth about botanicals is that some patients are quite interested in this approach. Addressing their interests and concerns can enhance patient retention and compliance.

Botanicals increase a physician's treatment options. Some patients are uncomfortable with the use of a particular medication, or even with the use of medication in general. Others may develop side effects or become unable to tolerate a particular drug. For example, hypertensive patients on medication may find the side effects unacceptable and request another approach.

Yet complementary medicine is not an approach that should be foisted on patients. These therapies are usually most appropriate for patients who express interest in self-care, lifestyle approaches, and integrative treatment. Patients who want to know what they can do in their own lives to improve their health are those most likely to want complementary medicine and to respond well to it.

Level 4. Comanaging patients with chronic illness. Along this continuum of interest, physicians may find that there are patients with extremely complex problems, such as fibromyalgia, which could be effectively comanaged with a skilled naturopathic physician. Other chronic disorders for which patients report seeking complementary medicine include allergies; anxiety and depression; arthritis; chronic pain, including back, neck, and joint pain; digestive disorders; fatigue; headaches; and insomnia (Eisenberg et al., 1998; Barnes et al., 2004).

Level 5. Inclusion of botanical practitioners into settings integrated with physicians. The questions that arise in this situation include how to find competent practitioners, and the most effective approach to this type of comanagement. Two professional associations that certify botanical knowledge via membership are the American Association of Naturopathic Physicians and the American Herbalists Guild. Most members of these associations will also be open to patient comanagement and naturopaths, in particular, are well-prepared for comanagement.

REFERENCES

Barnes PM, Powell-Griner E, McFann K, Nahin R. Complementary and alternative medicine use among adults: United States, 2002. *Adv Data.* 2004;343: 1–16.

Eisenberg D, Davis R, Ettner S, et al. Trends in alternative medicine use in the United States, 1990–1997: results of a follow-up national survey. *JAMA.* 1998;280(18):1569–1575.

NCCAM. R25-AT: CAM Education Project Grants. Available at: http://nccam.nih.gov/research/extramural/awards/2003/index.htm#8a. Accessed September 15, 2004.

Winslow LC, Shapiro H. Physicians want education about complementary and alternative medicine to enhance communication with their patients. *Arch Intern Med.* 2002;162:1176–1181.

CHAPTER 56

Overview of Botanical Therapy

Michael T. Murray, ND

THE ROLE OF HERBS IN MEDICINE

For the past two decades, about 25% of all prescription drugs in the United States have contained active constituents obtained from plants. Digoxin, codeine, colchicine, morphine, vincristine, and yohimbine are some popular examples. Many over-the-counter preparations are composed of plant compounds as well. It is estimated that more than $11 billion worth of plant-based medicines are purchased each year in the United States alone, and $43 billion worldwide (Fuchs, 1999).

Because a plant cannot be patented, very little research has been done in the 20th or 21st centuries on whole plants or crude plant extracts as medicinal agents, per se, by large American pharmaceutical firms. Instead, pharmaceutical firms screen plants for biological activity and then isolate the so-called active constituents (compounds). In fact, pharmacognosy, the study of natural drugs and their constituents, plays a major role in current drug development. If the compound

is powerful enough, the drug company will begin the formidable process of procuring Food and Drug Administration (FDA) approval—formidable because in the United States, FDA approval of a plant-based drug typically takes 10 to 18 years at a total cost of at least $230 million.

In contrast, European policies have made it economically feasible for companies to research and develop herbs as medicines. In Germany, herbal products can be marketed as medicines if they have been proven safe and effective (Keller, 1991). Actually, the legal requirements for herbal medicines are identical to those for all other drugs. Whether the herbal product is available by prescription or over-the-counter is based on its application and safety of use. Herbal products sold in pharmacies are reimbursed by health insurance if they are prescribed by a physician. The proof required by a manufacturer in Germany to illustrate safety and effectiveness for an herbal product is far less than the proof required by the FDA for drugs in the United States. In Germany, Commission E of the Federal Health Authority (comparable to the FDA) has developed a series of 200 monographs on herbal products. These reports, like the monographs produced in the United States by the FDA on over-the-counter medications, set standards for safety and efficiency (Kleijnen & Knipschild, 1993). An herbal product is viewed as safe and effective when a manufacturer meets the quality requirements of the Commission's standards or produces additional evidence of

---

Michael T. Murray, ND, is one of the leading researchers and lecturers in the field of natural medicine. He is author of more than 50 books, including *The Clinician's Handbook of Natural Medicine* and *The Encyclopedia of Nutritional Supplements*. With Joseph Pizzorno, ND, he is coeditor of *The Encyclopedia of Natural Medicine* and *The Textbook of Natural Medicine*, a two-volume professional reference.

safety and effectiveness, which can include data from the existing literature and anecdotal information from practicing physicians, as well as limited clinical studies.

The best single illustration of the difference in the regulatory issues on herbal products in the United States compared to Germany concerns *Ginkgo biloba*. In Germany, as well as France, extracts of *Ginkgo biloba* leaves are registered for the treatment of cerebral and peripheral vascular insufficiency (Kleijnen & Knipschild, 1993). Ginkgo products are available by prescription and over-the-counter purchase. Ginkgo extracts are among the three most widely prescribed drugs in both Germany and France, with a combined annual sales figure of more than $500 million. In contrast, in the United States, extracts identical to those approved in Germany and France are available as food supplements.

In the United States, no medicinal claims are allowed for most herbal products because the FDA requires the same standard of absolute proof required for new synthetic drugs. The FDA has rejected the idea of establishing an independent expert advisory panel for the development of standards similar to those of Germany's Commission E. Currently, herbal products continue to be sold as food supplements, and manufacturers are prohibited from making any diagnosis-relevant therapeutic claims for their products.

In the context of modern medicine, what advantages do herbal medicines possess over synthetic drugs? Generally, herbal preparations tend to be less toxic than their synthetic counterparts and offer less risk of side effects. (Obviously, there are exceptions to this rule.) In addition, the mechanism of action is often to correct the underlying cause of ill health. In contrast, a synthetic drug is often designed to alleviate the symptom or effect, but may not address the underlying cause. It has also

been demonstrated with many botanicals that the entire plant or crude extract is more effective than isolated constituents.

HERBAL MEDICINE AND THE PHARMACEUTICAL INDUSTRY

Since a plant cannot be patented, very little research has been done in the 20th century on plants as medicinal agents, per se, by the large American pharmaceutical firms. Instead, plants were screened for biological activity and the active constituents isolated. Researchers have been dismayed by the fact that in many instances the isolated constituent was less active biologically than the crude herb. Since the crude herb provided no economic reward to the American pharmaceutical firm, the crude herb or extract never reached the marketplace. In contrast, European policies on herbal medicines have made it economically feasible for companies to research and develop crude phytopharmaceuticals.

Another problem for herbal medicine in the United States has been the lack of standardization. The herb that best exemplifies this dilemma is digitalis. One batch of crude digitalis might have an extremely low level of active constituents, making the crude herb ineffective, while the next batch might be unusually high in active constituents, resulting in toxicity or even death when the standard amount is used. The lack of standardization made it easier for US pharmaceutical firms to rationalize their economic need to isolate, purify, and chemically modify the active constituents of digitalis so that they could market these compounds as drugs. The problem with using the pure active constituent is that the safe dosage range is smaller. Digitalis toxicity and death have increased dramatically as a result of purification. Toxicity was less of a factor when using the crude herb, because overconsumption of potentially toxic doses resulted in vomiting or diarrhea, thus avoiding the heart disturbance and death that occur now with pure digitalis cardiac glycoside drugs.

Fortunately, several European and Asian pharmaceutical firms began specializing in phytopharmaceuticals in the early part of the twentieth century. These companies have played a prominent role in researching, developing, and promoting herbal medicines.

Research is demonstrating that crude extracts often have greater therapeutic benefit than the isolated "active" constituent. This has been known for quite some time in other parts of the world, but in the United States isolated plant drugs are still thought of as having the greatest therapeutic effect. This myth is gradually eroding as our knowledge of herbal medicines increases. If current standardization techniques had been available earlier in the 20th century, it is possible that the majority of our current prescription drugs would be crude herbal extracts instead of isolated and modified active constituents.

HERBAL PREPARATION

Commercial herbal preparations are available in several different forms: bulk herbs, teas, tinctures, fluid extracts, and tablets or capsules. It is important for anyone who routinely uses or recommends herbs to understand the difference between these forms, as well as the methods of expressing strengths of herbal products. One of the major developments in the herb industry involves improvements in extraction and concentration processes.

Herbal Extracts

Extracts. Extracts are a concentrated form of the herb obtained by mixing the crude herb with an appropriate solvent (such as al-

cohol and/or water). When an herbal tea bag steeps in hot water, it is actually a type of herbal extract known as an infusion. The water serves as a solvent in removing some of the medicinal properties from the herb. Teas often are better sources of bioavailable compounds than the powdered herb, but teas are relatively weak in action compared to tinctures, fluid extracts, and solid extracts. Herbal practitioners often use these latter forms for medicinal effects.

Tinctures. Typically, tinctures are made by using an alcohol and water mixture as the solvent. The herb is soaked in the solvent for a specified amount of time, depending on the herb. This soaking lasts usually from several hours to a day, but some herbs may be soaked for much longer periods of time. The solution is then pressed out, yielding the tincture.

Fluid extracts. This type of extract is more concentrated than tinctures. Although they are most often made from hydroalcoholic mixtures, other solvents may be used (such as vinegar, glycerin, propylene glycol, and others). Commercial fluid extracts are usually made by distilling off some of the alcohol, typically by using methods that do not require elevated temperatures, such as vacuum distillation and countercurrent filtration.

Solid extracts. Further concentration of the fluid extract produces a solid extract, using the mechanisms described earlier for fluid extracts as well as other techniques such as thin-layer evaporation. The solvent is completely removed, leaving a viscous extract (soft, solid extract) or a dry, solid extract—depending on the plant, plant portion, or solvent used, and on whether a drying process was used. The dry solid extract, if not already in powdered form, can be ground into coarse granules or a fine powder. A solid extract can also be diluted with alcohol and water to form a fluid extract or tincture.

Analytical Methods

Improvements in analytical methods have led to definite improvements in cultivation techniques, harvesting schedules, storage, stability of active compounds, and product purity. For example, collection should be performed at a time when the active ingredient is present in the greatest amount. All of these gains have resulted in tremendous improvements in the quality of herbal preparations now available.

Methods currently utilized in evaluating herbs and their extracts include the following:

- Organoleptic
- Microscopic
- Physical
- Chemical
- Biological

Organoleptic analysis. Organoleptic analysis involves "the impression of the organs"—the application of sight, odor, taste, touch, and occasionally even sound, to identify the plant. The initial sight of a plant or extract may be so specific that it is sufficient for identification. If this is not enough, perhaps the plant or extract has a characteristic odor or taste. Organoleptic analysis represents the simplest, yet the most human, form of analysis.

Microscopic evaluation. This assessment is indispensable in the initial identification of herbs, as well as in identifying small fragments of crude or powdered herbs, adulterants (for example, insects, animal feces, mold, and other fungi), and characteristic tissue features of the plant. Every plant possesses a characteristic tissue structure, which can be demonstrated through the study of tissue arrangement, cell walls, and configuration when samples are properly stained and mounted.

Materials analysis. Physical methods are often used in crude plant evaluation to determine solubility, specific gravity, melting point, water content, degree of fiber elasticity, and other physical characteristics.

Chemical and biological methods. This methodology is used to determine the percentage of active principles, alkaloids, flavonoids, enzymes, vitamins, essential oils, fats, carbohydrates, protein, ash, acid-insoluble ash, or crude fiber present.

The analytical process requires more precise assays to determine quality. Sophisticated techniques, such as high-pressure liquid chromatography and nuclear magnetic resonance, are often used to separate molecules. The readings from these machines provide a chemical fingerprint as to the nature of chemicals contained in the plant or extract. These techniques are invaluable in the effort to identify herbs, as well as to standardize extracts. The plant or extract can then be evaluated by various biological methods, mostly animal tests, to determine pharmacological activity, potency, and toxicity.

HERBAL PRODUCTION

Collection and Harvesting

The range of sophistication in the processing of herbs is tremendous—from crude herb to highly concentrated standardized extracts. Nonetheless, there are some common stages (Bombardelli, 1991).

Wildcrafted. When plants are collected from their natural habitat, they are said to be wildcrafted. When they are grown, utilizing commercial farming techniques, they are said to be cultivated. When an herb is wildcrafted, there is a much greater chance that the wrong herb will be picked, a situation that could lead to serious consequences. The use of analytical methods can guarantee that the plant collected is the one desired.

Harvesting. The mode of harvesting varies greatly, from hand labor to the use of sophisticated equipment, but the mode is not as important as the time: a plant should be harvested when the part of the plant being used contains the highest possible level of active compounds. This is ensured by the use of analytical techniques.

Drying. After harvesting, most herbs have a moisture content of 60% to 80% and cannot be stored without drying. Otherwise, important compounds would break down or microorganisms would contaminate the material. Commercially, most plants are dried within a temperature range of 100°F to 140°F. With proper drying, the herb's moisture content will be reduced to less than 14%.

Garbling. Garbling refers to the separation of the portion of the plant to be used from other parts of the plant, dirt, and other extraneous matter. This step is often done during collection. Although there are machines that perform garbling, it is usually performed by hand.

Grinding or mincing. This process involves mechanically breaking down either leaves, roots, seeds, or other parts of a plant into very small units ranging from larger, coarse fragments to fine powder. The most widely used machine is the hammer mill. Other types of grinders include knife mills and teeth mills.

Extraction

The process of extraction is used in making tinctures, fluid extracts, and solid extracts. In this context, extraction refers to the separation by physical or chemical means of the desired material from a plant with the aid of a solvent. The US health food industry often uses alcohol and water mixtures as botanical solvents; occasionally extractions involve the use of oil-based (lipophilic) solvents or hypercritical carbon dioxide.

The simplest process consists of soaking the herb in the alcohol/water solution for a period of time, followed by filtering. Typically, this process will yield a lower quality extract at a higher price because the solvent, usually alcohol, cannot be reused. Since tinctures are 1:5 concentrates, this means 80% of the bottle's content is alcohol and water and only 20% herbal material. Tinctures are typically not as cost-effective or as stable as solid extracts.

Strength of Extracts

The potencies or strengths of herbal extracts are generally expressed in two ways. If they contain known active principles, their strengths are commonly expressed in terms of the content of these active principles. Otherwise, the strength is expressed in terms of concentration. For example, tinctures are typically made at a 1:5 concentration. This means 1 part herb (in grams) is soaked in 5 parts liquid (in milliliters of volume). This means that there is five times the amount of solvent (alcohol or water) in a tincture as there is herbal material.

A 4:1 concentration means that 1 part of the extract is equivalent to, or derived from, 4 parts crude herb. This is the typical concentration of a solid extract. One gram of a 4:1 extract is concentrated from 4 g of crude herb.

Typically, 1 g of a 4:1 solid extract is equivalent to 4 mL of a fluid extract (one seventh of an ounce) and 40 mL of a tincture (almost 1.5 oz). Some solid extracts are concentrated as much as 100:1, meaning it would take nearly 100 g of crude herb, or 100 mL of a fluid extract (approximately 3.5 oz), or 1000 mL of a tincture (almost 1 qt) to provide an equal amount of herbal material in 1 g of a 100:1 extract.

Larger manufacturers utilize more elaborate techniques to ensure that an herb is fully extracted and that the solvent is reused. For example, countercurrent extraction is often used. In this process, the herb enters into a column of a large percolator composed of several columns. The material to be extracted is pumped at a given temperature and rate of speed through the different columns, where it mixes continuously with solvent. The extract-rich solvent then passes into another column, and fresh solvent once again comes into contact with herbal material as it is passed into a new chamber. In this process, complete extraction of health-promoting compounds can be achieved. The extract-rich solvent is then concentrated through one of a variety of techniques.

Concentration. After extraction of the herb, the resulting solutions can be concentrated into fluid extracts or solid extracts. In large manufacturing operations, the techniques and machines used (such as thin-layer evaporators) ensure that the extracted plant components are not damaged. These machines work by evaporating the solvent, thus isolating the plant compounds. The solvent vapors pass into a condenser, in which they recondense to liquid form and can be used again. The result is separation of the extracted materials from the solvent, so that the final product is a pure extract, and the solvent can be used again and again.

Drying of extracts. Although a number of liquid-form extracts on the market can still be found (tinctures, fluid extracts, and soft extracts), a solid form is preferable. The primary reason is the greater chemical stability and reduced cost of the solid form (the alcohol in liquid-form extracts is often more expensive than the herb). In addition, tinctures, fluid extracts, and soft extracts are easily contaminated by bacteria and other microorganisms. Liquid forms of extracts also promote chemical reactions that break down the

herbal compounds. Consequently, a number of drying techniques are employed, including freeze-drying and spray-drying (atomization). The result is a dried, powdered extract that can then be put into capsules or tablets.

Excipients. An excipient is an inert substance added to a prescription to give it a certain form or consistency. The same excipients used in the manufacture of drug preparations and vitamin and mineral supplements are often used in the production of tablets and capsules containing herbs or herbal extracts. Many manufacturers will provide a list of excipients contained in their products.

Quality Control in Herbal Products

Quality control refers to processes involved in maintaining the quality or validity of a product. Regardless of the form of herbal preparation, some degree of quality control should exist. Currently, no organization or government body certifies the labeling of herbal preparations.

Without quality control, one cannot be sure that the herb contained in the bottle is the same as that stated on the label. Chemical analysis of over 35 different commercial preparations of feverfew (*Tanacetum parthenium*) and taheebo (*Taebuia avellanedae*) for active components (parthenolide and lapachol, respectively) found a wide variation in the amounts of parthenolide in commercial preparations (Heptinstall et al., 1992). The majority of products contained no parthenolide or only traces. Analysis of 12 commercial sources of taheebo could identify lapachol (in trace amounts) in only one product (Awang, 1988).

Determining Quality

In the past, the quality of the extract produced was often difficult to determine, as many of the active principles of the herbs were unknown. However, recent advances in extraction processes, coupled with improved analytical methods, have reduced this problem of quality control (Bonati, 1991a, 1991b; Karlsen, 1991). Expressing the strength of an extract by the concentration method does not accurately measure potency because there may be great variation among manufacturing techniques and raw materials. By using a high-quality herb (an herb high in active compounds), it is possible to create a more potent dried herb, tincture, or fluid extract compared to the solid extract that was made from a lower-quality herb. Standardization is the solution to the problem.

Standardization

The term "standardized extract" (or "guaranteed potency extract") refers to an extract guaranteed to contain a standardized level of active compounds. Stating the content of active compounds rather than the concentration ratio allows for more accurate dosages to be made.

The best way to express the quality of an herb is in terms of its active components. Regardless of the form, the herb should be analyzed to ensure that it contains these components at an acceptable standardized level. More accurate dosages can then be given. This form of standardization is generally accepted in Europe and is beginning to be used in the United States as well.

Standardization (i.e., stating the content of active constituents versus drug concentration ratio) allows the dosage to be based on active constituents (Bonati, 1991b). In Europe, dosage levels of extracts such as *Vaccinium myrtillus*, *Silybum marianum*, and *Centella asiatica* are based on their active constituent levels rather than drug ratio or total extract weight, for example, 40 mg of anthocyanosides for *Vaccinium myrtillus*, 70

mg of silymarin for *Silybum marianum*, and 30 mg of triterpenic acids for *Centella asiatica*. This type of dosage recommendation provides the greatest degree of consistency and assurance of quality.

Although these herbs are referred to in terms of their active constituents, it must be kept in mind that these are still crude extracts and not isolated constituents. An *Uva ursi* extract that has been standardized for its arbutin content, for example at 10%, still contains all of the synergistic factors that enhance the function of the active ingredient, arbutin.

THE FUTURE OF HERBAL MEDICINE

As more knowledge and understanding are gained about health and disease, medicine is adopting therapies that are more natural and less toxic. Lifestyle modification, exercise, stress reduction, meditation, dietary changes, and many other traditional naturopathic therapies are becoming much more valued in the mainstream. This illustrates the paradigm shift that is occurring as these therapies gain acceptance as effective clinical options.

Improvements in plant cultivation techniques and the quality of herbal extracts have led to the development of some very effective plant medicines. It is apparent that many of the wonder drugs of the future will be derived from plants, or plant cell cultures, and from cell cultures producing compounds naturally occurring in the human body (such as interferon, interleukin 2, various hormones, and others). Several herbal medicines described here may in fact already fulfill the role of wonder drug, for example, *Ginkgo biloba*, *Silybum marianum*, and *Panax ginseng*. The future of herbal medicine depends on several factors: continued research into botanical therapy, adoption of recognized standards of quality by manufacturers, continued existence of the naturopathic medical schools, and increased public awareness of the tremendous therapeutic value of herbs. Herbal medicine will undoubtedly play a major role in the medicine of the 21st century.

REFERENCES

Awang DVC. Commercial taheebo lacks active ingredient. *Can Pharmacol J.* 1988;121:323–326.

Bombardelli E. Technologies for the processing of medicinal plants. In: Wijeskera ROB, ed. *The Medicinal Plant Industry.* Boca Raton, FL: CRC Press; 1991: 96–98.

Bonati A. Formation of plant extracts into dosage forms. In: Wijeskera ROB, ed. *The Medicinal Plant Industry.* Boca Raton, FL: CRC Press; 1991a: 107–114.

Bonati A. How and why should we standardize phytopharmical drugs for clinical validation? *JEthnopharmacol.* 1991b;32:195–197.

Fuchs A. Annual industry overview. *Nutr Bus J.* 1999;IV(6):1–5.

Heptinstall S, Awang DV, Dawson BA, Kindack D, Knight DW, May J. Parthenolide content and bioactivity of feverfew (*Tanacetum parthenium* (L.) Schultz-Bip.). Estimation of commercial and authenticated feverfew products. *J Pharm Pharmacol.* 1992:44(5);391–395.

Karlsen J. Quality control and instrumental analysis of plant extracts. In: Wijeskera ROB, ed. *The Medicinal Plant Industry.* Boca Raton, FL: CRC Press; 1991:99–106.

Keller K. Legal requirements for the use of phytopharmaceutical drugs in the Federal Republic of Germany. *J. Ethnopharmacol.* 1991;32:225–229.

Kleijnen J, Knipschild P. Drug profiles—*Ginkgo biloba. Lancet.* 1993;340:1136–1139.

CHAPTER 57

Whole Complex Herbs

Francis J. Brinker, ND

In regard to its medical use, the term "herb" refers to any part of a plant used for its therapeutic properties. In this context, the word "herb" does not distinguish a non-woody plant from a woody-stemmed one, nor does it refer only to plants growing in soil rather than marine or hydroponic forms. The concept of herbs has even been broadened to include nonbotanical organisms such as mushrooms (fungi) that lack a plant's ability to photosynthesize and whose genetic similarities are in some aspects closer to animals than plants. The concept of which living entities should be called *herbs* is of technical significance in the study of botany, whereas in botanical medicine the practical distinction to be made is between a living plant and its derivatives.

The need to accurately characterize herbal products is necessary and is long overdue, if we are to appreciate the actual herbal preparation being discussed. A real herb is a whole living plant. A medicinal herb is the therapeutically active portion. When dead and dehydrated, it should be called a dried herb. If a tea is made, it is a native water extract of the plant, native in the sense of original and natural. Soaking in dilute alcohol results in a native hydroalcoholic extract, often referred to as a tincture, which is a fraction of the herb. With the water, alcohol, or other solvent removed, it becomes a solid extract. A specific portion removed from a native extract is a chemical subfraction of the herb. Isolating a specific component results in a purified compound, typically the form regulated in medicine as drugs. A purified compound, chemical subfraction, concentrated solid extract, or native liquid extract is not an herb; these are all more or less limited derivative fractions of the medicinal herb.

BIOAVAILABILITY OF WHOLE HERBS

In natural medicine, herbs are the medicinally active plant structures, distinct from plant extracts, concentrates, or active components that represent only a fraction of the activity present in the herb from which they are derived. In this sense, the phrase "whole herb" is used when referring to the medicinal portion of the plant with its fiber and its entire phytochemical composition. Likewise, the phrase "complex herb" is employed here to refer to the complete plant part used medicinally before extraction. Only in the whole complex herb is its chemical matrix intact.

The therapeutic and physiological activities are broader, while the impact is modified. Involving the whole herb alters the availability of some constituents. Absorption

Francis J. Brinker, ND, received his doctorate and postgraduate certification in botanical medicine from the National College of Naturopathic Medicine in Portland, Oregon. He is the author of several books on botanical medicine, including *Herb Contraindications and Drug Interactions*. He currently serves as clinical assistant professor for the Program in Integrative Medicine at the University of Arizona College of Medicine.

Source: Adapted from Brinker FJ. *Complex Herbs—Complete Medicines.* Sandy, OR: Eclectic Medical Publications; 2004.

may be slower for certain components, yet associated compounds may enable them to be more readily assimilated. The metabolic processing and elimination of constituents can be affected, depending on the influence of cofactors in the herb on enzyme systems and membrane transporters.

The whole herb and more complex (native or galenic) extracts generally have a much broader scope of application, compared to those products that are reduced to concentrated fractions of specific types of compounds. The narrowing of therapeutic uses is most typical for isolated components that have become the standard of conventional medical practice. The fact that the whole herb contains all of the active fractions and components suggests that it provides the complete medicinal effects when appropriate doses are utilized. It has been observed that, like nutrients available in whole foods, the therapeutic advantage can be equivalent even though less of an active component is available in the complexity of a complete herb, due to its additive and synergistic activities. On the other hand, sometimes a high dose provided by a concentrated extract or isolate is necessary to deliver the desired therapeutic effect. Each form deserves consideration when making a complete assessment and therapeutic judgment.

The complexity of an intact herb provides combined effects that cannot be achieved by separated fractions of the plant. Even conventional drying significantly impacts the effects of an herb by altering the complex interrelationships that exist chemically and energetically in the living, hydrated matrix. These complexes are expressions of the dynamic vitality of the plants.

Plants rarely produce static crystalline compounds. Exceptions involve structural and/or defensive compounds such as needle-like oxalic acid crystals.

Concentrations of substances not soluble in water typically occur on the surface of plants as nonliving resinous exudates, again to protect the plant or conserve its water to sustain the essential living dynamism. The difference in phytochemical expressions between a living plant and one that is dried is analogous to a living animal and one that has died. The means for functional activity are substantially altered. When natural phytochemical relationships in a live plant are reduced to dessicated, hardened, and/or crystalline forms, they have become essentially devitalized. The structural integrity of natural complexes can be relatively retained by flash-freezing.

Native extracts made with dilute alcohol can be expected to increase some effects, especially when utilizing fresh herbs, while losing other effects—more so when the herbs are dried. The concentrates of dried herbs with exaggerated pharmacological activity and reduced component content produce a stronger impact that may include excessive disruptive effects. Such focused influence may more readily overwhelm human physiology, which has become accustomed through the ages to the ingestion of fresh or dried complex herbs containing smaller amounts of bioactive compounds. These compounds occur in the context of each plant's complex chemical matrix. At times in severe illness a higher potency is necessary; therefore, a different standard can be applied to meet the requirements of ordinary maintenance or support.

DETERMINING THE APPROPRIATE FORM OF THE HERB

Empirical and scientific knowledge recognizes that each form of herbal preparation has distinct differences, advantages, and limitations that make one or several forms more appropriate than others for treating a particular individual's condition:

- The proper choice depends not only on the individual, but on a variety of factors affecting the availability of the active components.
- The relative solubility of the desirable compounds will depend on the solvent and temperature used. In the process of extraction such factors determine the presence and preservation of these constituents.
- Internally, their availability depends on alterations by digestion, metabolism by the intestinal bacterial flora, and assimilation from the gastrointestinal tract.
- Bioavailability is also affected by interactions with other components that affect their absorption, metabolism, and excretion on both organic and cellular levels.

These are the features that impact the pharmacokinetics of the active components. The pharmacodynamic interactions of components are likewise affected and reflect the changes in multiple component bioavailability due to these factors. Every variance produces changes of greater or lesser significance on the efficacy of the product consumed.

The intent of examining the different forms is to resist the notion that one type is always superior to the others. In fact each type of product has its own value and limitations. The factors that determine which is most appropriate involve both the patient's therapeutic requirements and personal preferences. Compliance is always a necessary consideration, since any medicine will fail to work if it remains in the bottle.

In general, a hierarchy of preference based on need and intent may influence choices. Remedies that are both medicinally effective and physiologically nourishing are typically botanicals closer to the whole natural state, or at least a traditional native extract. As with food, for prevention, maintenance, or tonic purposes those forms closest to the whole living plant are attractive. For nonthreatening subacute conditions, or when digestion is compromised, native liquid extracts also appear appropriate. In some acute illnesses or medical crises, more concentrated fractions, or even injectable isolates, are obviously advantageous. Yet no one rule of thumb applies to all cases and considerations.

CHAPTER 58

Interactions of Pharmaceuticals and Botanical Medicines

Francis J. Brinker, ND

INTRODUCTION

As the medicinal use of herbs becomes more common, an underlying issue is their possible interference with prescription drugs. The concerns of doctors and pharmacists are multiple. Will components of botanical remedies interfere with the kinetics of their prescriptions, such as absorption, metabolism, and/or excretion, rendering them less available or more so? Or will the effects of the herbs alter the effect of the drug through metabolic changes, antagonism, or additive effects? Naturopathic physicians and other health care providers who use herbal products medicinally often face these same quandaries in prescribing for patients on drug maintenance therapies who wish to explore other approaches for the same or different conditions. This chapter addresses some of the concerns shared by those who administer or provide pharmaceutical and/or botanical medicines and discusses certain benefits of using botanical remedies and drugs together. (For additional examples of synergistic use of botanicals and medications, also see Chapter 61 on herbs that enhance anti-inflammatory and analgesic drug effects while reducing risks.)

In herbs with primary active constituents, whose pharmacology has been elucidated, a fairly straightforward assessment of potential interactions can be made by those with standard medical/pharmacological training (for example, *Ephedra sinica* with its alkaloids ephedrine and pseudoephedrine). However, the case is not as simple with many herbs. Medicinal plants that have not attracted the attention of research scientists, as well as herbal remedies whose study has revealed a complexity that defies simplistic mechanistic explanations, can baffle even those clinicians who demonstrate an active interest in understanding the interplay of synthetic and natural medicinal agents. In an attempt to help bridge these gaps in knowledge, it is appropriate to address some general considerations and offer a variety of specific examples illustrating how botanical medicines may influence and modify the effects of common pharmaceuticals. Since the vast array of specific concerns cannot be addressed in a limited venue such as this, a practical reference source is needed. To supply this larger need, the author has compiled a more complete reference text from the scientific and medical literature (Brinker, 2001).

A brief biography of Francis J. Brinker, ND, appears in Chapter 57.

Source: Courtesy of Francis Brinker, ND, Tucson, Arizona. Adapted with permission from F. Brinker, ND, Interaction of pharmaceuticals and botanical medicines. *Journal of Naturopathic Medicine.* 1997;7(2):14–22. © 1997, American Association of Naturopathic Physicians.

COMPLEMENTARY COMBINATIONS

In some circumstances, the addition of botanical remedies to other medicines can improve the response or help protect from deleterious side effects of the pharmaceuticals.

This adjunctive approach to prescribing blends the best of both systems in cases in which the prescription drugs are deemed necessary for the patient's recovery or long-term maintenance. While the possibilities in this regard are many and varied, a few examples of how common medical prescriptions can be enhanced by the addition of botanical agents should suffice to illustrate such concomitant treatments.

Immune-enhancing botanicals. The standard medical approach to treating infections that led to the dominant success of pharmaceuticals in this field is the administration of antibiotics. The extensive use of these agents has led to a growing crisis, requiring the development of new forms of medication that overcome the increasing bacterial resistance to such compounds. The naturopathic approach has relied heavily on strengthening the body's resistance to infections by employing natural means and substances that enhance the immune response.

Among immune-enhancing botanicals, the American herb echinacea (purple cornflower) is considered foremost. European research on *Echinacea* species has identified a variety of nontoxic active constituents, among them high molecular weight polysaccharides, glycoproteins, isobutylamides, polyacetylenes, and caffeic acid derivatives that together enhance replication, phagocytosis, and cytokine production by various white blood cells. In addition, individual components have shown some antibacterial, antimycotic, and antiviral activities (Brinker, 1995a). In a clinical study on recurrent vaginal candidiasis, the re-currence rate after 6 months when using the topical antimycotic econazole nitrate alone for 6 days was 60.5% in 43 patients. The econazole treatment alone has been found markedly less effective (Coeugniet & Kuhnast, 1986), compared to the recurrence rate of 15.0% in 20 patients using both econazole topically and *Echinacea purpurea* pressed juice intravenously or subcutaneously as well as 16.7% in 60 patients using econazole topically and *E. purpurea* juice orally.

Other botanical remedies are known for immunomodulating benefits that enhance antimicrobial effects when treating infections.

Siberian ginseng (the root of *Eleutherococcus senticosus*) also contains high molecular weight heteroglycan polysaccharides that enhance phagocytosis in vitro and in vivo (Wagner et al., 1985). In addition, in a placebo-controlled study the alcoholic extract of eleutherococcus root given in 10 mL doses 3 times daily to 36 healthy humans for 4 weeks significantly increased the number of immunocompetent cells, especially T-cells (helper/inducer, cytotoxic, and natural killer cells), and generally enhanced the activation of T-lymphocytes with no side effects (Bohn et al., 1987). A study of children suffering from dysentery caused by *Shigella* species and enterocolitis caused by *Proteus* species compared the use of monomycin and kanamycin together with eleutherococcus and related *Echinopanax elatum* in 157 patients, while using antibiotics alone in 101 patients. The periods of disease decreased for children using the herbs together with the antibiotics (Vereshchagin et al., 1982).

MULTIPLE COMPLEMENTARY EFFECTS: TREATMENT OF BENIGN PROSTATIC HYPERPLASIA

Benign prostatic hyperplasia (BPH) is a condition that involves a number of different processes that seem amenable to treatment with complementary pharmaceutical approaches. Therefore, the smooth muscle relaxing 5α-adrenergic inhibitor terazosin (Hytrin), proven effective in relieving BPH symptoms, was combined with the 5α-reductase inhibitor finasteride (Proscar) in a clinical study. Though finasteride blocks conversion of testosterone to the more potent prostatic growth stimulator dihydrotestosterone, finasteride combined with terazosin proved no better than terazosin alone in treating BPH as documented by symptom scores in this study (Lepor et al., 1996).

Several botanical remedies have been shown in clinical studies to be effective in treating early stages of BPH. Of greatest benefit are three whose concentrated solid and liquid extracts are commonly used phytomedicinals in Europe: *Serenoa repens* (saw palmetto) fruit, *Pygeum africanum* (African prune) bark, and *Urtica dioica* (stinging nettle) root (Brinker, 1995b). Although the extracts of these herbs have only a mild 5α-reductase inhibitory activity compared to finasteride (Rhodes et al., 1993), the extracts impact the prostate by other means. Serenoa has shown some antiandrogenic effects (Brinker, 1995b), but it may be most useful due to its reduction of estrogen and androgen receptors in the nuclei of prostate cells (DiSilverio et al., 1992). In addition to mild 5α-reductase inhibition, pygeum and urtica extracts both demonstrated in vitro aromatase inhibition that reduces the conversion of androgens to estradiol, a contributing factor in BPH. While pygeum was the more potent of the two when used alone, together these extracts had a significantly stronger, synergistic aromatase-inhibiting effect (Hartmann et al., 1996). It is possible that the combined outcomes of these effective plant remedies together with terazosin would produce better clinical effects than when terazosin is taken alone, based upon the plant remedies' different mechanisms of action from each other and from finasteride.

Botanicals protective against drug side effects. Botanical medicines can offer protection from some of the undesirable side effects associated with liver compromise due to toxins or the use of pharmaceuticals.

Silybum marianum (milk thistle) fruit flavonolignans have been found to be protective against liver damage in rodents after exposure to a wide variety of xenobiotic hepatotoxins, including deoxycholate, acetaminophen, halothane, and ethanol due to the antioxidant and lipoxygenase-inhibiting activities of the flavonolignans (Brinker, 1995a). Clinical studies showed that using the flavonolignan extract silymarin with patients suffering from alcoholic cirrhosis decreased mortality and helped normalize serum enzymes indicative of liver damage (Brinker, 1995a; Fintelmann, 1986). Silymarin improves the metabolism of aspirin in cirrhotic rats and may thereby help prevent or reduce side effects from other medications metabolized in the liver of patients with liver disease. In a case of dilantin-induced hepatitis requiring dilantin as a maintenance therapy, liver enzymes normalized after silymarin was given (Fintelmann, 1986). In a double-blind, placebo-controlled study involving 60 patients chronically receiving the psychotropic drugs butyrophenones or phenothiazines, silymarin reduced lipoperoxidative hepatic damage (Palsasciano et al., 1994).

Botanical isolates enhancing medicinal effects. A number of botanically derived compounds have already been used in conventional medicine to enhance the medicinal effects of drugs.

Allantoin has been found to increase the healing of psoriasis when compared to coal tar alone. The cell-proliferant allantoin is found in yields of 1% to 2% in the leaves and roots of *Symphytum officinale* (comfrey);

the clinical research used allantoin in 2% concentration topically in a lotion or cream base (Brinker, 1995a).

The immune-stimulant polysaccharide lentinan from the *Lentinus edodes* (shitake) mushroom, when given by injection, increased the mean survival times in 77 patients over 100% compared to 68 patients given placebo in advanced recurrent stomach cancer patients receiving chemotherapy (Brinker, 1995a). The combination of isolated components from herbs with other pharmaceuticals is an established practice going back to the discovery of alkaloids. Using a more complex extract from a plant increases the number of interactive factors involved in combinations, but this type of botanical medicine is just as capable of increasing the therapeutic potential of other proven remedies.

BOTANICALS THAT REDUCE DRUG AVAILABILITY

There are several general categories of botanical medicines that need to be restricted when vital pharmaceutical drugs are being administered.

It is fairly obvious that if medicines, whatever their source, have antagonistic activities and are prescribed together, they will tend to hinder the effects desired from each one to a greater or lesser extent. The simultaneous prescription of antagonistic agents defies common sense and would be expected to occur only due to a lack of knowledge of the other medication being used. However, interference with medicinal effects not only occurs when two agents are directly antagonistic, but is more common when the absorption, metabolism, or excretion of a drug is compromised.

Delayed absorption. A delay in absorption of orally administered drugs and nutri-

ents can be caused by certain herbs that delay gastric emptying. This is particularly true of herbs that are high in water-soluble, hydrocolloidal fiber. The high viscosity of these herbs can also produce a semipermeable barrier over the gastrointestinal mucosa, another mechanism that may inhibit absorption.

This mechanism can cause positive or negative consequences, depending on the medical condition and the drug(s) and nutrient(s) involved. Since fiber (commonly referred to as gum or mucilage) is insoluble in alcohol, this effect is of greatest concern when certain powdered herbs, teas, juices, or dried aqueous extracts are taken orally in large quantities along with medications such as lithium salts, digoxin, or penicillin. Examples of these different types of hydrocolloidal preparations include powdered *Althaea officinalis* (marshmallow) root, cold infusion of *Ulmus fulva* (slippery elm) bark, *Aloe vera* (aloe) leaf gel, and alginate powder from brown algae. Many hydrocolloidal substances can be found in food items like okra and oats, or as food additives such as carrageenan, guar gum, locust bean gum, and pectin that are known to bind cholesterol. Bulk laxative herbs that can also interfere with cholesterol and drug absorption include *Linum usitatissimum* (flax) seed, *Trigonella foenum-graecum* (fenugreek) seed, and *Plantago psyllium* or *P. ovata* (psyllium) seed (Brinker, 2001).

Reduced absorption. Certain compounds found in botanical medicines can hinder absorption if they bind with alkaloidal medications such as atropine, codeine, ephedrine, and theophylline, which are susceptible to precipitation.

Tannins are the most common cause of this problem, although salicylates will also cause alkaloids to precipitate. Since tannins are present in some herbal powders, are extracted in hot water, and are soluble in alcohol, herbs that contain significant quantities of tannins should be avoided in all forms administered orally while taking alkaloid-containing medicines by mouth simultaneously. Tannins can also precipitate proteins and minerals such as iron or copper that may be important factors or cofactors in drug or nutritional therapies. Because the most commonly consumed plant high in tannins is *Camellia sinensis* (black, green, or oolong tea), a case history pertaining to the use of this recreational (and medicinal) beverage is important.

Other common beverage or medicinal teas that contain high amounts (over 10%) of tannins include *Arctostaphylos uva-ursi* (bearberry) leaves; *Juglans nigra* (black walnut) leaves, bark, and rinds; *Geranium maculatum* (cranesbill) rhizome; *Rubus* species (raspberry) leaves; *Quercus* species (oak) bark; and *Hamamelis virginiana* (witch hazel) leaves and bark. Common salicylate-containing herbs that may precipitate alkaloids include *Filipendula ulmaria* (meadowsweet) flowers, *Populus* species (poplar) bark and buds, *Salix* species (willow) bark, and *Gaultheria procumbems* (wintergreen) leaves (Brinker, 2001; Wagner et al., 1985). In summary, two mechanisms by which botanicals can reduce absorption are by reducing mucosal permeability and precipitating alkaloids.

Rapid elimination due to laxative effects. Botanical medicines can also reduce absorption of medicinal agents through their rapid elimination.

High doses of laxatives can lower absorption of orally administered medicinal compounds by increasing peristalsis and reducing the bowel transit time. Although naturopathic physicians tend to avoid the recommendation of herbs known for their excessive cathartic effects, it is still important to be aware of this mechanism. These herbs effectively lower absorption by diminishing the amount of available time and mucosal contact necessary for diffusion or transport to occur across the intestinal mucosa. Prolonged maintenance of such bowel stimulation would be termed abuse and is mostly encountered with self-administration of over-the-counter laxatives by bulimic patients. In cases of anthranoid-containing botanicals, chronic overuse is evidenced by a black discoloration of the rectal mucosa. The more common laxative herbs yielding anthroquinones are *Aloe* species (aloe) leave exudate, *Rheum* species (rhubarb) root, *Rhamnus purshiana* (cascara sagrada) bark, and *Cassia* species (senna) leaves and pods (Brinker, 2000, 2001).

Increased drug metabolism. The half-life of beneficial medications can also be decreased through the activity of herbs and botanicals that increase liver detoxification.

Many prescribed drugs are metabolized in liver microsomes. The rate of hepatic detoxification of environmental toxins (xenobiotics) can be increased. Herbs such as *Medicago sativa* (alfalfa) have been shown to increase metabolizing enzymes such as mixed-function oxidase in rodents (Brinker, 1995a, 2001). Indoles, produced enzymatically after consumption of glucosinolates found in various cruciferous vegetables and plants, have a similar effect and enhance the glutathione S-transferase activity (Sparnins et al., 1984). For example, indoles from *Brassica* species crucifers (cabbage, broccoli, etc.) increase the liver's metabolism of estradiol. Although increasing microsomal enzyme activity is useful as a means of detoxifying carcinogenic substances, the half-life of beneficial medications can also be decreased (Brinker, 1995a). In addition, high vitamin K intake from regular consumption of cruciferous vegetables can produce resistance to the effects of warfarin (Coumadin) (Walker, 1984).

Specific botanicals and nutrients are known to increase drug metabolism. St. John's wort (*Hypericum perforatum*) is the best documented for inducing cytochrome P450 3A4 metabolism of numerous drug substrates (Brinker, 2001).

Drug metabolism in rats and humans has been shown to increase through the use of the aromatic compound eucalyptol, found in cough drops and in the essential oil of *Eucalyptus* species used in volatile inhalant preparations for steam humidifiers. Eucalyptol decreased plasma and/or brain levels of amphetamine, zoxazolamine, pentobarbital, and aminopyrine in rats exposed to eucalyptol aerosol for 2 to 10 minutes per day for 4 days. In humans exposed to the aerosol for 10 minutes per day for 10 days, the rates of disappearance of plasma aminopyrine and of urinary excretion of 4-aminoantipyrine (its metabolite) were increased (Jori et al., 1970). Eucalyptol was also shown to increase liver metabolism of *p*-nitro-anisol and aniline. Given as an aerosol to rats for 4 days for either 5 to 10 or 15 to 30 minutes daily, eucalyptol significantly decreased pentobarbital levels in the brain and lowered the induced sleeping time when pentobarbital was given 18 hours after the last eucalyptol exposure (Jori et al., 1969).

Not all aromatic oils or terpenes induce microsomal enzyme activity. *Pinus pumilio* oil, guaiacol, menthol, α-pinene, and β-pinene were shown to be without effect (Jori et al., 1969). Aromatic substances that increase microsomal metabolism of drugs include those found in cedarwood (*Juniperus virginiana* and *J. ashei*) oil such as cedrol and cedrene. The inhaled aromatic oil with these components reduced hypnotic effects of hexobarbitone in mice and enhanced the removal of bishydroxycoumarin (Dicourmarol) from the blood in rats. The enzymes enhanced by the cedarwood volatiles were aniline hydroxylase, sulfanilamide acetylase, neoprontosil azoreductase, heptachlor epoxidase, and zoxazolamine hydroxylase (Corrigan, 1993).

INCREASED DRUG AVAILABILITY

Bioactivation. In contrast to the more common reduction of medicinal effects by botanicals that promote detoxification, an increase in metabolic conversion can occasionally result in increased toxicity and adverse effects. For example, absorption and/or inhalation of eucalyptol found in such over-the-counter preparations as analgesic balms—taken in combination with pyrrolizidine-containing herbs such as comfrey (*Symphytum officinale*) or coltsfoot (*Tussilago farfara*)—may increase the liver toxicity of the pyrrolizidine alkaloids. This phenomenon was demonstrated in research using medicinal *Eucalyptus globulus* leaves in combination with woolly groundsel (*Senecio longibus*) that contains pyrrolizidine alkaloids; the combination was found to produce greater and more rapid liver toxicity (White et al., 1983).

Reduced elimination. Increasing the activity of a pharmaceutical drug is a significant risk due to the side effects or toxicities normally associated with many of these potent synthetic medicines. One means by which this can occur is by increasing the half-life of a drug by slowing its breakdown or excretion. For example, the suppressive effect of the glycyrrhetinic acid component of *Glycyrrhiza glabra* (licorice) on 5β-reductase effectively delays the clearance of corticosteroids by the liver (Tamura et al., 1979).

POTENTIALLY HAZARDOUS ADDITIVE EFFECTS

The most common way that mixing medicines accentuates their effects is by combining two agents with similar activities.

There are a number of general categories of drugs for which this holds true. In many cases, botanical medicines with the same or similar effects as botanicals can be used to reduce the dosage of a toxic drug, or in some cases to replace a medicine that is not well tolerated. In either of these instances the gradual substitution of a botanical remedy for a prescription drug should only be done under a physician's close supervision and monitoring. The following are examples of serious overmedication resulting from combinations of medicines and botanicals with comparable effects.

Cardiotonic effects. A number of cardiotonic botanical medicines were traditionally used in combination with, or in place of, *Digitalis* species (foxglove) and their extracts. Since digitalis cardiac glycosides and their derivatives have become the standard agents for chronic treatment of cardiac insufficiency, the other botanical heart tonics, with the exception of *Strophanthus* species, have been mostly confined to naturopathic and herbal practice. Most of these remedies share with digitalis structurally similar steroidal glycoside components with comparable activity. Botanicals containing the types of compounds that strengthen the heart's contractions include *Convallaria majalis* (lily of the valley), *Adonis vernalis* (pheasant's eye), *Helleborus niger* (Christmas rose), and *Urginea maritima* (squill) (Brinker, 2001). *Selenicereus grandiflorus* (night-blooming cereus) lacks the steroidal glycoside components typical of this class of drug but acts as a cardiotonic agent nonetheless (Brinker, 1995a, 2001). Excessive amounts of these cardioactive medications alone or combined with digitalis could result in fatal arrhythmias or cardiac arrest (Brinker, 2000).

Anticoagulant and antiplatelet effects.
Some botanical remedies contain natural compounds that can result in a hemorrhagic diathesis with excessive consumption. These herbs can accentuate the effects of the prescription drug warfarin or other common anticoagulants enough to be of concern with regular consumption.

In one case report, plants possibly contributing to clotting problems in the past included *Melilotus officinalis* (sweet clover), *Asperula odorata* (woodruff), and *Dipteryx odorata* (tonka beans). Bromelain, the proteolytic enzyme from pineapple (*Ananus comosus*) is also believed to potentiate anticoagulant activity (Hogan, 1983). Other botanicals that may enhance the effects of warfarin include *Aesculus hippocastinum* (horse chestnut) bark due to the antiplatelet activity of its esculetin component, and *Cinchona* species (Peruvian bark) (Brinker, 2001). Garlic (*Allium sativum*) has been shown to inhibit platelet aggregation (Brinker, 1995a), and excessive consumption of garlic has resulted in spontaneous (Rose et al., 1990) and postoperative bleeding episodes (Burnham, 1995).

Sedative effects. Antianxiety, sedative, and central nervous system depressant medications are prescribed with the warning that they should not be mixed with alcohol due to the deleterious combined effects. A number of botanical medicines have also been shown through research to increase the effects of pharmacological sedatives, as demonstrated by increasing the sleeping time in animals induced by the drugs pentobarbital or hexobarbital.

These herbs and their extracts include *Melissa officinalis* (lemon balm), *Eschscholtzia californica* (California poppy), *Humulus lupulus* (hops), *Passiflora incarnata* (passion flower), and *Valeriana officinalis* (valerian) (Brinker, 1995a, 2001). Excessive sedation could result from the combination of these herbs with standard depressant drugs.

MAO inhibitor effects. Monoamine oxidase (MAO) inhibitors given mostly as antidepressant agents have long been known to interact with some drugs and foods that can result in a hypertensive crisis. This is most common with adrenergic agents. These adrenergic agents include the plant alkaloids ephedrine and pseudoephedrine obtained from *Ephedra* species (ephedra). (Though *Ephedra* species were banned by the FDA in 2004, the active components are still available in OTC drugs.)

Another familiar cause of this dangerous interaction are foods high in tyramine such as wine and cheese. The herb *Cytisus scoparius* (Scotch broom) also has a high tyramine content and can additionally aggravate high blood pressure due to the cardiac stimulant activity of its alkaloid sparteine. MAO inhibitors combined with excessive caffeine consumption from such sources as coffee (*Caffea* species), tea (*Camella sinensis*), cola (*Cola nitida*), or chocolate (*Theobroma cacao*) can also result in hypertensive episodes (Brinker, 2001).

Medicinal plants such as *Myristica fragrans* (nutmeg) and *Hypericum perforatum* (St. John's wort) act as MAO inhibitors in vitro (Brinker, 2001). Hypericum extract (from St. John's wort) is used effectively as an antidepressant in its own right (Brinker, 1995a). It not only performs as well as the standard tricyclic agents amitriptyline (Bergmann et al., 1993) and imipramine, and the tetracyclic antidepressant maprotiline, but was actually shown to be safer than the latter two drugs (Harrer et al., 1994; Vorbach et al., 1994). Due to its impressive clinical effects, it would be prudent to also avoid combining hypericum with other antidepressants, especially MAO inhibitors and those such as fluoxetine (Prozac) that act as selective serotonin reuptake inhibitors.

Hypoglycemic effects. Certain botanicals known to decrease blood sugar should be monitored to avoid hypoglycemic episodes in individuals with diabetes.

Insulin-dependent diabetics must monitor their blood sugar carefully to avoid hypoglycemic episodes. The combined effect of exogenous hypoglycemic agents with insulin treatment can disrupt the means by which diabetics maintain suitable blood sugar levels and avoid insulin shock. Although plant remedies are used to help control Type II diabetes mellitus, those under medication for Type I disease must be concerned about ingesting herbs that can have a significant impact on serum glucose. Certain plants have a well-documented ability to lower blood sugar levels through a variety of mechanisms. Since many hypoglycemic plants are also used as remedies for conditions unrelated to diabetes, their concomitant additive effect with insulin therapy would likely be inadvertent. Foremost among these plants is *Momordica charantia* (bitter melon), which contains a number of hypoglycemic constituents including the steroidal glycoside charantin, proteins p- and v-insulin, alkaloids, and others (Brinker, 2001; Raman & Lau, 1996; Bever & Zahnd, 1979).

Plants whose oral hypoglycemic activity has been confirmed and whose active constituents identified include *Allium sativum* (garlic) cloves, *Trigonella foenum-graecum* (fenugreek) seeds, *Vaccinium myrtillus* (bilberry) leaves (Bever & Zahnd, 1979), *Tecoma stans* (tronadora) leaves (Bever & Zahnd, 1979; Perez et al., 1980), and *Olea europaea* (olive) leaves (Gonzalez et al., 1992). Other botanical remedies whose activity has been more or less confirmed without identifying the specific active constituents include *Arctium lappa* (burdock) roots, *Fatsia horrida* (devil's club) root bark,

Gymnema sylvestre leaves, *Opuntia ficus-indica* (prickly pear) stems, *Syzygium jambolanum* (jambul) seeds, *Bidens pilosa* (aceitilla) plants, and *Turnera diffusa* (damiana) leaves (Bever & Zahnd, 1979; Perez et al., 1980). Hydrocolloidal fiber sources such as guar gum and psyllium taken in large quantities can delay gastric emptying and reduce the rate of absorption of dietary carbohydrates (Brinker, 2001).

Phototoxic effects. Certain botanicals have the capacity to act as phototoxic agents by increasing the skin's sensitivity to ultraviolet (UV) radiation.

Plants in the *Apiaceae* (carrot or parsnip) family typically contain components chemically categorized as furanocoumarins. These psoralen-like compounds can act as phototoxic agents by increasing the skin's sensitivity to ultraviolet radiation. Although occasionally problematic when used alone, the results are much more dramatic and damaging when these plants are taken simultaneously with 8-methoxypsoralen, prescribed to enhance UV therapy for hyperkeratotic conditions such as atopic eczema. Severe burns with swelling and blistering may occur. Those plants containing natural psoralens include *Angelica* species (angelica), *Apium graveolens* (celery), *Ammi visnaga* (khella), *Heracleum* species (hogweed), *Lomatium* species (wild parsnip), and *Daucus carota* (Queen Anne's lace). Plants outside of the *Apiaceae* family with components known to act as photosensitizers include *Ranunculus* species (buttercups), *Ruta graveolens* (rue), and *Hypericum perforatum* (Brinker, 2001).

Hypotension effects. Herbs that lower blood pressure may have an additive effect with pharmaceuticals used for this purpose.

Herbal diuretics that reduce fluid volume may also subsequently decrease cardiac output and blood pressure. Diuretic herbs include *Daucus carota* (wild carrot), *Agropyrum repens* (couch grass), *Galium aparine* (cleavers), and *Taraxacum officinale* (dandelion). Herbs used primarily for their hypotensive effects include *Crataegus oxycantha* (hawthorne), *Viscum album* (mistletoe), *Veratrum viride* (green hellebore), and *Rauwolfia serpentina* (snakewood) (D'Arcy, 1993).

Anticholinergic effects. A number of potent alkaloidal drugs are obtained from plant sources. The interactions involving the mother plant should be taken as equivalent to those of the isolated alkaloids. Therefore, plants that contain anticholinergic tropane alkaloids, such as atropine, can potentiate synthetic drugs having sedative, antihistaminic, or antispasmodic activities, and these combinations should be avoided. Atropine-containing plants include *Atropa belladonna* (deadly nightshade), *Datura stramonium* (Jimson weed), and *Hyoscyamus niger* (henbane) (D'Arcy, 1993).

Other adverse alkaloidal interactions. *Pausinystalia yohimbe* (yohimbe) is gaining popularity for use in cases of erectile dysfunction, based on the activity of its alkaloid yohimbine. The α_2-adrenergic antagonism by yohimbe alkaloids (yohimbine and extracts of the bark) would be toxic combined with tricyclic antidepressants and phenothiazides and could reverse the effects of antihypertensive drugs (DeSmet & Smeets, 1994).

The α_2-adrenergic antagonism of yohimbine and extracts of the bark would be toxic combined with tricyclic antidepressants and phenothiazides and could reverse the effects of antihypertensive drugs (DeSmet & Smeets, 1994).

The adverse interactions that may occur with *Rauwolfia serpentina* (Indian snakeroot) are the same as for its biogenic amine-depleting alkaloid reserpine. In addition to enhancing antihypertensives as mentioned above, *R. serpentina* can have a detrimental effect if used with depressants, MAO inhibitors, sympathomimetics, tricyclic antidepressants, or digitalis glycosides (Barnhart, 1991).

DIGITALIS COMBINATIONS WITH DISSIMILAR BOTANICALS

Besides the cardiotonic herbs already mentioned (such as *Strophanthus, Convallaria, Adonis, Helleborus, Urginea,* and *Selenicereus* species) that can have an additive effect with digitaloid cardiac glycosides, other herbal remedies can also affect the activity of digitalis constituents or their derivatives. Digitaloids are much prescribed drugs for atrial tachyrhythmia and congestive heart failure in our ever-aging population. Influencing the activity of these plant-derived medicines can have a profound impact on the life and health of the patient. Digitalis glycosides provide a useful example to illustrate the different types of interactions that may occur in conjunction with the use of herbs to the benefit and the detriment of those being medicated.

Besides cardiotonic effects, advantages that can be derived from phytotherapeutic agents in heart disease revolve mainly around the use of coronary vasodilators that improve the perfusion of the cardiac musculature and thereby enhance nutrient availability and metabolic waste removal. *Crataegus* species (hawthorne) leaves, flowers, and berries and their extracts have been shown to act therapeutically as vasodilators in relieving anginal pectoris, cardiac arrhythmias, and mild hypertension. A variety of active constituents, including triterpene acids, procyanidins, and flavonoids, help account for these benefits. The cardiotonic effect of *Digitalis, Convallaria,* and *Adonis* was increased by

Crataegus alcoholic extract in tests on guinea pigs. In cardiac failure, *Crataegus* functions well in conjunction with digitalis and digoxin. The *Crataegus* extracts increase the response and reduce the toxicity to the cardiac glycosides digoxin and digitoxin, as well as g-strophanthin, allowing a reduction of their doses.

Ammi visnaga (khella) is another botanical with coronary vasodilating components. The constituents khellin, visnadin, samidin, and dihydrosamidin obtained from khella have all shown this activity, with visnadin also producing positive inotropic effects. Visnadin given orally decreases the acute and chronic toxicity of digitoxin in mice by preventing bradycardia and reversing cardiac arrhythmias (Brinker, 1995a).

The absorption of digoxin is slowed by simultaneous consumption of guar gum, which reduces the plasma level temporarily. However, a more threatening interaction with digitaloids involves the use of botanical products that reduce blood potassium levels. Low serum potassium potentiates digitalis effects. The *Glycyrrhiza glabra* root component glycyrrhizin induces potassium excretion in conjunction with sodium and water reabsorption in the kidneys, resulting in hypokalemia and hypertension, if used in large amounts for prolonged periods (Brinker, 2001). However, licorice extracts are safer than consuming an equivalent amount of pure glycyrrhizin, due to modified intestinal absorption and bioavailability of the glycyrrhizin when it is combined with other licorice components (Cantelli-Fort et al., 1994).

Overuse of laxatives (such as the botanicals *Aloe, Rheum, Rhamnus,* or *Cassia* species) can also diminish blood levels of potassium, particularly when combined with potassium-depleting diuretics (Barnhart, 1991; Brinker, 2001). Although some herbal diuretics such as *Equisetum* species (horsetail) lead to significant potassium excretion (Perez Gutierrez et al., 1985), *Taraxacum officinale* (dandelion) leaves compensate for this excretory loss because of the leaves' high potassium content (Racz-Kotilla et al., 1994).

Since one of the uses of digitalis is to slow the contractile rate of the heart, plants with components that affect the autonomic control of this function can disrupt the digitaloid medication's influence. Anticholinergic atropine-containing botanicals (such as *Atropa*, *Datura*, and *Hyoscyamus* species) counteract the bradycardia, an effect that can be utilized in cases of digitalis toxicity (Brinker, 2000). *Ephedra* species containing the sympathomimetic ephedrine can induce tachyrhythmia in patients on digoxin as a result of enhanced ectopic pacemaker activity. The reserpine in *Rauwolfia* depletes sympathetic neurotransmitters, which may result in bradycardic arrhythmias for patients on digoxin (Barnhart, 1991). Consequently, it is important to monitor botanicals taken in conjunction with digitalis to avoid altering the intended effects of the medication.

CONCLUSION

Whether botanical medicines are complementary, reduce or increase bioavailability, or produce additive effects, their potential to modify the action of medication suggests the importance of identifying and monitoring herbal products taken in conjunction with pharmaceuticals. To safely prescribe botanicals for patients who are already taking other medicines requires not only a knowledge of the physiologic and pharmacologic effects of the herbal product, but also familiarity with the action of the pharmaceutical. All possible interactions cannot be addressed in a chapter of this scope. The considerations covered do suggest mechanisms of action and general tendencies for combinations of drugs from particular categories. However, each medicine, botanical or otherwise, needs to be studied for its own distinctive patterns of activity and interplay. In any case, an informed, careful approach must be the rule in prescribing all medicines, but most especially when the patient is already taking other medication.

REFERENCES

Barnhart ER, ed. Physician's Desk Reference. 45th ed. Oradell, NJ: Medical Economics Data; 1991.

Bergmann R, Nubner J, Demling J. Simple treatment of moderately serious depressions. *Therapie Neurol Psychitrie*. 1993;7:235–240.

Bever VO, Zahnd GR. Plants with oral hypoglycemic action. *Q J Crude Drug Res*. 1979;17:139–196.

Bohn B, Nebe CT, Birr C. Flow-cytometric studies with *Eleutherococcus senticosus* extract as an immunomodulatory agent. *Arzneim-Forsch*. 1987;37:1193–1196.

Brinker F. Botanical medicine research summaries. In: *Eclectic Dispensatory of Botanical Therapeutics*. Vol 2. Sandy, OR: Eclectic Medical Publications; 1995a.

Brinker F. An overview of conventional, experimental and botanical treatments of nonmalignant prostate conditions. In: *Eclectic Dispensatory of Botanical Therapeutics*. Vol 2. Sandy, OR: Eclectic Medical Publications; 1995b.

Brinker F. *Toxicology of Botanical Medicines*. 3rd ed. Portland, OR: Eclectic Medical Publications; 2000.

Brinker F. *Herb Contraindications and Drug Interactions*. 3rd ed. Sandy, OR: Eclectic Institute, Inc; 2001. [Updates and additions online at www.eclecticherb.com/emp.]

Burnham BE. Garlic as a possible risk for postoperative bleeding. *Plast Reconstr Surg*. 1995;95:213.

Cantelli-Fort G, Maffei F, Hrelia P, et al.. Interaction of licorice on glycyrrhizin pharmacokinetics. *Environ Health Pers*. 1994;102(suppl 9):65–68.

Coeugniet EG, Kuhnast R. Recurrent candidiasis: adjuvant immunotherapy with different formations of Echinacin. *Therapiewoche*. 1986;36:3352–3358.

Corrigan D. Juniperus species. In: DeSmet PAGM, et al., eds. *Adverse Effects of Herbal Drugs 2*. Berlin, Germany: Springer Verlag; 1993.

D'Arcy PF. Adverse reactions and interactions with herbal medicines. Part 2: drug interactions.

Adverse Drug React Toxicol Rev. 1993;12: 147–162.

DeSmet PAGM, Smeets OSNM. Potential risks of health food products containing yohimbe extracts. *BMJ.* 1994;309:958.

DiSilverio F, D'Eramo G, Lubrano C, et al.. Evidence that *Serenoa repens* extract displays an antiestrogenic activity in prostatic tissue of benign prostatic hypertrophy patients. *Eur Urol.* 1992;21:309–314.

Fintelmann V. Toxic metabolic liver damage and its treatment. *Zeit Phytother.* 1986;(3):65–74.

Gonzalez M, Zarzuelo A, Gamez MJ, Utrilla MP, Jimenez J, Osuna L. Hypoglycemic activity of olive leaf. *Planta Med.* 1992;8:513–515.

Harrer G, Hubner WD, Podzuweit H. Effectiveness and tolerance of the Hypericum extract LI 160 compared to maprotiline: a multicenter, double-blind study. *J Geriatr Psychiatr Neurol.* 1994;7(suppl I): S24–S28.

Hartmann RW, Mark M, Soldati F. Inhibition of 5α-reductase and aromatase by PHL-0080I (Prostatonin), a combination of PY 102 (*Pygeum africanum*) and UR 102 (*Urtica dioica*) extracts. *Phytomedicine.* 1996;3:121–128.

Hogan RP III. Hemorrhagic diathesis caused by drinking an herbal tea. *JAMA.* 1983;249:2679–2680.

Jori A, Bianchetti A, Prestini PE. Effect of essential oils on drug metabolism. *Biochem Pharmacol.* 1969; 18:2081–2085.

Jori A, Bianchetti A, Prestini PE, Garattini S. Effect of eucalyptol (1,8-cineole) on the metabolism of other drugs in rats and in man. *Eur J Pharmacol.* 1970;9:362–366.

Lepor H, Willford WO, Barry MJ, et al.. The efficacy of terazosin, finasteride, or both in benign prostatic hyperplasia. *N Engl J Med.* 1996;335:533–539.

Palsasciano G, Portincasa P, Palmieri V, Ciani D, Vendemiale G, Altomare E. The effect of silymarin on plasma levels of malon-dialdehyde on patients receiving longterm treatment with psychotropic drugs. *Curr Ther Res.* 1994;55:537–545.

Perez GRM, Ocegueda ZA, Munoz LJL, Avila AJG, Morrow WW. A study of the hypoglucemic (sic) effect of some Mexican plants. *J Ethnopharmacol.* 1980;12:253–262.

Perez Gutierrez RM, Yesca Laguna G, Walkowski A. Diuretic activity of Mexican Equisetum. *J. Ethnopharmacol.* 1985;14:269–272.

Racz-Kotilla E, Racz G, Solomon A. The action of *Taraxacum officinale* extracts on the body weight of laboratory animals. *Planta Med.* 1994;26:212–217.

Raman A, Lau C. Anti-diabetic properties and phytochemistry of *Momordica charantia L.* (Cucurbitaceae). *Phytomed.* 1996;2:349–362.

Rhodes L, Primka RL, Berman C, et al.. Comparison of finasteride (Proscar), a 5α-reducatase inhibitor, and various commercial plant extracts in in vitro and in vivo 5α-reductase inhibition. *Prostate.* 1993; 55:43–51.

Rose KD, Coisant PD, Parliament CF, Levin MB. Spontaneous spinal epidural hematoma with associated platelet dysfunction from excessive garlic ingestion: a case report. *Neurosurg.* 1990;26:880–882.

Sparnins VL, Venegas PL, Wattenberg LW. Gluthathione S-transferase activity: enhancement by compounds inhibiting chemical carcinogenesis and by dietary constituents. *J Natl Cancer Inst.* 1984; 68(3):373–376.

Tamura Y, Nichikawa T, Yamada K, Yamamoto M, Kumagai A. Effects of glycyrrhetinic acid and its derivatives on δ4-5α- and 5β-reductase in rat liver. *Arzneim-Forsch.* 1979;29:647–669.

Vereshchagin IA, Geskina OD, Bukhteeva RR. Increasing of antibiotic therapy efficacy with adaptogens in children suffering from dysentery and Proteus infections. *Antibiotiki.* 1982;27:65–69 (BA 75:32108).

Vorbach EU, Hubner WD, Arnold KH. Effectiveness and tolerance of the *Hypericum* extract LI 160 in comparison with imipramine: randomized, double-blind study with 135 outpatients. *J Geriatr Psychiatr Neurol.* 1994;7(suppl I):S19–S23.

Wagner H, Proksch A, Riess-Maurer I, et al. Immunostimulating polysaccharides (heteroglycans) of higher plants. *Arzneim-Forsch.* 1985;35:1069–1075.

Walker FB. Myocardial infarction after diet-induced warfarin resistance. *Arch Intern Med.* 1984;144: 2089–2090.

White RD, Swick RA, Cheeke PR. Effects of microsomal enzyme induction on the toxicity of pyrrolizidine (*Senecio*) alkaloids. *J Toxicol Environ Health.* 1983; 12(4–6):633–640.

CHAPTER 59

Botanical Treatment Strategies: Migraine Case Studies

Jill Stansbury, ND

IDENTIFYING MIGRAINE ETIOLOGY

A complementary medicine approach to the treatment of migraine headaches focuses on the underlying factors that trigger vascular phenomena. The following three cases exemplify common migraine presentations and how each might be treated specifically using botanicals:

- Allergy-induced migraines
- Muscle tension migraines accompanied by anxiety
- Hormonally triggered migraines

ALLERGY-INDUCED MIGRAINES

When treating patients with migraines, the initial step is to ascertain whether the complaint might be related to underlying allergic hypersensitivity. A simple history and review of physiological systems will typically reveal concomitant allergic and/or atopic phenomena. If there are symptoms of chemical sensitivity, hay fever, eczema or skin reactivity, food allergies, or bowel reactivity the migraines are likely to be an allergic phenomena and should be treated accordingly.

History, Diagnosis, and Treatment

History: The first case involves a 30-year-old woman who experiences migraines weekly, sometimes with no apparent trigger, and sometimes following exposure to perfumes or fumes. She also has exercise-induced asthma, hay fever, eczema, and irritable bowel syndrome.

Diagnosis: Hypersensitivity allergy-induced migraines.

Treatment: The herbal formula includes agents known to be helpful in cases of asthma, allergies, blood histamine phenomena, and related conditions:

- *Tanacetum parthenium* (feverfew)—Reduces allergic responses via platelets and blood vessels
- *Curcuma longa* (turmeric)—Antioxidant that provides liver support to remove antigens from blood
- *Ginkgo biloba*—Stabilizes blood platelets and blood vessels; provides antiallergy and antioxidant effects
- *Crataegus oxyacanthaor* or *monogyna* (hawthorne)—Stabilizes blood vessels, reduces histamine, anti-inflammatory effects

Jill Stansbury, ND, received her doctorate from National College of Naturopathic Medicine; she is currently chairwoman of the Botanical Medicine Department and has been a professor there since 1991. Licensed as a naturopathic physician in Washington state, she has maintained a private practice in southwestern Washington for more than 20 years. She also writes, lectures, teaches workshops, and serves on the editorial and advisory boards of several publications and organizations.

Courtesy of Jill Stansbury, ND, Battle Ground, Washington.

Adjunctive Protocol

Antioxidant protection. The intervention for allergic patients also typically includes the use of antioxidants, the primary nutrients responsible for subduing free radicals (oxidizing agents) in our bodies. Oxidizing agents abound in our world and include internal toxins such as normal metabolic waste, chemicals such as pesticides, food additives, household products, perfumes, and deodorants, as well as toxins from smoke, car exhaust, photocopier fumes, new synthetic building materials, and carpeting. When these types of toxins bind onto any type of cellular membrane, the toxins usually destroy the cell. The presence of oxidizing agents in the blood can also trigger the release of histamines and serotonin from blood platelets and initiate allergic and inflammatory reactions throughout the body.

When our bodies have plentiful levels of antioxidant nutrients, toxins to which we are exposed in our daily environment are less likely to trigger the allergic inflammatory cascade. Important antioxidant nutrients include beta carotene, vitamins C and E, lipoic acid, selenium, zinc, and many naturally occurring plant constituents. Antioxidants bind to toxins and escort them out of the body so that the toxins do not bind to tissues or cells. Other nutrients and plant constituents also aid the liver in detoxification, enabling the body to eliminate toxins before they become harmful.

Minimizing allergic reactivity. Antioxidants provide nutritional support to stabilize blood vessels and decrease allergic phenomena. Some of the most powerful antioxidants are flavinoids, found in botanicals that are brightly pigmented, with beneficial effects on vasculature and blood cells. For example, the botanical turmeric is an intense yellow-orange color, high in antioxidant flavonoids

with anti-inflammatory activity. Colorful vegetables and fruits are also rich sources of these compounds, including beets, cabbage, spinach, squash, and berries.

Lowering levels of allergens. Specific food sensitivities can be a factor in migraines, so allergy testing or an elimination diet can be beneficial.

Promoting detoxification. Since the skin functions as a secondary organ of elimination, activities that open the pores and cleanse the body will tend to remove toxins and lighten the burden on the kidneys and liver. Effective approaches include exercise, skin brushing, and saunas.

Specific Botanicals

Tanacetum Parthenium (Feverfew)

This herb is classic for migraine headaches, particularly those that involve hyperreactive blood cells such as occurs in allergies. Tanacetum is less effective for headaches that are triggered by hormones, stress, or muscular tension.

Vascular phenomena. *Tanacetum* is useful for any kind of vascular phenomenon that involves acute hypersensitivity or allergic response. The research on this botanical indicates that it stabilizes platelets, histamine release, and reactivity of blood vessels. It also has known effects on prostaglandins.

Curcuma Longa (Turmeric)

Curcuma is the Latin name for the whole herb, while its active constituent, a flavonoid, is referred to as curcumin.

Anti-inflammatory. *Curcuma* has been well researched and is documented to decrease inflammation via a number of prostaglandin pathways. This botanical is also a powerful antioxidant, an anti-inflammatory, and supports liver function, helping to cleanse the blood of pro-inflammatory substances.

Liver support. *Curcuma* supports the detoxification of antigens and oxidants via the glutathione pathway, which converts fats and fat-soluble toxins and wastes into a more water-soluble form, assisting their elimination from the body.

Blood cleansing. *Curcuma* provides benefits in blood cleansing, a term from traditional herbalism that implies supporting the organs of elimination and digestive function: the pancreas, gall bladder, liver, and intestinal tract. This also entails promotion of beneficial bacteria and the health of the intestinal ecosystem, as well as the mucous membranes of the gastrointestinal tract, which all play a role in removing toxins.

Specific constituents. Curcumin, one of the most studied active constituents of curcuma, is sometimes concentrated and dispensed in capsules or included in lesser quantities in formulas for liver and antioxidant support.

Ginkgo biloba

This circulatory herb was historically used for millenia in China, where it is indigenous.

Circulatory effects. *Gingko* is well documented to improve circulation to the brain, heart, and limbs, and is given for cerebral vascular insufficiency as well as other circulatory and cardiac applications. For the elderly it is indicated for complaints related to poor cerebral circulation, ringing in the ears, dizziness, loss of focus, confusion, senility, and Alzheimer's. *Gingko* has also been used to improve poor circulation in the limbs in conditions such as Raynaud's syndrome or arterial insufficiency, as a heart tonic, and for blood pressure.

Anti-inflammatory and blood thinner. There is extensive molecular research on *Ginkgo's* effect on inflammatory phenomena via platelets. It has been found to inhibit PAF (platelet activating factor), a type of messenger chemical that induces platelets to clump together. Because platelets often initiate both clotting and the inflammatory cascade, inhibiting PAF will reduce allergic hypersensitivity as well as moderately thin the blood.

Vascular stabilizer. The blood vessel lining—the endothelium—also plays a role in allergic phenomena by reacting to antigens or other offenders in the blood. *Gingko* has been shown to have a stabilizing effect on the endothelium through numerous mechanisms, each affecting nitric oxide and its associated enzymes housed in blood vessel walls.

Crataegus oxycantha (Hawthorne)

This nourishing herb is a tree of the rose family, native to Europe. The bright red berries have powerful effects as anti-inflammatory, antioxidant, and tissue stabilizers, particularly for the heart and blood vessels.

Circulatory effects. *Crataegus* was historically used as a tonic for heart or circulatory complaints. It improves circulation to the heart and coronary arteries, strengthening the heart muscle and lowering blood pressure. It is included in this formula because it also decreases the inflammatory process in the blood and reactivity in blood vessel walls. This botanical can be used for people who are prone to varicosities or fragile veins. Although it is difficult to reverse varicosities, research on the bioflavonoid content of *Crataegus* has found that it strengthens blood vessel walls, through collagen-stabilizing effects. *Crataegus* also helps to strengthen connective tissue elsewhere in the body and protects it from oxidative damage.

Effects on allergic phenomena. This herb decreases endothelial reactivity to some degree, stabilizing platelets, histamine, and mast cells. *Crataegus* has been found to prevent the conversion of histidine to hyperinflammatory histamines, although this effect tends to be weaker than the action of other herbs known for this effect, and it is not a pharmaceutical-like antihistamine.

Improving endothelial dysfunction. *Crataegus* is utilized for allergic phenomena that occur when microcapillaries become hyperpermeable. If bioflavonoid levels are insufficient to repair connective tissue, these tissues develop weakened areas that leak blood and its components into the body's tissues. The result can be swelling or a tendency to bruising; this phenomenon can also trigger asthma, eczema, irritable bowel syndrome, or other inflammatory phenomena. The resultant scarring of the microendothelia decreases circulation over time. Although it appears that we are able to generate new capillaries when existing ones are destroyed, that regeneration cannot be sustained indefinitely. There can be permanent consequences to scarring both the larger blood vessels and the microcapillaries. This type of endothelial dysfunction has been implicated in many forms of chronic vascular and inflammatory disorders and may be an underlying factor that sustains these conditions.

Outcome

Allergy-related migraine symptoms usually improve over 2 to 3 months' time as the allergic phenomena gradually lessen. Typically, the patient who has weekly headaches finds that the headaches decrease to every other week within the first month or so. It may take a few months for the full effects of dietary changes to become apparent.

STRESS-RELATED MIGRAINES

Headaches associated with stress usually involve acute muscular contraction due to physical tension or an emotional trigger such as anxiety. Tension in any of its forms in the mind or body can cause a shift in brain biochemistry and the balance of neurotransmitters. Herbs specific for this type of headache can be taken to address muscular tension, reduce elevated cortisol levels that occur with stress, and produce a calming effect on the mind and emotions. For many patients, these herbs can be used in times of stress, on an as-needed basis for insomnia or tension. For individuals who are prone to stress and headaches, some of these herbs can be taken in low doses on an ongoing basis.

History, Diagnosis, and Treatment

History: The second case involves a 30-year-old woman who has episodic migraines that are extremely incapacitating, associated with tightness in the back, shoulders, neck, and scalp, and throbbing pain in the entire crown and forehead. The headaches do not occur in association with her menses or any pattern other than stress. She also suffers from frequent insomnia and occasional panic attacks.

Diagnosis: Stress/anxiety-related muscular tension that extends to the muscular layer of the vasculature

Treatment: Botanicals indicated for stress:

- *Cimicifuga racemosa* (black cohosh)—Counters anxiety (anxiolytic) and is an anti-inflammatory specific for muscular contraction headaches
- *Piper methysticum* (kava)—Anxiolytic, antispasmodic, pain relief (anodyne)
- *Withania somnifera* (ashwagandha)—Adrenal support for chronic stress reaction, gamma-aminobutyric acid (GABA) agonist, improves insomnia

Specific Botanicals

Cimicifuga racemosa (Black Cohosh)

This herb is well known in botanical medicine as a woman's herb. *Cimicifuga* has documented hormonal effects due to its isoflavone constituents. This herb is effective for menopausal symptoms, including hot flashes, and has been investigated for osteoporosis, due to its weak estrogenic-like effects. In this particular formula, *Cimicifuga* is used due to its effects in moderating muscular contraction headaches and anxiety. Molecular research has shown it to affect neurotransmitters as well as.

Piper methysticum (Kava)

Kava has been used in the United States in herbal medicine for decades without problem. Many people appreciate it as an aid in relieving stress, nervous tension, or muscle cramping.

Contraindications. Liver cautions associated with kava are a concern. Use of kava should be avoided for patients with known liver disease such as hepatitis C and those on liver-toxic medications. In the Fiji Islands, where kava is used as alcohol or coffee is in the West, heavy consumers are known to develop elevated liver enzymes and in some cases jaundice and scaly rashes. At high doses kava's hepatic effects are comparable to those of alcohol. However, at moderate doses, many individuals can use kava safely. When used occasionally for concerns such as acute muscle tension and headaches, almost everyone can tolerate it for a day without harm.

Pain management. Kava can be a useful tool for addressing chronic pain, for example, for patients with spinal injuries that cause muscle pain and contractions. For these pain patients, narcotics, sedatives,

morphine, or opiates would be the primary pharmaceutical options, so kava offers a reasonable alternative. For a few specific patients, kava may be appropriate for long-term use. These patients should be monitored frequently and their liver enzymes checked every 3 to 6 months or annually, and all known hepatotoxins should be avoided. Certainly kava can be omitted altogether whenever it does not seem like a wise choice for the patient.

Anxiolytic. Kava can be used at the time of an emerging headache, when people begin to experience muscle tension, stress, or anxiety. This herb is somewhat like a pharmaceutical in its action, in that it comes on rapidly (within a half hour or so) and wears off rapidly. For an occasional bad day, it can be taken every half hour to relax muscles and prevent a headache.

Stress management. In general, kava is taken on an as-needed basis. This herb can also be taken at a lower, adjusted dose or combined with black cohosh or other nervines and used in moderation long-term for stress management. The mild calmative effects are indicated for people who are prone to stress associated with physical tension, particularly muscle tension.

Nervine. In traditional herbology, a *nervine* is a plant having a tonifying effect on the nervous system. Kava appears to decrease nerve excitability, which may be why it seems to moderate stress, anxiety, and pain. It is known to decrease the excitability of nerves through the potassium-gated channels on the nerves themselves. The research on kava indicates that it also binds to GABA receptors in the brain. It can be used in combination with other herbs depending on the circumstances, to provide a calming, relaxing, anxiolytic effect.

Withania somnifera (Ashwagandha)

Withania is the Latin name for the Ayurvedic herb ashwagandha. Interestingly, ashwagandha has been used to both improve sleep and promote energy. This herb is sometimes referred to as Indian ginseng, although it is not a true ginseng. Like ginseng, it is thought to be useful in managing stress.

Adaptogen. Ashwagandha is an adrenal tonic, moderating adrenaline and cortisol responses. Herbs that provide this type of balancing effect on adrenal function are described as *adaptogens*. When we are under long-term stress and function constantly in the sympathetic mode, the increased production of cortisol and adrenaline helps us sustain the pace. However if that pace is maintained month after month, year after year, the way many of us live, the adrenal glands eventually "down-regulate," becoming less responsive to ACTH (adrenocorticotropic hormone) and other stress-induced chemicals released by the brain. Then one is less able to tolerate stress, one's energy output tends to wane, and steroid output decreases as well.

Ashwagandha, like other adaptogens, can improve energy by increasing adrenal output. It is also known to bind to GABA receptors; consequently, it provides a balance between managing adrenalin and cortisol output, while calming the mind and emotions.

Tonic. Ashwagandha is known as a tonic herb and the term ashwagandha means, "like a horse." A debate within the herbal community is whether that implies that it makes one strong as a horse, provides the stamina of a horse, or supports the fertility or virility of a horse, as is often attributed to adrenal tonics and adaptogens.

Outcome

These herbs can be used in combination, periodically when stress is elevated, or they can be taken in smaller doses long-term to moderate tension for anxiety-prone individuals. This formula is appropriate for acute tension, such as muscle contraction headaches, because it is fast acting and relaxes the mind as well as the muscles. Kava may be omitted and other botanicals substituted— muscle relaxers such as *Valerian*, or nervines such as *Hypericum*, depending on the patient and the circumstance.

HORMONALLY TRIGGERED MIGRAINES

Migraines triggered by hormonal phenomena are experienced by some women premenstrually. Although they may also experience these symptoms at other times in their cycle, typically these responses are associated with the menses. Research has not fully confirmed the factors that cause the blood vessels to constrict, dilate, and then progress to the entire inflammatory cascade (the sequence of events that precedes migraines). However, a hormonal trigger to migraines is logical since we now know there are estrogen receptors on the blood vessels and adrenergic receptors on both the blood vessels and the uterus.

History, Diagnosis, and Treatment

History: The third case involves a 30-year-old woman who experiences headaches premenstrually. Her headaches are accompanied by abdominal heaviness, some bloating, and breast tenderness. Headaches are typically right sided and accompanied by sensitivity to light, visual changes, and mild nausea. She has never had a migraine away from her menses.

Diagnosis: Vasomotor phenomena with a hormonal trigger

Treatment: Botanicals indicated:

- *Vitex agnes castus*—A progesteronic fluid retention may trigger migraines and progersterone may reduce this; estrogen receptors on blood vessels may be implicated.
- *Taraxicum officinalis*—Promotes diuresis and liver metabolism of estrogen.
- *Sanguinaria canadense*—Specific for vasomotor disorders, used only in small doses because it is potentially caustic.

Hormonal Etiology

We tend to see symptoms of fluid retention most frequently in women who have high estrogen relative to progesterone, since estrogen tends to promote fluid retention. In selecting a botanical protocol for these patients, two strategies come to mind. One approach is to assist the body in excreting estrogen more efficiently. The other is to improve hormone balance by supporting the body's production of progesterone when estrogen levels are normal, but progesterone is low to suboptimal.

Specific Botanicals

Vitex agnes castus (Chasteberry)

If progesterone is insufficient, the herb *Vitex* may be appropriate. This is a classic herb recommended for premenstrual migraines, mentioned in herbals hundreds of years old for menstrually related migraines and women's hormone issues.

Promoting progesterone production. For many women with hormonal concerns, normalizing low progesterone can balance out excessive estrogen and abolish symptoms of PMS and fluid retention. *Vitex* has been shown to affect the release of gonadotropins via dopamine. Gonadotropins are hormone-like agents released by the pituitary (LH—luteinizing hormone and FSH—follicle stimulating hormone). Gonadotropins act on the ovaries and adrenals (and testes in men) to stimulate estrogen, progesterone, and testosterone output. Overall, *Vitex* affects the brain in a manner that promotes LH and supports increased progesterone levels; this serves to "oppose" estrogen, which is commonly in excess.

Systemic support. *Vitex* is typically taken all month to increase a woman's progesterone, rather than simply taking it at the time of a headache. Symptoms such as headaches or fluid retention are less likely to develop if progesterone-enhancing herbs are taken on an ongoing basis.

Lowering estrogen levels. The other approach to hormonal migraines is to lower excessive estrogen in the tissues by assisting the body in excreting or metabolizing it more efficiently. Many herbs are known to have this effect—particularly the *alterative* roots, which are somewhat bitter and act on the liver.

Taraxicum officinalis (Dandelion)

This is a classic remedy with liver supportive effects, like many roots in the aster or compositaea family. Although burdock and chicory have similar mechanisms, taraxicum is also known to be a diuretic and a cholagogue, promoting bile release from the liver.

Improving estrogen metabolism. Any substance that promotes bile production tends to enhance liver activity, particularly the ability of the liver to emulsify fats. Estrogens, like all steroids, are built on cholesterol molecules, so estrogen metabolism can be promoted by supporting bile production. This improves not only fat metabolism, but also more efficient excretion of estrogen from the system through liver detoxification (via the process of conjugation).

Supporting estrogen detoxification. The normal life of estrogen in the body is quite short: It is released from the ovaries into the bloodstream and removed from systemic circulation as soon as that blood reaches the liver. Once estrogen is conjugated, it is less active, and is transported to the intestines for elimination from the system. Estrogen disposal can be compromised if there is constipation or poor elimination of wastes.

Minimizing toxic load. Estrogen detoxification may also be compromised when the liver is inundated with substances to process and detoxify, which is quite common. Detoxification is necessary whenever we take medication, have too much to drink, do heavy cleaning, or spray the garden with pesticides. A slowdown in detoxification can lead to excessive levels of estrogen in the body. Furthermore, many chemicals and pesticides are known to bind to estrogen receptors and elicit an estrogenic effect. This is another reason why so many people have elevated estrogen levels. In this particular botanical protocol, dandelion or some other bitter herb is selected to enhance estrogen elimination from the system via the liver and promote better hormone balance. Minimizing exposure to environmental chemicals and toxins can also help the liver and actually reduce the estrogen load in the body.

Sanguinaria Canadense

In cases of hormonal migraine, the ideal formula includes an herb specific for vascular phenomena, such as *Sanguinaria*.

Addressing vascular phenomena. *Sanguinaria* is indicated for vasomotor blood vessel activity such as hot flashes and migraines. It is specific for heat, perspiration, or flushing and associated headaches. This herb is especially appropriate for one-sided headaches, typical of some migraines. This is also the herb of choice when there is acute vascular phenomena, such as blind spots in the visual field.

Formulation

Both *Vitex* (chasteberry) and *Taraxicum* (dandelion) are typically taken all month long. For the convenience of the patient, *Sanguinaria* could also be taken all month, but in extremely small amounts. This botanical is so strong and caustic, it can burn the mouth when taken repeatedly over time. Consequently, it is only appropriate for use in highly dilute form, in a formulation prepared by a skilled herbalist. In this migraine protocol, *Sanguinaria* is combined with *Vitex* and *Taraxicum*, but in extremely small amounts. A 2-ounce bottle holds approximately 64 ml, so a good ratio would be 30 ml *Vitex*, 30 ml *Taraxicum*, and 4 ml *Sanguinaria*. In that concentration, the *Sanguinaria* would be diluted to a safe dosage that could be used during the entire month.

Outcome

Typically women will see improvements after a month of use, by the next menses. If no changes are observed within 2 or 3 months, the formula should be changed.

PROMOTING HORMONE PRODUCTION

Research. Studies on hormonal agonists have revealed complex underlying issues in the workings of receptors and their agonists/antagonists.

One good example is that hormonal agents from plants, such as isoflavones from soy, are known to bind to estrogen receptors. Some saponins and other steroidal compounds in plants are also known to bind to estrogen receptors. If these constituents bind to an estrogen receptor and have a stimulating effect, we describe it as an agonist. Many plant constituents act as weak agonists compared to the estrogens produced by a woman's own body. (Estrogenic hormones that are endogenously produced include estradiol, estriol, and estrone.)

When relatively weak plant agonists bind to an estrogen receptor, these agonists can crowd out or compete for binding sites with a woman's own more powerful endogenous estrogen. By this mechanism, some plant-based estrogen agonists reduce estrogenic effects in the body when estrogen levels are high, yet provide a weak estrogenic effect when estrogen levels are low. This ability to work in both directions, either raising estrogen or lowering it depending on the situation, is known as an *amphoteric* action in herbalism.

Competing hormones. The laboratory identification of a substance as an estrogen agonist *in vitro* does not indicate the action which that particular weak agonist will have within the body—in the context of a living, physiologically active system. When a very weak estrogen agonist in the bloodstream is competing with the body's more powerful endogenous estrogens, this creates competition for binding sites, ultimately reducing the binding of estrogen. In that situation, providing a supplement to increase estrogen actually decreases overall estrogen stimulation and subsequently estrogen levels in the tissues. Yet in isolation—*in vitro*—the isoflavone acted as a stimulus. Essentially, these molecular mechanisms of action can be surprisingly subtle.

Adaptogenic hormonal effects. Among the botanicals that support women's health, we find that herbs tend to be effective yet moderate in their action. Botanicals bind to estrogen receptors in the vasculature and decrease inflammatory phenomena, but do not seem to be overstimulating to breast or uterine tissue. These botanicals do not lead to increased hyperplasia of the uterine lining like many pharmaceutical hormones, but tend to be highly selective in their activity.

CONCLUSION

These are sample formulas—the author customizes formulas for all patients individually, depending on their needs and the causal factors involved (for example, adrenal issues, muscle spasms, vasomotor phenomena, hormonal triggers, or stress and tension). For allergy-induced migraines, herbs that stabilize the blood vessels are very specifically selected to assure that they do not cause allergenic effects as well. All these formulas can be amended or fine tuned, depending on the requirements of the individual.

The more we learn about botanicals, the more we come to realize their subtlety and complexity, which is the beauty and mystery of biochemistry and organic phenomena.

CHAPTER 60

Assessing the Effectiveness of Naturopathic Medicine

Carlo Calabrese, ND, MPH

In the current discussion surrounding the integration of complementary medicine in health care, the first and most frequent question is: Do these treatments alleviate symptoms and cure disease? Naturopathic medicine is one of the practices under consideration. An analysis of the effectiveness of this discipline illustrates some of the difficulties in answering this question for health care providers, consumers, third-party payers, and policy makers. The intent of this brief discussion is to offer an approach for estimating the potential efficacy of naturopathic medicine (hypothesis generating) and provide additional methodology for its successful investigation (hypothesis testing).

OVERVIEW

Naturopathy is a primary health care profession that includes the promotion of health, and the prevention, diagnosis, and treatment of disease. The practice is licensed in 12 states and 3 Canadian provinces. In Arizona and British Columbia, acupuncture is a part of the regulated practice; elsewhere, naturopathic physicians must obtain an additional license to practice acupuncture. The license typically is broad, allowing naturopathic doc-

tors (NDs) to diagnose any disease and treat it using any natural means. There are perhaps 4000 licensed naturopathic physicians in the United States who have been trained in accredited 4-year postbaccalaureate institutions. There may be several thousand more unlicensed naturopaths whose training is highly variable.

Licensed naturopaths are considered by many to be among the most broadly educated in complementary practices and are well prepared for integration into the mainstream health care system due to their training in the basic and diagnostic sciences of biomedicine and their broad range of practice.

CURRENT STATE OF RESEARCH

Biomedical research methods that are considered a gold standard by the scientific community have been typically developed to provide reliable data on a single therapeutic intervention for a specific Western diagnosis/disease. However, these research methods are not designed to assess a multifactorial approach to a given condition. As a result, the research does not usually encompass the full scope of clinical practice or the potential therapeutic benefits of naturopathic treatment. Rather, studies to date tend to represent naturopathy as apparently less effective than it may actually be. In addition, evaluations with a single-agent and single-problem focus

A brief biography of Carlo Calabrese appears in Chapter 55.

Courtesy of Carlo Calabrese, ND, MPH, Portland, Oregon.

do not take into account the residual benefits to the range of health problems of the patient nor on distal effects, such as future health status and health care utilization.

Consequently, there is limited research on practices that encompass whole medical systems such as naturopathy, Oriental medicine, and Ayurveda. All three of these approaches are characterized by treatment through multiple modalities with a global approach to individuals and their unique constellation of physical and mental constitutions, stressors, and symptoms.

Although the most useful approach would be to determine whether naturopathic medicine in its entirety is effective, the body of evidence on the whole practice of naturopathic medicine is as scarce as it is for other non-dominant whole systems of practice. Research in whole practices is only recently gaining interest at the National Institutes of Health. New tools for research are also beginning to be accepted with the development of methodologies in practice-based and health services research.

METHODOLOGY

Comparison trials between different systems of practice are needed for holistic disciplines such as naturopathic medicine. In order to more accurately reflect the benefits of this approach, outcome measures would be not only disease-specific, but also both broad and long-term including health status, well-being, utilization, and cost. Only then can the relative utility of the various approaches to health care be determined.

Compounding the methodological difficulties of research in this practice, there are structural obstacles as well. There are only 2 decades of research history at the academic centers of this profession. Practitioners who are expert in naturopathic medicine and the individualization of treatment are typically not trained in rigorous comparative trials. Even if the infrastructure and training were in place, sources of funding remain few, and most funding agencies make their decisions on the basis of biomedical theories of a very different nature than those of naturopathy.

In the extant research of naturopathic treatment, most studies are focused on single substances rather than the combinations of agents, procedures, and lifestyle changes of naturopathic practice. Without the economic incentives that favor the in-depth study of patentable drugs, trials in naturopathic therapeutics tend to be smaller and with fewer replications. In addition, many practices present special methodological or ethical problems for control, randomization, or blinding, thereby making it more difficult to perform studies as rigorously as desired. In sum, there have not been comparative trials to date that are designed to assess the practice of naturopathic medicine in its entirety, as a holistic, multidisciplinary practice.

EVALUATING EFFECTIVENESS

The large trials needed to assess naturopathic medicine have not yet been performed. In lieu of multidisciplinary research, an approach to the existing evidence is offered here that suggests the efficacy of naturopathy as a systemic intervention. There are currently numerous clinical trials that have evaluated the effect of specific individual treatments applied in naturopathic clinical practice and this research has yielded positive results. A pattern of such positive results can be assembled, encompassing various naturopathic treatment modalities, as seen in the two research reviews that follow. This provides a matrix of clinical trial evidence that may suggest the possibility of marked efficacy in naturopathic medicine as a system.

Some variations in the clinical knowledge bases distinguish naturopathic and conventional medicine and should also be considered in any discussion of comparative research.

Supporting healthy function. Naturopathic practice addresses not only disease entities, but also prevention and health enhancement. In a naturopathic approach, the aim is to support healthy function. A naturopathic physician may arrive at a functional and constitutional assessment as well as a disease diagnosis. Treatment is individualized for the particular patient's condition rather than for a disease entity. Frequently, a combination of treatments is applied and is continuously adjusted over time as the patient's condition changes.

Prescribing for subsets of patients. Consonant with the principle of seeking the cause, the treatment is individualized in a more subtle fashion than just by disease. Many interventions are used by naturopathic physicians only in a carefully selected subset of patients displaying particular symptoms. For example, about half of depressed women on birth control pills show vitamin B_6 (pyroxidine) deficiency, and most of these will improve with pyroxidine supplementation (Adams et al., 1974). Concomitantly, evidence of beneficial effects from pyroxidine supplementation on undifferentiated depression in such women is mixed.

Secondary health benefits. Naturopathic interventions, often aimed at inadequate basic physiological functions or at dysfunctional behaviors, frequently promote improvement in more than one disease simultaneously. It is common for practitioners to choose among therapeutic options that will yield an efficient outcome as well as an effective response, maximizing the cost-benefit ratio.

Drawing on an extensive clinical foundation. Experimental evidence is not the only form of evidence, and sometimes not the best evidence for particular interventions or therapeutic questions. Validation for pharmaceutical science is now based on double-blind, controlled clinical trials. However, the literature on this type of research has not served as the primary repository for the practice wisdom of naturopathy, a discipline that has developed empirically more through clinical processes than by formal academic and regulated epistemological processes.

Many naturopathic treatments are based on a long history of human use and comprise the body of expertise of many generations of healers. These treatments are less likely than patentable drugs to be formally tested in comparison trials. However, because of the relatively benign nature of the agents used, therapeutic trials are very common in naturopathic practice and lead to a rapid accumulation of clinical experience.

Combining therapies with synergistic effects. Naturopathic physicians combine many of these relatively nontoxic treatments but, with few exceptions, trials in combination treatment are infrequent. It may be that even when the right criteria are specified, the benign single agents used do not demonstrate a statistically significant therapeutic difference if used alone. The bioactivity of most nutrients and botanicals is mild and diffuse compared to that of molecularly identified pharmaceutical agents. However, used in combination, they may have additive or synergetic effects, particularly when the individual remedies work via differing mechanisms. An example is the treatment of back pain using an herbal muscle relaxant combined with manipulation. With a well-chosen strategy, the beneficial effects may be amplified. This type of potential benefit is missed in the literature of controlled trials. While therapeutic combinations may also be common in conventional medicine, they are nearly universal in naturopathic care.

Applying lifestyle as a therapeutic. There are similarities and differences between naturopathy and conventional medicine. Certain interventions within the naturopathic repertoire are much more frequently used among NDs than among medical doctors. In other cases, the treatment approach may be similar. For example, the management of diabetic nephropathy by protein restriction or of atherosclerosis with a low-saturated fat diet may be just as common among allopathic physicians as among naturopathic ones, though naturopaths may be more assiduous in their application.

Prevention and health promotion. In naturopathic practice, prevention and health promotion constitute primary treatment strategies. Review of the literature here focuses on the treatment of two disease states. Some of the treatments cited later for osteoarthritis and migraine in fact have side effects that are positive rather than negative. Still, the critical prevention and health promotion goals of ordinary naturopathic practice are not reflected in the evidence following.

Having touched on these issues, it may be clear that randomized, controlled clinical trials and the extant literature will not tell the whole story of efficacy in naturopathic medicine. In the absence of studies that offer a profile of the whole practice, the literature on controlled clinical trials can, however, provide a good suggestion of the potential benefit. One may look at the range of treatments within the scope of naturopathic clinical practice that have been tested in randomized, controlled clinical trials for an orthodox disease classification. Such an analysis would involve reviewing the medical literature of randomized trials for each of the naturopathic modalities used to treat a given condition, primarily diet therapy, nutritional supplementation, botanical medicine, homeopathy, physical medicine (physical therapy, hydrotherapy, and manipulation), and mind-body medicine (such as counseling and psychotherapy, biofeedback, hypnosis, imagery, and others). The criterion for the selection of these treatments is whether there have been clinical trials of acceptable design for which there is no significant evidence controverting the hypothesized effect at the time of this writing.

To offer an overall sense of the generalized efficacy of naturopathic medicine, different diseases that span the range of age, gender, chronicity, severity, and mortality could be chosen for review. However, due to space limitations, only two conditions are reviewed here. Most other conditions are similarly available to treatment with multiple therapeutic approaches. The treatments described here would by no means represent complete, or even actual, treatment regimens, but rather possible interventions that have fairly strong experimental evidence in treating the particular disease within the treatment options of naturopathic physicians.

Clinical experience confirms that coordinated combination therapy with several interventions, each of which is supported by good evidence and works via different pathways, is likelier to work than a single agent. Identifying treatments for which current evidence is strongly positive, and which are likely to be used in conjunction with each other, gives a sense of the possible magnitude of benefit with naturopathic medicine if it were practiced under a treatment selection criterion of randomized trial evidence.

RESEARCH ON OSTEOARTHRITIS INTERVENTIONS

Nutritional Supplements

Caruso I, Pietrogrande V. Italian double-blind multicenter study comparing Sadenosymethionine (SAMe), naproxen, and placebo in the treatment of degenerative joint disease. *Am J Med.* 1987;83(5A):66–71. Seven hundred forty-three patients received 1200 mg SAMe, 750 mg naproxen, or placebo daily. SAMe exerted the same analgesic activity as naproxen; both were more effective than placebo (p < .01). SAMe tolerability was better than that of naproxen.

Machtey I, Ouaknine L. Tocopherol in arthritis: a controlled pilot study. *J Am Geriatr Soc.* 1978;26:328. A double-blind, crossover study in which 29 subjects received 600 mg tocopherol or placebo for 10 days in random order. Fifty-two percent had "marked improvement" in pain while on tocopherol versus 4% during placebo (p < .01).

Rovat LC. Clinical research in osteoarthritis design and results of short-term and long-term trials with disease modifying drugs. *Int J Tissue Reactions.* 1992;14(5):243–251. Report of three double-blind, randomized trials of oral glucosamine sulfate compared to placebo and ibuprofen. Glucosamine was more effective than placebo (N = 252, p < .025) and as effective as ibuprofen (N = 200, p = .77). The glucosamine sulfate was as well tolerated as placebo, with fewer adverse reactions than ibuprofen (p < .001).

Bruyere O, Pavelka K, Rovati LC, Deroisy R, Olejarova M, Gatterova J, Giacovelli G, Reginster JY. Glucosamine sulfate reduces osteoarthritis progression in postmenopausal women with knee osteoarthritis: evidence from two 3-year studies. *Menopause.* 2004; 11(2):138–43. Studies of glucosamine sulfate for OA continue to accumulate including both symptomatic and disease progression measures. A report on two randomized trials on glucosamine sulfate monitored effects on symptoms and joint structure in 319 post-menopausal women with knee OA. Minimal joint space width was assessed at baseline and after 3 years from standing anteroposterior knee radiographs. The glucosamine group showed no joint space narrowing, whereas the placebo group showed a narrowing of −0.33 mm (p < 0.0001).

Rejholec V. Long-term studies of antiosteoarthritic drugs: an assessment. *Semin Arthritis Rheum.* 1987;17(2, suppl 1):35–53. One hundred forty-seven patients received either cartilage extracts or placebo. Placebo patients were permitted to use nonsteroidal anti-inflammatory drugs (NSAIDs) during exacerbations. After 5 years, pain scores in the cartilage patients dropped 85% versus 5% in controls. With cartilage, joint deterioration was 37% less, and less time was lost from work.

Botanical Medicine

Deal CL, Schnitzer TJ, Lipstein E, Seibold JR, Stevens RM, Levy MD, Albert D, Renold F. Treatment of arthritis with topical capsaicin: a double-blind trial. *Clin Ther.* 1991; 13(3):383–395. A randomized study of a constituent of cayenne in 70 patients versus placebo showed a reduction in subjective pain (p < .003).

Kulkarni RR, Patki PS, Jog VP, Gandage SG, Patwardhan B. Treatment of osteoarthritis with a combination herbomineral formulation: a double-blind, placebo controlled, crossover study. *J Ethnopharmacol.* 1991;33(1–2):91–95. Trial of a combination of *Boswellian serrata, Curcuma longa, Withania somnifera,* and zinc in 42 patients showed a reduction in pain severity (p < .001) and disability (p < .05).

Physical Medicine

Trock D, Bollet AJ, Dyer RH Jr, Fielding LP, Miner WK, Markoll R. A double-blind trial of the clinical effects of pulsed electro-magnetic fields (PEMF) in osteoarthritis. *J Rheumatol*. 1993;20(3):456–460. Twenty-seven patients were randomized to PEMF or sham treatment; in PEMF patients, 23% to 61% improvement was observed in clinical outcome variables versus improvement of 2% to 18% with sham treatment.

Stener-Victorin E, Kruse-Smidje C, Jung K. Comparison between electro-acupuncture and hydrotherapy, both in combination with patient education and patient education alone, on the symptomatic treatment of osteoarthritis of the hip. *Clin J Pain*. 2004; 20(3):179–185.

In a small study, 45 patients with radiographically demonstrated osteoarthritis of the hip, pain related to motion, pain on load, and ache were randomized to electro-acupuncture (EA) or hydrotherapy (both in combination with patient education), or patient education alone. Assessments were done at baseline, end of treatment, and 1, 3, and 6 months after treatment. Pain related to motion, pain on load, and ache during the night were reduced up to 3 months after the last treatment in the hydrotherapy group and up to 6 months in the EA group. Ache during the day was significantly improved in both the EA and hydrotherapy group up to 3 months after the last treatment. Disability in functional activities was improved in EA and hydrotherapy groups up to 6 months after the last treatment. There were no changes in the education group alone.

Mind-Body Medicine

Gay MC, Philippot P, Luminet O. Differential effectiveness of psychological interventions for reducing osteoarthritis pain: a comparison of Erickson hypnosis and Jacobson relaxation. *Eur J Pain*. 2002; 6(1):1–16. Patients reporting pain from hip

or knee OA were randomly assigned to eight sessions of Erickson hypnosis, Jacobson relaxation, or a wait-list control. The two experimental groups had a lower level of subjective pain than the control group, and the level of subjective pain decreased with time. Benefits of hypnosis appeared more rapidly than relaxation. Both of the treatment groups were associated with reductions in analgesic medication taken.

RESEARCH ON MIGRAINE INTERVENTIONS

Diet

Egger J, Carter CM, Wilson J, Turner MW, Soothill JF. Is migraine food allergy? A double-blind, controlled trial of oligoantigenic diet treatment. *Lancet*. 1983;344:865–869. Of 88 children with severe frequent migraines, 93% recovered on an oligoantigenic diet. Of the 82 who improved, all but 8 relapsed on reintroduction of 1 or more foods. Of the 82, 40 completed a follow-up with test foods disguised in an oligoantigenic base. There were highly significant relationships between the active material and symptoms.

Nutritional Supplements

Schoenen J, Jacquy J, Lenaerts M. Effectiveness of high-dose riboflavin in migraine prophylaxis. A randomized controlled trial. *Neurology*. 1998;50(2):466–470. In a 3-month trial of 400 mg vs. placebo in 55 migraine patients, riboflavin was superior in reducing attack frequency (p = 0.005) and headache days (p = 0.012). The proportion of patients who improved by at least 50% (responders) was 15% for placebo and 59% for riboflavin (p = 0.002). Other studies show the safety profile of riboflavin to be wide.

Faccinetti F, Sances G, Borella P, Genazzani AR, Nappi G. Magnesium prophylaxis of menstrual migraine: effects on intracellular magnesium. *Headache.* 1991;31:298–301. In 20 patients, duration and intensity of migraines were significantly lower in subjects given 360 mg of elemental magnesium daily for 2 months compared with those in the placebo group.

Botanical Medicine

Murphy JJ, Heptinstall S, Mitchell JRA. Randomized double-blind placebo-controlled trial of feverfew in migraine prevention. *Lancet.* 1988;2:189–192. Symptoms were significantly reduced in the group receiving herbal treatment compared to those receiving placebo (N = 72; p < .005).

Homeopathy

Brigo B, Serpelloni G. Homeopathic treatment of migraines: a randomized double-blind study of 60 cases (homeopathic remedy versus placebo). *Berlin J Res Homeopathy.* 1991;1(2):98–106. Over 4 months, 80% of patients improved with homeopathy versus 13% on placebo; on a visual analog scale for pain, the mean decrease in symptom score for those treated with homeopathy was 6.2 versus 0.6 cm for those receiving the placebo.

Physical Medicine

Solomon S, Guglielmo KM. Treatment of headache by transcutaneous electrical stimulation. *Headache.* 1985;25:12–15. Subjects treated with transcutaneous electrical stimulation had significantly greater improvement than those receiving placebo.

Nelson CF, Bronfort G, Evans R, Boline P, Goldsmith C, Anderson AV. The efficacy of spinal manipulation, amitriptyline, and the combination of both therapies for the prophylaxis of migraine headache. *J Manipulative Physiol Ther.* 1998;21(8):511–519. Patients with migraine headache (N = 218) were studied in a randomized comparison of manipulation, amitriptyline, or a combination of the two for 8 weeks of treatment. All study groups showed improvement. There was no advantage to combining amitriptyline and spinal manipulation for the treatment of migraine headache; spinal manipulation seemed to be as effective as a well-established and efficacious treatment (amitriptyline) and, on its safety profile, should be considered a treatment option for patients with frequent migraines.

Mind-Body Medicine

Fentress DW, Maske BJ, Mehegan JE, Benson H. Biofeedback and relaxation-response training in the treatment of pediatric migraine. *Med Child Neurol.* 1986; 28(2):139–146. In 18 children assigned to one of three treatment groups, those receiving electromyography (EMG) biofeedback or relaxation-response training experienced a significant reduction in headache symptoms compared to controls, a difference that was sustained after 1 year.

REFERENCE

Adams PW, Wynn V, Seed M, Folkand J. Vitamin B_6, depression, and oral contraception. [Letter]. *Lancet.* 1974;2:516–517.

CHAPTER 61

Enhancing Anti-inflammatory Drug Effects with Botanicals

Francis J. Brinker, ND

OVERVIEW

Scientific studies that investigate the anti-inflammatory effects of herbs in humans often do so while the patients are concurrently receiving a maintenance dose of conventional medications to provide baseline control of pain and inflammation. In these human studies, combinations of anti-inflammatory drugs with stinging nettle, willow, devil's claw, bromelain, and thunder god vine products have shown improved therapeutic outcomes, while cat's claw, ginger, and frankincense may also help prevent ulcerogenic effects from nonsteroidal anti-inflammatory drugs (NSAIDs) based on animal studies. Capsicum and licorice extracts have been shown to reduce the gastric ulceration commonly associated with excessive use of NSAIDs. Herbs with potential antiplatelet effects like feverfew and ginger, but especially concentrated products like bromelain and curcumin from turmeric, must be carefully monitored when given in conjunction with aspirin or other NSAIDs associated with bleeding difficulties. The combined use of proper products made from these herbs with comparable anti-inflammatory drugs offers advantages that frequently surpass the use of either alone.

Acute and chronic inflammation, and its accompanying pain, is one of the most common conditions for which people have traditionally sought medical treatment. Along with physical therapy and appropriate exercises, prescription and over-the-counter (OTC) drugs are the standard means by which people control their pain and discomfort. It is estimated that almost 175 million Americans use OTC painkillers. After recognition of serious sequelae to the long-term use of corticosteroids to counter inflammation, nonsteroidal anti-inflammatory drugs (NSAIDs) have become the mainstay in providing on-going relief. Often, one form of medication proves inadequate (Wolfe et al., 1999; Mease, 2003).

NSAID risks involve multiple systems of the body and are well known, especially gastric ulceration and bleeding, which increase with advanced age (Wolfe et al., 1999; Fung & Kirschenbaum, 1999). To help reduce these occurrences, selective cyclooxygenase (COX)-2 inhibitors were developed, but additional adverse effects and a potential for drug interactions make these agents less than ideal (Fung & Kirschenbaum, 1999). Additionally, topical analgesics and/or local steroid applications or injections are used in many cases. For rheumatoid arthritis (RA) and

A brief biography of Francis Brinker appears in Chapter 58.
Courtesy of Francis Brinker, ND, and InnoVision Communications. This chapter is adapted from Brinker F. Enhancing anti-inflammatory and analgesic drug effects while reducing risks with herbs and their derivatives. *Integrative Medicine*. 2004;3(1):24–42. © 2004.

spondyloarthropathies, disease-modifying agents including methotrexate, sulfasalazine, hydroxychloroquine, cyclosporine, D-penicillamine, and gold are specifically employed. So called "biological response modifiers," which inhibit leukocytes or cytokines, such as tumor necrosis factor-alpha (TNF-α) or interleukins, are considered "new" means of treating this especially challenging autoimmune arthropathy (Mease, 2003; Cannella & O'Dell, 2003). Inconsistent results with all of these approaches have led to a return (at lower doses) to prescribing prednisone for intractable cases (Conn & Lim, 2003).

Each of these common pharmaceutical approaches has it own inherent drawbacks. In 1994, the number of American deaths from gastrointestinal complications related to NSAIDs was about 15,000, the same as the combined deaths due to malignant melanoma, asthma, and cervical cancer (Fung & Kirschenbaum, 1999). In 1997, there were approximately 16,500 deaths in the United States from NSAID toxicity in arthritis patients. This number is nearly equivalent to the number of deaths from AIDS (16,685), 50% more than deaths from multiple myeloma, 300% more than deaths from asthma, 350% more than deaths from cervical cancer, and 1100% more than deaths from Hodgkin's disease (Wolfe et al., 1999). Newly recognized risks of NSAID use are regularly being reported. While NSAIDs and COX-2 inhibitors have not been clinically shown to favorably affect cartilage integrity, some, such as indomethacin, appear to accelerate damage to joint structures (Ding, 2002). Nonaspirin NSAIDs tend to increase systolic blood pressure, and antihypertensive prescriptions in the elderly increase proportionately to the dose of these drugs when they are prescribed (Townsend, 2002). NSAIDs also appear to increase the risk of miscarriage during pregnancy (Nielsen et al., 2001), while some OTC NSAIDs (indomethacin, salicylates) and analgesics (acteminophen) produce adverse fetal effects (Anon, 2000).

A survey of 4300 adults by the National Consumers League, as reported in *U.S. News and World Report* (Hobson, 2003), revealed a significant contributor to these risks. More than one third of those questioned admitted using OTC painkilling medications more frequently than recommended, and 29% took more pills than the label directed. Overuse seemed particularly pronounced among users of ibuprofen and naproxen. Analgesics such as acetaminophen are often used during acute exacerbations of chronic inflammation to keep NSAID doses at levels that reduce the risk of adverse effects. Acetaminophen hepatotoxicity from acute overdose was associated with 112,809 calls to 64 poison control centers in the United States in 2001, of which 59,087 were treated and 238 resulted in death. Although, in many cases the drug was used in suicide attempts, almost half of the deaths were associated with coingestion of other drugs (Kociancic & Reed, 2003).

USING HERBS WITH ANALGESICS

It is no wonder that when health professionals consider using herbs with analgesic and/or NSAID drugs, they consider the risk of adverse interactions. However, in assessing these interactions, the vast majority are described as "potential," or in other words, theoretical.

Potential Concerns

The greatest area of concern is enhancement of the antiplatelet activity of aspirin and increasing possible gastric hemorrhage induced by NSAIDs. Some herbs like garlic or concentrated extracts like standardized ginkgo extract appear to have induced hemorrhage in some individuals with or without concomitant aspirin use (Abebe, 2002). However, these and most other herbs in question are of greater concern when combined with anticoagulants like warfarin. In addition, herbs containing natural prodrugs like salicin and coumarin do not have the same anti-platelet or anti-coagulant effects of their respective synthetic derivatives, aspirin or warfarin. The metabolism of these natural phytochemicals in humans results in different chemical forms of salicylate and coumarin compounds that lack an influence on platelets and coagulation, though some natural coumarins do possess antiplatelet, rather than anticoagulant, effects (Norred & Brinker, 2001). Some others used as anti-inflammatories—like ginger, feverfew, turmeric, and willow—have demonstrated antiplatelet activity, but have not been associated with hemorrhagic drug interactions in humans. Salicylate-containing herbs have been purported to increase toxicity of acetaminophen to the kidneys, but no documentation confirms this as anything more than speculation (Abebe, 2002).

Utilization

In comparison with prescription and OTC anti-inflammatory use, current employment of herbs to treat conditions such as arthritis appears to be very limited. In 1994, a questionnaire mailed to 3384 arthritis patients in the United Kingdom received 1020 responses to questions about their use of complementary remedies such as herbs and food supplements (Ernst, 1998). Of these respondents, 23.5% identified one to three herbs they believed helped, while 16.3% also listed one to three herbal products they had tried that were not helpful. Those most often listed as helpful were devil's claw (*Harpagophytum*

procumbens) by 1.3% and feverfew (*Tanacetum parthenium*) by 0.6%; each was considered by 0.6%, respectively, to be ineffective. (Devil's claw liquid was specified as ineffective.) Only 17 respondents reported adverse effects after using herbals and/or nutritional supplements. In spite of limited application of botanical and nutritional products in Great Britain at that time, in less than a decade a number of published clinical studies that used herbal products for osteoarthritis (OA) or rheumatoid arthritis (RA) found evidence that some are effective, relatively safe, and associated with the reduced consumption of anti-inflammatory drugs (Loing et al., 2001; Soeken et al., 2003).

Positive Outcomes

Inflammatory disorders are typified by elevations in cyclooxygenase and lipoxygenase products. Yet other significant biomarkers that contribute to these complex processes are also being identified, and herbs have been shown to favorably affect the broad panoply of associated inflammatory factors. Herbs from all around the world, and their extracts/fractions/components, are discussed here in the context of primary anti-inflammatory drugs in humans. In addition, some of these adjuvant herbs and/or their derivatives protect against the ulcerogenic effects of anti-inflammatory drugs in animal studies. Some herbs or their components that primarily protect against ulcers caused by NSAIDs in humans have also been shown to produce anti-inflammatory and/or analgesic effects with drugs when certain active isolates are applied topically. These types of complementary effects make the use of specific herbal products together with some drugs already widely used for inflammation an attractive means of improving outcomes and allaying adverse effects.

Table 61–1 Orally Effective Herbal Anti-inflammatory/Analgesic Primary Adjuvants

Herb	Study and Length[a]	N	Condition	Dosage Form
Stinging Nettle (*Urtica dioica*) leaves	O, R[6] 2W	36	Acute arthritis	Stewed leaves
Willow (*Salix spp.*) bark	O, C[6] 78W	451	Low back pain	Standardized bark extract
Willow	R, PC, DB[9] 4W	191	Low back pain	Standardized bark extract
Feverfew (*Tanacetum parthenium*) leaves	PC, DB[16] 6W	40	Rheumatoid arthritis	Leaf powder
Devil's claw (*Harpagophytum procubens*) root rhizome	R, C, DB[17] 4W	122	Osteoarthritis	Cryo-ground root powdered
Devil's claw	R, PC, DB[18] 4W	109	Low back pain	2:5:1 root concentrated extract
Devil's claw	O[19] 8W	227	Low back pain or osteoarthritis	Standardized root extract
Bromelain-pineapple (*Ananas comsus*)	R, PC, DB[23] 0.5W	160	Episiotomy	Standardized stem extract
Bromelain	PC, DB[24] 1W	59	Cataract surgery	Standardized stem extract
Thunder god vine (*Trypterygium wilfordii*) roots	O[25] 76W	13	Rheumatoid arthritis	Standardized root extract
Thunder god vine	PC, DB[27] 20W	21	Rheumatoid arthritis	Standardized root extract

Study and Length
    a: C = controlled, DB = double-blind, O = open, PC = placebo-controlled, R = randomized, SB = single-blind; W = weeks

continues

Table 61-1 continued

Daily Dose	Drug Combination	Outcome	Mechanisms of Action[b]
2.3 gm (dry wt.)	Diclofenac	Reduced drug dosage equally effective	Decreased TNF-α, IL-1β, IL-2, IF-γ, AP-1, NF-κB, LT-B4[1–5]
120 or 240 mg salicin	NSAIDs, acetaminophen	High dose pain relief, cost-effective	Inhibits COX[8]
120 or 240 mg salicin	Tramadol	Dose-dependent tramadol reduction	Same as above
70–86 mg	NSAIDs, analgesics, corticosteroids	Improved grip strength	Inhibits COX-2, LOX, phospholipase-A2, TNF-α, IL-1[10–15]
2.6 gm (57 mg harpagoside)	Dicilofenac and/or acetaminophen with caffeine	Safer and as effective as diacerhein; lowers drug use	Undetermined
2.4 gm (50 mg harpagoside)	Tramalol	More pain free with same drug dose	Same as above
60 mg (harpagoside)	NSAIDs	Reduced NSAID use	Same as above
400,000 RU (160 mg)	Aspirin and either codeine or propoxyphene	Better recovery, less aspirin/ codeine	Decreases KN, BK, PGE$_2$ TXB$_2$[20–22]
160 mg (400,000 RU)	Aspirin or propoxyphene	Less inflammation, more bleeding	Same as above
< 575 mg	NSAIDs, prednisone	Improved pain, ESR, swelling, stiffness, CRP, RFC	Indirectly decreases expression of COX-2, PGE$_2$[26]
180 or 350 mg	NSAIDs, prednisone	Symptoms, lab improved, more side effects	Same as above

Mechanisms of Action

b: AC = anti-complement; AP = activator protein; 11β-OHSD = 11 beta-hydroxysteroid dehydrogenase; BK = brandykinin; COX = cyclooxygenase; CRP = C reactive protein; ESR = erythrocyte sedimentation rate; GP = glycoprotein; HETE = hydroxy-eicosatetraenoic acid; IF = interferon; IL = interleukin; KN = kininogen; LOX = lipoxygenase; LT = leukotriene; MAP = major acute phase protein; MG = macroglobulin; NF = nuclear factor; PG = prostaglandin; RF = rheumatoid factor; TNF = tumor necrosis factor; TX = thromboxane

c: ESR = erythrocyte sedimentation rate; CRP = C-reactive protein; RF = rheumatoid factor

Table 61–2 Primary Anti-inflammatory Adjuvants, Secondary Anti-ulcer Agents

Herb	Study and Length[a]	N	Condition	Dosage Form
Cat's claw (*Uncaria tomentosa*) bark	R, PC, DB[32] 28–52W	40	Rheumatoid arthritis	Aqueous-acid extract
Ginger (*Zingiber officinale*) rhizome	O[39] 12W	6	Rheumatoid arthritis	Fresh or dried rhizome (root)
Ginger (3.25 parts) and galanga (*Alpinia galanga*) rhizome (1 part)	R, PC, DB[40] 6W	247	Osteoarthritis	Standardized extracts
Frankincense (*Boswellia serrata*) gum resin	Meta-analysis of 11 trials[47] 4–26W	375	Rheumatoid arthritis and osteoarthritis	Standardized dried lipophilic extract
Ginger, frankincense, turmeric (*Curcuma longa*) root, ashwagandha (*Withania somnifera*) root	R, PC, DB[49] 16W	165	Rheumatoid arthritis	Standardized combination extract

Study and Length
  a: C = controlled, DB = double-blind, O = open, PC = placebo-controlled, R = randomized, SB = single-blind; W = weeks

continues

Table 61–2 continued

Daily Dose	Drug Combination[c]	Outcome	Mechanisms of Action[b]
60 mg (1.5% pentacyclic oxindoles)	1. NSAIDs prednisolone 2. Indomethacin[29,30]	Fewer painful, swollen joints	Decreases COX-2, TNF-α, NF-κB)[28,30–31]
5.0 gm fresh or 0.5–1.0 gm dried	1. NSAIDs	Less pain, stiffness, swelling, stopped NSAIDs	Inhibits COX-2, decreased TXB_2, PG[33,34–38]
510 mg	1. Acetaminophen 2. Aspirin, Indomethacin (ginger)[41]	13% with less pain standing, 13% with GI upset	Same as above
600 mg to 3.6 gm	1. NSAIDs	Less pain, stiffness, swelling, less NSAIDs	Inhibits LOX; decreases LTB_4, 5-HETE; AC[42–46]
444 mg to 592 mg	1. Prednisone 2. Indomethacin[29,30] (turmeric)[51]	Less pain, swelling, tenderness, rheumatoid factor	(turmeric) Inhibits LOX, COX-2; Decreases PGE_2, NF-κB binding[44,48,50]
			(ashwagandha) Decreases α2-GP, α1-MAP, α2-MG[52,53]

Mechanisms of Action

   b: AC = anti-complement; AP = activator protein; 11bβ-OHSD = 11 beta-hydroxysteroid dehydrogenase; BK = brandykinin; COX = cyclooxygenase; GP = glycoprotein; HETE = hydroxy-eicosatetraenoic acid; IF = interferon; IL = interleukin; KN = kininogen; LOX = lipoxygenase; LT = leukotriene; MAP = major acute phase protein; MG = macroglobulin; NF = nuclear factor; PG = prostaglandin; TNF = tumor necrosis factor; TX = thromboxane

Drug Combination

   c: 1 = as anti-inflammatory adjuvant in human studies
      2 = as anti-ulcer agent in animal studies

Table 61–3 Primary Oral Anti-ulcer Agents and Topical Anti-inflammatory Adjuvant Isolates

Herb	Study and Length[a]	N	Condition	Dosage Form
Chili/cayenne (*Capsicum frutescens*) pepper fruit	C[54] 0.15W	18	Healthy	Fruit powder
Capsaicin	R, PC, DB[55] 4W	101	Rheumatoid arthritis and osteoarthritis	0.025% capsaicin cream
Licorice (*Glycyrrhiza glabra*) root	C, DB[56] 5W	9	Aspirin-damaged stomach	Deglycyrrhizinated extract
Licorice	C, SB[58] 12W	100	Benign gastric ulcers	Deglycyrrhizinated extract
Glycyrrhetinic acid (GA)	C, DB[59] 0.15W	23	Healthy	95% ethanol solution

Study and Length
  a: C = controlled, DB = double-blind, O = open, PC = placebo-controlled, R = randomized, SB = single-blind; W = weeks

continues

Table 61–3 continued

Daily Dose	Drug Combination[c]	Outcome	Mechanisms of Action[b]
20 gm	1. Aspirin	Less stomach mucosal damage	Increased mucosal blood flow
Applied 4 times	2. NSAIDs, analgesics, corticosteroids	Burning, less pain	Depletes substance P
1.05 gm	1. Aspirin	Reduced fecal blood	Increases gastric mucin[57]
6 tablets	1. NSAIDs, corticosteroids	88% ulcers healed	Same as above
0.2 mg GA	2. Hydrocortisone	Increased cutaneous vasoconstriction	Inhibits 11β-OHSD

Mechanisms of Action
   b: 11β-OHSD = 11 beta-hydroxysteroid dehydrogenase
   c: 1 = as protectant in human studies
      2 = as adjuvant in human studies

Drug Combination
   c: 1 = as anti-ulcer agent in human studies
      2 = as anti-inflammatory adjuvant in human studies

In many of the studies involving chronic inflammation due to arthritis, the inclusion criteria allow for ongoing use of a steady maintenance dose of analgesics, disease-modifying drugs, and/or NSAIDs. Improvements in symptoms can then be recognized as an enhancement of baseline conventional therapy. A few studies specifically measure the reduction of NSAID or corticosteroid use as the research outcome of combining herbal products with these drugs. This drug intake reduction effect is desirable from the standpoint of reducing the risk of adverse effects. Established knowledge of toxicity and cumulative individual patient responses provide an appropriate baseline with which to assess any advantages from these integrative applications. Outcomes are considered beneficial when herbs effectively reduce the dose or side effects, or replace, complement, or enhance the therapeutic effects of conventional medications.

These benefits are not limited to combinations of drugs with herbal products. Botanical anti-inflammatory preparations have been found effective when used alone in clinical studies. Activity of herb fractions and/or components has also been demonstrated in laboratory research, which has aided in the delineation of mechanisms involved. An in-depth evaluation of these botanicals allows an appreciation of the potential complementary effects on the basis of both direct clinical studies and supportive mechanistic evidence. The complementary effects of herbal preparations used with drugs as primary adjuvants, as adjuvants with potential anti-ulcer effects, and as primary anti-ulcer protectants are summarized in Tables 61–1, 61–2, and 61–3, respectively.

CONCLUSIONS

There is a great need for published case studies and clinical trials. Findings from private open-label trials deserve communication in letters and journals when pertinent clinical observations are made. Preliminary findings such as these, supported by background pharmacological studies and knowledge of traditional applications, serve as an impetus for more extensive clinical studies. For herbs with established safety records, which lack evidence of adverse interactions as currently employed, their incorporation to improve patient care may be advanced through simple methods that hopefully attract positive scientific, public, and media interest.

(For specific in-depth information on the botanicals described in the tables, readers are referred to the original article and the books and other publications of Francis Brinker.)

TABLE REFERENCES

1. Teucher T, Obertreis B, Ruttkowski T, et al. Cytokine secretion in whole blood of healthy volunteers after oral ingestion of an *Urtica dioica L* leaf extract. *Arzneimittelfarschung*. 1996;46: 906–910.
2. Obertreis B, Ruttkowski T, Teucher T, et al. Ex-vivo in-vitro inhibition of lipopolysaccharide stimulated tumor necrosis factor-α and interleukin-1β secretion in human whole blood by extractum *Urticae dioicae foliorum*. *Arzneimittelforschung*. 1996;46:389–394.
3. Klingelhoefer S, Obertreis B, Quast S, et al. Antirheumatic effect of IDA 23, a stinging nettle leaf extract, on in vitro expression of T helper cytokines. *J Rheumatol*. 1999;26:2517–2522.
4. Riehemann K, Behnke B, Schulze-Osthoff K. Plant extracts from stinging nettle (*Urtica dioica*), an antirheumatic remedy, inhibit the proinflammatory transcription factor NF-κB. *FEBS Lett*. 1999;442:89–94.
5. Obertreis B, Giller K, Teucher T, et al. Antiphlogistic effects of *Urtica dioica folia* extract in

comparison to Caffeic Malic Acid. *Arzneimittelsorschung*. 1996;46:52–56.

6. Chrubasik S, Enderlein W, Bauer R, et al. Evidence for antirheumatic effectiveness of *Herba Urticae dioicae* in acute arthritis: a pilot study. *Phytomedicine*. 1997;4(2):105–108.

7. Meier B, Sticher O, Julkunen-Tiitto R. Pharmaceutical aspects of the use of willows in herbal remedies. *Planta Med*. 1988;54:559–560.

8. Schmid B, Kotter I, Heide L. Pharmacokinetics of salacin after oral administration of a standardized willow bark extract. *Eur J Clin Pharmacol*. 2001;57:387–391.

9. Chrubasik S, Kunzel O, Black A, et al. Potential economic impact of using a proprietary willow bark extract in outpatient treatment of low back pain: an open non-randomized study. *Phytomedicine*. 2001;8(4):241–251.

10. Heptinstall S, White A, Williamson L, et al. Extracts of feverfew inhibit granule secretion in blood platelets and polymorphonuclear leucocytes. *Lancet*. 1985;1(8437):1071–1074.

11. Makheja AN, Bailey JM. A platelet phospholipase inhibitor from the medicinal herb feverfew (*Tanacetum parthenium*). *Prostagland Leukot Med*. 1982;8:653–660.

12. Capasso F. The effect of an aqueous extract of *Tanacetum parthenium L.* on arachidonic acid metabolism by rat peritoneal leukocyctes. *J Pharm Pharmacol*. 1986;38:71–72.

13. Sumner H, Salan U, Knight DW, et al. Inhibition of 5-lipoxygenase and cyclo-oxygenase in leukocytes by feverfew. *Biochem Pharmacol*. 1992;43:2313–2320.

14. Williamson LM, Harvery DM, Sheppard KJ, et al. Effect of feverfew on phagocytosis and killing of *Candida guiltermondii* by neutrophils. *Inflammation*. 1988;12(1):11–16.

15. Hwang D, Fischer NH, Jang BC, et al. Inhibition of the expression of inducible cyclooxygenase and proinflammatory cytokines by sesquiterpene lactones in macrophages correlates with the inhibition of MAP kinases. *Biochem Biophys Res Comm*. 1996;226:810–818.

16. Pattrick M, Heptinstall S, Doherty M. Feverfew in rheumatoid arthritis: a double blind, placebo controlled trial. *Ann Rheum Dis*. 1989;48:547–549.

17. Chantre P, Cappelaere A, Leblan D, et al. Efficacy and tolerance of *Harpagophytum procumbens* versus diacerhein in treatment of osteoarthritis. *Phytomedicine*. 2000;7(3):177–183.

18. Chrubasik S, Zimpfer C, Schutt U, et al. Effectiveness of *Harpagophytum procumbens* in treatment of acute low back pain. *Phytomedicine*. 1996;3(1):1–10.

19. Chrubasik S, Thanner J, Kunzel O, et al. Comparison of outcome measures during treatment with the proprietary *Harpagophytum* extract doloteffin in patients with pain in the lower back, knee or hip. *Phytomedicine*. 2002;9:181–194.

20. Maurer HR. Bromelain: biochemistry, pharmacology and medical use. *Cell Mol Life Sci*. 2001;58:1234–1245.

21. Lotz-Winter H. On the pharmacology of Bromelain: an update with special regard to animal studies on dose-dependent effects. *Planta Med*. 1990;56:249–253.

22. Vellini M, Desideri D, Milanese A, et al. Possible involvement of eicosanoids in the pharmacological action of Bromelain. *Arzneimittelforschung*. 1986;36:110–112.

23. Zatuchni GI, Columbi DJ. Bromelains therapy for the prevention of episiotomy pain. *Obstet Gynecol*. 1967;29(2):275–278.

24. Spaeth GL. The effect of Bromelains on the inflammatory response caused by cataract extraction: a double-blind study. *The Eye, Ear, Nose and Throat Monthly*. 1968;47:26–33.

25. Tao X, Cush JJ, Garret M, et al. A phase I study of ethyl acetate extract of the Chinese antirheumatic herb *Triptergium wilfordii Hook F* in rheumatoid arthritis. *J Rheumatol*. 2001;28(10):2160–2167.

26. Maekawa K, Yoshikawa N, Du J, et al. The molecular mechanism of inhibition of interleukin-1 beta-induced cyclooxygenase-2 expression in human synovial cells by *Tripterygium wilfordii Hook F* extract. *Inflamm Res*. 1999;48:575–581.

27. Tao X, Younger J, Fan FZ, et al. Benefit of an extract of *Triterygium wilfordii Hook F* in patients with rheumatoid arthritis. *Arthritis Rheum*. 2002;46(7):1735–1743.

28. Piscoya J, Rodriguez Z, Bustamante SA, et al. Efficacy and safety of freeze-dried cat's claw in osteoarthritis of the knee: mechanisms of action of the species *Uncaria guianensis*. *Inflamm Res*. 2001;50:442–448.

29. Sandoval M, Okuhama NN, Zhang XJ, et al. Anti-inflammatory and antioxidant activities of cat's claw (*Uncaria tomentosa* and *Uncaria guinensis*) are independent of their alkaloid content. *Phytomedicine*. 2002;9:325–337.

30. Sandoval-Chacon M, Thompson JH, Zhang XJ. Antiinflammatory actions of cat's claw: the role of NF-κB. *Aliment Pharmacol Ther.* 1998;12: 1279–1289.

31. Sandoval M, Charbonnet RM, Okuhama NN, et al. Cat's claw inhibits TNFα production and scavenges free radicals: role in cytoprotection. *Free Radic Biol Med.* 2000;29(1):71–78.

32. Mur E, Hartig F, Eibl G, Schirmer M. Randomized double-blind trial of an extract from the pentacyclic alkaloid-chemotype of *Uncaria tomentosa* for the treatment of rheumatoid arthritis. *J Rheumatol.* 2002;29(4):678–681.

33. Srivastava KC. Effect of onion and ginger consumption on platelet thromboxane production in humans. *Prostaglandins Leukot Essent Fatty Acids.* 1989;35:183–185.

34. Kiuchi F, Shibuya M, Kinoshita T, et al. Inhibition of prostaglandin biosynthesis by the constituents of medicinal plants. *Chem Pharm Bull.* 1983;31: 3391–3396.

35. Tjendraputra E, Tran VH, Liu-Brennan D, et al. Effect of ginger constituents and synthetic analogues on cyclooxygenase-2 enzyme in intact cells. *Bioorg Med Chem.* 2001;29:156–163.

36. Kiuchi F, Shibuya M, Sankawa U. Inhibitors of prostaglandin biosynthesis from ginger. *Chem Pharm Bull.* 1982;30(2):754–757.

37. Srivastava KC. Aqueous extracts of onion, garlic and ginger inhibit platelet aggregation and alter arachidonic acid metabolism. *Biomed Biochem Acta.* 1984;43:S335–S346.

38. Srivastava KC. Isolation and effects of some ginger components on platelet aggregation and eicosanoid biosynthesis. *Prostagland Leukot Med.* 1986;25:187–198.

39. Srivastava KC, Mustafa T. Ginger (*Zingiber officinale)* and rheumatic disorders. *Med Hypotheses.* 1989;29:25–28.

40. Altman RD, Marcussen KC. Effects of a ginger extract on knee pain in patients with osteoarthritis. *Arthritis Rheum.* 2001;44(11):2531–2538.

41. Al-Yahya MA, Rafatullah S, Mossa JS, et al. Gastroprotective activity of ginger, *Zingiber officinale Rosc*, in albino rats. *Am J Chin Med.* 1989;17(1–2):51–56.

42. Kimmatkar N, Thawani V, Hingorani L, et al. Efficacy and tolerability of *Boswellia serrata* extract in treatment of osteoarthritis of knee: a randomized, double-blind, placebo-controlled trial. *Phytomedicine.* 2003;10:3–7.

43. Safayhi H, Boden SE, Schweizer T, et al. Concentration-dependent potentiating and inhibitory effects of boswellia extracts of 5-lipoxygenase product formation in stimulated PMNL. *Planta Med.* 2000;66:110–113.

44. Ammon HPT, Safayhi H, Mack T, et al. Mechanism of antiinflammatory actions of curcumin and boswellic acids. *J Ethnopharmacol.* 1993;38: 113–119.

45. Singh GB, Singh S, Bani S. Anti-inflammatory actions of boswellic acids. *Phytomedicine.* 1996; 3(1):81–85.

46. Knaus U, Wagner H. Effects of boswellic acid of Boswellia serrata and other triterpenic acids on the complement system. *Phytomedicine.* 1996; 3(1):77–81.

47. Safayhi H, Mack T, Ammon HPT. Protection by boswellic acids against galactosamine/endotoxin-induced hepatitis in mice. *Biochem Pharmacol.* 1991;41(10):1536–1537.

48. Jobin C, Bradham CA, Russo MP, et al. Curcumin blocks cytokine-mediated NF-κB activation and proinflammatory gene expression by inhibiting inhibitory factor 1-κB kinase activity. *J Immunol.* 1999;163:3474–3483.

49. Chopra A, Lavin P, Patwardhan B, et al. Randomized double-blind trial of an Ayurvedic plant derived formulation for treatment of rheumatoid arthritis. *J. Rheumatol.* 2000;27:1365–1372.

50. Zhang F, Altorki NK, Mestre JR, et al. Curcumin inhibits cyclooxygenase-2 transcription in bile acid and phorbol ester-treated human gastrointestinal epithelial cells. *Carcinogenesis.* 1999; 20(3):445–451.

51. Rafatullah S, Tariq M, Al-Yahya MA, et al. Evaluation of turmeric (*Curcuma longa*) for gastric and duodenal antiulcer activity in rats. *J Ethnopharmacol.* 1990;29:25–34.

52. Anbalagan K, Sadique J. Influence of an Indian medicine (ashwagandha) on acute-phase reactants in inflammation. *Indian J Exp Biol.* 1981;19: 245–249.

53. Anbalagan K, Sadique J. *Withania somnifera* (ashwagandha), a rejuvenating herbal drug which controls alpha-2-macroglobulin synthesis during inflammation. *Int J Crude Drug Res.* 1985;23(4): 177–183.

54. Yeoh KG, Kang JY, Guan R, et al. Chili protects against aspirin-induced gastroduodenal mucosal injury in humans. *Dig Dis Sci.* 1995;40(3):580–583.

55. Deal CL, Schnitzer TJ, Lipstein E, et al. Treatment of arthritis with topical capsaicin: a double-blind trial. *Clin Ther.* 1991;13(3):383–395.

56. Rees WDW, Rhodes J, Wright JE, et al. Effect of deglycyrrhizinated liquorice on gastric mucosal

damage by aspirin. *Scand J Gastroenterol.* 1979;14;605–607.

57. Goso Y, Ogata Y, Ishihara K, et al. Effects of traditional herbal medicine on gastric mucin against ethanol-induced gastric injury in rats. *Comp Biochem Physiol.* 1996;113C(1):7–21.

58. Morgan AG, McAdam WAF, Pacsoo C, et al. Comparison between cimetidine and Caved-S in the treatment of gastric ulceration, and subsequent maintenance therapy. *Gut.* 1982;23:545–551.

59. Teelucksingh S, Mackie AD, Burt D, et al. Potentiation of hydrocortisone activity in skin by glycyrrhetinic acid. *Lancet.* 1990;335: 1060–1063.

CHAPTER REFERENCES

Abebe W. Herbal medication: potential for adverse interactions with analgesic drugs. *J Clin Pharm Ther.* 2002;27:391–401.

Anon. OTC drugs can be harmful to the unborn child. *Drug Ther Perspect.* 2000;16(3):12–14.

Cannella AC, O'Dell JR. Is there still a role for traditional disease-modifying antirheumatic drugs (MDARDs) in rheumatoid arthritis? *Curr Opin Rheumatol.* 2003;15(3):185–192.

Conn DL, Lim SS. New role for an old friend. Prednisone is a disease-modifying agent in early rheumatoid arthritis. *Curr Opin Rheumatol.* 2003;15(3): 193–196.

Ding C. Do NSAIDs affect the progression of osteoarthritis? *Inflammation.* 2002;26(3):139–142.

Ernst E. Over-the-counter complementary remedies used for arthritis. *Pharm J.* 1998;260:830–831.

Fung HB, Kirschenbaum HL. Selective cyclooxygenase-2 inhibitors for the treatment of arthritis. *Clin Ther.* 1999;21(7):1131–1157.

Hobson K. Overdoing it (Health & Medicine: Vital Signs). *U.S. News and World Report.* February 10, 2003. Available at: www.usnews.com/usnews/health/articles/030210/10healthbrf.lede.htm. Accessed December 1, 2004.

Kociancic T, Reed MD. Acetaminophen intoxication and length of treatment: how long is long enough? *Pharmacotherapy.* 2003;23(8):1052–1059.

Long L, Soekenk K, Ernst E. Herbal medicines for the treatment of osteoarthritis; a systematic review. *Rheumatol.* 2001;40:779–793.

Mease PJ. Disease-modifying antirheumatic drug therapy for spondyloarthropathies: advances in treatment. *Curr Opin Rheumatol.* 2003;15(3): 205–212.

Nielsen GL, Sorensen MT, Larsen H, et al. Risk of adverse birth outcome and miscarriage in pregnant users of non-steroidal anti-inflammatory drugs: population based observational study and case-control study. *BMJ.* 2001;322:266–270.

Norred CL, Brinker F. Potential coagulation effects of preoperative complementary and alternative medicines. *Altern Ther Health Med.* 2001;7(6): 58–67.

Soeken KL, Miller SA, Ernst E. Herbal medicines for the treatment of rheumatoid arthritis: a systematic review. *Rheumatology.* 2003;42:652–659.

Townsend RR. Non-aspirin nonsteroidal anti-inflammatory drugs. *J Clin Hypertens.* 2002;4(6): 436–440.

Wolfe MM, Lichtenstein DR, Sing G. Gastrointestinal toxicity of nonsteroidal anti-inflammatory drugs. *New Engl J Med.* 1999;340(24):1888–1899.

PART X

Models of Integrative Medicine

CHAPTER 62

The Healing Power of Relationship-Centered Care

David Rakel, MD

The patient–practitioner relationship is integral to effective complementary medicine. This support can be vital, particularly when patients develop serious illness—then the relationship between patient and health care practitioner becomes central. Patients whose health is vulnerable want and need highly knowledgeable guidance, whether they have a life-threatening disorder or a chronic condition. Effective treatment is facilitated by a relationship with a practitioner who can provide patients with a sense of control and empowerment, through a collaborative approach to partner in their care (Tresolini & Pew-Fetzer Task Force, 1994).

The effect of expectation. The body's ability to heal itself is based in part on belief and expectancy (Moerman & Jonas, 2002). Once we have the expectation that we will get better, the body often responds (Benedetti, 2002). The power of belief, reflected in the placebo effect, is a familiar strategy in research methodology (de Craen et al., 1999). Typically inert medications serve as placebos, but other aspects of a health care encounter can also have this effect, including various treatment techniques, medical information, and the patient's own belief in various aspects of treatment. We know from the research that placebo effects can also result from the interaction with a health care practitioner (Thomas, 1978; Di Blasi et al., 2001). The medical literature supports the existence of "physician effects," including enhanced patient–doctor interaction effects. In the context of clinical practice, this means that as a health care practitioner, your interaction with your patients is an important aspect of the healing equation.

PHYSICIAN EFFECTS

There is a substantial amount of research that explores the importance of interactions between patients and health care providers, usually physicians (Bass et al., 1986; Roter et al., 1995; Latham, 1998; Di Blasi et al., 2001; Pappas & Perlman, 2002). Although much of the literature focuses on subjective outcomes such as patient satisfaction, there are a number of studies that point toward more objective, health-related outcomes. For example:

- In 1995 Stewart reported the results of a systematic review of studies assessing health outcomes of physician–patient communication. Of 21 studies meeting the criteria, 16 reported positive health outcomes. Reported benefits ranged from decreased anxiety, distress, and pain, to improvements in blood pressure, mobility, and general health-related quality of life. Effect sizes ranged from 20% to 40% for anxiety scores, to a three-fold difference in resolution of headache (Stewart, 1995).
- In 1998 Roter and colleagues published a meta-analysis of 153 studies "that evaluated the effectiveness of interventions to improve patient compliance with medical regimens." They found significant benefit for good patient–provider

A brief biography of David Rakel appears in Chapter 1.

communication, ranging from improved compliance with medication and more consistent follow-up visits to better outcomes on laboratory tests and general health assessments. Effect sizes ranged from 0.17 to 0.60, with most in the 20% to 30% range (Roter et al., 1998).

- In 2001 Di Blasi and colleagues published a systematic review of "context effects on health outcomes." They reviewed 25 randomized trials, reporting generally positive results. Positive and negative studies were noted, with effect sizes ranging from small to large. Researchers noted, "one relatively consistent finding is that physicians who adopt a warm, friendly, and reassuring manner are more effective than those who keep consultations formal and do not offer reassurance" (Di Blasi et al., 2001).

Courtesy of Bruce Barrett MD, PhD

The relationship contributes to healing. The patient–practitioner relationship can build the confidence that patients need in order to take action to improve their health. In fact, it is difficult for the patient's medical care to progress without that relationship, which can be a factor in communication, compliance, and fundamental attitudes toward healing. Continuity of care with the primary care practitioner also allows for the deeper understanding of the patient and the etiology and progression of his or her condition. The greatest benefit arises when patients have a practitioner who understands them well and then suggests treatment or an appropriate referral, based on that individual's diagnosis, constitution, and preferences for care. Consequently, even referrals require careful analysis and are ideally strategic and central to the patient's treatment.

TREATING COMPLEX CONDITIONS

When patients develop chronic illness, it can be challenging to identify the actual underlying cause. The process is like being asked to solve a mystery novel in the first couple of pages. In many cases, the solution is not apparent for some time. A good working relationship helps to provide a point of stability for patients while the evaluation of their illness proceeds. One way to support the patient is not to focus on the answer, but rather on establishing a good working relationship and open communication. This allows the answer to unfold much more efficiently. Then patients are more likely to develop a sense of trust and divulge their story, which holds clues to unraveling the mystery of their illness.

A focus on the patient's story. Physician and patient, working in collaboration, piece together the patient's story to explore the underlying root cause(s) or etiology. Telling the story serves a number of purposes. As practitioners, we listen to the words, but also make it a point to notice nonverbal cues that reflect vitality or depletion, including tone of voice, body language, and emotions. This information processing allows for more accurate assessment of the individual's needs. Careful listening does more than show respect for the patient—it also provides information essential to the analysis of the patient's condition. The process of telling this story to a compassionate listener also brings emotion-laden information into focused coherence. This creates the opportunity to draw meaning from disparate pieces, giving the patient a greater sense of control and understanding (Langer, 1983).

This is the art of medicine—which involves more than just stating the evidence. It is through the relationship that we develop the understandings, intuitions, and insights from fragments of apparently unrelated information that allow us to perform a logical analysis and draw accurate and meaningful conclusions. Relationship-centered care also enables us to use an integrative process more efficiently and make the most appropriate decisions or referral, with the best possible result for that patient.

THE DYNAMIC PROCESS OF HEALING

The process of evaluation and treatment is dynamic and multifactorial:

1. Good communication in the patient-practitioner relationship creates rapport and empathy, which supports the diagnostic process of evaluation and understanding. This insight enables the physician to develop the most efficient treatment plan possible.
2. Treatment options are considered in the context of the patient's belief system and the culture in which they live. The evidence and science inform the decision of which therapeutic modalities best match the diagnosis and other requirements of the individual.
3. The physician and the patient agree upon a plan of action that both believe will lead to improved health. In integrative practice, this is a collaborative approach that may involve both conventional and complementary referrals. For example, a patient with cancer may have a team that includes the primary care physician, an oncologist, a nutritionist, a traditional Chinese medicine practitioner, and a chaplain. The primary practitioner is in the best position to organize a collaborative team that will support the patient's needs. In a truly integrative approach, the patient is an active participant in the team decision-making process.
4. Healing is a dynamic, evolving process that requires continuous reevaluation. What works at one time may need modification and adaptation in the future.

These four steps occur within an environment of constant change. As this process continues to unfold, physician and patient are constantly learning from past experiences and developing new insights on how to maintain the balance of health. In doing so, we also develop a deeper understanding of our core needs. This is a journey inward—ideally one that leads to an understanding of why a symptom may be present. For example, does it reflect a genetic aberration, a lifestyle stressor, an underlying functional issue such as inflammation, a nutritional deficiency, or is it filling a psychological need?

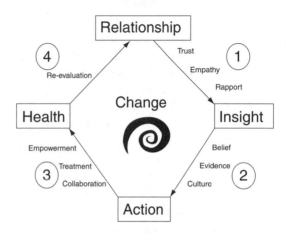

If this inner process is never explored, an individual will continue to rely on external influences to reduce the severity of symptoms without learning what the symptoms can teach us. A symptom can often be a red flag to alert us to lifestyle habits or situations that are not conducive to health and well-being. If we simply treat or suppress the symptom without fully understanding it, we will not have the opportunity to learn what is required to fully resolve it.

If we first focus on what is needed for the body to heal, we will require fewer therapies to promote healing, resulting in lower health care costs and improved quality of life for our patients.

RELATIONSHIP-CENTERED CARE

Uniqueness of the individual. In this process, it is also essential that we retain a focus on the individuality of the patient. Ten people with the same disease may have 10 different paths toward health. The treatment plan will be reflective of the patient's physiological health, his or her diagnosis, and also the approach to treatment with which the patient is most comfortable, as a result of culture and personal beliefs (Tresolini & Pew-Fetzer Task Force, 1994).

The value of an ongoing patient–practitioner relationship. The physician–patient relationship can be a stabilizing factor in patients' lives, particularly those with chronic illness. This relationship has been aptly described using a kaleidoscope as a metaphor (Thomas, 1981). Many genetic and environmental factors enter into the equation. While some factors are more important than others, there is an overall pattern that determines the outcome. During the course of our lives, the kaleidoscope turns a little as each new positive or negative factor is added. The pattern is constantly changing and susceptible to future change. The persistence of good health or the development of disease depends upon a particular configuration of factors in a given individual at a given time. It is most ideal if patients have someone to whom they can always turn, to partner with in support of their health, because what works today may be different than what has worked in the past (House et al., 1988).

The role of intention. What matters is not just the patient's intention, but also the practitioner's intention and awareness. Is the practitioner truly present with the patient—or is he or she thinking about all the patients in the waiting room and the paper that has to be written that evening? The practitioner's mindful presence plays a role in how the patient perceives the interaction and responds to the therapy prescribed. Being present with intent enhances the relationship, rapport, and joy of the encounter. (Suchman et al., 1997; Epstein, 1999).

The role of the evidence. There are important junctures in the process of decision making when our patients need us to revisit and scrutinize the research to make the best recommendations based on that evidence. Patients who seek care for cancer, for example, want the best information and the best evidence possible to help them understand how they should proceed in treatment. Patients want someone to help them through the vast number of options, ranging from surgery, chemotherapy, radiation, and pharmaceuticals, to diets, nutraceuticals, botanicals, and adjunctive complementary therapies.

For many patients with chronic disorders, there are no obvious answers, and numerous multifaceted approaches to treatment. Patients need someone who is comprehensively knowledgeable to coach them—to provide them with better understanding of the most effective options.

As in other areas of life, it is the pairing of compassion and knowledge that is most effective, because one without the other would not provide the full potential for healing. Often the relationships we build are one of the most rewarding aspects of our work, which make it all worthwhile. Frequently, this is also the aspect of medicine that brings us the most joy.

REFERENCES

Bass MJ, Buck C, Turner L, Dickie G, Pratt G, Robinson HC. The physician's actions and the outcome of illness in family practice. *J Fam Pract.* 1986;23:43–47.

Benedetti F. How the doctor's words affect the patient's brain. *Eval Health Prof.* 2002;25:369–386.

de Craen AJ, Kaptchuk TJ, Tijssen JG, Kleijnen J. Placebos and placebo effects in medicine: historical overview. *J R Soc Med.* 1999;92:511–515.

Di Blasi Z, Harkness E, Ernst E, Georgiou A, Kleijnen J. Influence of context effects on health outcomes: a systematic review. *Lancet.* 2001;357: 757–762.

Epstein RM. Mindful practice. *JAMA.* 1999;282(9): 833–839.

House J, Landis KR, Umberson D. Social relationships and health. *Science.* 1988;241:540–545.

Langer EJ. *The Psychology of Control.* Beverly Hills, CA: Sage; 1983.

Latham CE. Is there data to support the concept that educated, empowered patients have better outcomes? *J Am Soc Nephrol.* 1998;9:Suppl-4.

Moerman DE, Jonas WB. Deconstructing the placebo effect and finding the meaning response. *Ann Int Med.* 2002;136:471–476.

Pappas S, Perlman A. The importance of doctor-patient communication. *Complement Altern Med.* 2002;86:1–10.

Roter DL, Hall JA, Kern DE, Barker LR, Cole KA, Roca RP. Improving physicians' interviewing skills and reducing patients' emotional distress. A randomized clinical trial. *Arch Int Med.* 1995;155:1877–1884.

Roter DL, Hall JA, Merisca R, Nordstrom B, Cretin D, Svarstad B. Effectiveness of interventions to improve patient compliance: a meta-analysis. *Med Care.* 1998;36:1138–1161.

Stewart MA. Effective physician-patient communication and health outcomes: a review. *Can Med Assoc J.* 1995;152:1423–1433.

Suchman AL, Markakis K, Beckman HB, Frankel R. A model of empathic communication in the medical interview. *JAMA.* 1997;277:678–682.

Thomas CB. Stamina: the thread of life. *J Chronic Dis.* 1981;34:41–44.

Thomas KB. The consultation and the therapeutic illusion. *BMJ.* 1978;1:1327–1328.

Tresolini CP and Pew-Fetzer Task Force. *Health Professions Education and Relationship-Centered Care.* San Francisco, CA: Pew Health Professions Commission; 1994.

ADDITIONAL BIBLIOGRAPHY

Brody H. The doctor as therapeutic agent: a placebo effect research agenda. In Harrington A, ed. *The Placebo Effect: An Interdisciplinary Exploration.* Cambridge, MA: Harvard University Press; 1997: 77–92.

Charon R. The patient-physician relationship. Narrative medicine: a model for empathy, reflection, profession and trust. *JAMA.* 2001;286:1897–1902.

Gotler RS, Flocke SA, Goodwin MA, Zyzanski SJ, Murray TH, Stange KC. Facilitating participatory decision-making: what happens in real-world community practice? *Med Care.* 2000;38:1200–1209.

Guadagnoli E, Ward P. Patient participation in decision-making. *Soc Sci Med.* 1998;47:329–339.

Hrobjartsson A, Gotzsche PC. Is the placebo powerless? Update of a systematic review with 52 new randomized trials comparing placebo with no treatment. *J Int Med.* 2004;256(2):91–100.

Kaplan SH, Greenfield S, Ware JE. Assessing the effects of physician-patient interactions on the outcomes of chronic disease. *Med Care.* 1989;27:S110–S127.

Krupat E, Bell RA, Kravitz RL, Thom D, Azari R. When physicians and patients think alike: patient-centered beliefs and their impact on satisfaction and trust. *J Fam Pract.* 2001;50:1057–1062.

Moerman DE. *Meaning, Medicine and the Placebo Effect.* Cambridge, MA: Cambridge University Press; 2002.

Savage R, Armstrong D. Effect of a general practitioner's consulting style on patients' satisfaction: a controlled study. *BMJ.* 1990;301:968–970.

Shapiro AK, Shapiro E. *The Powerful Placebo: From Ancient Priest to Modern Physician.* Baltimore, MD: Johns Hopkins University Press, 1997.

Simpson M, Buckman R, Stewart M et al. Doctor-patient communication: the Toronto consensus statement. *BMJ.* 1991;303:1385–1387.

Starfield B, Wray C, Hess K, Gross R, Birk PS, D'Lugoff BC. The influence of patient-practitioner agreement on outcome of care. *Am J Pub Health.* 1981;71:127–131.

CHAPTER 63

Completing Your Patient Referral Network

John C. Reed, MD, MD(H)

INTRODUCTION

With the increased inclusion of complementary therapies in health care, physicians will play an expanded role in the integration of complementary services. The physician is ideally placed within the system to encourage appropriate utilization. A doctor's level of comfort with referrals to CAM practitioners will depend on his or her level of exposure, education, and knowledge of these specialties. Patients will appreciate physicians who are able to effectively refer to and involve complementary practitioners in care planning, and the practitioners who can integrate complementary health care and traditional services will find they have a valued niche within their professions.

, Most primary care medical practitioners (family doctors, internists, gynecologists, and pediatricians) have a panel of well-established specialists in their community to whom they refer patients. These specialists typically include general and specialty surgeons, psychologists and psychiatrists, ophthalmologists and optometrists—and various medical sub-specialists such as endocrinologists, gastroenterologists, and neurologists. Physicians build their preferred referral lists based on the medical needs of their immediate patient population for adjunctive diagnostic and treatment services.

With the broadening of interest in preventive care and outpatient management of chronic illness, we now need a new referral panel model. Ideally, this model will address ongoing health and wellness care in a manner that integrates the full range of patient needs, including those that can be effectively met by various complementary service providers.

INTEGRATIVE HEALTH PRACTICE MODEL

One model for integrative care reflects the functional causes of personal health problems that most individuals experience. This model (Figure 63–1) focuses on three essential—and interrelated—aspects of good health: biochemical/metabolic, psychological, and biomechanical function. Health service providers can also be grouped according to their expertise in addressing these functional areas. The advantage of this model to the medical practitioner is to suggest aspects of health promotion and treatment intervention that may be outside one's usual practice model, but that may be of genuine interest to one's patients. For the professional in complementary medicine, this model can serve as a reminder that no one can address all aspects of care and that building relationships with other health specialists is an important aspect of a truly holistic health care model.

Biochemical function. The first factor consists of healthy biochemical functioning (function of the body's organs, immune cells, hormones, nutrition, and the generation of

A brief biography of John Reed appears in Chapter 8.
Courtesy of John C. Reed, MD, MD(H), Sterling, Virginia.

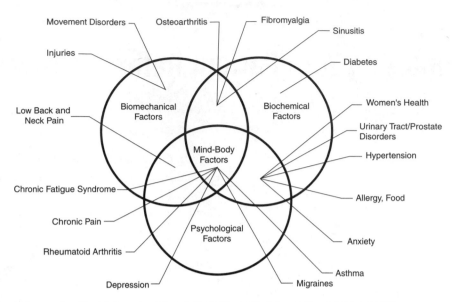

Figure 63–1 Integrative Health Practice Model. © 1995, 2005, John C. Reed, MD, MD(H).

metabolic energy). This area is the focus of most modern allopathic care, which involves using medications to correct unhealthy chemical disturbances (or substituting synthetic chemicals for deficiencies in the naturally occurring ones). This area is also the province of preventive nutrition and natural medicine—the prescription of herbs, homeopathics, and nutraceuticals to prevent or address ailments.

Psychological function. The second area—psychological factors—is one in which our society has become quite astute. We have developed the understanding that human life encompasses biopsychosocial experiences, which can lead to healthy or unhealthy beliefs, relationships, and emotional patterns that contribute to health and illness.

Biomechanical function. The third area has been largely underrepresented in the orthodox medical model, while being maintained in the chiropractic and osteopathic professions. This aspect of the model recognizes that humans

are designed to move in space and gravity. The health of our body's biomechanical system of bones, joints, nerves, and muscles enables us to move, work, play, and love with ease and joy. Sports medicine is a modern reflection of this health need in our society, addressed by medical doctors, orthopedic specialists, chiropractors, exercise physiologists, and personal/athletic trainers. Traditional practices such as yoga, tai chi, and the martial arts also support this aspect of health.

Figure 63–1 relates the functional model of health to chronic medical problems. This diagram indicates health issues most frequently treated at an American WholeHealth integrative medicine center in Chicago in 1996 (original unpublished data).

Three functional areas overlap in a holistic model. For example, joint inflammation (chemistry) affects joint movement and body posture. Muscle holding patterns (biomechanics) can reflect psychological factors such as chronic fear or depressed mood. Chemical imbalances ranging from gross deficiencies of B vitamins to subtle genetic variations in brain chemistry can manifest as mental disorders ranging from depression to dementia. Each individual's mind and body—mind-body system—reflects and responds to the environment, which also has physical, chemical, and cultural effects on well-being.

The powers of the mind are not just processes that create or undo psychological problems; we now know how to develop and integrate the capabilities of mind and body to enhance health maintenance and recovery from illness. For example mind-body methods have been shown to improve human athletic performance. These methods have also been found to improve the effectiveness of chemotherapy and, as a result, cancer outcomes in patients using chemotherapy. This suggests the value of a health care management strategy that addresses and supports these interacting components of health—as well as the treatment of disease and specific disease "entities." This functional model can provide the context for the integration of a diversity of health and disease specialists in the management of personal health issues.

Medical care also can be organized according to specialists that treat specific aspects of physiology, such as dental care, eye care, and skin care, and specialists that work with target populations, such as women's health and geriatrics, as well as pain management, and emergency care. Within each of these specialty areas the multifactor model comes into play, reflecting typical health fac-

tors and interventions in that medical specialty. In an integrative model, for example, modern pain management involves close cooperation between oral and injectable pain medication management, manual therapy, acupuncture for the neuromusculoskeletal system, and psychological management of mood, emotion, and post-traumatic stressors that could contribute to pain problems. To apply this model to your own practice, we have provided two tables for your review.

The first table, 63–1, is an inventory designed to help you evaluate your own practice, and how you currently relate to different types of patient problem areas:

- Are you a specialist or a generalist?
- Do you treat most of the problems patients bring to you by yourself, or do you treat some problems and refer others to specialists in your field or practitioners in supportive specialties?
- Which types of specialists are on your current referral panel?

The second table, 63–2, is a planning reference that indicates various types of practitioners—medical doctors, allied health professionals, and complementary providers—who might be useful in addressing health issues in each of these areas.[*] Your priorities will be different if you are a generalist—a primary care practitioner who does a wide range of diagnosis and referral services—or if you are a disease management specialist, who refers to skilled practitioners with very specific technical expertise to meet the needs of your clientele. Completing this exercise will prepare you to apply some of the approaches in this book and help you identify the types of complementary medicine practitioners that you consider a high priority for your personal "virtual integrative health team."

---

[*] The suggestions here reflect both the growing body of evidence-based criteria for use of the complementary medicine specialties and the author's experience in designing care pathways and credentialing programs in more than 20 years of integrative general practice, pain management practice, and health care administration.

Table 63–1 Health Care Practice Inventory

		Services in General Practice	Services as a Specialist/ Consultant
Health Issues I Treat	*Services I Provide*	[Check those applicable]	
Biochemical/internal medicine disorders	Perform evaluations and management for patients in my practice		
	Drug management		
	Nonpharmaceutical measures: vitamins, nutraceuticals herbs, etc.		
	Dietary and nutritional counseling		
	Subspecialty medical care: skin, GI tract, eyes, endocrine function, etc.		
	General surgical care		
	Specialty surgical care: ENT, eye, gynecology, cancer, heart conditions, etc.		
	Other		
Biomechanical/ neuromusculo- skeletal disorders	Perform evaluations and management for patients in my area or specialty		
	Outpatient procedural care: injections, physical modalities, acupuncture		
	Hands-on manual therapy for joints, muscles, and fascia		
	Exercise/movement and fitness instruction		
	Specialty surgical care: orthopedics, neurologic, podiatric		

Table 63–1 continued

Provided/ Referred Out	Services Referred Out	Practitioners to Whom I Currently Refer	Types of Specialists I Would Like to Add (see 63–2)
		[Enter names/types of practitioners]	

continues

Table 63–1 continued

		Services in General Practice	Services as a Specialist/ Consultant
Health Issues I Treat	*Services I Provide*	*[Check those applicable]*	
Biopsychosocial disorders	Perform evaluations and management in my practice		
	Individual counseling, psychotherapy		
	Specialty psychiatric care		
	Spiritual/pastoral counseling and support		
	Mind-body skills instruction, coaching, and support		
Special patient care populations	Pain management, pain medicine		
	Women's or men's health		
	Pregnancy care and childbirth support		
	Pediatric and adolescent health		
	Developmental delay, learning problems/ disabilities		
	Geriatric health		
	Cancer care		
	Cardiovascular care		
	Dental health		

Table 63–1 continued

Provided/ Referred Out	Services Referred Out	Practitioners to Whom I Currently Refer	Types of Specialists I Would Like to Add (see 63–2)
	[Enter names/types of practitioners]		

Table 63–2.1 Integrative Practice Planning Reference

		Medical and Osteopathic Practitioners	Conventional Allied Health Practitioners
Issues Treated	*Services Needed*	*Typical Medical Referral Panel*	
Biochemical/internal medicine disorders	Perform diagnostic evaluations and management for patients	Family practice, internal medicine, gynecology, pediatrics	Physician assistant, nurse practitioner, clinical nurse specialist
	Drug management	Same as above	Same as above, plus clinical pharmacist
	Nonpharmaceutical measures: vitamins, herbs, nutraceuticals	Holistic medicine, medical acupuncturist	Holistic nurse practitioner
	Dietary and nutritional counseling	Holistic medicine	Registered dietician
	Subspecialty medical care: skin, GI tract, eyes, endocrine function, etc.	Dermatologist, gastroenterologist, ophthalmologist, endocrinologist	Optometrist
	General surgical care	General surgeon, anesthesiologist	n.a.
	Specialty surgical care	ENT specialist, ophthalmologist, gynecologist, urologist, oncologist, cardiologist	n.a.
	Other		

Table 63–2.1 continued

Licensed Complementary Practitioners	Nonlicensed CAM/Wellness Services	Practitioners to Whom I Refer for These Services	Types of Specialists I Would Like to Add
Complementary Referral Resources		*[Enter names/types of practitioners]*	
Naturopathic physician, Oriental medicine doctor			
Naturopathic physician (in states where scope of practice allows)			
Chinese herbal medicine, licensed acupuncturist, clinical nutritionist	Herbalist, Ayurvedic practitioner, electrotherapy		
Same as above	Holistic health counselor		
n.a.	n.a.		
Naturopathic physician (in states where scope of practice allows minor outpatient surgery)	n.a.		

continues

Table 63–2.2 Integrative Practice Planning Reference

		Medical and Osteopathic Practitioners	Conventional Allied Health Practitioners
Issues Treated	*Services Needed*	*Typical Medical Referral Panel*	
Biomechanical/ neuromusculo- skeletal disorders	Perform diagnostic evaluations and physical medicine care for patients	Orthopedist, physiatrist, osteopathic manual specialist	Physical therapist, occupational therapist
	Outpatient care: injections, physical modalities, acupuncture	Physiatrist, medical acupuncturist, podiatrist, pain specialist	Physical therapist, occupational therapist
	Hands-on manual therapy for joints, muscles, and fascia	Osteopathic manual specialist	Physical therapist, occupational therapist
	Exercise/movement and fitness instruction	Physiatrist, sports medicine specialist	Physical therapist, occupational therapist
	Specialty surgical care: orthopedics, neurologic, podiatric	Orthopedic surgeon, neurosurgeon, podiatrists	n.a.
	Other		

continues

Table 63–2.2 continued

Licensed Complementary Practitioners	Nonlicensed CAM/Wellness Services	Practitioners to Whom I Refer for These Services	Types of Specialists I Would Like to Add
Complementary Referral Resources		*[Enter names/types of practitioners]*	
Chiropractic physician	n.a.		
Acupuncturist, chiropractic and naturopathic acupuncturist			
Chiropractor, naturopathic physician, clinical massage therapist, acupuncturist with Asian bodywork training	Rolfing, Hellerwork, and other structural integration practitioners; Trager practitioner		
Chiropractic physician, massage therapist, acupuncturist with tai chi or Qigong training	Instructors: Feldenkrais, Alexander, Pilates, yoga, tai chi, Qigong; personal trainer		
n.a.	n.a.		

Table 63–2.3 Integrative Practice Planning Reference

		Medical and Osteopathic Practitioners	Conventional Allied Health Practitioners
Issues Treated	*Services Needed*	*Typical Medical Referral Panel*	
Biopsychosocial disorders	Perform diagnostic evaluations and mental health care management	Psychiatrist, primary care physician	Psychologist, behavioral counselor, nurse practitioner
	Individual counseling, psychotherapy	Same as above	Same as above plus licensed social workers
	Specialty psychiatric care	Psychiatrist, medical hypnotherapist	Psychiatric nurse
	Spiritual/pastoral counseling and support	n.a.	Pastoral counselor
	Mind-body and relaxation skills instruction, coaching, and support	Physicians specializing in mind-body coaching	Psychologist, behavioral health counselor, hypnotherapist
	Other		

continues

Table 63–2.3 continued

Licensed Complementary Practitioners	Nonlicensed CAM/Wellness Services	Practitioners to Whom I Refer for These Services	Types of Specialists I Would Like to Add
Complementary Referral Resources		*Enter names/types of practitioners*	
Naturopathic physician			
Naturopathic physician	Health coach, stress management, support groups		
Biofeedback therapist	n.a.		
n.a.			
Biofeedback therapist	Music, art, and drama therapists; mindfulness meditation; hypnotherapist; stress management		

Table 63–2.4 Integrative Practice Planning Reference

		Medical and Osteopathic Practitioners	Conventional Allied Health Practitioners
Issues Treated	*Services Needed*	*Typical Medical Referral Panel*	
Special patient care populations	Pain management, pain medicine	Pain specialists, physiatrist, anesthesiologist, medical acupuncturist, osteopathic manual specialist, psychiatrist	Physical therapist, occupational therapist, psychologist, behavioral health counselor, hypnotherapist
	Women's health	Family practice, internal medicine, gynecologist, holistic physician	Physician assistant, nurse practitioner, clinical nurse specialist
	Men's health	Family practice, internal medicine, urologist, holistic physician	Physician assistant, nurse practitioner, clinical nurse specialist
	Pregnancy care and childbirth support	Obstetrician, family physician, medical acupuncturist	Nurse-midwife
	Pediatric and adolescent health	Pediatrician, family physician	Nurse practitioner, behavioral counselor
	Developmental delay, learning problems/ disabilities	Pediatrician, neurologist, holistic physician	Speech therapist, physical therapist, psychologist
	Geriatric health	Medical internist, geriatrician, holistic physician	Registered dietician
	Cancer care	Oncologist, internist, holistic physician	Behavioral health counselor, registered dietician
	Cardiovascular care	Cardiologist, internist, surgeon, holistic physician	Physical therapist, rehab physiatrist, registered dietician
	Dental health	Dentist, holistic dentist	Dental hygienist
	Other		

continues

Table 63–2.4 continued

Licensed Complementary Practitioners	Nonlicensed CAM/Wellness Services	Practitioners to Whom I Refer for These Services	Types of Specialists I Would Like to Add
Complementary Referral Resources		*Enter names/types of practitioners*	
Chiropractor, acupuncturist, naturopathic physician/ acupuncturist, clinical massage therapist	Instructors of mindfulness meditation, yoga, tai chi, and Qigong; Rolfing, Hellerwork, and Trager		
Naturopathic physician, Oriental medicine doctor, massage therapist	Herbalist		
Naturopathic physician, Oriental medicine doctor	Herbalist		
Naturopathic physician, licensed acupuncturist	Midwife, doula, childbirth ed., lactation consultant		
Chiropractic and naturopathic doctor			
Acupuncturist (auriculotherapy), biofeedback, clinical nutritionist	Feldenkrais instructor, sound therapy		
Nutritionist, Oriental medicine doctor, naturopath	Tai chi, yoga, Feldenkrais teachers		
Nutritionist, acupuncturist, naturopath	Meditation, mind-body skills, guided imagery		
Clinical nutritionist, naturopathic physician	Tai chi, Qigong, yoga, trainer for cardio rehab		
Acupuncturist			

CHAPTER 64

Credentialing Complementary Practitioners

John C. Reed, MD, MD(H) and Vickie Ina, MBA

THE CREDENTIALING PROCESS

In the modern US health care system, the credentials of potential practitioners are evaluated through a formal credentialing process. There are several factors, such as program design, liability, and marketing strategy, that determine the level of simplicity or sophistication of the credentialing programs operated by health plans, hospitals, and medical groups. The credentialing process provides an organization with the ability to systematically assess the training, experience, practice history, and skills of their potential providers. Credentialing standards may incorporate both recognized benchmarks of the professional specialty and the contracting organization's self-defined quality standards.

Credentialing provides an organizational screening process or "seal of approval" by the membership organization, hospital, or heath plan. This process ensures that some standard professional criteria have been used to review the characteristics of providers. For a practitioner-managed organization, such as a group practice, or a specialty practice association that contracts to provide services to health plans, credentialing is an evaluation and screening tool that defines quality standards and the organization's exposure to professional and operational liability. [A group practice or hospital will be responsible to the public (to its patients) if it recruits and employs a health care provider with a poor track record.] For the health plan, credentialing is an evaluation process that allows the health plan to minimize its exposure to liabilities, such as financial penalties, adverse public relations, and practitioner or member complaints.

The credentialing process also allows many plans to comply with quality standards such as those of the National Committee on Quality Assurance (NCQA) and various state regulatory agencies. These compliance requirements are sometimes necessary to maintain a managed care license and to meet mandated service requirements. If credentialing services are delegated by the health plan to an outside vendor, the health plan monitors these delegated services by periodically auditing the vendor's performance. For the consumer, credentialing or qualifying standards provide a level of trust and comfort that the practitioners being recommended are qualified to provide quality service.

A brief biography of John Reed, MD, MD(H) appears in Chapter 8.

Vickie Ina, MBA, is former senior vice president of product development at Consensus Health dba OneBody.com, where she developed and managed the CAM networks. She has more than 15 years of senior management experience in managed care environments, including positions as director of Network Development at OnCare Health, director of provider relations at Foundation Health/Managed Health Network, and director of professional relations at Blue Shield of California. Ms. Ina's responsibilities have encompassed negotiation of provider contracts, establishment of performance structures, management of credentialing, and involvement with regulatory and legal issues surrounding network management.

Courtesy of John C. Reed, MD, MD(H), Sterling, Virginia and Vickie Ina, MBA.

The credentialing of complementary and alternative medicine (CAM) practitioners will vary from organization to organization. Credentialing is also defined by the nature of the service provided. For example, if an organization is simply offering a referral service or a directory of discounted services, a basic level of credentialing may be performed. If the organization is offering panels of practitioners to provide "carve-out" specialty services (such as chiropractic or acupuncture care) that are paid for by the health plan, it sets standards for complementary practitioners that ideally mirror all the review standards the national managed care plans apply to their panels of medical and osteopathic physicians. Health plans want to be able to assure employers who contract with them that their credentialing "report cards," created by NCQA and similar bodies, are reflective of the care the health plan takes in choosing providers of complementary therapies. Organizations such as the NCQA have established specific requirements for medical, behavioral health, and chiropractic providers. NCQA's standards can (and should) be mirrored in the screening process for other licensed complementary providers whenever the insurer is assuming the risk of necessary health care and paying for the complementary practitioner's services. Although many factors can be considered in credentialing, all credentialing programs should be checking licensure status, specialty training and experience, malpractice insurance coverage, and practitioner sanctions history.

National Practitioner Data Bank

The National Practitioner Data Bank (NPDB) can be researched by a qualified organization for malpractice claims history against a particular provider. Complaints

COMPONENTS OF THE CREDENTIALING PROCESS

A typical credentialing process for physicians takes 90 to 120 days and involves a structured review and verification process of submitted documents and information chosen from the following:

- A contract specifying professional and business duties of the practitioner and the contracting organization, including terms and conditions, grievance and appeals process, and termination process
- Comprehensive provider application outlining training, experience, licensure sanctions, and malpractice history
- Release form to verify insurance and claims history with malpractice insurance carriers
- An attestation statement by the practitioner, verifying his or her physical and mental capability to provide the required services
- Professional license and/or certification documents
- Records indicating satisfactory completion of specialty training programs
- Required professional, business, and premises liability insurance policy coverage
- Documentation of employment and practice experience since professional graduation
- Practitioner capabilities for data reporting and profiling
- Thorough on-site review of provider offices, records, and operations
- Independent review of registries of sanctions or convictions such as the National Practitioner Data Bank (NPDB), insurance carriers, Medicare/Medicaid, and state police records
- Peer review of the practitioner's application and all related documents to identify past events that might predict poor future performance

about quality of care that have resulted in state board sanctions or judgments against providers are filed with the NPDB. In addition to medical doctors and chiropractors, acupuncturists are also listed in this database, particularly physicians who provide acupuncture. Due to the confidential nature of the information, access is restricted to organizations holding risk for the care provided by the practitioner, performing an evaluation for quality management, or for other appropriate reasons. These organizations typically include health maintenance organizations (HMOs), health plans, management services organizations, and medical groups. The data bank can be accessed and queried in a number of ways, including mail, fax, or Internet.

The NPDB does not cover everyone. For example, malpractice suits or sexual misconduct actions against massage and body-work practitioners are not required to be reported to this data bank.

Malpractice Insurance

Malpractice insurance companies typically require a statement of claims history upon initial policy application. If the practitioner provides a release, the credentialing organization can query the malpractice insurance carrier to determine whether there are pending, past, or current suits that have been filed against the practitioner. Any existing claims are indicated in the insurer's background information on the practitioner. The fact that a practitioner may have had a malpractice claim filed against him or her does not automatically disqualify the practitioner, nor necessarily reflect the quality of the practitioner. The malpractice claims are typically evaluated through a credentialing committee peer-review process to determine if the incident(s) in question are a predictor of future poor performance.

LICENSING AND LEGAL REQUIREMENTS

Licensure is an important form of professional recognition for complementary providers. State licensure allows a greater level of public confidence in the practitioners and in the health plans offering their services. The license indicates that the profession and the practitioners have gone through a certain level of review, and that the state is now involved in the liability exposure by licensing them. By issuing the license, the state board has taken a level of responsibility to verify the training and quality of service of these practitioners. However, licensing and legal requirements vary from state to state. Each state can also have significantly different standards of practice for complementary health care providers. The following table (Table 64–1) contains a review of state licensure for familiar complementary health professionals conducted by a credentialing organization in 2003. State licensure provides the legal basis for professional privileges that allow the rendering of services by licensed practitioners. Since laws continue to change, check your state's current regulations on complementary health services.

Training and Experience

When a state has no licensing procedure for the practitioners of a complementary health specialty, the task of an independent credentialing organization is to define the standards for competence and excellence within that field. This is best done by engaging the participation of capable practitioners and national membership or certifying organizations in that particular specialty (see respective resource chapters in this book).

Table 64–1 Complementary Practitioners: Licensing by State—2003

State	DC [1]	LMP/ LMT [3]	CN/RD [1]	ND [1]	ND acu [3]	LAc [1]	MD/DO acu [3]
Alabama	Other Bd	Lic/Reg	—	—	—	Other Bd	Lic/Reg
Alaska	Other Bd	—	Other Bd	Other Bd	—	Other Bd	Lic/Reg
Arizona	Other Bd	—	Other Bd	Regulated	Lic/Reg	Regulated	Lic/Reg
Arkansas	Other Bd	Lic/Reg	Other Bd	—	—	Other Bd	na
California	Other Bd	—	Other Bd	—	—	Other Bd	Lic/Reg
Colorado	Other Bd	na	—	—	—	Regulated	Lic/Reg
Connecticut	Other Bd	Lic/Reg	Regulated	Other Bd	Lic/Reg	Regulated	Lic/Reg
Delaware	Other Bd	Lic/Reg	Other Bd	Regulated	na	Regulated	Lic/Reg
Florida	Other Bd	Lic/Reg	State Bd	Other Bd	na	Other Bd	Lic/Reg
Georgia	Other Bd	—	Other Bd	—	—	State Bd	Lic/Reg
Hawaii	Other Bd	Lic/Reg	—	Other Bd	na	Other Bd	—
Idaho	Other Bd	—	Other Bd	—	—	Other Bd	na
Illinois	State Bd	—	Other Bd	—	—	Other Bd	Lic/Reg
Indiana	Other Bd	—	Other Bd	—	—	State Bd	Lic/Reg
Iowa	Other Bd	Lic/Reg	Other Bd	Regulated	Lic/Reg	State Bd	Lic/Reg
Kansas	State Bd	—	Other Bd	Regulated	na	Regulated	Lic/Reg
Kentucky [2]	Other Bd	—	—	—	—	—	Lic/Reg
Louisiana	Other Bd	Lic/Reg	Other Bd	—	—	State Bd	Lic/Reg
Maine	Other Bd	Lic/Reg	Other Bd	Other Bd	Lic/Reg	State Bd	Lic/Reg
Maryland	Other Bd	Lic/Reg	Other Bd	—	—	State Bd	Lic/Reg
Mass.	Other Bd	—	Other Bd	Regulated	na	State Bd	—
Michigan	Other Bd	—	—	—	—	—	Lic/Reg
Minnesota [2]	Other Bd	—	Other Bd	—	—	State Bd	Lic/Reg
Mississippi	Other Bd	Lic/Reg	Other Bd	—	—	—	Lic/Reg
Missouri [2]	Other Bd	Lic/Reg	—	—	—	—	Lic/Reg
Montana	Other Bd	—	Other Bd	Other Bd	na	State Bd	—
Nebraska	Other Bd	Lic/Reg	Other Bd	—	—	Other Bd	Lic/Reg
Nevada	Other Bd	—	—	—	—	State Bd	Lic/Reg
New Hamp.	Other Bd	Lic/Reg	Other Bd	Other Bd	na	Other Bd	Lic/Reg
New Jersey [2]	Other Bd	—	—	—	—	Other Bd	Lic/Reg
New Mexico	Other Bd	Lic/Reg	Other Bd	—	—	Other Bd	Lic/Reg
New York	Other Bd	Lic/Reg	Other Bd	—	—	Other Bd	Lic/Reg
North Car. [2]	Other Bd	Lic/Reg	—	—	—	Other Bd	Lic/Reg
North Dakota	Other Bd	Lic/Reg	Other Bd	Regulated	na	Regulated	Lic/Reg
Ohio	Other Bd	Lic/Reg	Other Bd	—	—	State Bd	Lic/Reg
Oklahoma	Other Bd	—	State Bd	—	—	—	Lic/Reg

continues

Table 64–1 continued

State	DC [1]	LMP/ LMT [3]	CN/RD [1]	ND [1]	ND acu [3]	LAc [1]	MD/DO acu [3]
Oregon	Other Bd	Lic/Reg	Other Bd	Other Bd	—	State Bd	Lic/Reg
Pennsylvania	Other Bd	—	—	—	—	State Bd	Lic/Reg
Rhode Island	Other Bd	Lic/Reg	Other Bd	Regulated	—	Regulated	na
South Car.	Other Bd	Lic/Reg	—	—	—	State Bd	Lic/Reg
South Dak. [2]	Other Bd	—	Other Bd	—	—	—	Lic/Reg
Tennessee	Other Bd	Lic/Reg	Other Bd	—	—	State Bd	Lic/Reg
Texas	Other Bd	Lic/Reg	Other Bd	Regulated	na	State Bd	Lic/Reg
Utah	Other Bd	Lic/Reg	Other Bd	Other Bd	Lic/Reg	Other Bd	Lic/Reg
Vermont	Other Bd	—	Other Bd	Other Bd	Lic/Reg	Other Bd	na
Virginia	State Bd	Lic/Reg	State Bd	—	—	State Bd	Lic/Reg
Washington	Other Bd	Lic/Reg	Regulated	Regulated	—	Regulated	Lic/Reg
West Va.	Other Bd	Lic/Reg	Other Bd	—	—	Other Bd	Lic/Reg
Wisconsin	Other Bd	Lic/Reg	Other Bd	—	—	Regulated	Lic/Reg
Wyoming	Other Bd	—	Other Bd	—	—	—	na
DC	Other Bd	Lic/Reg	Other Bd	Other Bd	na	State Bd	na

1. Source of data in columns 2, 4, 5, and 7: Federation of State Medical Boards of the United States (FSMB). Health professions regulated and legislative schedules. In: *Licensing Boards, Structure and Disciplinary Functions. 2003 Exchange.* Dallas, TX: FSMB. 2003; 67–68.

2. Source of data on specific states. Federation of State Medical Boards of the United States (FSMB). Health professions regulated by States. In: *1999–2000 Exchange.* Dallas, TX: FSMB. 1999; vol. 3: 86–87.

3. Source of content in columns 3, 6, and 8: American Whole Health; © 2003.

Practitioner abbreviations: DC—Doctor of Chiropractic; LMP—Licensed Massage Practitioner; LMT—Licensed Massage Therapist; CN—Certified Nutritionist; RD—Registered Dietician; ND—Naturopathic Doctor; ND acu—Naturopathic Doctor acupuncturist; LAc—Licensed Acupuncturist; MD/DO acu—Medical Doctor/Doctor of Osteropathy acupuncturist.

Licensure: State Bd—regulated by state medical board; Other Bd—regulated by separate/other board; Regulated—regulated but under no board; Lic/reg—some form of licensure or regulation in place; — no state regulation; na—information not available.

The standards for appropriate education in complementary therapies tend to be less clearly defined than those in medical education. Medical schools are accredited based on review by independent evaluating institutions. These institutions set standards for the content of a medical education curriculum that will prepare doctors to practice in the health care system. Training at a nationally accredited program is one of the requirements for state licensure.

This is not the case in some complementary professions. For example, massage therapy schools are largely proprietary, and graduation from a training institution ap- proved by COMTA (Commission on Massage Training Accreditation) is not required for massage licensure in many states or local jurisdictions. States that license naturopathic physicians usually require graduation from an accredited biomedical naturopathic medical school program. However there are many practitioners who have undertaken to learn "traditional naturopathy," by correspondence courses or self-directed training programs. Their practice may be legal in some states that do not have ND practice acts, but their clinical exposure and preparation is by no means standardized. In certain states the acupuncture licensing laws may allow acupuncturists to prescribe herbs, homeopathy, or nutritional supplements, but the qualifying standards in that state may not include any training or examination standards for such ancillary health care practices.

Some chiropractic physicians are oriented toward acute outcomes-based musculoskeletal treatment in a rehabilitative model (such as seen in an interdisciplinary specialty spine center). Others are more oriented to a wellness care or maintenance care model that enrolls patients for long-term treatment.

The variation of training and experience in the nonlicensed professions can be even greater. Due to this wide range of variability in the quality of different professional training programs for complementary practitioners, credentialing organizations need to develop their standards by working with practitioners and leaders knowledgeable within each specialty. A number of recognized national organizations and training programs are currently in the process of creating basic national professional standards for nonlicensed health and wellness practitioners; for example, the Pilates Method Alliance is developing standards for Pilates instructors.

Although the number of formal credentialing programs for complementary health professionals is increasing, the average medical practitioner cannot assume the same uniform clinical background among these practitioners as among the more established medical subspecialists and allied health professionals. Creating an effective virtual health care team for your practice will involve interviewing practitioners, and reviewing their background, experience, and practice philosophy.

CHAPTER 65

Health Promotion, Wellness, and Complementary Medicine

Roger Jahnke, OMD

CONSUMERS WANT A FOCUS ON WELLNESS EVEN MORE THAN ALTERNATIVE THERAPIES

When the research on utilization of complementary and alternative medicine was first published, most of us assumed that consumer use of complementary medicine focused primarily on therapies such as acupuncture, chiropractic, massage, and other provider-rendered services. However, a closer reading of the data suggests that the largest percentage of consumer activity in this area has involved self-care for wellness and prevention, rather than treatment. The data indicate that as much as two thirds of this utilization (or more) occurs in activities such as exercise, nutrition, and stress reduction (Eisenberg et al., 1993, 1998, Astin, 1998; Barnes et al., 2004).

Health promotion programming integrates quite logically with both complementary medicine and conventional medicine. This same congruence is evident for health promotion derivatives, including wellness, health enhancement, disease management, longevity medicine, behaviorally based health improvement, and mind-body healing.

The seminal survey of Eisenberg and colleagues (1993) provides indications that more than two-thirds of the responses re-

flected the use of self-care activities. Data from a follow-up study led by Eisenberg (1998) revealed comparable trends, with increased utilization of wellness and prevention reported. Similar findings resulted from a Stanford survey in the *Journal of the American Medical Association* (Astin, 1998). In that study, again more than two thirds of respondents reported using self-care activities to complement mainstream medical care.

This trend continues to grow. Analysis of data from a survey conducted by the National Health Service and NCCAM in 2002 (Barnes et al., 2004), suggests that lifestyle approaches constitute more than 70% of complementary and alternative utilization. Based on the results of that survey, it appears that less than 30% of consumer utilization involved treatment provided by practitioners. The lifestyle approaches, in order of prevalence, included:

- Therapeutic exercise such as deep breathing, yoga, tai chi, and Qigong
- Methods of stress reduction including meditation, relaxation, and imagery
- Special diet and the use of supplements such as vitamins and herbs

Findings from the major studies on complementary medicine consistently reflect a high level of consumer interest in health, fitness, and prevention. Despite the consumer and media focus on complementary therapies, there is actually far greater demand for

---

A brief biography of Roger Jahnke appears in Chapter 4.

Courtesy of Roger Jahnke, OMD, Santa Barbara, California.

self-care activities and products focused on health improvement. Services and programs that accurately reflect consumer interest and utilization trends ideally include an emphasis on self-care, health promotion, and lifestyle change.

Case Study: Wellness Programs in Health Systems

California Pacific Medical Center and Kaiser Permanente Medical Center of San Francisco both offer a rich array of courses, workshops, and support groups that include all these examples and more. The Riverside System in Virginia, with several hospitals and ambulatory care centers, includes six fitness centers that are available to both patients and the community. The Mercy System in Cincinnati has also opened several impressive healthplex facilities that offer a comprehensive and diverse menu of health improvement programming. Low-tech health enhancement programs such as nutritional counseling, therapeutic exercise, stress reduction, and support groups are proliferating in health care programs throughout the United States.

EXPANDING THE CONTINUUM OF CARE

Our understanding of the role of lifestyle in health continues to increase. The research has found that even in populations already receiving treatment for disease, lifestyle approaches can be applied to improve patient outcomes, reduce medical costs, and enhance quality of life. The well-documented Ornish program for the reversal of heart disease has demonstrated these benefits, with an average savings of $30,000 per patient per year (Ornish, 1998). Outcomes in prevention are also impressive, as demonstrated in recent diabetes research such as the Diabetes Prevention Program (2003) and the Finnish Diabetes Prevention Study (Lindstrom et al., 2003). These expanded applications of lifestyle-based therapies make it clear that health improvement can be adapted to the needs of individuals across the entire continuum of care, in services for:

- Consumers who are well
- Those at risk
- Early intervention
- Chronic illness
- Disease treatment and rehabilitation

Case Study: Reversing Heart Disease

The Ornish Program for Reversing Heart Disease is an example of health promotion principles applied to the needs of high-risk patients with heart disease symptoms. Yet the program costs approximately 20% of typical expenditures for coronary artery disease (Ornish et al., 1998), with an accompanying decrease in human cost. The program involves careful screening, medical and case management, health education, and coaching. Participants learn new ways of eating, exercising, and reducing stress. They also participate in support groups with others, reinforcing their efforts. Many patients in the program have experienced not only improved health and quality of life, but also the actual regeneration of heart tissue, documented on PET scans (Koertge et al., 2003).

The Ornish program has also been applied in a large clinical trial focused on prostate cancer (Ornish et al., 2001; Block et al., 2004). The lifestyle approach developed in these programs is currently being offered at 15 medical centers and hospitals in the eastern United States (Highmark et al., 2004). These programs are an example of an innovation that meets consumer demand for lifestyle options.

Case Studies: Diabetes Prevention

Extensive research has focused on the prevention and management of diabetes, including the Pima Indian Study, the Iowa Women's Health Study, and the Physicians' Health Study. Three recent studies that have reevaluated the role of lifestyle factors in diabetes include the Finnish Diabetes Prevention Study (Tuomilehto et al., 2001; Lindstrom et al., 2003), the Diabetes Prevention Program at George Washington University (2002, 2003), and the Da Qing Study in Da Qing, China (Pan et al., 1997; Li et al., 2002). This research tracked participants with insulin resistance to determine the most important factors in delaying the onset of Type 2 diabetes. Primary factors identified included:

- Moderate weight loss: research found benefit from as little as 5% reduction in body weight
- Moderate diet: less fat, increased fiber, possibly a low glycemic index diet, and increased omega-3 fatty acids (Steyn et al., 2004)
- Moderate exercise: for example, 140 minutes per week

These factors were found to decrease the incidence of diabetes by 58% in the Finnish and American studies, which followed participants for 3 years. The Da Qing study reported a 42% prevention rate in the incidence of diabetes through diet and exercise over the 6-year period of the study. The Finnish study also compared the efficacy of lifestyle and medication in delaying the onset of diabetes and found medication to decrease the incidence of diabetes by 31%, compared with 58% through lifestyle (Scheen et al., 2003).

The Diabetes Prevention Program (2002), which involved 1079 participants, reported that success involved a number of key elements (comparable to those of the Ornish program) including clinical support, case management, supervised physical activity, and patient education.

TEN ACTUAL LEADING CAUSES OF DEATH

Lifestyle and prevention have become a pervasive theme in contemporary health care. In recent decades, health care biostatistics have expanded to encompass the role of behavioral and lifestyle factors in mortality. These analyses suggest that the leading given causes of death are secondary to actual underlying causes of death (McGinnis & Foege, 1993; McGinnis et al., 2002; Mokdad et al., 2004). Preventable behavioral factors are now believed to cause the major diseases of industrial nations. While the 10 leading causes of death imply that we are the victims of disease, the 9 underlying causes reflect the more accurate idea that we frequently choose behaviors that cause disease (see Table 65–1). Depending on one's perspective, perhaps 6 or even all 9 of these "actual causes" are preventable. The data provide a clear rationale for expanding the continuum of care to include health promotion and prevention.

From this perspective, it also becomes appropriate to ask, What are the underlying causes of high-risk behaviors? What causes a person to choose to smoke, overuse alcohol, use recreational drugs, indulge in junk food, neglect exercise, agree to high-risk sex, carry firearms, or neglect seat belt use? The answer to these questions is even more provocative, and far less medical—and includes causative factors such as internal and external stress, low self-esteem, poor communication skills, lack of access to information, and social or peer pressure. Many of these behaviors also involve an addictive

Table 65–1 Leading Causes of Morbidity in the United States

10 Leading Causes of Death, 2000[1]	9 Actual Causes of Death, 2000[2]
Heart disease	Tobacco
Cancer	Obesity and inactivity
Cerebrovascular disease	Alcohol
Chronic lower respiratory disease	Conditions due to microbial agents
Accidents (unintentional injuries)	Motor vehicle accidents
Diabetes	Toxic agents (pollutants, etc.)
Pneumonia/influenza	Firearms
Alzheimer's disease	Sexual behavior (associated infectious
Kidney disease	diseases)
Septicemia	Illicit drug use

Sources of content:

1. U.S. Department of Health and Human Services, CDC. Table 1. Deaths, percent of total deaths, and death rates for the 10 leading causes of death in selected age groups, by race and sex: United States, 2000. *National Vital Statistics Report.* 2002;50(16):13.

2. Mokdad AH, et al. Actual causes of death in the United States, 2000. *JAMA.* 2004;291(10):1238–1241.

component. Smoking, alcohol use, and eating disorders can reflect stress responses, imbalances in neurochemistry, genetic influences, or all of these factors.

NEW TOOLS FOR HEALTH PROMOTION AND WELLNESS

The most effective programs addressing these factors involve a multidisciplinary approach. Successful interventions, such as Ornish programs, bariatric obesity management, addictions programs, and the management of chronic illness typically include:

- Promotion of a healthy lifestyle
- Interventions that address medical conditions or biochemical imbalances through medication or nutritional therapy
- Behavioral support, such as case management or health coaching
- Group support to sustain motivation

Case Study: Innovative Group Support Services

St. Charles Hospital in Bend, Oregon, has offered symptom reduction support groups for people with chronic illness, focused on reducing medical symptoms through basic health enhancement activities such as good nutrition, breath practice, meditation, exercise, and massage. The program serves people with a range of conditions, all working together in a single group, each focusing on his or her own individual health improvement. The program functions as a form of social support for participants, to reinforce the behavioral goals they set for themselves. Outcomes data indicate that these clients experienced measurable improvements in their health and, on average, a 37% reduction in their use of medication and medical care (Jahnke, 2001).

As the health care continuum expands, a range of new programs will continue to emerge to meet consumer expectations for wellness, empowerment, life extension, and health longevity. In this context, earlier disease-based health promotion interventions will be complemented with mind-body methods and programs (see Table 65–2).

THE CASE FOR HEALTH PROMOTION

The emerging models for the delivery of health care—comprehensive delivery, complementary medicine, holistic health care, integrative medicine, and others—have one thing in common: The models all involve expanding the continuum of care. The new paradigm includes health promotion as a foundational element.

The evolution of health care delivery is likely to include a major focus on health improvement in its many permutations. We also predict that complementary medicine will rarely emerge in isolation from health promotion. For example, acupuncture is just a clinical tool without a wide array of supporting lifestyle components (such as therapeutic diet, Qigong, tai chi, and meditation). Acupuncture in complement to these behavioral endeavors becomes a complete system: traditional Chinese medicine.

Health promotion will eventually be viewed as essential if we are to maximize outcomes and manage costs. Preventive and self-care programs that address both health and illness are critical to demand management, risk management, new forms of disease management, wellness, and performance enhancement. Although complementary therapies are the current focus of much attention, in the evolution of health care health promotion may actually be the more powerful tool.

Table 65–2 Complementary Systems of Health Promotion

Mainstream Health Promotion	Complementary Approaches to Health Promotion
Health risk appraisals	Lifestyle appraisals, nutritional appraisals
Preventive health screenings	Biomarkers in serum and in saliva; antibody testing
Risk reduction programs	Health coaching and group support, biofeedback, stress reduction
Smoking cessation programs	Group support, behavioral approaches, auricular acupuncture, nutrient therapy
Drug and alcohol management	Support groups and 12 Step programs, acupuncture, and nutrient therapy
Preventive and therapeutic nutrition	Biochemical and functional nutrition and herbal formulas
Fitness and exercise	Yoga, tai chi, and Qigong
Progressive relaxation	Visualization and imagery, meditation, spirituality
Health education	Consumer-driven information resources: self-help books, radio, the Internet

Courtesy of Roger Jahnke, OMD, © 2005, Santa Barbara, California.

Contemporary data suggest that this could become one of the most effective frameworks for achieving critical health care goals: de-

creasing risk, enhancing access, minimizing costs, expanding revenue, and improving clinical outcomes.

REFERENCES

Astin J. Why patients use alternative medicine: results of a national study. *JAMA*. 1998;279(19): 1548–1553.

Barnes PM, Powell-Griner E, McFann K, Nahin R. Complementary and alternative medicine use among adults: United States, 2002. *Adv Data*. 2004;(343): 1–16.

Block KI, Cohen AJ, Dobs AS, Ornish D, Tripathy D. The challenges of randomized trials in integrative cancer care. *Integr Cancer Ther*. 2004;3(2):112–127.

Diabetes Prevention Program (DPP) Research Group. The Diabetes Prevention Program (DPP): description of lifestyle intervention. *Diabetes Care*. 2002; 25(12):2165–2171.

Diabetes Prevention Program Research Group. Within-trial cost-effectiveness of lifestyle intervention or metformin for the primary prevention of type 2 diabetes. *Diabetes Care*. 2003;26(9):2518–2523.

Eisenberg D, Davis R, Ettner S, et al. Trends in alternative medicine use in the United States, 1990–1997: Results of a follow-up national survey. *JAMA*. 1998;280(18):1569–1575.

Eisenberg DM, Kessler RC, Foster C, et al. Unconventional medicine in the United States. *N Engl J Med*. 1993;328(4):246–252.

Highmark, Ornish D. *Lifestyle Advantage*. Available at: www.lifestyleadvantage.org. Accessed July 15, 2004.

Jahnke R. Phasing in integrative medicine. In: Faass N, ed. *Integrating Complementary Medicine into Health Systems*. Sudbury, MA: Jones and Bartlett/ Aspen; 2001.

Koertge J, Weidner G, Elliott-Eller M, et al. Improvement in medical risk factors and quality of life in women and men with coronary artery disease in the Multicenter Lifestyle Demonstration Project. *Am J Cardiol*. 2003;91(11):1316–1322.

Li G, Hu Y, Yang W, et al. Effects of insulin resistance and insulin secretion on the efficacy of interventions to retard development of Type 2 diabetes mel-

litus: the DA Qing IGT and Diabetes Study. *Diabetes Res Clin Pract*. 2002;58(3):193–200.

Lindstrom J, Louheranta A, Mannelin M, et al., and the Finnish Diabetes Prevention Study Group. The Finnish Diabetes Prevention Study (DPS): lifestyle intervention and 3-year results on diet and physical activity. *Diabetes Care*. 2003;26(12):3230–3236.

McGinnis JM, Foege WH. Actual causes of death in the United States. *JAMA*. 1993;270(18):2207–2212.

McGinnis JM, Williams-Russo P, Knickman JR. The case for more active policy attention to health promotion. *Health Aff*. 2002;21(2):78–93.

Mokdad, AH, et al. Actual causes of death in the United States, 2000. *JAMA*. 2004;291(10):1238–1241.

Ornish D. Avoiding revascularization with lifestyle changes: the Multicenter Lifestyle Demonstration Project. *Am J Cardiol*. 1998;82(108):72T–76T.

Ornish D, Scherwitz LW, Billings JH, et al. Intensive lifestyle changes for reversal of coronary heart disease. *JAMA*. 1998;280(23):2001–2007.

Ornish DM, Lee KL, Fair WR, Pettengill EB, Carroll PR. Dietary trial in prostate cancer: early experience and implications for clinical trial design. *Urology*. 2001;57(4 Suppl 1):200–201.

Pan XR, Li GW, Hu YH, et al. Effects of diet and exercise in preventing NIDDM in people with impaired glucose tolerance. The Da Qing IGT and Diabetes Study. *Diabetes Care*. 1997;20(4):537–544.

Scheen AJ, Letiexhe MR, Ernest P. Prevention of type 2 diabetes: lifestyle changes or pharmacological interventions? [Article in French] *Rev Med Liege*. 2003;58(4):206–210.

Steyn NP, Mann J, Bennett PH, et al. Diet, nutrition and the prevention of type 2 diabetes. *Public Health Nutr*. 2004;7(1A):147–165.

Tuomilehto J, Lindstrom J, Eriksson JG, et al., and the Finnish Diabetes Prevention Study Group. Prevention of type 2 diabetes mellitus by changes in lifestyle among subjects with impaired glucose tolerance. *N Engl J Med*. 2001;344(18):1343–1350.

CHAPTER 66

Evolution of an Integrative Practice

Brian Bouch, MD

Hospital-based emergency medicine and family practice medicine were the primary focuses of my medical practice from 1973 until 1984, and I am board-certified in emergency medicine.

In 1985, I began the formal study of acupuncture, then opened a small practice, initially providing family medicine and acupuncture. Gradually, the practice expanded into other areas of complementary medicine as I brought in practitioners with various types of training. A skilled osteopath joined me, enabling us to offer osteopathic manipulation, and I associated with a licensed acupuncturist, who has been active in the practice for the past 17 years.

Once I had gained the initial formal training, my own skills in the use of complementary therapies developed as I continued to learn from my colleagues. Working with the acupuncturist, who is highly knowledgeable in Chinese herbal therapy, I expanded my knowledge of botanicals. I have also obtained training in the use of herbal therapies and read extensively in this area. My knowledge

Brian Bouch, MD, a graduate of Dickinson College, summa cum laude, Phi Beta Kappa, and University of Pennsylvania School of Medicine, has had careers in family practice, public health medicine, emergency medicine (board certified), and complementary medicine practice. He divides his time between complementary medicine practice in northern California and teaching acupuncture to physicians. Dr. Bouch was the first medical director of Commonweal, a self-help retreat and information center for cancer patients, and medical director of Consensus Health and One Body Inc., which brought complementary insurance benefits to major health plan subscribers and created one of the most respected Internet sites on CAM.

of homeopathy is focused on a practical level—not through a formal study of classical homeopathy, but rather by learning how to use first-aid homeopathic remedies for acute conditions. Coursework in osteopathic theory and technique has further expanded my knowledge base. Having a massage practitioner in the office that provides deep-tissue work has given me the opportunity to learn the value of that discipline's contribution to holistic healing.

Nutritional therapy is the other area in which I have spent time in intensive study and have gained additional training. The use of nutrition in my practice includes not only diet recommendations, but also the focused use of nutritional supplements and megavitamin and mineral therapy through both oral supplementation and intravenous administration. Functional medicine is a related field, which includes an emphasis on digestive ecology and treatment of leaky gut syndrome, based on the work of Jeffrey Bland, PhD (see Chapters 13 and 67). These perspectives grow out of the Western paradigm and can be found in mainstream literature but are addressed in functional practice through diet and nutrient therapy, as well as occasional use of prescription medication.

The development of my practice as a complementary provider has entailed a great deal of self-education through workshops, in-depth reading, and conversations with colleagues about what is effective and what works. Everything I learn brings me back to the question of what will have the greatest impact on patient care problems with the least potential for harm. Complementary therapies have provided me with a skill set of low-risk approaches to many of the chronic problems that constantly surface in my clinical practice.

Over the past 15 years, my medical practice has evolved into an integrative medicine clinic, Hillpark Medical Center. Typically there are four to six practitioners: myself and another physician acupuncturist who is also a yoga instructor, two licensed acupuncturists/herbalists, an osteopathic physician specializing in manipulation, a massage therapist, and a nutritional counselor specializing in weight management.

Teaching and consulting are other meaningful aspects of my work in integrative medicine. Since 1987, I have taught UCLA's course, "Medical Acupuncture for Physicians," serving as one of the primary instructors. More recently I have added a consulting service for patients with life-threatening disorders providing personalized medical searches and advocacy. This service is available to patients nationwide, and it has given me the opportunity to provide in-depth research to patients with difficult health conditions.

CHAPTER 67

Functional Medicine in Integrative Practice

Institute for Functional Medicine

FUNCTIONAL MEDICINE DEFINED

Functional medicine is a dynamic approach to assessing, preventing, and treating complex chronic disease. A functional approach helps clinicians identify and ameliorate dysfunctions in the physiology and biochemistry of the human body as a primary method of improving patient health. Specific clinical applications of functional medicine evolve as emerging research and clinical experience combine to shape more effective interventions, yet the mission of · functional medicine remains the same—to help patients achieve optimal health by improving the underlying functionality of the human body.

Functional medicine is not a unique and separate body of knowledge. It is grounded in scientific principles and research widely available in medicine today, but applied through a different model. Functional medicine is dedicated to prevention, early assessment, and improved management of complex, chronic disease by intervening at multiple levels to address core clinical imbalances and to restore each patient's functionality and health. It is a clinician's discipline, and any clinician with good grounding in Western basic and medical sciences can learn and apply it.

A profile of the Institute for Functional Medicine appears in Chapter 13.

Courtesy of David S. Jones, MD, Sheila Quinn, and the Institute for Functional Medicine, Gig Harbor, Washington.

THE SCIENCE BEHIND FUNCTIONAL MEDICINE

Functional medicine incorporates work that is emerging within the field of functional genomics, which is anchored in the basic sciences of cellular biology, modern nutritional biochemistry, and genetics (Hieter & Bogoski, 1997; Kohler, 2001).

The fundamental physiological processes that must function well for the patient to achieve and sustain health include:

- Communication, both outside and inside the cell
- Bioenergetics, or the transformation of food into energy
- Replication, repair, and maintenance of structural integrity, from the cellular to the whole body level
- Elimination of waste
- Protection and defense
- Transport and circulation

Environmental inputs and these physiological processes interact with the patient's genetic strengths and vulnerabilities; if something goes awry at any point, and the patient is vulnerable to those malfunctions, core clinical imbalances can arise.

Recognizing that clinicians need concepts that are workable at the point of care, the virtually infinite ways in which imbalances can develop have been condensed to the following six general areas:

- Hormonal and neurotransmitter imbalances
- Oxidation-reduction imbalances and mitochondropathy
- Detoxification and biotransformational imbalances
- Immune and inflammatory imbalances
- Digestive, absorptive, and microbiological imbalances
- Structural imbalances, from cellular membrane function to the musculoskeletal system

These imbalances are precursors to the signs and symptoms by which we detect and diagnose organ system disease. They arise from dysfunction or defect within the fundamental physiological processes that cut across all organ systems, and they alert the health care provider to pay attention to the full expression of disease and dysfunction. Improving balance—in the patient's environmental inputs and in the body's fundamental physiological processes—is the precursor to restoring health, and it involves much more than treating symptoms. Each of these imbalances is explored in considerable detail in the process of applying the functional medicine matrix to patient assessment.

CORE PRINCIPLES OF FUNCTIONAL MEDICINE

1. Biochemical Individuality

Lifestyle translates into quantifiable effects on health through well-known biochemical and genetic mechanisms. An individual's genetic profile will set the stage for a range of possible induction scenarios, and lifestyle factors will modify expression within that range of possibilities (Ambrosone et al., 1996; Lin, 1996; Cross et al., 1998). For example, among apparently healthy people, the activity of liver enzymes involved in

detoxification, measured through caffeine clearance studies, may vary among individuals by 4- to 7-fold (Wahllander et al., 1990). Individualized therapy using appropriate nutritional support may result in improvement and normalization of enzyme activity (Coughtrie et al., 1994).

Some studies suggest that individuals who develop Parkinson's and Alzheimer's diseases may have detoxification impairments that increase their susceptibility to the neurotoxic effects of certain chemicals (Steventon et al., 1989; Heafield et al., 1990). Adverse drug reactions are indicators that biochemical individuality can be a life and death matter (Severino & Del Zompo, 2004) with special relevance for the aged (McLean & Le Couteur, 2004). Finally, biochemical individuality may well explain inconsistent research findings about important factors in the development of disease (Ambrosone et al., 1996).

2. Patient-Centered Care

From a functional medicine point of view, patients must be seen in the context of their unique biochemistry, embedded in an environmental context that continuously washes over their genetic landscape. Recognition of three factors distinguishes the patient-centered approach from a disease-centered one: antecedents, triggers, and mediators.

- Antecedents—Various antecedents to imbalance include genetic susceptibilities, lifestyle habits, and psychosocial and emotional factors; they shape the patient's strengths and vulnerabilities, and thus are an important focus of functional medicine evaluation and treatment.
- Triggers—When the individual is in a vulnerable or imbalanced state, triggers such as infection, toxic insult, and emotional or physical trauma can set in motion an inflammatory cascade.

• Mediators—Physiological chemical mediators, such as cytokines or prostaglandins, can perpetuate a disease process or pathological condition indefinitely unless prevented by compensatory mechanisms within the body itself (Givertz & Colucci, 1998), or by skilled clinical intervention.

A clinician using integrative functional medicine principles realizes it is not enough to "name" a disease (find a diagnosis) without also examining the unique set of antecedents, triggers, and mediators that set the stage for, and perpetuate, the underlying mechanisms of each patient's presenting signs and symptoms. The practitioner must focus directly on the unique set of circumstances and dysfunctions that must be addressed to reverse or ameliorate the patient's complaints (Satyanarayana & Shoskes, 1997; Astin, 1998).

3. Dynamic Balance of Internal and External Factors

Findings in molecular medicine suggest that modifiers of gene expression are ubiquitous in the food we eat, the air we breathe, and the water we drink. Our diet and our environment are, in effect, constantly communicating and interacting with our genes to modify their expression as part of the body's inherent physiological response. Such external cues can have a profound effect on biological function. Integrative functional medicine practitioners address lifestyle habits that impact the internal milieu and assess the dynamic interaction between internal and external environment. For example, evidence continues to accumulate that oxidative stress from external triggers (such as immune response to infection) and defects in energy metabolism (within the mitochondria) may contribute to a number of dysfunctional processes, including neurodegenerative diseases (Beal, 1995).

Another noteworthy area that has had a great deal of recent study involves the development of Type 2 diabetes mellitus. The interplay of nurture (external lifestyle habits and emotional context) and nature (internal response) are well represented in the progression from leptin resistance to hyperinsulinemia, insulin resistance, and the expression of upper body obesity. This imbalance of external and internal factors sets the stage for the progression to diabetes and its complications (Kaplan, 1989). In addition, metabolic changes that may account for the development of diabetes in nonobese patients ("metabolically obese") are now being explored. If these factors are identified early, physicians may be able to help patients prevent the onset of noninsulin-dependent diabetes mellitus (NIDDM) (Ruderman et al., 1998).

4. Complex Physiological Relationships and Connections

Functional medicine implies a profound awareness of the human being as a complex, adaptive system. The antecedents of dysfunction rest within the complex web of biology, genetics, and environment. Within that web, the role of nutrients in balancing a patient's complex physiological processes is central. A few examples of interesting research on that subject include:

Oxidative stress. Oxidative stress continues to be recognized as a key influence in myriad disease processes; in particular, it can lead to the induction of mediators of inflammation and a cascade of injury and biological damage. Antioxidants normally used by the body in countering the effects of oxidative stress may be lowered by an ongoing inflammatory process, and supplementation may be beneficial (Inserra et al., 1997). Oxidative damage to sperm cell DNA has been studied in young smoking men who are deficient in folate and vitamin C. The children of these men showed a significant increase in cancer when matched with a nonsmoking cohort (Lykkesfeldt et al., 2000).

Influences on the endocrine system. Nutrition can play a vital role in reducing the risk of disease in the presence of genetic deviations—polymorphisms—that affect complex processes such as oxidative stress (Ambrosone et al., 1999).

- Nutrition is central to the maintenance of a healthy endocrine system (an extremely complex, interconnected system). Undernutrition may contribute to detrimental alterations in the pituitary-adrenal axis (Pugliese, 1990).
- Key nutrients can assume pivotal importance in function. The mineral chromium, for example can be effective in improving glucose tolerance (a complex process), and may be beneficial in controlling diabetes mellitus (Fox & Sabovic, 1998).

5. Health as Positive Vitality

Health is more than the absence of disease; it involves the key role of organ reserve. Loss of function as a result of disease or aging is generally a gradual phenomenon. Individuals do not suddenly cease to function adequately. The process is progressive and long-term. The loss of function associated with disease among older individuals is now believed to be a consequence of the progressive loss of organ reserve (Fries, 1980). Stresses that could at an earlier time be accommodated now exceed the organism's resilience, which results in a health crisis. Organ reserve is related to biological age. Measures of function have been shown to be important in predicting mortality for older, hospitalized patients (Ikegami, 1995). We can modify how quickly we lose organ reserve and undergo biological aging through changes in lifestyle,

environment, and nutrition. It is now recognized that 75% of our health and life expectancy after age 40 is modifiable on the basis of such choices (Vita et al., 1998; Fries, 1996; Murray & Lopez, 1997).

APPLYING FUNCTIONAL MEDICINE IN PATIENT CARE

An examination of the core clinical imbalances that underlie the expression of disease is a critical step in a functional medicine evaluation. Imbalances arise as environmental inputs are processed by one's body, mind, and spirit through a unique set of genetic predispositions, attitudes, and beliefs. When we talk about influencing "gene expression," we are interested in the interaction between "environment" in the broadest sense and the patient's genetic predispositions. Many environmental factors that affect genetic expression are (or appear to be) a matter of choice (such as diet and exercise), but others are very difficult for the individual patient to alter or escape (air and water quality, toxic exposures); still others may be the result of unavoidable accidents (trauma, exposure to harmful microorganisms in the food supply through travel). Finally, socioeconomic, emotional, and spiritual issues may play a significant role in health and must be taken into account.

The influence of these "environmental inputs" on the human organism is indisputable, and they are often powerful agents in the search for health. The functional medicine practitioner, as part of the cycle of evaluation within the functional medicine matrix (see the following), takes these inputs into consideration when working with a patient to reverse dysfunction or disease, and to restore health:

- Diet (type and quantity of food, food preparation, calories, fats, proteins, carbohydrates)
- Nutrition (both dietary and supplemental)

- Air and water
- Physical exercise
- Environmental toxins (xenobiotics) and radiation
- Psychosocial factors (including family, work, community, economic status, stress)
- The emotional, mental, and spiritual context of the patient's life

THE FUNCTIONAL MEDICINE MATRIX

Evaluation of the complex system described above is accomplished through the use of the functional medicine matrix, which combines environmental inputs (diet, nutrition, and exercise) and mind/body/spirit issues with the six core imbalances to create an organizing structure within which all the information about the patient can be collected, sorted, and analyzed. Once learned, the matrix (see Figure 67–1) becomes an efficient and effective tool for delivering patient-centered care according to functional medicine principles and processes.

Where is functional medicine most useful?

Treatment of complex, chronic disease. Functional medicine directly addresses the restoration of health, looking for common

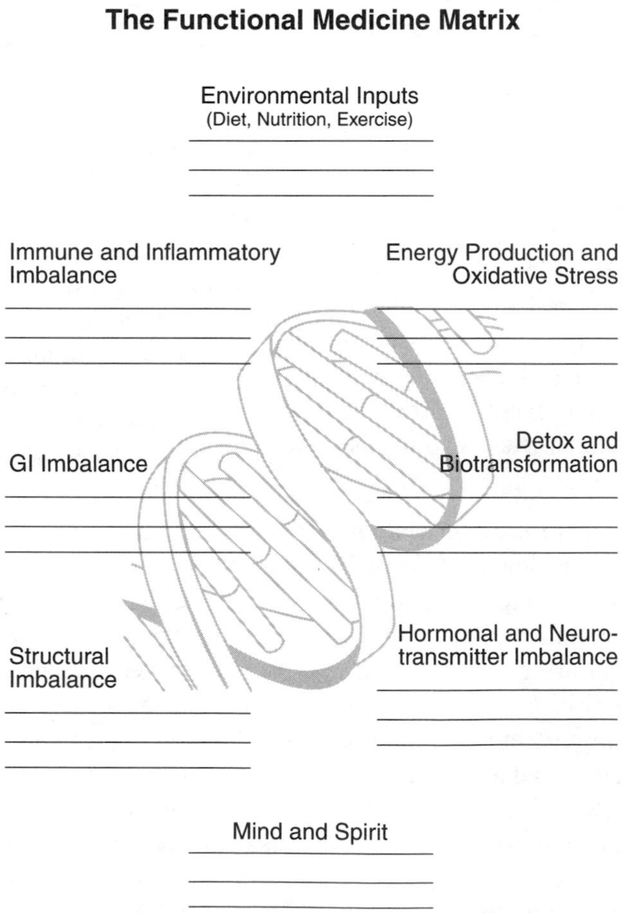

The Functional Medicine Matrix

Figure 67–1 The Functional Medicine Matrix

factors among various symptoms, diagnoses, and comorbidities that can be affected by intervening to improve function at the cellular level and the organ level. The functional medicine matrix takes into direct consideration the patient's lifestyle and diet, genetic predispositions, and core clinical imbalances—seeking a multifactorial and individualized approach that will reach beneath symptoms to restore function and generate momentum toward health.

Support for healthy aging. A growing body of research emphasizes that loss of function over a lifetime is gradual and modifiable, a central principle in functional medicine. Many of us assume that sickness is a natural consequence of the aging process (senescence), but no studies have validated this assumption. It is true that with every decade we live beyond age 30 our probability of death increases. It is true that older people are generally sicker than younger people. It is also true that aging is associated with decreased functional organ reserve. However, none of these associated facts proves that it is actually aging itself that causes a person to become ill. The association between age and sickness does not demonstrate that aging initiates the specific physiological mechanisms that lead to disease (McMurdo, 2001).

Assessing the effects of lifestyle and environment. There is compelling evidence that lifestyle and environment play a very significant role in the development of many of the chronic diseases that are associated with aging. With certain diseases, lifestyle may turn out to be more important than aging or genes. "The etiologic foundations of most modern chronic diseases are considered heterogeneous and highly dependent on the environment . . . 100% of the increase in prevalence of Type 2 diabetes and obesity in the US during the latter half of the 20th century must be attributed to a changing environment interacting with genes, since 0% of the human genome has changed during this time period" (Booth et al., 2000).

Exploring genetic influences. Genes do not code for specific diseases of aging. Instead, they code for various strengths and weaknesses in the human constitution that give rise to resistance or susceptibility factors for age-related diseases. We now know that even diseases such as cancer that we once thought were "all in the genes" are caused by interactions between our gene matrix and environmentally derived signals transduced at the cell membrane interface and then translated through genetic processing. Some people get the luck of the draw and have more resistance genes to environmental factors. For most people, however, the occurrence of illness as we age is a result of the blending of genetic susceptibility factors with environmental exposures (Subramanian et al., 2002).

"Genetic and environmental factors, including diet and life-style, both contribute to cardiovascular disease, cancers, and other major causes of mortality, but various lines of evidence indicate that environmental factors are most important" (Willet, 2002). The multifactorial "genes for heart disease" or "genes for cancer" may never be expressed as the disease unless the individual plunges these less resistant genes into an environment that is harmful for his or her unique constitution. For example, the susceptibility within the array of "genes for heart disease" may not result in heart disease until the person eats a diet rich in saturated fat, smokes, lives a lifestyle that enhances frequent high tides of his or her stress hormones, and/or has inadequate levels of the B vitamins in his or her diet to appropriately respond to these environmental stressors (Willett, 2002). "Nutritional support can be tailored to the individual genotype to favor beneficial phenotypic expression or to suppress processes that lead to later pathology" (Abumrad, 2001). Following this recognition gives individuals much greater control over their health as they age than they would have if all sickness were simply a natural consequence of advancing age. Our lives depend on the vast array of information within our genome and how/what signals are—and have been—generated to induce expression from our genome.

Doctors of the 21st century will soon need to understand how to assess patients' genotypes (Gerling et al., 2003) and how to personalize treatment for individual needs, but the evidence is convincing that they need to know right now how to help patients improve lifestyle and environment, apply dietary and nutritional interventions, and manage genetic vulnerabilities to minimize the risks of age-related debility and chronic disease.

INTEGRATED CARE

Functional medicine is discipline neutral—the field is accessible to any health practitioner who has a fairly standard Western medical science background. There are significant advantages to this "neutrality," particularly as the nation's health care system becomes more and more open and adaptive to integrated care concepts:

- Further development of universal concepts and vocabulary—Patients with chronic disease often see multiple practitioners from a variety of fields. It is extremely valuable to the patient (and to the efficient delivery of care) when those practitioners have a common "language" for discussing patient health. Functional medicine creates a unifying conceptual framework, mind-set, and information architecture about health and disease, regardless of widely varied clinician training and skills.

- Providing a rational basis for integrative treatment—Although the science underlying functional medicine is complex, the application of therapeutic and prevention-oriented approaches is often relatively straightforward; patients can understand it and so can practitioners from many different backgrounds. Functional medicine creates a more level playing field between and among patients and providers.

Functional medicine is firmly grounded in scientific principles and data but does not adopt a rigid perspective on medicine. The use of dietary interventions, clinical nutrition, exercise therapy, mind-body-spirit support, botanical medicines, physical medicine, and energy medicine such as acupuncture can all be integrated into functional medicine teaching and practice when the science warrants it. The use of drugs and/or surgery does not disappear, but lifestyle interventions assume a certain primacy because of their lower cost and their long-term role in the restoration of health and prevention of disease (or complications of disease).

Conventional providers and alternative providers alike are able to integrate functional medicine thinking and concepts into their existing knowledge base because these concepts are based on international research in biochemistry and cellular physiology. This medical basis underlies the theory and super-structures of the many professions. Funtional medicine does not take credit for this body of science, but it has organized this information to make it more widely accessible, by focusing on:

- Basic processes such as inflammation and the role of the inflammatory cascade in the etiology of health disorders
- Cellular dynamics, such as the function of the mitochondria in energy production

- The status of organ function, for example liver function, long before there is end-state disease
- The role of systems, for instance the importance of digestive health in general physical well-being

Among the health care professions, an abiding interest in "functionality"—how things work and what to do when they don't—is a shared terrain. Consequently, functional medicine helps create a bridge between conventional and complementary practitioners and approaches—promoting mutuality of ideas and interests, always in the context of the patient's needs. This common ground can enhance the delivery of integrated care and contribute to the development of respectful and productive professional relationships among health care providers.

REFERENCES

Abumrad N. The gene-nutrient-gene loop. *Curr Opin Nutr Metab Care.* 2001;4:407–410.

Ambrosone CB, Freudenheim JL, Graham S, et al. Cigarette smoking, N-acetyltransferase 2 genetic polymorphisms, and breast cancer risk. *JAMA.* 1996;276(18):1494–1501.

Ambrosone CB, Freudenheim JL, Thompson PA, et al. Manganese superoxide dismutase (*Mn*SOD) genetic polymorphisms, dietary antioxidants, and risk of breast cancer. *Cancer Res.* 1999;59:602–606.

Astin JA. Specialist delivery of primary care [Letter]. *JAMA.* 1998;280(19):1661.

Beal MF. Aging, energy, and oxidative stress in neurodegenerative diseases. *Ann Neurol.* 1995;38:357–366.

Booth FW, Gordon SE, Carlson CJ, Hamilton MT. Waging war on modern chronic diseases: primary prevention through exercise biology. *J Appl Physiol.* 2000;88:774–787.

Coughtrie M, Bamforth K, Sharp S, et al. Sulfation of endogenous compounds and xenobiotics: interactions and function in health and disease. *Chemico-Biological Interactions.* 1994;92:247–256.

Cross CE, van der Vliet A, Eiserich JP. Cigarette smokers and oxidant stress: a continuing mystery. *Am J Clin Nutr.* 1998;67:184–185.

Fox GN, Sabovic Z. Chromium picolinate supplementation for diabetes mellitus. *J Fam Pract.* 1998;46:83–86.

Fries JF. Aging, natural death, and the compression of morbidity. *NEJM.* 1980;303:130

Fries JF. Physical activity, the compression of morbidity, and the health of the elderly. *J R Soc Med.* 1996;89:64–68.

Gerling IC, Solomon SS, Bryer-Ash M. Genomes, transcriptomes, and proteomes. *Arch Intern Med.* 2003;163:190–198.

Givertz M, Colucci W. New targets for heart failure therapy: endothelin, inflammatory cytokines, and oxidative stress. *Lancet.* 1998;352(suppl I):34–38.

Heafield MT, Fearn S, Steventon GB, et al. Plasma cysteine and sulfate levels in patients with motor neuron, Parkinson's and Alzheimer's disease. *Neuroscience Letters.* 1990;110:216–220.

Hieter P, Boguski M. Functional genomics: it's all how you read it. *Science.* 1997;278:601–602.

Ikegami N. Functional assessment and its place in health care [Letter]. *NEJM.* 1995;332(9):598–599.

Inserra PF, Ardestani SK, Watson RR. Antioxidants and immune function. In: Garewal HS, ed. *Antioxidants and Disease Prevention.* Boca Raton, FL: CRC Press; 1997:19–29.

Kaplan NM. The deadly quartet: upper-body obesity, glucose intolerance, hypertriglyceridemia, and hypertension. *Arch Intern Med.* 1989;149:1514–1520.

Kohler P. From theory to practice in the genomics era. *Physicians Practice Digest.* 2001:A6–A7.

Latchman DS. Mechanisms of disease: transcription-factor-mutations and disease. *NEJM.* 1996;334(1):28–32.

Lin H. Smokers and breast cancer: "chemical individuality" and cancer predisposition [Editorial]. *JAMA.* 1996;276(18):1511.

Lykkesfeldt J, Christen S, Wallock LM, Chang HH, Jacob RA, Ames BN. Ascorbate is depleted by smoking and repleted by moderate supplementation: a study in male smokers and nonsmokers with matched dietary antioxidant intakes. *Am J Clin Nutr.* 2000;71(2):530–536.

McLean AJ, Le Couteur DG. Aging biology and geriatric clinical pharmacology. *Pharm Rev.* 2004;56:163–184.

McMurdo M. A healthy old age: realistic or futile goal? *BMJ.* 2001;321:1149–1151.

Murray CJL, Lopez AD. Alternative projections of mortality by cause 1990–2020: global burden of disease study. *Lancet.* 1997;349:1498–1504.

Pugliese MT. Endocrine function adaptations in undernutrition. *World Rev Nutr Diet.* 1990;62:186–211.

Ruderman N, Chisholm D, Pi-Sunyer X, Schneider S. The metabolically obese, normal-weight individual revisited. *Diabetes.* 1998;47(5):699–713.

Satyanarayana K, Shoskes D. A molecular injury-response model for the understanding of chronic disease. *Molecular Medicine Today.* 1997;3:331.

Severino G, Del Zompo M. Adverse drug reactions: role of pharmacogenomics. *Pharmacol Res.* 2004; 49(4):363–373.

Steventon GB, Heafield MT, Waring RH, Williams AC. Xenobiotic metabolism in Parkinson's disease. *Neurology.* 1989;39:883–887.

Subramanian G, Adams M, Venter JC, Broder S. Implications of the human genome for understanding human biology and medicine. *JAMA.* 2002; 286(18):2296–2307.

Vita AJ, Terry RB, Hubert HB, et al. Aging, health risks, and cumulative disability. *NEJM.* 1998;338: 1035–1041.

Wahllander A, Mohr S, Paumgartner G. Assessment of hepatic function: comparison of caffeine clearance in serum and saliva during the day and at night. *J Hepatol.* 1990;10(2):129–137.

Willett, WC. Balancing life-style and genomics research for disease prevention. *Science.* 2002;296: 695–697.

CHAPTER 68

Interprofessional Referral Protocols

Robert D. Mootz, DC

REFERRALS IN INTEGRATIVE PRACTICE

Although there is a culture of patient referral and reporting within mainstream medicine, similar protocols and written communication have often been less common in complementary care disciplines (Barnett, 1998). Recent surveys of general medical practitioners suggest an increasing interest and willingness to accept and make referrals to complementary practitioners such as chiropractors (Ko & Berbrayer, 2000; Priotta et al., 2000; Rooney et al., 2001; Langworthy & Birkelid, 2001). However, a clearer understanding of relevant clinical issues in complementary care management and specific treatment plans is needed by conventional practitioners and payers (Brussee et al., 2001, Mootz & Bielinski, 2001). Interdisciplinary communication in complementary care is frequently provided by patients or through informal messages from the provider, rather than through direct communication or written reports (Brussee et al., 2001, Thomas et al., 2001). Written professional communication from complementary providers appears to

occur infrequently, but can be a source of better understanding and more effective care comanagement (Triano et al., 1998; Breen et al., 2000, 2004; Langworthy & Birkelid, 2001). Following basic protocols can facilitate integrative comanagement—particularly the management of complex cases—and foster better interprofessional interaction.

Referral Direction

When a practitioner sends a patient to another specialist, it is important to communicate the nature of the referral. Since most specialists are extremely busy, a brief written report letter is most useful. A short, explicit report is more likely to be read by the specialist. However, when a patient referral is received, the optimal response following evaluation is a more detailed report of findings and recommendations. However, it is also essential that communication be concise and efficient. In summary, the need to have a permanent record of interventions and recommendations for the chart of the other provider is essential for both clinical management and medicolegal considerations.

Referral Purpose

There are several reasons for making a referral (Mootz, 1990). The referring provider may want a second opinion about a case, help in the management of a case, or the transfer of complete management of a case to another practitioner. It is important that the referring provider make the purpose for the referral

---

Robert D. Mootz, DC, is associate medical director for chiropractic at the Department of Labor and Industries in Washington State. He has coauthored and edited several texts on chiropractic care, including a monograph for the Agency for Health Care Policy and Research on the chiropractic profession and a report for the RAND Corporation on cervical manipulative therapy. His current research focuses on best practices in the treatment and management of occupational injuries; he recently participated in a Washington State workgroup exploring barriers to insurance coverage for CAM services and interdisciplinary communication.

clear. If referrals are made without a clear understanding of the purpose, it is possible that future problems between the clinicians could develop. For example, without a letter of introduction explaining what has been done previously for the patient and the reason for the referral, the specialist may recommend a course of care that has already proven ineffective. This can usually be prevented through communication with the specialist in advance regarding case response and management approaches to date (including what has been attempted by others seeing the patient earlier).

When a practitioner wants another doctor to evaluate a patient (review the case, update the history, or perform an examination) and report observations and recommendations, that practitioner should request a consultation and evaluation. If the referring practitioner requires that the other doctor provide treatment, he or she should request a consultation for evaluation, and treatment. By being clear about this in advance, there is little doubt as to the purpose of the referral, thereby minimizing potential misunderstandings. For the same reasons, it is important that the referring practitioner be clear about the continuing role that he or she will have in the management of the case. It is the responsibility of the primary treating practitioner to ensure that all care being provided is coordinated and that no clinician counteracts the efforts of other clinicians involved in the case. In addition to actual treatment, this includes recommendations for home care, such as exercises, work restrictions, self-care, or nutritional advice.

If the doctor accepting the referral understands the referring practitioner's rationale for care, any differences of opinion can be worked out, preventing frustration for the patient when conflicting advice is given. Although it is typical for specialists to report

back, it is a good idea to request that the doctor report back on his or her findings at the time the referral is made. These days, unpaid time for written reporting is harder to come by, and follow-up with other doctors may sometimes be needed, particularly if there is some uncertainty regarding care planning.

OUTGOING REFERRAL PROTOCOL

The following steps should be taken when making a referral to another clinician. Any provider can follow these guidelines when referring to another, as well as to practitioners in another discipline. Chiropractors tend to refer patients to other practitioners regularly, and some studies have suggested that those who also send written reports receive more direct referrals from others (Mootz and Meeker, 1990).

MAKING REFERRALS

In the referral process, the role of the practitioner is to:

1. Identify the services that the patient needs and clarify the need for referral with the patient. This can help to prevent apprehension on the part of the patient.
2. Identify a clinician who can provide these services. If the practitioner has not established an interreferral relationship previously, he or she should personally telephone the clinician and very briefly describe what is needed, and ask whether the clinician would be willing to accept the referral. If the other clinician agrees, the practitioner should proceed with the next step. Should a doctor be unable to accept (for example, too busy or outside of his or her area of expertise), the practitioner should request the name of someone the other specialist would recommend and proceed to make contact with that person or with the referring practitioner's next choice.

3. Have the office staff contact the other clinician's office and arrange for scheduling the patient. It is extremely helpful, as well as professional, to provide the other office with the patient's entrance data (name, address, phone, insurance information, and other essential specifics). Often, it is most convenient for the other office to call the patient directly to schedule exact appointment times.

4. Write a letter briefly describing the reason for the referral and provide a short summary of the history, findings, and past treatment. The referring practitioner should be sure to indicate what role, if any, he or she intends to play in the continuing care and further management of the patient.

5. Follow-up on the progress of the patient with the other provider. Even if the specialist fails to report back to the referring practitioner, politely following up with a letter or a phone call conveys genuine interest that engenders respect.

As the primary provider of record, the referring practitioner should play an important role in overall management and follow-up of the patient, especially when two or more providers are directly involved in the ongoing care of a patient (Mootz, 1987).

RESPONDING TO REFERRALS

The following steps summarize the procedures for reporting back on patients referred to a practitioner.

1. When a referred patient has been scheduled, a brief letter on letterhead stationery thanking the doctor should be sent, confirming the date and time of the appointment. Generally, correspondence on professional letterhead regarding patients is more likely to be read and even kept in the patient chart. The practitioner should indicate that he or she will report back after the evaluation.

Before beginning the case, the practitioner should determine whether the patient is being sent for evaluation only or for evaluation and treatment. If it is unclear what the referring physician wants when the patient is initially referred, the practitioner should call the doctor, briefly summarize his or her findings and recommendations, and ask whether the referring physician is in agreement with the planned course of action.

2. Upon completion of the evaluation, a fairly detailed report should be sent, summarizing the practitioner's findings (history, examination, and any special studies, such as laboratory and X-rays), clinical impressions, and recommendations. This should be done even if the practitioner has verbally outlined the findings, as described in the previous step. It is common courtesy to close by thanking the referring physician for the opportunity to assist in the evaluation and/or care of the patient.

It is recommended that this initial report be sent in the form of a narrative on letterhead—but again, clearly organized and concise. The use of a form specifically designed for this purpose may be adequate, as well. These typically have sections for notations about findings and recommendations. However, handwritten entries need to be legible, and details such as abbreviations or the names of tests must be clear because they may not be meaningful to anyone outside that discipline.

3. If it is determined that the practitioner will be providing treatment, a very brief letter indicating progress should be sent to the referring physician at periodic intervals (for example, following a reexamination). It is perfectly acceptable for a progress report to be brief, for example, a one-page letter or preformatted form.

4. When care is complete, a brief final report should be sent, summarizing progress and indicating that the patient has been discharged. Any recommendations given to the patient for future self-care or follow-up should also be noted.

INCOMING REFERRAL PROTOCOL

When referrals come to a practitioner, the procedures and expectations differ somewhat. Receiving a complete and timely report back from a specialist is a satisfying experience and makes a practitioner feel comfortable to refer patients again. Therefore, when that same practitioner receives patients from others, he or she should respond in the same way. Doing so communicates the practitioner's expertise in a professional manner and increases the comfort level of the referring physician. This can be particularly true for traditional medical providers who may have limited training or experience in alternative therapies.

Just as the practitioner is the primary provider of record when referring a patient out, a doctor who refers a patient to that practitioner is the primary physician of record. Therefore, professional courtesy dictates that the referring doctor's concerns be addressed. The patient should never be involved in a difference of opinion between the two practitioners. Every effort should be made to articulate the contribution to care in a manner that is competent and appropriate to the physician of record. By following these steps, this can be readily accomplished. Undoubtedly, at times not all recommendations will be followed by the physician of record. However, in the long run, it is most important to develop a foundation of trust and cooperation with other practitioners, always in a context of maximizing benefit for the patient. These interdisciplinary linkages provide the opportunity to work collegially, bringing expanded resources to bear on complex conditions.

It is important to recognize differences in practice philosophy. For example, lifestyle therapies tend to receive greater emphasis in the treatment protocol of complementary practitioners. When referrals are received, it is wise to determine and communicate recommendations for both immediate and long-term therapy. The treatment should include recommendations for the specific situation (such as acute low-back pain) as well as any relevant discussion of a more lasting lifestyle intervention.

CONCLUSION

Any practitioner is likely to find it frustrating when another provider manages the case without communicating clearly. Referral protocol is most effectively aimed at setting the stage for clear and comfortable collaboration to increase the number of therapeutic options available.

The clinician who refers the patient out is considered the provider of record (Mootz, 1990). By communicating and coordinating approaches, the patient will receive consistent care, and the referring provider will not have the sense that the patient is being co-opted. Since these referral protocols require some extra work, it is helpful to develop an office routine for efficent, consistent follow-up. This supports effective professional communication and fosters greater respect from patients and colleagues alike (Mootz, 1987). Most importantly, when practitioners coordinate and cooperate with one another, patients benefit.

Proper referral protocol may not be followed by all providers. This, however, should not deter practitioners from behaving professionally. Many allied health professionals and general practitioners tend to treat referrals in a very casual manner. The provider who functions with timely, thorough, and consistent communication to peers is identified in the community as competent, qualified, and concerned. This communication provides the basis for contacts and procedures that can facilitate involvement with other health care modalities, medical specialties, or institutions (Triano et al., 1998). Successful interaction with other providers can contribute ultimately to better understanding and cooperation between the disciplines.

REFERENCES

Barnett PB. Clinical communication and managed care. *Med Group Manage J*. 1998;45(4):60–66.

Breen A, Carr E, Mann E, Crossen-White H. Acute back pain management in primary care: a qualitative pilot study of the feasibility of a nurse-led service in general practice. *J Nursing Management*. 2004;12: 201–209.

Breen A, Carrington M, Collier R, Vogel S. Communication between general and manipulative practitioners: a survey. *Complementary Therap Med*. 2000:8:8–14.

Brussee WJ, Assendelft WJ, Breen AC. Communication between general practitioners and chiropractors. *J Manipulative Physiol Ther*. 2001;24(1):12–16.

Ko GD, Berbrayer D. Complementary and alternative medicine: Canadian physiatrists' attitudes and behavior. *Arch Phys Med Rehabil*. 2000;81(5):662–667.

Langworthy JM, Birkelid J. General practice and chiropractic in Norway: how well do they communicate and what do GPs want to know? *J Manipulative Physiol Ther*. 2001;24(9):576–581.

Mootz RD. Interprofessional referral protocol: how to make referrals that benefit all parties. *Today's Chiropract*. 1987 September/October;37–40.

Mootz RD. Interprofessional relations: appropriate referral protocols. *Am Back Soc Newsletter*. 1990;6(4).

Mootz RD, Bielinski LL. Issues, barriers, and solutions regarding integration of CAM and conventional health care. *Top Clin Chiropr*. 2001;8(2): 26–32.

Mootz RD, Meeker WC. Referral patterns of California Chiropractic Association members. *Am Back Soc Newsletter*. 1990;6(3):17.

Priotta MV, Cojen MM, Kotsirilos V, Farish SJ. Complementary therapies: have they become accepted in general practice? *Med J Aust*. 2000; 172(3):102–103.

Rooney B, Fiocco G, Hughes P, Halter S. Provider attitudes and use of alternative medicine in a Midwestern medical practice in 2001. *WMJ*. 2001; 100(7):27–31.

Thomas KJ, Nicholl JP, Fall M. Access to complementary medicine via general practice. *Br J Gen Pract*. 2001;51(462):25–30.

Triano JJ, Raley B. Chiropractic in the interdisciplinary team practice. *Top Clin Chiropract*. 1994;1(4): 58–66.

Triano JJ, Rashbaum RF, Hansen DT. Opening access to spine care in the evolving market: integration and communication. *Top Clin Chiropract*. 1998;5(4): 44–52.

CHAPTER 69

Program in Integrative Medicine, University of Arizona

Victoria Maizes, MD

The Program in Integrative Medicine, founded by Dr. Andrew Weil in 1994, leads the nation in the range and depth of educational programs in integrative medicine. Four comprehensive fellowships are now offered at the University of Arizona and a wide range of additional learning opportunities are currently being developed. In addition, medical students and residents from around the nation come to learn from the program's faculty.

PROGRAMS IN INTEGRATIVE MEDICINE

Residency Programs

Residential Fellowship

This 2-year residential fellowship, developed for physicians by the Program in Integrative Medicine, is the first comprehensive educational program of its type in the world. The goal of the fellowship is to train leaders in integrative medicine who will create similar programs at other academic institutions and influence policy or the future training of physicians.

The program has graduated 23 fellows in integrative medicine and 5 in pediatric integrative medicine research, as of 2004. Of the program's 28 graduates, 17 are in academic centers developing integrative medicine programs, performing research, and teaching medical students, residents, and physicians. Graduates have authored four textbooks, speak at national conferences, and sit on a number of NIH review committees, editorial boards, and the boards of national organizations.

The residential fellowship will undergo a major change in 2005. It will begin with a 9 month distance learning component (the Associate Fellowship) followed by a 10-month sabbatical experience in Tucson. The program continues to include clinical, leadership, and research components, and is intended to train physicians in integrative medicine who will take on leadership roles in academic institutions.

Integrative Family Medicine

This four-year pilot program integrates training in integrative medicine with three-year conventional family practice residencies, sponsored by six participating family medicine residency programs across the country: Albert Einstein College of Medicine (New

Victoria Maizes, MD, is executive director of the Program in Integrative Medicine at the University of Arizona and associate professor of Medicine, Family and Community Medicine, and Public Health. A graduate of the University of California, San Francisco and fellow of the University of Arizona, Dr. Maizes is a national leader in the field of integrative medicine and has helped develop comprehensive curriculum for medical students, fellows, and family medicine residents.

Source: Courtesy of Victoria Maizes, MD, and the University of Arizona Program in Integrative Medicine, Tucson, Arizona.

York), Maine Medical Center (Portland), Middlesex Hospital Family Practice Residency Program (Middletown, Connecticut), Oregon Health Sciences University (Portland), the University of Arizona (Tucson), and the University of Wisconsin (Madison). A hybrid of our residential and associate fellowships, the residencies offer supervision at integrative medicine clinics by family practice residency faculty. This program is the first comprehensive integrative medicine curriculum within conventional training.

Research Programs

NIH-Supported Research Fellowship

This two-year research fellowship is currently in its second year with six research fellows, in a training program designed to prepare research scientists for academic careers in integrative medicine. The conceptual foundation for this program is a systems theory–driven approach to the investigation of processes and outcomes of integrative clinical care and mechanisms of healing. Training will also focus on preparation in methodological rigor and study design to develop state-of-the-science research. In addition to PIM research faculty, the faculty includes members from diverse disciplines, such as medicine, nursing, pharmacology, various complementary medicine modalities and systems, psychology, anthropology, epidemiology, nutrition, and public health.

Electives and Seminars

Elective Rotation in Integrative Medicine

This four-week rotation provides medical students and residents the opportunity to become familiar with a range of complementary therapies and to evaluate these systems critically. The rotation includes supervised observation of patient treatment in the Integrative Medicine Clinic and precepting with a variety of practitioners in the Tucson area, which include osteopaths, naturopaths, homeopaths, and traditional Chinese medicine practitioners. Through these experiences, students gain an increased understanding of how and when complementary therapies can interface most effectively with conventional approaches. Over a period of 6 years, this program has served approximately 30 University of Arizona medical students, 30 medical residents, and 80 visiting medical students from other universities.

Integrative Medicine Enrichment Elective and Interdisciplinary Seminar

Enrichment electives and interdisciplinary seminars have been taught by program faculty and residential fellows to University of Arizona medical students since 1997. The electives introduce first- and second-year students to basic concepts of integrative medicine, focusing on specific modalities and the evidence that supports their use. Two areas are addressed each semester from topics that include: nutrition, mind-body medicine, herbal medicine, acupuncture, manual medicine, and others. For third-year medical students, interdisciplinary seminars provide a deepened understanding of the components of integrative medicine and treatment characteristics of key complementary therapies.

Distance Learning Programs

Associate Fellowship (AF)

This two-year distance learning program is designed to teach physicians, nurse practitioners, and physician's assistants how to incorporate the philosophies and techniques of integrative medicine into their practices. The fellowship includes 3 residential weeks in Tucson, offering an opportunity to study within a vibrant learning community. More than 50 adjunct faculty members join PIM faculty and staff to teach the program. Course content is modeled on the residential fellowship and is presented via the Web and online dialogues, as well as in articles, books, videos, and audio recordings.

The program includes access to an extensive database of the research evidence and content that fellows use initially for learning, but can also use for review and future reference. Web-based interactive case studies provide the opportunity to apply an integrative approach to patient care, focused on the treatment and prevention of specific diseases and conditions. Each scenario incorporates expertise from several treatment modalities. However, rather than merely teaching facts, the program uses Web-based discussions moderated by expert practitioners to support new approaches to clinical problem solving. Additionally, these discussions tend to build a virtual community of physicians working toward the same goal. All modules and learning can be paced by participants. As of 2005, 236 physicians have enrolled in 5 classes and 83 have graduated.

Online Courses: Nutrition and Health and Botanical Studies

A series of three-month online courses in nutrition and botanical medicine have been developed by the Program in Integrative Medicine. Nutrition and Cardiovascular Health is the first of these modules available via the Internet to all health care professionals. The content covers the fundamentals of diet and nutrition for heart health, including: macro- and micronutrients, fad diets, supplements, phytonutrients, motivating patient change, the state of the research in this field, and more. Virtual case histories are provided as learning tools. Continuing education credits of 16.5 hours are provided to physicians, nurses, and registered dieticians. A series of other clinical topics are also available, including Botanical Foundations and Nutrition and Cancer.

Department of Defense Distance Learning Fellowship

This one-year, online fellowship program is currently in development.

For additional information on all these programs, see the Program's Web site at www.integrativemedicine.arizona.edu.

CHAPTER 70

Implementing and Evaluating Optimal Healing Environments

Wayne B. Jonas, MD, and Ronald A. Chez, MD

OVERVIEW

Healing is defined as the process of recovery, repair and return to wholeness. It is the foundation for a vision of medicine in which the focus is the alleviation of suffering, the enhancement of well-being and the treatment of chronic illness. The incorporation of new approaches to healing is important for the management of chronic illness and the development of sustainable approaches in health care. A new model of healing (and a better scientific foundation for that model) is needed—one that integrates diverse healing philosophies from around the world. We believe that developing inner and outer environments that optimize the inherent healing capacities of individuals, social systems, and the physical environment is an important step in achieving that vision.

We define an optimal healing environment (OHE) as one in which the social, psychological, spiritual, physical, and behavioral components of health care are oriented toward support and stimulation of healing and the achievement of wholeness. In our opinion, these components include at least five domains plus the physical and organizational structures that support them. The five core domains of an optimal healing environment are:

1. Conscious development of intention, awareness, expectation, and belief in improvement and well-being
2. Self-care practices that facilitate the experience of wholeness and well-being, and that foster greater compassion, love, and awareness of interconnectivity
3. Development of listening and communication skills and service-oriented, altruistic behaviors that cultivate social support and trust, including the "therapeutic alliance"—in the health care setting
4. Instruction and practice in health promoting behaviors in lifestyle to support self-healing such as proper diet, exercise, leisure and work balance, and addiction management
5. Responsible use of integrative medicine via the collaborative application of con-

A biography of Wayne Jonas appears in Chapter 7.

Ronald A. Chez, MD, founding Deputy Director of the Samueli Institute, has served as a practitioner, researcher, professor, educator, author, and administrator in some of the nation's most prestigious medical institutions. Board certified in obstetrics and gynecology with a subspeciality in maternal-fetal medicine, he has authored more than 530 research articles and public and physician audiovisual learning aids in the areas of physician–patient relationship, maternal and fetal physiology, clinical obstetrics, nutrition, and biophysics. Since 2000, his writing and lecturing has focused on topics in complementary medicine.

Source: Courtesy of Wayne B. Jonas, MD, and Ronald A. Chez, MD, Samueli Institute, Alexandria, Virginia. From: Jonas WB, Chez RA. Implementing and evaluating optimal healing environments. *Wellness Management.* 2004;20(2): 1–5. National Wellness Institute member e-newsletter. Available at: www.nationalwellness.org.

Table courtesy of Mary Ann Liebert, Publishers. From: Jonas WB, Chez RA. Introduction. In: Toward Optimal Healing Environments in Health Care. Supplement 1. 2004;10;S2.

ventional and complementary practices in a manner supportive of healing processes

These five domains need support from the physical space in which healing is practiced, including characteristics of light, music, architecture, and color. These domains also need supportive organizational structures including leadership, mission focus, and evaluation and reward policies among other elements that can create a healing environment. Health care managers and leaders ideally should have personal experience in these environmental domains, and practice self-care, personal wellness, and preventive approaches in their own lives.

DESCRIBING OPTIMAL HEALING ENVIRONMENTS

Here we provide a short summary of the healing domains, and speculate on how they can be built from current foundations in health care. These domains, and their supporting physical and organizational environments, are represented in Table 70–1.

1. Developing Intention and Awareness

Our current health care system has primary focus on treatment and cure of disease. Thus, patients and their families are oriented toward getting procedures that can "fix" their problems. Often with chronic disease, patients' expectations are low for any fundamental healing in the midst of their condition. In addition, patients may not be prepared to engage in self-care activities that facilitate healing. Thus educational programs that orient people to the perspective of healing are needed. These programs should educate and enhance expectations about the possibilities of wellness, wholeness, and improved functioning.

Often people can obtain feelings of peace, meaning, and purpose in life when they perceive a personal connection and contribution to something larger than themselves. This sense of coherence can be fostered with various psychological, spiritual, and/or traditional religious practices. In the latter case, it is termed religiosity. However, frequently the experience of connection or spirituality does not occur within the context of formal religions, or individuals choose to keep it outside such domains. Thus, experientially based programs that foster this sense of expanded awareness and connectivity, with or without the context of spirituality, may be added to basic educational programs on the healing process.

2. Experiencing Personal Wholeness

A cognitive understanding of healing and the development of healing intention is crucial, but insufficient for stimulating healing behavior and experience. Patients also need to have an experience of wholeness and well-being. Some patients with chronic disease may not recall ever feeling well. Well-being does not depend on cure and can be fostered with various mind-body-energy practices. It is in these areas of psychophysiological practices and their effects that a sense of wholeness is experienced and developed; this may include an experience of healing presence or healing energy. Both arise from a sense of personal integration or wholeness, and can be fostered with mind-body practices through personal growth sessions and workshops, a common approach in the West, or through practices such as yoga, tai chi, and meditation, commonly used in the East.

3. Cultivating Healing Relationships

Immersion in healing relationships is one of the most powerful ways to stimulate,

Table 70–1 Optimal Healing Environments

Building Healing Spaces	Developing Awareness and Intention	Experiencing Personal Wholeness	Cultivating Healing Relationships	Practicing Healthy Lifestyles	Applying Collaborative Medicine	Creating Healing Spaces
Nature • Color • Light • Fine Arts • Architecture • Aroma • Music	*Enhance belief* • Expectation • Hope • Understanding • Love	*Enhance integration* • Mind • Body • Emotion • Energy	*Enhance caring* • Compassion • Communication • Empathy • Social support	*Enhance health habits* • Diet • Exercise • Relaxation • Balance	*Enhance medical care* • Conventional • Complementary • Traditional • Alternative	Leadership • Mission • Culture • Teamwork • Technology • Evaluation • Service
	Achieved with Learning programs • Mindfulness practice	*Achieved with* Personal growth • Mind-body practices	*Achieved with* Communication skills • Community support	*Achieved with* Family education • Support groups	*Achieved with* Clinical teams • Person-centered care	

Table courtesy of Mary Ann Liebert, Publishers. From: Jonas WB, Chez RA. Introduction. In: *Toward Optimal Healing Environments in Health Care.* Supplement 1. 2004;10;S2.

support, and maintain wellness and recovery. Family, friends, and community generally form the primary relationships. The work site, school, community, and health care settings can also facilitate relationships that support healing and wellness. Characteristics of such interactions involve empathy, compassion, beneficence, caring, love, reassurance, comfort, warmth, trust, confidence, credibility, honesty, courtesy, respect, harmony, challenge, and communication. Cultivating these characteristics requires skills in listening and communication, and can be fostered by engaging in social service, and through family and community activities. An optimal healing environment should incorporate training in these characteristics and develop opportunities for such activities in educational and group programs.

4. Practicing Healthy Lifestyles

Health promotion and disease prevention involves behavioral and lifestyle activities targeted toward establishing habitual behaviors that support well-being, facilitate healing, and prevent or treat illness. These programs are often established at work sites, schools, community centers, churches, or hospitals and clinics. They typically involve five behavioral areas:

1. Management of negative addictions (smoking, alcohol, drugs, unhealthy sexual behavior, violence) and fostering positive habits (relaxation methods, healthy sexual behavior, establishment of social support networks)
2. Healthy eating
3. Regular and appropriate physical exercise
4. Stress management techniques and attending to attaining balance between work, leisure, and family activities
5. Screening for preventable disease

Optimal healing environments should provide services that foster and maintain healthy lifestyles.

5. Applying Collaborative Medicine

Complementary and alternative medicine is popular among the public and is increasingly used in mainstream health care institutions. Integrative medicine is the coordinated application of a variety of complementary and conventional modalities in therapeutic settings. The coordinated, appropriate preventive and therapeutic approaches are important for obtaining and maintaining wellness and healing. From the perspective of optimal healing environments, approaches that support and stimulate the inherent healing and self-recovery capacities of a person are primary, but curative treatments are needed as well. The ideal system would match the individual patient or client and support persons with the most appropriate treatment strategy derived from the variety of global health care systems and the preferences and capabilities of the patient.

Collaborative medicine requires the coordination of multiple service components. These components include:

1. The availability of knowledgeable and competent practitioners
2. Appropriate facilities, equipment, and supplies for practice
3. Reliable, quality products
4. Supportive organizational and professional settings
5. Information about safety, effectiveness, and interactions of treatment modalities
6. Training in appropriate communication and partnership skills for the appropriate selection of interventions
7. Economic resources for delivery and availability of services

6. Healing Places and Spaces

Both the physical space and the leadership environment (the place) are crucial for the successful creation of effective healing environments. Healing spaces may contain a variety of components that foster or detract from wellness and recovery including architecture, nature, color, sound, music, art, and light. Designing community, personal, and sacred spaces that incorporate the aspects of a healing environment are integral to the support of health and well-being. Healing places require the understanding, experience, and support of the leadership and organizational decision makers for successful implementation of a healing environment. Health care managers and leaders ideally should have personal experience in these environmental domains.

7. Implementing Optimal Healing Environments in Health Care Settings

Clinical, work site, school, and health care settings are busy places. The people involved in these settings have goals of productivity, service, and quality parameters. Time is precious and often short—a factor that itself may influence healing and its optimization. How the core domains of healing might be implemented in a manner within the context of normal health care and other settings is the focus of our research interests. Many of these domains have been partially implemented in a variety of settings. Work site health promotion programs have successfully implemented many behavioral and lifestyle changes in ways that impact health and productivity. Healing-oriented clinics and hospitals have been developed and have demonstrated their ability to deliver quality treatment. Integrative medicine programs are developing models for appropriate use of complementary and alternative medicine. Patient education programs teaching self-care, including support groups, have an impact on chronic disease management and its outcomes. The addition of social support to standard care, such as a visit or phone call from a nurse after treatment, has shown improved clinical outcomes and reduced mortality in several clinical populations.

Can a health care program efficiently maximize the components of optimal healing? What impact would an optimal healing environment have on morale, practitioner-patient interactions, patient satisfaction and empowerment, clinical outcomes, and costs? The components in Table 70-1 under the heading "achieved with" may provide guidelines for the development of such programs. A comprehensive environmental program might include the following as a minimum:

1. Education about healing, its capacity, expectation, and implementation
2. Instruction in ways to expand awareness, manage beliefs, and improve emotions
3. Practice in enhancing mind-body integration through self-applied skills
4. Opportunities for cultivation of interpersonal communication, social support, and service
5. Education and engagement in core healthy lifestyle choices
6. Provision of quality health care delivery with collaborative and integrative components
7. Attention to the physical and organizational structures that facilitate healing

ASSESSING AN OPTIMAL HEALING ENVIRONMENT

The competent, rigorous, and effective performance of clinical research in the area of healing environments requires appropriate tools for measurement. Ways to assess the elements and outcomes of an optimal healing environment can be extrapolated from existing assessment and evaluation scales, which have been validated. A healing environment measuring tool should include a focus on three main areas: health and disease outcomes, process outcomes, and financial outcomes. Another facet of measurement would be the linking of biologic, physiologic, and disease-specific markers. These measures should include tangible outcomes such as money, value, health behaviors, measurements of quality of life and pain, functional status, and patient satisfaction for quantitative analyses. Each of these, and others, would then be directed toward the communities being explored: work sites, medical practices, hospitals, schools, health maintenance organizations, and the patient–provider dyad or therapeutic alliance.

It is our belief that the development and evaluation of optimal healing environments can provide a model for the effective management of chronic illness, the improvement of well-being, and the integration of prevention with treatment. These environments are complementary to conventional medicine. The ability to conceive of, design, create, and implement healing environments will always begin with the individual, whether it be the healer, the one who is healed, a significant other, organizational leaders, and/or the community as an entity.

Index

NOTE: tables are denoted by *t*